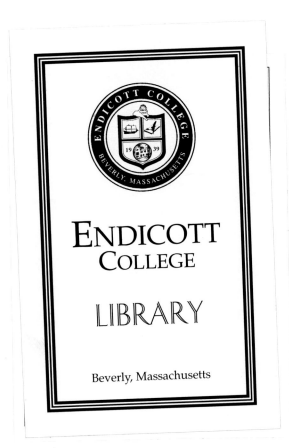

Brain Asymmetry

edited by Richard J. Davidson and Kenneth Hugdahl

A Bradford Book
The MIT Press
Cambridge, Massachusetts
London, England

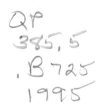
This book was set in Palatino by Asco Trade Typesetting Ltd., Hong Kong and was printed and bound in the United States of America.

Library of Congress Cataloging-in-Publication Data

Brain asymmetry / edited by Richard J. Davidson and Kenneth Hugdahl.
    p.   cm.
 "A Bradford book."
 Includes bibliographical references and index.
 ISBN 0-262-04144-8
 1. Cerebral dominance.   2. Laterality.   I. Davidson, Richard J.
II. Hugdahl, Kenneth.
QP385.5.B725   1994
612.8'2—dc20   94-10554
                                      CIP

We dedicate this book to our families:
Susan, Amelie, and Seth; and Maerit, Anna, and Emilia

Contents

Preface

The study of brain asymmetry has had a long tradition in the behavioral and biomedical sciences. The fact that the vertebrate nervous system is divided in half has attracted the attention and has sparked the speculation of numerous generations of scientists. Of particular note in the history of research on this topic was the once held presumption that brain asymmetry was a property of only human brains, since such asymmetry was linked to handedness and language. This presumption gave rise to a flurry of pronouncements about the role of lateralized brain function in complex mental processes. Many of these early forays, fueled by issues salient in the popular culture, terminated in scientific dead ends (see Harrington's review in this volume). However, one characteristic that was central to the early theorizing on brain asymmetry that is still apparent today is the emphasis on hierarchical integration across multiple levels of the neuraxis and types of processes. Related to this is the recognition of the importance of asymmetries at all levels of the central and peripheral nervous systems. Not only are there two cerebral hemispheres, there are also right and left halves of most central structures including the thalamus, amygdala, hippocampus, caudate, and many other subcortical sites of major importance to higher mental processes. In addition, the peripheral nervous system has a right and left branch.

The study of brain asymmetry continues to attract unique forms of integration in the biobehavioral sciences. We see evidence of methodological integration across behavioral and biological measures. There is also a steady stream of integration across basic and applied levels of analysis. Finally, many different types of psychological processes have been usefully related to brain asymmetry including sensory, perceptual, cognitive, and attentional processes, learning, and emotion. We cannot identify any other construct that forms the focus of such a diverse array of behavioral processes. Traditional views of asymmetry as only reflecting differences between the hemispheres in the processing of language and visuospatial stimuli are today replaced by a much more elaborated concept where brain asymmetry is associated with such constructs as approach versus withdrawal behavior, maintenance versus interruption of ongoing activity, tonic versus phasic aspects of behavior, positive versus negative emotional valence, high versus low spatial resolution gradients, to mention just a few. The two divisions of the nervous system may also have differential effects on peripheral processes; for example, effects of the vagus nerve on the heart may be regulated more from the right than from the left hemisphere.

Because of the extraordinarily diverse range of phenomena studied within the context of brain asymmetry, the extant literature is spread across a number of different disciplines including psychology, cognitive science, neurology, the neurosciences, psychiatry, anatomy, and endocrinology. Investigations of different aspects of brain asymmetry are published in myriad journals that span these disciplines. It is thus extremely difficult to obtain an overview of the entire area. It is our hope that this volume serves such a function. We mean for it to be representative and not exhaustive in its coverage of modern laterality research. The topics we chose to include illustrate the scope of modern research on brain asymmetry. We strove to highlight the diverse range of conceptual and methodological approaches that appear most promising in contemporary studies of brain asymmetry.

In our selection of contributors, we wished to feature those investigators with active research programs. It goes without saying that there are many talented investigators in this area who could not be included. It is equally important to note that we could not include all areas of modern research on this topic. To do so would also have made the volume unwieldy. We therefore chose a range of both long-standing as well as relatively recent topic areas to showcase those issues that we consider to be the most promising. Thus, the principal aim has been to survey research on brain asymmetry in its widest context, from sociocultural influences to basic physiology. The present volume includes a wide spectrum of phenomena and processes in the social, cognitive, emotional, and physiological domains that are relevant for an understanding of the functional significance of cerebral asymmetry.

In our invitations to authors to contribute to this volume, we requested that each author address a set of common questions in her or his chapter. These questions included:

1. Is the research described predicated on a particular model of cerebral lateralization? If so, what is that model?

2. What is the relation between the model of cerebral lateralization implicit or explicit in your research and other extant models?

3. What are the methods or approaches you use to study whatever aspect of laterality you describe? What are the advantages and disadvantages of the methods/approaches you adopt?

4. What are the major unanswered questions in the research that you have reviewed? What should the research agenda in your area be for the next decade?

Although not all of the authors provide explicit answers to these questions, most chapters do, at least implicitly, address the questions.

Our hope in undertaking this project was to gather in a single volume the most exciting and influential work on brain asymmetry. We did not expect a single unifying theory or conceptual approach to emerge from this effort. Rather, it will be clear to the reader how diverse and wide ranging is the modern study of brain asymmetry. It will also be apparent that research on brain asymmetry is highly relevant to many different subdisciplines in the biobehavioral sciences including cognitive science, affective science, perception, learning, developmental studies, comparative psychology and evolutionary theory, psychopathology, and behavioral neurology. The methods used by various investigators are equally wide ranging and include anatomical studies of cytoarchitecture in animal brains, assessment of patients with localized brain damage using traditional neuropsychological tests, behavioral techniques involving the lateralization of sensory input and/or motor output to make inferences about asymmetrical functioning, neuroimaging procedures including electrophysiology, positron emission tomography, and magnetic resonance imaging to make inferences about the regional structure and function of the living human nervous system. In short, the study of brain asymmetry provides a paradigm for what we believe to be the future trends in the study of brain/behavior relations from both an experimental and clinical perspective.

This volume is divided into sections, each section dealing with a particular aspect of laterality. Harrington provides a historical overview of how the concept of laterality and brain asymmetry has been treated from the first proposals in the nineteenth century. Lewis and Diamond, and Galaburda provide evidence for both phylogenetic and anatomical substrates of laterality. Perceptual-attention, cognitive, and motor laterality are discussed in several chapters, focusing on recent research developments and clinical applications. Peters also provides an update on recent views of handedness and its relation to other indices of laterality, and Hugdahl presents a new model on laterality and learning, focusing on how basic associations are formed in the brain. Lane and Jennings, and Wittling describe research on central-autonomic integration, and how the cardiovascular system is differently regulated from the left and right hemispheres. New views on the lateralization of emotions and affect are presented by Davidson, and Liotti and Tucker, and focus on individual differences in lateralized central nervous system activity as predictors of affect and the role of corticolimbic networks in emotions. The important issue of communication between the hemispheres, interhemispheric interaction, is treated at length in the chapters by Banich, Liedermann, and Zaidel, while developmental issues in laterality research are discussed by Hiscock and Kinsbourne, Segalowitz and Berge. Pathologies of development are treated in chapters by Hynd et al. and Boliek and Obrzut on dyslexia and brain asymmetry. Finally, Bruder, and Robinson and Dowhill link laterality to psychopathology and to focal brain injury, respectively, providing a clinical perspective on recent trends in laterality research.

It is our hope that by seeing the broad spectrum of research on brain asymmetry within a single volume, readers can appreciate the breathtaking scope of modern inquiry in this area. Research on brain asymmetry touches almost every substantive topic in the biobehavioral science, and the study of its functional significance facilitates the development of theories of mental processes and behavior that honor the underlying biological architecture.

I Historical Overview

1 Unfinished Business: Models of Laterality in the Nineteenth Century

Anne Harrington

FUNDAMENTAL ASSUMPTIONS OF LOCALIZATION THEORY: THE PHRENOLOGIC CONNECTION

In his *Science and the Modern World*, the philosopher Alfred North Whitehead (1925) declared:

When you are criticizing the philosophy of an epoch, do not chiefly direct your attention to those intellectual positions which its exponents feel it necessary chiefly to defend. There will be some fundamental assumptions which adherents of all the variant systems within the epoch unconsciously presuppose. Such assumptions appear so obvious that people do not know what they are assuming because no other way of putting things has ever occurred to them. With these assumptions a certain limited group of types of philosophic systems are possible, and this group of systems constitutes the philosophy of the epoch.

Many of the fundamental assumptions—the unquestioned truths—that provide the tacit grounding for modern laterality research have their source in an early nineteenth-century approach to visualizing mind-brain relations called localization theory. This has become such a familiar approach to brain research that it would be useful to try to recapture a sense for the original high stakes driving the venture. Debates about the localizability of functions in the brain have always been more than just debates about structure-function correlation. They have been—and remain today—a critical part of the story of how human beings have attempted over the past two centuries to apply the categories of scientific understanding to *themselves*: minds and brains caught somehow between a universe of social and moral realities, and a universe that seems to stand outside of such realities, and that they choose to call "natural."

Conventionally, the story of cerebral localization begins with the work of Franz Joseph Gall, at the start of the nineteenth century. Although Gall was a distinguished neuroanatomist, he would become much better known for his system of "organology" or phrenology. This system was rooted in three fundamental principles: (1) the brain is the organ of the mind (*not* an obvious proposition at the time); (2) the brain is a composite of parts, each of which serves a distinct mental faculty; and (3) the size of the different parts of the brain, as assessed chiefly by examining the bumps on the skull, corresponds to the relative strength of the different faculties served (Spurzheim, 1908).

Gall was certainly not the first to interest himself in the relationship between organic structure and different aspects of psychic activity in the brain. Before Gall, the physiologist Charles Bonnet had gone so far as to declare that anyone who thoroughly understood the structure of the brain would be able to read all the thoughts passing through it "as in a book." Bonnet, though, had imagined the brain's presumed different organs as vehicles which the immaterial soul manipulated at will, like a pianist at the keyboard. Where Gall most clearly broke from his predecessors was in his decision to eliminate this pianist, this overruling soul, and posit instead a brain composed of some 30 self-animated organs that together somehow added up to the totality of human mind and personality. Within Gall's system, the piano was to play itself.

This first naturalization of the human mind was accomplished, then, through a model that made *division of labor* a framing principle of brain function. A corollary principle, whose legacy would leave clear traces on later discussions of lateralized functioning, was *hierarchy*. In finding differences between parts of the brain, Gall simultaneously asserted their *unequal* worth. His system made a distinction between lower, "animal" propensities, instincts, and emotions (reproductive instinct, aggressiveness, and so forth), and more refined intellectual faculties and sentiments (notably "verbal memory," but also faculties like calculation, spatial recognition, etc.). The less exalted animal instincts were located in the lower, posterior lobes of the brain (the sexual instinct as low down as the cerebellum) and the higher intellectual faculties were localized in the frontal lobes. A prominent forehead had long been considered a mark of nobility and superior intelligence, while the beetle brow was regarded with distrust and derision; Gall now "naturalized" these cultural biases by locating them in brain structure, where, in a range of guises, they would persist through the nineteenth century and recognizably into our own era.

But Gall did not just give brain science an attractive model rooted in certain already persuasive traditions. He also helped establish several heuristic principles still largely operational today. It was he who helped teach scientists that *to locate the material base for a piece of mind is to claim it for science.* And it was he who insisted on the corollary principle that *to break mind down into its brain-based building blocks is to know it.* This way to truth was not a necessary one—different choices could have been made (as were in fact made by evolutionary biology)—but the principles would facilitate a highly practical and productive style of research and justification that has not yet been superseded.

The whole enterprise, of course, took a gamble on a bold assumption: namely, that human scientists and human brains had similar strategies for conceptualizing the building blocks of the mind. That is to say, localization theory began with historically conventional categories of mind like "language," "aggression," "emotion," and hoped that these would turn out in fact to represent distinct natural entities that could fairly be traced to circumscribed brain areas. The gamble helped launch neuropsychology—but was it rooted in a true premise? Nothing revealed in the brain itself, even today, could guarantee that Sir Charles Scott Sherrington would not yet have the last word, when he predicted that the contributions made by the cortex to human behavior would actually, "when they are ultimately analyzed, resolve into components for which at present we have no names" (Sherrington, 1955).

In the early nineteenth century, however, other aspects of Gall's system rankled more. Beginning in the 1820s, the French experimental physiologist Jean-Pierre-Marie Flourens used a combination of animal experimentation and the testimony of "inner sense" to discredit the entire phrenologic premise that the mind was a mosaic of isolated functions. Slicing systematically through the brains of a variety of laboratory animals (mostly birds, with the odd rodent or rabbit), he had found no evidence that specific cortical areas subserved different functions: instead, all functions seemed to grow gradually weaker and weaker as more and more brain matter was removed, until at length the animal sank into dementia. This was interpreted as a triumph for the idea that the brain in fact functioned as a unity. A lot was riding on this refutation of Gall's modular, self-regulating mind-brain: in Flourens' 1846 critique of phrenology (dedicated to Descartes), Gall and his followers were declared guilty of undermining the unity of the soul, human immortality, free will, and the very existence of God! (Flourens, 1846).

Flourens' influence on orthodox physiology was to be profound: partly because there was a limited amount of counterevidence available at the time, and certainly partly also because a unitary conception of mind and brain seemed as theologically essential to most of Flourens' colleagues as to Flourens himself. If, though, by the 1820s, Flourens appeared to have won the battle for antilocalization and the unified soul, the outcome of the war remained undetermined. Gall's candle would be kept burning into the 1860s by the French neurologist Jean-Baptiste Bouillaud, at which point the whole question of cerebral localization—and, close in its wake, laterality—would be thrown wide open.

THE LOCALIZATION OF LANGUAGE

Bouillaud's importance for the history of localization theory lies in his unswerving conviction during a skeptical time that there was something to the whole phrenologic approach after all, and that, above all, Gall had been right to put his faculty of "verbal memory" in the frontal lobes. Over a period of almost 40 years, Bouillaud (1825) collected and presented more than 100 cases of frontal lobe damage resulting in loss of speech. Yet, in the climate of the time, he would only be able to convince a minority of his colleagues. The turning point would not come until 1861, the year the neuroanatomist and anthropologist Paul Broca resolved to test Bouillaud's claims himself.

By the time of Broca's entry onto the scene, the authority of traditional institutions and traditions was coming under increasing pressure, and the medical profession's original united stance against brain localization was beginning to crumble and polarize. At stake was not only the scientific truth or clinical usefulness of different approaches to brain functioning but the continuing validity of the belief in the transcendent unity and immateriality of the human spirit. A decision on this point of theology was perceived to have direct political consequences. At a time in French history when a conservative monarchy had entered into an alliance with a conservative Catholic Church, science and naturalist philosophies seemed an obvious way of challenging and undermining traditional authorities. For many frustrated republicans and freethinkers, the bottom line was clear: if everything in the universe, including the human soul, was natural, then the Church and her political allies were stripped of their claims to transcendent authority, and must give way to a new rational order (Jacyna, 1981).

Knowing this, it is useful to know as well that the traditional founder of modern localization theory, Paul Broca, was also the founder of the Paris Society of Anthropology, well-known in French intellectual circles as a focus for left-wing, anticlerical activity. One of its chief aims was to bring French philosophy back down to earth by grounding it firmly in a material base (Hammond, 1980). Obviously, if neurology were to establish a principle of brain functioning that involved breaking up the soul and localizing the different pieces in different parts of the cortex, that would go some way toward the goal of "materializing" French philosophy. Broca was fully aware of this (Broca, 1861a, chapter 2).

The fact that the debate over localization now focused on *language* is also significant. Broca was strongly predisposed to believe that, if this highest intellectual faculty were to be localized *anywhere* in the cortex, it would be in the frontal lobes. Gall's original claim for a link between intelligence and frontal lobe functioning (and, conversely, between instinct, passion, and posterior lobe functioning) had been buttressed since the early nineteenth century by a wide range of studies that compared the brains of different human racial groups with their "known" intellectual capacities. Virtually all of these had concluded that the white European races, which everyone "knew" stood biologically and culturally at the peak of human evolution, also possessed a considerably more developed frontal area than the "primitive" nonwhite human races. The French neuroanatomist Pierre Gratiolet had even gone so far as to classify the Caucasian, Mongoloid, and Negroid races in terms of their alleged dominant brain regions; viz., "frontal race," "parietal race," and "occipital race," respectively (Harrington, 1987, p. 42). Given this, one can begin to see why it would have been hardly conceivable to a European scientist such as Broca that a lofty intellectual faculty like language—used to such good effect by such fellow Europeans as Shakespeare, Voltaire, and Goethe—could have its seat anywhere *other* than in the frontal area.

Against this background, the specific clinical circumstances of Broca's investigation into the problem of language localization can be quickly reviewed. His first—and most famous—patient (known as "Tan" because that was the only word he could say) suffered from loss of speech even though his tongue and lips were not paralyzed, and even though he still seemed to understand what was said to him. At the autopsy, just 6 days later, it was indeed found that the frontal lobes of the brain were damaged, particularly the third frontal convolution (a different place than Gall's model had predicted). However, portions of the parieto-temporal lobes in the rear of the brain were also damaged. Broca got around this complication by arguing that the appearance of the patient's brain suggested that the posterior damage dated back to a period before the patient had lost his speech and was therefore irrelevant to the matter at hand. He then went on to affirm a link between Tan's frontal lobe damage and his speech loss, which Broca understood as a peculiar form of memory disorder involving loss of memory of the movements needed to pronounce words (Broca, 1861a).

The case of Tan did not at once turn the tide of scientific and medical opinion in favor of localization theory, but it represented a critical first step, and would soon be followed by a number of corroborating cases from a range of sources (Broca, 1861b). In very short order, Broca's claims for a center in the brain for the functioning of speech would slip on the mantle of a scientific fact, heralded as the first big success story in the history of cerebral localization. This is an intriguing development in more ways than one. What allowed Broca to accomplish something in a couple of years that Bouillaud—no less distinguished as an authority—had failed to accomplish in over 40? What made Broca's assertions count for more than those of his critics? It is notable that at the time when public opinion was swinging more and more in favor of Broca's views, another French physician, Armand Trousseau, had gathered information on 135 cases of speech loss that he felt largely *failed* to confirm the localizationist model, while Broca had a mere 32 cases in favor, many of them equivocal (Ryalis, 1984).

This all suggests that the triumph of localization theory cannot be understood by reference to the excellence of Broca's clinical work alone, but must take into account a range of other factors. Space does not allow a complete analysis here; however, the recollections of a leading French neurologist who lived through these times, Pierre Marie, may be of interest. Marie recalled how students living in the Third Republic in the 1860s seized upon the then-new doctrine of brain localizationism, because, by its materialistic radicalness and distastefulness to the older generation, it seemed to represent scientific progress. As such, according to Marie, it would also be adopted as a symbol of free thought and liberal politics. In Marie's words: "For a while, among the students, faith in localization was made part of the Republican credo" (Marie, 1906, p. 570). A comparison here with the enthusiastic response in the late 1960s—especially among politically liberal younger researchers—to the original laterality model of bimodal (logical/intuitive) consciousness may not be amiss.

LEFT-SIDED SPEECH, AND THE PROBLEM OF HEMISPHERIC ASYMMETRY

Most of Broca's cases not only seemed to confirm a connection between frontal lobe damage and speech loss, they also seemed to point to a link between speech loss and damage to the *left* side of the brain. The discovery of the unilateral or asymmetric nature of language's localization was to produce shock waves in medical thinking that would ultimately extend far beyond the narrow confines of clinical neurology. Initially, the fact that lesions causing speech disorders were found almost exclusively on the left side of the brain (and rarely the right) had been seen as an unexpected—and thoroughly unwelcome—complication of the main business at hand, which was to localize speech in the frontal lobes. Nevertheless, by the end of the 1860s, the asymmetry problem would transform the way neurologists regarded higher mental functioning in the human brain.

Things developed in the following way: although he saw that he would have to account for the clinical data, Broca was not prepared to accept the idea that nature could create two (apparently) identical structures that functioned differently. Belief in the innate functional symmetry of bilateral organs of the body was deeply embedded in French physiologic thinking. Speaking before the Society of Anthropology in 1865, Broca thus recalled the belief of neuro-anatomist Pierre Gratiolet that there were developmental differences between the two sides of the brain (caused by differential nutrition), with the left frontal lobe growing slightly faster than the right. In childhood then, Broca now proposed, when we are forced to master the complex manual and intellectual skills that characterize civilized human life—articulate language being preeminent among them—we tend to rely on our slightly more mature left frontal lobe. In other words, developmental predisposition means that we learn to speak with *half* our brain only, just as we learn to write with our right hand (the left brain half controlling the right body half). At the same time, some exceptional people—those we call left-handers—learn to talk with their right hemispheres (Broca, 1865).

This proposal of Broca's, that functional asymmetry was not inborn, but was an artifact of education and civilization upon the human mind, is remarkable for the way it discovers a virtue in necessity. From being a physiologic absurdity, functional asymmetry was suddenly declared "one of the principal traits of the human brain" (Broca, 1869, p. 392), a reflection of man's (particularly *man's*) capacity to lift himself by his own efforts beyond mere animal existence into a civilized, human state (Bérillon, 1884; Ball, 1884; Bastian, 1880; Delaunay, 1874). Because mid–nineteenth century neurologists believed that the effects of education upon the brain were inheritable, it was also argued that the more motivated races—those capable of what Broca (1860) called "perfectibility" or continuing self-improvement—would tend to develop more and more asymmetric brains as time went on. It is not surprising, therefore, that by 1869 Broca "had been able to assure" himself that asymmetry was less pronounced in the brains of blacks than in those of whites (Broca, 1869). Similarly, the French biologist Gaétan Delaunay (1874) argued that women's brains were less asymmetric than those of men, resembling in that respect the relatively symmetric brains of savages and young, uneducated children. In short, under Broca, asymmetry not only became a distinguishing mark of humanity in general, but a means of distinguishing the "better" vintage lineages of humankind from the substandard.

LATERALIZED FUNCTIONING IN THE NINETEENTH CENTURY: UNFINISHED BUSINESS

One of the first effects of this interpretation of brain asymmetry was to encourage a view of the left side of the brain as the intelligent, educated "human" side. This was accompanied by the growth of a certain suspicion toward the speechless right hemisphere, which seemed to be allowed to remain in an uneducated, animalistic state. Then, out of a variety of questions and observations inspired by the basic template of brain asymmetry, a more comprehensive view of the differences between the two hemispheres began to emerge. Let us briefly review some of the key themes.

Anatomic Asymmetries

Comparisons between the two sides of the brain took their point of origin from the fact that Gratiolet had not only argued that the left *frontal* lobe grew in advance of the right; he had equally made the case that the right *posterior* (occipital) lobe grew in advance of the left, so that in the end a kind of balance was achieved between the two sides of the brain. Broca, having seized upon the first part of this passage from Gratiolet to account for language asymmetry, did not neglect the second part either. In 1866, he reported on the work of a German osteologist, Hans Carl Barkow (1864), who had found a tendency in a number of human skulls for the frontal region to be slightly more pronounced on the left side, and the posterior region to be slightly more pronounced on the right side. Praising the exactness of Barkow's results, Broca (1866) then mentioned that he had had the opportunity to confirm them himself on two series of 20 brains, male and female respectively. All this new evidence made him increasingly confident that Gratiolet had been right, and that there was "a sort of compensation between the weight of the two frontal lobes and the two occipital lobes" (p. 196). Three years later, these alleged frontal-posterior differences between the hemispheres were given an explicitly functional cast, with the reported finding that the left frontal lobe was more abundant in gray matter than the right (gray matter being seen as the stuff of intellect), while the right occipital lobe was more abundant in gray matter than the left (Roques, 1869, p. 728).

Later, as aphasiology developed to a point where attention was no longer so exclusively riveted on the role of the frontal lobes in speech, the neuroanatomist Jules Bernard Luys (1879) would contend that structural asymmetries between the two hemispheres actually tended to be most pronounced in the "sphenotemporal regions." Not widely seized upon, this proposal would receive a measure of support in 1890 from a Viennese anatomist, O. Eberstaller, who found that the left sylvian fissure in human brains tended to be slightly longer than the right. Research by D. J. Cunningham (1892) published 2 years later in Ireland corroborated Eberstaller's findings. Cunningham, however, denied that these differences in fissure length had any implications for understanding the structural conditions underlying speech and handedness. This is because he had found the same asymmetries in the brains of various higher apes, and he did not believe that apes displayed any evidence of right-handedness (Cunningham, 1902, p. 293). The idea that hemispheric functional asymmetry might in some way be explicable in terms of temporal lobe asymmetries then went underground for some 80 years, to be resurrected in the 1960s with the work of Norman Geschwind and his colleagues (1968) in the United States.

In a 1972 article, Arthur Benton would rightly stress that the nineteenth century by and large failed to consider the possibility of right hemisphere involvement in certain visuospatial tasks, which would, in the 1970s, be perceived as one of its chief functional strengths. Given all these associations between the right hemisphere and occipital lobe functioning, the omission might seem surprising. It is true that John Hughlings Jackson would argue, beginning as early as 1864, for the existence of special "visuo-perceptive" functions in the right hemisphere, but his claims were not based on a view of the occipital area as "visual cortex" (Jackson, 1876; Harrington, 1987, chapter 7). Munk in fact did not localize his "visual center" in the occipital lobes until 1877 (correcting David Ferrier's earlier localization in the supramarginal and angular gyrus). In a paper published in 1895, an American physician from Philadelphia, Th. Dunn, also did suggest that there might exist "a center (which may, for convenience, be named the geographic center) on the right side of the brain for the record of optical images of locality, analogous to the region of Broca for that of speech on the left side in right-handed persons" (Dunn, 1895, p. 54). Dunn's views, however, were similarly not based on a consideration of any possible anatomic differences between the two occipital lobes, but were derived from clinical observation.

Still, the fact that the possibility of special right brain visual capacities was mostly overlooked in no sense means (as twentieth-century reigning wisdom used to have it) that the nineteenth century dismissed the right hemisphere as "merely a weaker version of the left" (Benton, 1972) or ignored it altogether.

If the anterior lobes were identified with human intelligence and reason, the posterior lobes —ever since Gall—had remained the presumed site of affect and instincts. Thus it was argued that the right hemisphere played a predominant role in sensibility, emotion, and activities related to vegetative, instinctual life—in this sense, neatly complementing the intellectual activities of the talking, manually dextrous left hemisphere.

Sensorimotor Asymmetries

But beliefs about posterior vs. frontal lobe functioning were just a starting point for this emerging "first" model of cerebral laterality. It became known, beginning in the 1870s, that there were cortical sensory centers located predominantly in the posterior regions of the brain, and motor centers in the frontal regions (Fritsch and Hitzig, 1870; Ferrier, 1876). The Viennese physiologist Sigmund Exner compared motor and tactile representation in the human brain for various parts of the body, and came to the conclusion that motor representation was both more intensive and extensive on the left side, while sensory representation was more intensive and extensive on the right side (Exner, 1891, pp. 64–65). Various clinical evidence seemed to offer some support to this claim. In France, Armand de Fleury (1872) had concluded that left brain damage tended to cause disorders of movement, while right brain damage was much more frequently associated with disorders of the sensibility (p. 840). Pierre Janet, studying disorders associated with the unilateral physical symptoms of hysteria, found—in a sample of 388 cases—a much greater tendency for patients with hysterical paralyses and anesthesias on the right side of their body to suffer globally from various motor disturbances: 71% of right-sided hysterics had movement disorders vs. only 37.8% of left-sided hysterics (Janet and Raymond, 1899).

The Right Hemisphere and Emotional Disorders

With a basic theoretical template of lateralized hemispheric functioning in position, people began to see things in ways that might not have been possible before. In 1881, Jules Bernard Luys, a neuroanatomist who had done important work on the thalamus, published a paper arguing for an "emotion" center in the right hemisphere which would complement the "intellectual" centers already established in the left hemisphere. He had been struck by the fact that there seemed to be definite and consistent personality differences between those of his patients suffering from right hemiplegia and those suffering from left hemiplegia. Whereas the former, he said, were "more or less apathetic, more or less silent, passive and stricken with hebetude," the latter were emotionally volatile, suffered from maniclike symptoms and delusions of persecution. Luys thought that these affective abnormalities might be explained on the hypothesis that some normal inhibiting center for emotion in the right hemisphere had been destroyed by a lesion supplementary to that responsible for the left hemiplegia—a lesion which he tentatively localized in the temporal area of the brain (Luys, 1881a).

This emerging case for a special right hemisphere role in emotion was given an additional boost by repeated observations that hysterical disorders —above all, the characteristic anesthesias and paralyses alluded to above— tended to manifest their symptoms unilaterally on the left side of the body (implying, according to French theory at the time, a "functional" lesion of the right hemisphere). Paul Briquet's (1859) *Traité clinique et thérapeutique de l'hystérie* noted that hysterical hemianesthesia had been observed three times more frequently on the left side than the right, and hysterical hemiparalysis was found by later researchers to follow a similar pattern (Richer, 1881, pp. 530, 552). Brown-Séquard (1874) examined 121 cases of hysterical hemiplegia and found a ratio of 4:1 in favor of the left side. In discussing the issue, Paul Richer went so far as to call hysteria's predilection for the left side of the body "Charcot's rule," although he warned that there were several exceptions. That the rule was nonetheless widely accepted right up into the early twentieth century can be seen from the number of authors cited by the British psychoanalyst Ernest Jones in a 1908 article which claimed to refute the old belief that hysteria favors the left side of the body (Jones, 1908).

The Right Hemisphere as the "Organic" Side of the Brain

Charles Edouard Brown-Séquard agreed with his colleagues that the left hemisphere was primarily concerned with communication and intellectual activity while the right hemisphere served chiefly in "the emotional manifestations, hysterical manifestations included." He added, though, that the right cerebral hemisphere also played a role in "the needs of the nutrition of the body in various parts" (Brown-Séquard, 1874). His claim here was primarily based upon comparisons of symptoms produced by organic lesions to the left and right sides of the brain. Various "troubles in the realm of nutrition"— bedsores, edema, pulmonary congestion, involuntary evacuation of feces and urine—more frequently accompanied right sided lesions than left, and physical symptoms from right brain lesions generally were more severe and apt to result in death than left-sided ones (Brown-Séquard, 1871, 1874; but see the contradictory conclusions by de Fleury, 1872). Charcot had also reported his clinical impression that the right hemisphere was more directly involved in "nutritional functions of the skin": in studies of bedsores developing in conjunction with hemiplegia, more cases were found to result from lesions of the right hemisphere than from the left (Bérillon, 1884, p. 100).

The Right Hemisphere and Psychopathology

Not only was the right hemisphere seen as the "emotional" and "organic" side of the brain; it also was believed to harbor basic irrationalist tendencies that could lead to madness. The immediate rationale for this idea was rooted in the evolutionary thinking of the time. People had always known that the mad were in some sense like animals (which is one of the reasons that they had previously been chained and beaten). Before the mid–nineteenth century, however, their animality had generally been held to be a sign of their fall from God's grace, or of their essential "otherness." The message of the new evolutionary thinking was much more alarming: the mad were like animals because, on some level, *all* of us were like animals; madness was the ultimate revenge of the "animalistic other" lurking in all our brains, wresting control over the once-civilized human.

Now if, as Broca had suggested, only the *left* half of our brain was truly civilized—if we were only half human—then it became possible to envision the "brute brain within the man's" (the phrase is Maudsley's) as lying on the right side of the skull. In 1879, Jules Bernard Luys became the first implicitly to argue along those lines with his declaration that, in the insane, the assumed natural disparity in weight between the hemispheres was increased to pathologic proportions and "completely reversed." Instead of the left lobe slightly outweighing the right as (he believed) in the sane, "nutrition" was guided in the opposite direction to favor the right hemisphere (Luys, 1879). Two years later, Luys (1881b) published the results of an examination he had carried out on 55 brains of persons judged insane at death; the right lobe was said to outweigh the left in 71% of them. Montyel (1884), whose later sample of 89 brains excluded cases of general paralysis (which he felt were an exception to the rule), pushed the figure up to 81%. Corroborating data on 400 brains had been published across the Channel by Crichton-Browne (1878). The question of a link between the right brain and madness continued to be debated throughout the century (Lyon, 1895); indeed, in 1887, Montyel would go so far as to declare that, ever since Luys had published his 1881 statistics, it "had not ceased to be the order of the day" (Montyel, 1887).

Gender and Racial Considerations

The same belief in the right hemisphere's animal nature that made it possible to assign it a causal role in madness also inspired inquiries into its differential functioning in men and women, who were believed to stand on distinctly different rungs of the evolutionary ladder. Among Broca's group, Gustav le Bon (1879) had declared that the brains of many Parisian women actually resembled more closely those of gorillas than those of adult white males. He admitted that there did exist a few intelligent women in the world, some of whom were even superior to the average male, but he argued that they were monstrosities, like a gorilla with two heads. Consequently they need not be taken into consideration (pp. 60–61). How to account for this female inferiority? For some scientists and physicians, the idea of hemisphere-lateralized functioning would prove a seductive resource. Thus it was suggested that "the terms 'male hemisphere' and 'feminine hemisphere' should render rather well the differences in nature between the two brains, of which one, more intellectual, is more stable, and of which the other, more excitable, is also more readily exhausted" (Klippel, 1898, pp. 56–57). Gaétan Delaunay (1874), a French comparative biologist, argued extensively for "remarkable" parallels between the right and left side of the brain and body, and "known" physical and mental differences between men and women. His claims and evidence were a source of considerable discussion for several decades (Klippel, 1898; Urquhart, 1879–1880; Descourtis, 1882; Hall and Hartwell, 1884; Manacéïne, 1894; Lombroso, 1903).

In a later publication, Delaunay (1878–1879) would futher suggest that the primary reason for the relative right-brainedness of women and left-brainedness of men was embryologic. Since every embryo was a fusion of a mother and father, it could be supposed that the "male element" always developed into the right side of the body (governed by the left half of the brain), while the "female element" always developed into the left side of the body (pp. 72–75). Although Delaunay was content to stop with that, several decades later Wilhelm Fliess (1906), close friend and inspiration for Sigmund Freud, would move the basic idea of a male/female lateralized brain in heady new directions: linking a theory of bisexuality to a theory of bilateral dominance. In both men and women, Fliess argued, the right side of the body (and, presumably, left hemisphere) served as the anatomic locus for the dominant sex, while the left side (and right hemisphere) served the opposite sex. Left-handedness was a sign of incomplete sexual dominance. As he noted, "effeminate men and masculine women are [always] entirely or partly left-handed" (p. 260–262).

As Gould points out (1951, p. 102) "inferior" groups are often interchangeable with one another within the framework of biological determinism. Thus, the last decades of the nineteenth century found Delaunay in Paris, seeking to prove further that the left hemisphere predominated in groups at a superior level of evolution, while the right took the lead in persons at an inferior level of evolution: these included white women, adult male members of nonwhite races, children, and the lower classes. Delaunay believed himself to have observed, for example, a tendency for members of superior groups to gravitate toward the right in walking, while members of inferior groups, dominated by their right hemisphere, tended to direct themselves to the left (Delaunay, 1879). Similarly, superior races tended to rotate to the right ("In France, in all our national dances, we turn to the right"), while middling inferior races (the Chinese, Japanese, Turks, Mexicans) turned toward the left, and the most inferior races of all (Africans, for example) just jumped up and down without turning at all! (Delaunay, 1883, 1884).

The reception of Delaunay's work, all published in the prestigious *Lancette française*, is an important illustration of one way in which a society's values can become so rooted in its way of looking at scientific questions that scientists cannot even see anything operating beyond the data. None of Delaunay's peers ever raised questions about biases in his data, because, in their world-view, the inferiority of certain human groups, like nonwhites and women, was as much a matter of observable "fact" as the most solid descriptive claims of neuroanatomy.

Sleep, Dreaming, and Other Altered States

Late in the century, Marie de Manacéïne, a (woman!) psychologist from St. Petersburg, performed some experiments which she took to mean that the left hemisphere was primarily concerned with waking existence, while the right was especially involved in sleep and dreaming. In a series of experiments performed on 52 subjects, Manacéïne found that tickling a sleeper's face on the right side of the median line always caused him to brush at himself with his left hand, even when he was lying on his left side and the action of that hand was impeded. Significantly, left-handed people (of which she had a small sample) always brushed at their faces with the right hand, even when the left was lying free. "These facts," Manacéïne believed, "may be explained on the hypothesis that the most active cerebral hemisphere is resting during the hours of deep sleep" (Manacéïne, 1897).

Although he did not refer to Manacéïne's work, the prominent psychologist and rival to Freud, Pierre Janet, would 2 years later give further credence to this view of the right hemisphere as the brain half that was active during sleep in his analysis of the relationship between the episodic symptoms of hysteria and the side of the body afflicted with the permanent stigmata (Janet and Raymond, 1899). In a pool of 388 cases, incidents of spontaneous somnambulism, fugue, and attacks of pathologic sleep were significantly more frequently found in cases of hysteria where the stigmata were restricted to the left side than in cases of right-sided hysteria (72.2% in left-sided-hysteria vs. 48% in right-sided-hysteria).

Frederick Myers (1885) took up this ball and went still further with it, proposing that something he called the "subliminal self"—a sort of unconscious mind with paranormal access to spiritual realms—had its primary focus in the right hemisphere. He pointed out that the writing and speech of mediums and other entranced people often resembled the distorted language of patients with damage to their left hemispheres and presumed to be "talking" out of their right brains; i.e., speech was often emotionally disinhibited and formally distorted, with written words sometimes in mirror image or reversed. In a variation on this idea, the Italian criminal anthropologist Cesare Lombroso (1909) pointed to parallels between the left-sidedness of symptoms seen in hysteria and the left-sidedness of mediumistic "symptoms," i.e., the fact that the "spiritistic phenomena" seen in séances (apparitions, rappings, etc.) often took their point of origin from the left side of the medium's body (p. 117). Lombroso also called attention to the supposedly high incidence of actual left-handedness among mediums. All this seemed, in his words, "to indicate the increased participation of the right lobe of the brain in mediumistic states, as occurs with hypnotized persons, and would explain the concomitant unconsciousness" (Lombroso, 1908, p. 378).

BRAIN DUALITY AND DIVIDED CONSCIOUSNESS, NINETEENTH-CENTURY STYLE

Lateralized hemispheric functioning, by definition, seemed to imply a certain natural tendency for the two sides of the brain to function independently. As the French physiologist Brown-Séquard put it in 1874, "the very fact that the loss of speech depends on a disease of the left side of the brain ... is extremely important in showing that the two sides of the brain may act independently of each other" (Brown-Séquard, 1874). Was it possible that, under certain conditions, this natural independence could be exaggerated to pathologic proportions? If so, could one have here the makings of an explanation for a range of psychiatric conditions suggestive of split or double consciousness? In a time in European cultural history when "the entire nineteenth century was preoccupied with the problem of the coexistence of ... two minds [within one person] and of their relationship to each other" (Myers, 1885, p. 145), more than a few medical men were prepared to play with the idea that brain duality did in fact mean literally that we each had "two minds" within one skull, minds that could sometimes get out of sync and struggle against each other.

The possibilities suggested by this notion provided an intriguing new lens for viewing old clinical phenomena. Some of the resulting attempts to map "divided consciousness" onto the two brain halves would reveal an infant neuropsychiatry at its most naked and vulnerable. A patient's ("subjective") sense that he or she was "two people" would be seized upon by the doctor as a key piece of evidence in support of the physiologic ("objective") hypothesis that the patient's two hemispheres had fallen into a state of pathologic independence or disequilibrium. The double-brain hypothesis would then be used by the doctor to explain that same subjective state and provide an allegedly deeper-level, "objective" account of the patient's condition. It is a fascinating sort of mirror logic.

The case of "D," recounted in an influential 1882 medical dissertation by the French physician Gabriel Descourtis, is typical here:

D ... always speaks using the pronoun "we"; "we will go," "we have walked a great deal." He says that he speaks like this "because there is someone with him"; at meals, he says: "I've had enough but the other has not." He begins to run; he is asked why, and he replies that he would prefer to stay [where he is], but it is the "other" who forces him on, even though he holds him back by his coat. One day, he hurls himself upon a child in order to strangle it, saying that it is not he but the "other." Finally he tries to commit suicide, "to kill the other," whom he believes to be hidden in the left part of his body; he also calls him "left D ..." and names himself "right D ...," bad D ... and good D ..., etc. The patient falls little by little into dementia. Autopsy reveals a considerable difference between the two halves of the brain.... It is evident that the unilateral seat of these lesions was the cause, if not unique, at least essential of the double personality delirium; the individual was different on each side, he felt himself double. (Descourtis, 1882)

In another case, a young man began to receive visits from an apparition that dressed in a hunting outfit and called itself "M. Gabbage." As time went on, Gabbage increasingly tormented the young man with incessant questions, and later forced him to commit senseless and violent acts. The physician Benjamin Ball (1884) recalled the way in which the original diagnosis implicating independent hemispheric action was made:

One day, when conversing with him on the subject of his impulsions, he said to me: "You are not up to date in science; you seem to be unaware that one often has two brains in one's head. This is precisely the case with me. Gabbage has the left brain and I possess the right brain. Unfortunately, it's always the left side that gets the better of me, and this is why I cannot resist the advice of this man who appears to be an evil spirit or at least a malevolent fellow." … Here we have then a brain whose functions seem to be quite clearly doubled, and one can readily believe, following the theory of the patient himself, that one of the hemispheres is fully delirious, while the other regards it with compassion. (p. 37)

Persuasive as they may have seemed to some, there were others who sharply criticized diagnoses like these, made without an "iota of proof" (Bruce, 1897). The Scottish physician Lewis Bruce took pride in his use of the more "objective" evidence of handedness in implicating the double brain in cases of divided consciousness. In one case of his, for example, a patient alternated between periods in which he spoke English and was right-handed, and periods in which he spoke a rather incoherent form of Welsh, and used only his left hand. In this second state, he was also "shy and suspicious" and appeared "to be constantly on the lookout for unseen danger" (Bruce, 1895, pp. 60–62).

As one would expect, it was usually the right hemisphere (subjectively experienced on the left side) that was perceived to support the "crazy" self in cases of divided personality, but there were exceptions. In 1902, Eugen Bleuler reported a case of "unilateral delirium," complicated, he believed, by a callosal disconnection between the two hemispheres (see Interhemispheric Crosstalk, below). The patient's right hand grabbed at ropes, chopped things with an axe, sowed seeds, and slung away unwanted invisible objects with great vigor. Sometimes it would seize hold of the blankets or the pillow and try to yank them away, and once it upset the patient's dinner. When this happened, the sane left hand readjusted the bedclothes, wiped the patient's mouth, and gave every appearance of remaining in contact with reality. The consciousness associated with the delirious right-handed activities of the patient had full command of language; the rational consciousness corresponding to the patient's left-handed activities seemed to be occasionally able to speak, but was considerably more limited in this respect (Bleuler, 1902–1903).

Manipulating the Hemispheres in vivo

Now isolated clinical cases like these were all very well, but some people at the time wanted more systematic, controlled evidence. They were to find it, as they thought, in an unlikely tactic: hysteria research using hypnosis and related manipulations. The story behind this development began in 1876 when an elderly doctor, Victor Burq, wrote to Claude Bernard, then president of the Paris Biological Society. Burq explained that, for the past 25 years, he had been curing women suffering from hysterical hemianesthesia by applying metallic discs to the afflicted side of their bodies. He asked Bernard if the society would be willing to investigate and confirm the genuineness of his findings. Bernard agreed, and appointed a committee to the task which consisted of three leading neurologists: Jean Martin Charcot, Amedée Dumontpallier, and Jules Bernard Luys. After a year of study at Charcot's Salpêtrière, the committee reported back, full of praise for Burq. Not only were the so-called metalloscopic effects genuine, but a new discovery had been made in the course of investigation. It seemed that when sensibility was returned to one side of the body, the normal sensibility on the other side of the body was lost. This was called the "law of transfer" and implied, according to French theory at the time, that metals (and by now also magnets and electric currents) were able to effect a displacement of function from one hemisphere of the brain to the other (Dumontpallier, Charcot, and Luys, 1877). As Charcot put it at the time: "It appears that with these hysterics, the nervous fluid, if one will pardon the expression, does not transport itself to one side until after it has in part abandoned the other" (Féré, 1902, p. 108).

Matters got even more interesting when researchers started claiming that it was possible to transfer, not just hemianesthesia and hemiparalysis, but voluntary actions and intellectual activity as well. This was called "psychic transfer." One subject, for example, was made to write numbers on a page in the normal way using her right hand, while a magnet was secretly put by her left elbow. It was said that she was able to write only as far as the number 12 before she was compelled to stop and transfer the pen to her left hand with which she continued to write, but in mirror image (mirror-writing being widely seen as a product of the right brain), and was furthermore agraphic or incapable of writing with her right hand (Binet and Féré, 1885).

From here, one sees a situation in which the interest in hemispheric functional independence aroused by the "transfer" studies was carried over into a closely related research venture that used, not magnets and metals, but hypnotic induction techniques to manipulate the nervous systems of hysterics (on the relationship between metalloscopy and hypnosis, see Harrington, 1988a,b). Quite simply, it turned out that one could hypnotize the brain's two hemispheres separately (Charcot and Richer, 1878). You could hypnotize a patient and then wake up only half her brain (doctors then commented on the "cold-blooded" manner in which the patient noticed she was "cut in two" [Luys, 1890]). You could invoke unilateral hypnosis and "transfer" it. You could bring about a state of functional aphasia by plunging the left brain into a state of catalepsy; because similar right brain manipulations were said not to have any effect on speech, this last was offered as a "new experimental proof" of Broca's left-sided localization of language (Ballet, 1880).

Most dramatic of all, though, were the experiments that involved simultaneous but separate (and generally opposing) hallucinations in each hemisphere. It was Amedée Dumontpallier at La Pitié hospital who pioneered this line of research, and for a while he became quite renowned for his studies in which it was claimed (for example) that half a patient's face smiled as its corresponding hemisphere hallucinated a pleasant country fair and the other half grimaced in terror as it recoiled from an attack by an hallucinated dog (Dumontpallier, 1882; Bérillon, 1884). Jean Martin Charcot (1883) also experimented with this form of hemihypnosis. An English visitor to the Salpêtrière, George Robertson, declared, after being shown Charcot's version of this trick: "I had before me a person angry with one side of the face and laughing with the other" (Robertson, 1892, pp. 505–506).

It all seemed compelling for a while, but ultimately experiments like these —along with a more general tendency of advocates to exaggerate the explanatory power of the double brain—began to undermine the overall credibility of this line of speculation and inquiry. Theodule Ribot (1891) spoke disdainfully of those authors who indulged in "a kind of psychological manichaeism," claiming that "cerebral dualism suffices to explain every discrepancy in the mind, from simple hesitation between two resolves, to the complete duplication of personality" (p. 109). Pierre Janet (1889) also failed to find much explanatory value in the idea. "In fact," he said, "we have, all of us, two brains, and we are neither madmen, nor somnambulists, nor mediums" (p. 414). Charles Mercier (1901) in England put it quite unequivocally that "an hypothesis of so wild a character, and so utterly unsupported by evidence, does not merit serious discussion" (p. 509).

The perceived likelihood that the double brain had much to do with divided consciousness also grew more tenuous as it became increasingly clear (in the words of a critic) that "[we] are not bound to the number two in considering the mass of conscious, subconscious, and unconscious states that may succeed one another in our body" (Rosse, 1892, p. 187). At an 1885 congress on psychiatry and neuropathology at Antwerp, a Dr. Verriest presented a patient suffering from "double consciousness." He then revealed that this woman could also be thrown into a *third* state of consciousness through "hypnotic passes." "In such a case as this," he asked, "what becomes of Luys' hypothesis of the functional alternation of the two cerebral hemispheres?" (Congress of Psychiatry and Neuro-pathology at Antwerp, 1885–1886, pp. 621–622).

INTERHEMISPHERIC CROSSTALK: NINETEENTH-CENTURY VIEWS OF THE CORPUS CALLOSUM

Doubt was also thrown upon the entire argument linking hemispheric independent action to pathologic splits of consciousness by uncertainty surrounding the functions of the corpus callosum, the huge bundle of fibers joining the two sides of the brain. Most advocates for dual hemisphere action believed that the healthy person experienced a sense of unified consciousness because the corpus callosum provided a bridge of conduction between two psychic realms. Yet there were numerous cases on record in which the corpus callosum had been lacking or damaged without producing any discernible "split" in consciousness, or any discernible mental symptoms at all. In England, William Ireland (1886) spoke of the work of Eduard Hitzig in Germany, "who has studied the question carefully, [and] observes that no well-marked disorder of motion or sensation follows atrophy of the corpus callosum, nor is there any characteristic mental defect attendant upon this lesion" (pp. 317–318; for a variety of puzzling cases, see Bruce, 1889; Erb, 1885; Ransom, 1895).

Yet, even in the midst of a sea of uncertainty, an oddly isolated island of clarity and conviction began emerging. The hero in this story is the German neurologist Hugo Liepmann, well-known for his development of the diagnostic category of "apraxia" or inability to perform purposive movements (for the paradigmatic case, see Bruce, 1889). In 1905, Liepmann reviewed the results for 89 patients tested for signs of apraxia following unilateral hemiplegia, and found a compelling pattern. Whereas the *right* brain–damaged patients all performed promptly and well with their right hands (their left hands being paralyzed), about half of the left brain–damaged patients showed signs of severe apraxia or dyspraxia when attempting to function with their left hands (which they used since their right hands were paralyzed). Through various tests, Liepmann ruled out any possibility that this left-sided apraxia was simply due to some sort of failure to understand instructions. The remaining conclusion was radical: an intact left hemisphere was not only necessary for proper functioning of *right*-sided movements (as everyone had long known), but was important as well for the execution of willed actions on the *left* side; in other words, it played an executive role in voluntary motor function for the entire body, both the right and left sides (Liepmann, 1900).

This expansion of the classic doctrine of left brain domination to include voluntary or purposive movements (*Zweckbewegungen*) not only raised some intriguing questions of its own, it also opened the door to an important new view of the corpus callosum. Liepmann argued that, on the highest levels of voluntary motor functioning, it served as a channel through which the left side of the brain (especially the frontal or motor region controlling the limbs) could work its "will" on the right side. From this, at least two important clinical predictions followed:

Lesions which affect the arm center in the left hemisphere itself or its projection fibers as well as the callosal fibers, cut off the arm center in the right cerebral hemisphere from this dominance, and simultaneously paralyze the right upper extremity.... A lesion which only affects the corpus callosum ... would cause left-sided dyspraxia by cutting off the right-sided hand center from its dominance by the left side, while the right hand would not necessarily be either paralyzed or apraxic. (Liepmann, 1905, p. 38)

In 1905, Liepmann's second postulated clinical syndrome—left-sided dyspraxia resulting from a callosal lesion alone—was still just that, a postulated or theoretical entity. This unsatisfactory situation, however, was remedied remarkably quickly. A mere 2 years later, when Liepmann (1907) sat down to write an updated theoretical paper on matters concerning the corpus callosum, he was able to point to no less than three recent case studies which essentially conformed to the clinical picture outlined in the 1905 paper (van Vleuten, 1907; Hartmann, 1907; Liepmann and Maas, 1907). Two more clinical reports bearing favorably on the model and expanding on it were to follow very close on the heels of these first three (Maas, 1907; Goldstein, 1908). One is struck not only by the speed with which apparent confirmation followed in the wake of prediction but also by how much of an "in-house" job the process of confirmation seems to have been. All the key actors were German neurologists thoroughly familiar with Liepmann's recent views on the functioning of the corpus callosum and all (except possibly Hartmann) knew Liepmann personally. One need not suspect any of these men of bad faith to wonder a bit about this phenomenon. Are we simply dealing here with a group of exceptionally talented clinicians who knew (better than anyone else) what to look for, or are there ways in which institutionalized methods and theoretical biases can influence not only how science explains its observations but the act of clinical observation—of "seeing"—itself?

CONCLUSION

The laterality research program of the nineteenth century, of course, is not ours. The first venture was largely shaped by French and, to a lesser extent, by German researchers during a time when the brain sciences were fascinated by problems in comparative neuroanatomy, (racialist) anthropology, and the unusual consciousness associated with what would today be called dissociative personality disorder, but was then called hysteria or dual personality. Research questions at the time took their starting point and justification from a tendency to turn to classic brain localization theory as a basic approach to most questions about mind-brain relations, from differences in intelligence, to outright madness, to subtle personality changes (Harrington, 1989, 1991).

Early in the twentieth century, the literature of the nineteenth-century laterality and asymmetry research effort largely fell into obsolescence for reasons ranging from a growing skepticism about much of the relevant hysteria and hypnosis research (which grew increasingly occult and fantastic as the 20th century proceeded [Harrington, 1988b]), to the outbreak of World War I (an event that shifted the intellectual focus of brain research from Europe to the United States). As is well known, in the 1960s a new generation of researchers, with an initial home base in the western United States, would rediscover brain asymmetry and laterality as a problem, largely through the stimulus provided by the dramatic behavior of so-called split-brain patients. These were, of course, the group of epileptic patients whose corpora callosa were severed (for therapeutic reasons) by neurosurgeons Joseph Bogen and Philip Vogel, and who were then studied by Roger Sperry and a group of his graduate students (for this history, see Harrington, 1987, chapter 8). Even as much data were gathered in these years that would be critical in developing and refining later theories about the significance and etiology of brain asymmetry and lateralized functioning, the new research also proved to have a powerful popular appeal, and a startling capacity to resonate with cultural preoccupations of the day. The concept of dual lateralized functioning—with the left hemisphere being seen as the site of analytic, verbal cognition, and the right hemisphere as the site of more "holistic," affective, and perceptual processes—became an apparently inexhaustible source of cultural and psychological speculation, and (for some) an inspiration for moralistic critique. Western society was accused of having overdeveloped its rational "left brain" at the expense of the "other side of the brain," whose modes of processing were said to be better developed in Oriental cultures (Bogen, 1969; Ornstein, 1972; Harrington and Oepen, 1989). One 1970s German article, borrowing from the rhetoric and conviction of the American laterality brain research program, went so far as to suggest that the essence of National Socialism had lain in its neglect of the "holistic" right hemisphere and its cultivation of what were basically "left hemisphere" values and habits of thought: "... the Nazis with their calculating, bookkeeping rationality were trained in piecemeal thinking to an extreme degree and viewed people as clumps [Stücke]. It is simply false to dismiss the other form of thinking, the thinking mode of the nondominant brain half as irrational; thinking holistically is not irrational" (Portele, 1979).

Today, some 30 years down the road, claims tend to be less bombastic (at least within the mainstream community) and methods considerably more refined. New imaging technologies are allowing for considerably more precise information about the workings of the brain in vivo. Categorical generalizations about lateralized functioning have given way to more systematic attention to individual differences. Studies on the functional significance of the right-left lateral axis tend more often to be qualified along frontal-caudal and cortical-subcortical axes. There is more appreciation of the likely role of neurochemistry in both the development and expression of lateralized functioning. Still, we of course do not know how far the questions we ask today will make sense to neuroscientists a century from now, what they will find valuable in our results, or what ingrained cultural values and inherited intellectual assumptions will be discovered to have shaped our own readings of the data.

As we continue to develop the laterality paradigm as a probe into mind-brain relations, some awareness of the unfinished business of the history of this problem field is one important resource that can help us hedge our bets. It is not simply that knowledge of a neglected body of literature may provide new data or serve as a conceptual stimulus for current research (although both of these benefits are possible). Rather, the history of a scientific discipline or problem field matters because history is the best observational laboratory the scientific community has available for testing hypotheses about science and the factors that foster its success in the complex context of the real world. Why—and to what ends—have models of the brain historically been constructed in the ways they have? Why does an idea fail to rally enduring support in one time only to succeed in another? Why does one group "see" things another group does not even know to look for? Asking questions like these may begin to help us to discover patterns in our own research agendas that are problematic or, conversely, needlessly confining, and may encourage us to think afresh about avenues rejected for reasons we might not consider relevant today. Whether we usually give much thought to the fact or not, we are all involved in "writing" the present history of brain laterality research. One additional challenge we may choose to take on would be to become more conscious authors of our own legacy.

REFERENCES

Ball, B. (1884). Le dualisme cérébral. *Revue Scientifique. Série III, 7,* 33–37.

Ballet, G. (1880). Nouveau fait à l'appui de la localisation de Broca. Demonstration expérimentale de la localisation de la faculté du langage dans l'hémisphère gauche du cerveau. *Le Progrès Médical, 8,* 739–741.

Barkow, H. C. (1864). *Bemerkungen zur pathologischen Osteologie.* Breslau: Ferdinand Hirt's Königliche Universitäts Buchhandlung.

Bastian, H. C. (1880). *The brain as an organ of mind.* London: Kegan Paul.

Benton, A. (1972). The 'minor' hemisphere. *Journal of the History of Medicine and Allied Sciences, 27,* 5–14.

Bérillon, E. (1884). *De l'indépéndance fonctionnelle des deux hémisphères cérébraux.* Paris: A. Parent.

Binet, A., and Féré, C. (1885). L'hypnotisme chez les hystériques. I. Le transfert psychique. *Revue Philosophique de la France et de l'Étranger, 19,* 1–25.

Bleuler, E. (1902–1903). Halbseitiges Delirium. *Psychiatrisch-neurologische Wochenschrift, 4*(34), 361–367.

Bogen, J. E. (1969). The other side of the brain II: An appositional mind. *Bulletin of Los Angeles Neurological Societies, 34,* 135–162.

Bouillaud, M. J. (1825). *Traité clinique et physiologique de l'encéphalité ou inflammation du cerveau, et de des suites.* Paris: J.-B. Baillière.

Broca, P (1860). Discussion sur la perfectibilité des races. *Bulletins de la Société d'Anthropologie, 1,* 337–342.

Broca, P. (1861a). Remarques sur le siège de la faculté du langage articulé, suivies d'une observation d'aphémie (perte de la parole). *Bulletins de la Société Anatomique, 36,* 330–357.

Broca, P. (1861b). Nouvelle observation d'aphémie produite par une lésion de la moitié posterieure des deuxième et troisième circonvolutions frontales. *Bulletins de la Société Anatomique. Série II, 6,* 398–407.

Broca, P. (1865). Du siège de la faculté du langage articulé. *Bulletins de la Société d'Anthropologie, 6,* 377–393.

Broca, P (1866) [index title]. Poids comparé des lobes frontaux et occipitaux, et des deux hémisphères. In Correspondance, *Bulletins de la Société d'Anthropologie. Série II, 1,* 195–196.

Broca, P. (1869). L'ordre des primates. Parallèle anatomique de l'homme et des singes. XI. Le cerveau. *Bulletins de la Société d'Anthropologie. Série II, 4,* 374–395.

Brown-Séquard, Ch. E. (1870). Symptômes variables suivant le côté de l'encéphale qui est le siège des lésions. *Comptes rendus de la Société de Biologie. Série V, 2,* 27–28, 96–97.

Brown-Séquard, Ch. E. (1871). Parallèle des phénomènes différents observés dans les lésions des hémisphères droits et gauches du cerveau. *Comptes rendus de la Société de Biologie. Série V, 3,* 96.

Brown-Séquard, Ch. E. (1874). Dual character of the brain (Toner lecture). *Smithsonian Miscellaneous Collections Washington, DC, 1878, 15*, 1–21.

Bruce, A. (1889). On the absence of the corpus callosum in the human brain, with the description of a new case. *Brain, 12*, 171–190.

Bruce, L. (1895). Notes of a case of dual brain action. *Brain, 18*, 54–65.

Bruce, L. (1897). On dual brain action and its relation to certain epileptic states. *Transactions of the Medical Chirurgical Society of Edinburgh, 16*, 114–119.

Charcot, J., and Richer, P. (1878) Catalépsie et somnambulisme hystériques provoqués. *Le Progrès Médical, 6*, 973–975.

Charcot, J. M. (1883). *Exposé des titres scientifiques du M. J. M. Charcot.* Paris: Victor Goupy et Jourdan.

Congress of Psychiatry and Neuro-pathology at Antwerp [Notes and News] (1885–1886). *Journal of Mental Science, 31*, 621–622.

Crichton-Browne, J. (1878). On the weight of the brain and its component parts in the insane. *Brain, 1*, 504–518.

Cunningham, D. (1892). *Contributions to the surface anatomy of the cerebral hemispheres.* Dublin: Royal Irish Academy.

Cunningham, D. (1902). Right-handedness and left-brainedness [the Huxley lexture for 1902]. *Journal of the Royal Anthropological Institute of Great Britain and Ireland, 32*, 273–296.

de Fleury, A. (1872). Du dynamisme comparé des hémisphères cérébraux dans l'homme. *Association française pour l'avancement des sciences, 1*, 834–845.

Delaunay, G. (1874). *Biologie comparée du côté droit et du côté gauche chez l'homme et chez les êtres vivants.* Paris: A. Parent.

Delaunay, G. (1878–1879). *Études de biologié comparée,* 2 vols. Paris: V. Adrien Delahaye.

Delaunay, G. (1879). De la tendance des individus à se diriger à gauche ou à droite. *Lancette française: Gazette des hôpitaux, 52*, 253–254.

Delaunay, G. (1883). De la rotation. *Lancette française: Gazette des hôpitaux, 56*, 970–971.

Delaunay, G. (1884). Du croisement des membres et de la façon de s'asseoir. *Lancette française: Gazette des hôpitaux, 57*, 332–333.

Descourtis, G. (1882). *Du fractionnement des opérations cérébrales et en particulier de leur dédoublement dans les psychopathies.* Paris: A. Parent.

Dumontpallier, A. Charcot, J. M., and Luys, J. B. (1877). Rapport fait à la Société de Biologie sur la métalloscopie du docteur Burq. *Comptes rendus de la Société de Biologie (sec. mémoires). Série VI, 4*, 1–24.

Dumontpallier, A. (1882). Indepéndance fonctionnelle de chaque hémisphère cérébral—illusions, hallucinations unilatérales ou bilatérales provoquées. *Comptes rendus de la Société de Biologie. Série VII, 4*, 786–797.

Dunn, Th. D. (1895). Double hemiplegia with double hemianopsia and loss of geographical center. *Transactions of the College of Physicians of Philadelphia. Third Series, 17*, 45–55.

Erb [no initial] (1885). A case of hemorrhage in the corpus callosum. *The Journal of Nervous and Mental Diseases, 12*, 121.

Exner, S. (1881). Untersuchungen über die Localisation der Functionen in der Grosshirnrinde des Menschen. Vienna: Wilhelm Braumuller.

Féré, Ch. (1902). L'alternance de l'activité des deux hémisphères cérébraux. *L'anneé psychologique, 8,* 107–149.

Ferrier, D. (1876). *The functions of the brain.* London: Dawsons of Pall Mall, 1966.

Fliess, W. (1906). *Der Ablauf des Lebens.* Leipzig: Franz Deuticke, 1923.

Flourens, J. P. M. (1846). *Phrenology examined,* C. L. Meigs (Trans.). Philadelphia, PA: Hogan & Thompson.

Fritsch, G., and Hitzig, E. (1870). Über die elektrische Erregbarkeit des Grosshirns. In *Some papers on the cerebral cortex,* G. von Bonin (Trans.). Springfield, IL: Chartes C Thomas, 1960.

Geschwind, N., and Levitsky, W. (1968). Human brain; left-right asymmetries in temporal speech region. *Science, 161,* 186–187.

Goldstein, K. (1908). Zur Lehre von der motorischen Apraxie. *Journal für Psychologie und Neurologie, 11,* 169–270.

Gould, S. J. (1981). *The mismeasure of man.* New York: W. W. Norton Co.

Hall, G. S., and Hartwell, E. M. (1884). Research and discussion, bilateral asymmetry of function. *Mind, 9,* 93–109.

Hammond, M. (1980). Anthropology as a weapon of social combat in late nineteenth century France. *Journal of the History of the Behavioral Sciences, 16,* 118–132.

Harrington A. (1987). *Medicine, mind and the double brain: A study in nineteenth-century thought.* Princeton, NJ: Princeton University Press.

Harrington, A. (1988a) Metals and magnets in medicine: Hysteria, hypnosis, and medical culture in fin-de-siècle Paris. *Psychological Medicine, 18,* 21–38.

Harrington, A. (1988b). Hysteria, hypnosis and the lure of the invisible: The rise of neo-mesmerism in fin-de-siècle french psychiatry. In W. F. Bynum, R. Porter, and M. Shepherd (Eds.), *The anatomy of madness: Essays in the history of psychiatry,* Vol. 3, *The asylum and its psychiatry* pp. 226–246. London: Tavistock Press.

Harrington, A. (1989). Psychiatrie und die Geschichte der Lokalisation geistiger Funktionen. *Nervenarzt, 60,* 603–611.

Harrington, A. (1991). Beyond phrenology: Localization theory in the modern era. In P. Corsi (Ed.), *The enchanted loom: Chapters in the history of neuroscience,* New York, NY: Oxford University Press.

Harrington, A., and Oepen, G. (1989). "Whole brain" politics and brain laterality research. *Archives of European Neurology, 239*(3), 141–143.

Hartmann, F. (1907). Beiträge zur Apraxielehre. *Monatsschrift für Psychiatrie und Neurologie, 21* (Jan–June), 97–118, 248–270.

Ireland, W. (1886). The blot upon the brain: Studies in history and psychology (pp 317–318). New York, NY: G. P. Putnam's Sons.

Jackson, J. H. (1876). Case of large cerebral tumour without optic neuritis and with left hemiplegia and imperception, In J. Taylor (Ed.), *Selected writings of John Hughlings Jackson,* Vol 2 (pp 146–152). London: Hodder & Stoughton, 1931.

Jacyna, L. S. (1981). The physiology of mind, the unity of nature, and the moral order in Victorian thought. *British Journal History of Science, 14,* 109–132.

Janet, P. (1889). L'automatisme psychologique, ed 7. Paris: Librairie Felix Alcan, 1913.

Janet, P., and Raymond, F. (1899). Note sur l'hystérie droite et sur l'hystérie gauche. *Revue neurologique, 7,* 851–855.

Jones, E. (1908). Le côté affecté par l'hémiplégie hystérique. *Revue neurologique, 16,* 193–196.

Klippel, M. (1898). La non-équivalence des deux hémisphères cérébraux. *Revue de Psychiatrie,* pp 52–57.

le Bon, G. (1879). Variations du volume du cerveau et sur leurs relations avec l'intelligence. *Revue d'Anthropologie, 8,* 27–104.

Liepmann, H. (1900). Das Krankheitsbild der Apraxie (motorischen Asymbolie) auf Grund eines Falles von einseitiger Apraxie. *Monatsschrift für Psychiatrie und Neurologie, 8,* 15–44, 102–132, 182–197.

Liepmann, H. (1905). Die linke Hemisphäre und das Handeln [orig. pub. in *Münchener medizinische Wochenschrift,* No. 48, 49]. Reprinted in *Drei Aufsätze aus dem Apraxiegebiet (neu durchgesehen und mit Zusatzen versehen)* (pp 17–50). Berlin: Karger, 1908.

Liepmann, H. (1907). Über die Funktion des Balkens beim Handeln und die Beziehungen von Aphasie und Apraxie zur Intelligenz. [orig. pub. in *Münchener medizinische Klinik,* No. 25, 26] Reprinted in *Drei Aufsätze aus dem Apraxiegebiet (neu durchgesehen und mit Zusatzen versehen)* (pp 51–80). Berlin: Karger, 1908.

Liepmann, H., and Maas, O. (1907). Fall von linksseitiger Agraphie und Apraxie bei rechtsseitiger Lähmung. *Journal für Psychologie und Neurologie, 10,* 214–227.

Lombroso, C. (1903). Left-handedness and left-sidedness. *North American Review, 177,* 440–444.

Lombroso, C. (1908). Psychology and spiritism [review of Enrico Morselli's Psicologia e 'spiritismo']. *The Annals of Psychical Science, 7,* 376–380.

Lombroso, C. (1909). *After death—what?,* W. S. Kennedy (trans). Boston, MA: Small, Maynard & Co.

Luys, J. B. (1879). Études sur le dédoublement des opérations cérébrales et sur le rôle isolé de chaque hémisphère dans les phénomènes de la pathologie mentale. *Bulletin de l'Académie de Médecine. Serie II, 8,* 516–534, 547–565.

Luys, J. B. (1881a). Recherches nouvelles sur les hémiplégies émotives. *Encéphale, 1,* 378–398.

Luys, J. B. (1881b). Contribution à l'étude d'une statistique sur les poids des hémisphères cérébraux à l'état normal et à l'état pathologique. *Encéphale, 1,* 644–646.

Luys, J. B. (1890). Faits tendant à démontrer que le lobe droit joue un rôle dans l'expression du langage articulé. *Revue d'hypnologie theorique et pratique, 1,* 134–146.

Lyon, S. B. (1895). Dual action of the brain. *New York Medical Journal, 62,* 107–110.

Maas, O. (1907). Ein Fall von linksseitiger Apraxie und Agraphie. *Neurologisches Centralblatt, 26,* 789–792.

Manacéïne, M. de (1894). Suppléance d'un hémisphère cérébral par l'autre. *Archives italiennes de biologie, 21,* 326–332.

Manacéïne, M. de (1897). *Sleep: Its physiology, pathology, hygiene and psychology.* London: Walter Scott, Ltd.

Marie, P. (1906). Revision de la question de l'aphasie: l'aphasie de 1861 à 1866; essai de critique historique sur la genèse de la doctrine de Broca. *Semaine médicale,* pp 565–571.

Mercier, C. A. (1901). *Psychology, normal and morbid.* London: George Allen & Unwin.

Montyel, M. de (1884). Contribution à l'étude de l'inegalité de poids des hémisphères cérébraux dans la folie nevrosique at la démence paralytique. *Encéphale, 4,* 574–589.

Montyel, M. de (1887). Contribution à l'étude du poids des hémisphères cérébraux chez les aliénés. *Annales Médico-Psychologiques. Serie I, 6,* 364–382.

Myers, F. W. H. (1885). Automatic writing II. *Proceedings of the Society for Psychical Research, 3,* 23–63.

Ornstein, R. (1972). *The psychology of consciousness.* San Francisco, CA: W. H. Freeman & Co.

Portele, G. (1979). Gestalttheorie und Wissenschaftstheorie. Pläyoder für eine alternative Wissenschaft. *Gestalt Theory, 1*(1), 26–38.

Ransom, W. B. (1895). On tumours of the corpus callosum, with an account of a case. *Brain, 18,* 531–550.

Ribot, T. (1891). *The diseases of personality, authorized translation,* ed 4. Chicago, IL: Open Court Publishing Co, 1910.

Richer, P. (1881). Études cliniques sur l'hystéro-épilepsie ou grande hystérie. Paris: Delahaye et Lecrosnier.

Robertson, G. M. (1892). Hypnotism at Paris and Nancy. Notes of a visit. *Journal of Mental Science, 38,* 494–531.

Roques, F. (1869). Sur un cas d'asymétrie de l'encéphale, de la moelle, du sternum et des ovaires. *Bulletins de la Société d'Anthropologie. Série II, 4,* 727–732.

Rosse, I. C. (1892). Triple personality. *Journal of Nervous and Mental Diseases, 19,* 186–191.

Ryalls, J. (1984). Where does the term "aphasia" come from. *Brain and Language, 21,* 358–363.

Sherrington, C. S. (1955). *Man on his nature.* Cambridge, England: Cambridge University Press.

Spurzheim, J. G. (1908). *Phrenology or the doctine of the mental phenomena,* ed 2. Philadelphia, PA.: J. B. Lippincott Co.

Urquhart, A. R. (1879–1880). On the habitual tendency of individuals to direct themselves to the right or left [abstract of communication by M. Delaunay, May 18, 1879]. *Brain, 2,* 291–292.

van Vleuten, C. F. (1907). Linksseitige motorische Apraxie: Ein Beitrag zur Physiologie des Balkens. *Allgemeine Zeitschrift für Psychiatrie und Psychisch-gerichtliche Medizin, 64,* 203–239.

Whitehead, A. (1925). *Science and the modern world.* Cambridge, England: Cambridge University Press.

II Phylogenetic Antecedents and Anatomic Bases

2 The Influence of Gonadal Steroids on the Asymmetry of the Cerebral Cortex

David Warren Lewis and
Marian Cleeves Diamond

Today, with a known number of factors influencing the structure and function of the cerebral cortex, it is difficult to imagine that we once thought this remarkable part of the brain was immutable. Both internal and external environmental components are continuously, directly or indirectly, altering the cerebral cortex. With the myriad of sensory receptors receiving the numerous kinds of stimuli, as well as the various enzymes, hormones, immune, and dietary elements constantly impinging on cortical cells, how does one know for certain the role of one specific component acting alone? In order to understand brain function in general, what other choice do we have than to study separately one or two variables at a time? Hopefully, in the future, the individual elements can be integrated better to provide a more holistic functional picture.

At one time we thought that both cerebral hemispheres were quite similar in morphology, and in turn function, and that gonadal steroids acted primarily on the hypothalamus, but now, from many investigations, we know differently. In this chapter we have chosen to illustrate that the asymmetric pattern of the cerebral cortex is influenced by gonadal steroids, realizing that many other factors, including adrenocortical steroids, affect asymmetry as well.

More and more evidence is accumulating to indicate the role of gonadal steroids in the determination of cerebral cortical asymmetry. Several behaviors observed in rats, including male-typical sexual behaviors, some forms of aggression, and some maze-learning skills, appear to be dependent on the presence of estrogen in the male brain during critical periods in late gestation and early postnatal life. The source of this estrogen in males, is, paradoxically, conversion of testosterone produced in the fetal testes into estrogen by an aromatizing enzyme localized in neural tissues. It is well documented that males whose testosterone is depleted, or in whom the conversion of testosterone to estrogen is inhibited, or whose estrogen receptors are blocked, display less male-typical behavior and more female-typical behavior. These behavioral changes correlate with steroid-dependent anatomic and morphologic changes in specific hypothalamic nuclei. In this chapter, however, we investigate whether there are similar steroid-dependent patterns of growth in the cerebral cortex, and specifically in developing cerebral cortical asymmetry.

In previous experiments, we have observed that in male Long-Evans rats, the right cerebral cortex is statistically significantly thicker than the left in most regions. The cortex of the female rats is more symmetric, but when asymmetry is observed, the left side tends to be thicker than the right, although the differences are rarely statistically significant (Diamond, Johnson, and Ingham, 1975). That the sex steroid hormones play some role in determining asymmetry in the cerebral cortex was demonstrated by experiments in which the gonads were removed (Diamond, 1984). With further investigations, we have shown that these left-right and male-female differences are related to the differential and asymmetric distribution of estrogen receptors in the cortex. From the results of our previous studies we hypothesize that limiting the conversion of testosterone to estrogen by administering 1,4,6-androstatriene-3,17-dione, (ATD) (a competitive inhibitor of aromatase, the enzyme that converts testosterone to estrogen) will alter the usual sexually dimorphic pattern of growth and asymmetry in the cerebral cortex in a manner similar to that found in the hypothalamus.

There is ample evidence illustrating that the aromatization hypothesis applies to the hypothalamus. There are anatomic sex differences in several specific hypothalamic nuclei that are involved in reproductive behavior, including the sexually dimorphic nucleus (SDN) of the preoptic area (POA) (Gorski et al., 1978), the ventromedian nucleus (Dorner and Staudt, 1969a,b), and the suprachiasmatic nucleus (Robinson et al., 1986). Sexual differentiation of the rat hypothalamus occurs during a specific critical period of development (Rhees, Shryne, and Gorski, 1990), and perinatal interventions have more profound effects than interventions in mature animals (Jacobson, Davis, and Gorski, 1985; Dohler et al., 1986). The aromatization hypothesis formulated by McDonald and Doughty (1974) is that testosterone induces sexual differentiation in the hypothalamus through interactions with estrogen receptors, after being converted to estrogen by local aromatase. Sex differences in the hypothalamus therefore depend not only on the presence of testosterone but on the expression of estrogen receptors in specific regions (Leiberburg et al., 1978; MacLusky, Chaptal, and McEwen, 1979), the presence of aromatase in specific regions (Reddy, Naftolin, and Ryan, 1974) and its activity (George and Ojeda, 1982), and the accessibility to estrogen receptors of circulating estrogen or locally generated estrogen derived from testosterone (Plapinger, McEwen, and Clemens, 1973; McEwen et al., 1975). Estrogen in appropriate doses is as effective as testosterone in masculinizing the hypothalamus (Christiansen and Gorski, 1978; Dohler et al., 1984), whereas nonaromatizable androgens are ineffective (McDonald and Doughty, 1974). Estrogen receptor blockers attenuate the effects of testosterone (Dohler et al., 1986), and so does inhibition of aromatase (McEwen et al., 1977, 1979). Estrogen actions on the hypothalamus are associated with sex differences in the size and cellularity of specific regions (Jacobson et al., 1981), in synaptogenesis (Raisman and Field, 1973), in expression of cellular progestin receptors (Parsons, Rainbow, and

McEwen, 1984) and in serotoninergic (Handa et al., 1986) and cholecystokininergic innervation (Micevych, Matt, and Go, 1988).

From the above, it is clear that sexual differentiation of the hypothalamus depends on local aromatization of testosterone to estrogen. The next question is, Do the same biological mechanisms contribute to sex differences in the cerebral cortex? How well do current knowledge and experimental data provide answers to the following six questions?

1. Is the rat cerebral cortex sexually dimorphic in morphology, histology, biochemistry, and function?

2. When do sex differences in the rat cerebral cortex develop?

3. Is testosterone responsible for sexual differentiation of the rat cerebral cortex?

4. Does testosterone act on the developing cerebral cortex primarily by conversion to estrogen and interactions with estrogen receptors?

5. Does testosterone act on the developing cerebral cortex by interaction with androgen receptors?

6. Is aromatase activity present in rat cerebral cortex during the appropriate developmental periods?

THE RAT CEREBRAL CORTEX IS SEXUALLY DIMORPHIC

The cerebral cortex in rats is, like the hypothalamus, sexually dimorphic. In male Long-Evans rats, the right cerebral cortex is, in general, thicker than the left (Diamond, Johnson, and Ingham, 1975; Diamond, Johnson, and Ehlert, 1979; Diamond, Dowling, and Johnson, 1980; Diamond, 1983, 1984, 1987, 1988). This asymmetry is present at birth (Diamond, 1983) and continues throughout life, with the statistically significant differences disappearing in very old age (Diamond et al., 1975, 1983). Long-Evans females have more symmetric cortices, and when asymmetry is present in females, it tends to be left-greater-than-right asymmetry (Diamond et al., 1979, 1980, 1983; Diamond, 1984, 1985, 1987, 1988). In the very old female, the cortical pattern is more male-typical in the occipital cortex, a pattern not seen in the young adult Long-Evans females (Diamond, 1985, 1987). Patterns similar to those found in Long-Evans young adult rats have been identified in cerebral cortical thickness of Sprague-Dawley male and female rats at 90 days (Stewart and Kolb, 1988) and males at 130 to 140 days (Fleming et al., 1986), in neocortical volume of 7-month-old Purde-Wistar rats (Sherman and Galaburda, 1985), in orbital prefrontal cortical volume of Wistar rats at various ages (Van Eden, Uylings, and Van Pelt, 1984) and in hemispheric dimensions of male adult Long-Evans rats and male mongrel cats (Kolb et al., 1982). A variety of asymmetries, some of them sexually dimorphic, are present in the human brain (Geschwind and Galaburda, 1985; Habib, 1989).

Differences in cortical thickness and volume reflect differences in cell size or number, or both. In male rats, the thicker right cortex has more neurons, oligodendroglia, and total glia per unit area than the left; females have more neurons and glia in the left cortex per unit area than in the right (McShane et al., 1988). In general, direct comparisons *between* males and females have not demonstrated a sex difference in cortical neuron number (Pfaff, 1966; Yanai, 1979b), although males have larger cortical cell diameters (Gregory, 1975; Yanai, 1979b), larger nucleolar areas (Pfaff, 1966), and greater occipital cortex RNA content (Soriero and Ford, 1970) than females. Following [^{3}H]-thymidine injection of Wistar rats on day 7, at day 60 more cells are labeled in males than in females (Yanai, 1979b), indicating that there are differences in the rate of cell maturation and timing of neural cell division between the sexes.

Hemispheric asymmetries in cortical biochemistry also have been reported. In female C3H/He mice, focal cortical lesions on the right side have different immunologic effects than left-sided lesions (Renoux et al., 1983; Barneoud et al., 1987). Asymmetries in male rats are seen in cortical aminopeptidase activity (Alba et al., 1985) and in serotoninergic response to focal cortical lesions (Mayberg, Moran, and Robinson, 1990).

Cerebral cortical asymmetry also can be approached from the perspective of sex differences in behavior. While sex differences in reproductive behavior often are associated with asymmetries in subcortical structures such as the hypothalamus, a large number of nonreproductive behaviors also are sexually dimorphic and may reflect cortical asymmetries (Denenberg, 1981; reviewed in Hines and Gorski, 1985; Juraska, 1986; Hellige, 1990).

In summary, the cerebral cortex in the rat is sexually dimorphic. Males show an asymmetry between the right and left sides that differs in direction and degree from that of females. The difference in thickness reflects both structural and biochemical differences between the right and left sides, and these differences may be associated with sexually dimorphic and lateralized behaviors.

CORTICAL ASYMMETRY IS ALTERED BY BOTH PRENATAL AND EARLY POSTNATAL INTERVENTIONS

Specific critical periods for sexual differentiation of the SDN of the POA have been identified in rats (Rhees et al., 1990) and guinea pigs (Byne and Bleirer, 1987). Less data are available concerning the timing of interventions that alter cerebral cortical asymmetry. Cortical asymmetry in males has been demonstrated at birth (Diamond, 1983) and at 6 days of age (Diamond, Dowling, and Johnson, 1980). Males gonadectomized at birth lose their usual right-greater-than-left asymmetry and are left-greater-than-right asymmetric in some cortical regions, whereas females ovariectomized at birth show an opposite shift in cortical asymmetry to the right (Diamond, Johnson, and Ehlert, 1979). Exposing dams to stressful conditions during pregnancy lowers fetal serum testosterone in male progeny (Ward and Weisz, 1980), but not in females (Ward and Weisz, 1984). Prenatal maternal stress causes male progeny to shift from right-greater-than-left to left-greater-than-right in somatosensory cortical asymmetry (Anderson et al., 1986).

That both prenatal stress and day 1 gonadectomy alter cortical asymmetry indicates that the critical period for establishing asymmetry begins prior to birth and extends into early postnatal life. This interval is similar to the period for sexual differentiation of the hypothalamus and of reproductive and non-reproductive behaviors, which also are modified by these interventions. Although the cortex remains plastic in adulthood to influences such as environmental enrichment (Smith, 1934; Diamond et al., 1964; Bennett et al., 1974) and adrenalectomy (Fisher et al., unpublished data), it has been our experience that such interventions affect cortical thickness bilaterally more often than asymmetrically (Diamond, 1985).

THERE ARE SEX DIFFERENCES IN SERUM TESTOSTERONE DURING CEREBRAL CORTICAL DIFFERENTIATION, AND INTERVENTIONS THAT ALTER TESTOSTERONE LEVELS ALTER CORTICAL ASYMMETRY

Differences in serum testosterone levels between male and female rats have been identified both prenatally and postnatally. Males have been reported to have higher levels than females on gestational day 18 only (Ward and Weisz, 1980, 1984), or on gestational days 19, 20, and 21 (Slob et al., 1980). Postnatally, male rats experience a testosterone surge within 1 to 3 hours after birth (Corbier, Roffi, and Rhoda, 1983), a condition which is not present in females. Male rats generally have higher levels of testosterone (George and Ojeda, 1982) from birth through approximately day 20 (Lieberburg, Wallach, and McEwen, 1977; Lieberburg et al., 1978; Lieberburg, MacLusky, and McEwen, 1980). Nonetheless, female rats are exposed to significant amounts of testosterone, which may be as high as those in males on several prenatal days (Ward and Weisz, 1980) and about 50% as high as male littermates in the immediate postnatal period (Slob et al., 1980).

Interventions that alter cortical asymmetry alter gonadal steroid levels as well. Prenatal stress lowers fetal serum testosterone (Ward and Weisz, 1980), but not in females (Ward and Weisz, 1984), and decreases aromatase activity in brains of males and females (Weisz, Brown, and Ward, 1982). Prenatal stress alters cortical asymmetry (Fleming et al., 1986), size of the SDN-POA (Anderson et al., 1986), and reproductive and nonreproductive behaviors (Ward, 1971; Archer and Blackman, 1971) in males. Prenatal stress does not have similar effects on females, although it may increase female-typical reproductive behavior (Ward, 1977).

Like prenatal stress, early gonadectomy reduces testosterone levels in male pups and has similar effects on male cortical asymmetry (Diamond, 1985), hypothalamus (Jacobson et al., 1981), and behavior (Corbier et al., 1983;

Heinsbroeck et al., 1987). Early ovariectomy alters female cortical asymmetry in Long-Evans rats (Pappas, Diamond, and Johnson, 1978), but not Sprague-Dawley rats (Stewart and Kolb, 1988). The reason for this strain difference is not clear. Ovariectomy apparently does not alter differentiation of the female hypothalamus or the "organizational" components of female behavior, although there is some controversy on this point (Dohler et al., 1986).

Morphine inhibits testicular steroidogenesis and lowers serum testosterone in males (Cicero et al., 1976); endogenous opioids play a role in sexual differentiation (Ward, Orth, and Weisz, 1983). Naloxone and naltrexone block the actions of endogenous opioids and prevent their mediation of testosterone-negative feedback on luteinizing hormone (LH) secretion (Cicero, Schainker, and Meyer, 1979), maintaining or increasing serum testosterone levels. Thus concurrent treatment with naltrexone prevents the effect of prenatal maternal stress on male sexual behavior (Ward, Monaghan, and Ward, 1986), and postnatal naltrexone (P1-21) increases brain weight and somatosensory cortical thickness in Sprague-Dawley rats (Zagon and McLaughlin, 1983a,b) and somatosensory cortical thickness in Long-Evans rats, with altered cortical symmetry (Reyes, 1993). In naltrexone-treated animals, "enlarged brain size was accompanied by an increase in the number of neurons and glia, particularly those arising postnatally" (Zagon and McLaughlin, 1983), just as in normal males compared to females, as discussed previously.

In summary, there is a good deal of indirect evidence that exposure to testosterone prenatally and postnatally is responsible for the sexually dimorphic asymmetry of the cerebral cortex, but direct proof is still lacking. Such proof might come from examination of females exposed to testosterone in utero from adjacent males, or of females exposed to exogenous testosterone prenatally or postnatally. It would be helpful to know if exogenous testosterone restores male-typical cortical asymmetry in neonatally gonadectomized males, or increases cortical asymmetry in normal males. Until such experiments are done, we still can say with confidence that prenatal stress and early gonadectomy reduce testosterone levels in male rats and opioid blockade increases them, and that these interventions are associated with sex-specific changes in cortical thickness and asymmetry.

DOES TESTOSTERONE ACT ON THE DEVELOPING CEREBRAL CORTEX PRIMARILY BY CONVERSION TO ESTROGEN AND INTERACTIONS WITH ESTROGEN RECEPTORS?

We have noted the paucity of direct observations of the effects on cortical asymmetry of testosterone deprivation in males and of testosterone exposure in females. There is a similar lack of information on the effects of estrogen on cerebral cortical development. Estrogen agonists such as diethylstilbestrol and MER-17, which are effective in masculinizing hypothalamic morphology and function in females (Tarttelin and Gorski, 1988), have not been investigated in the developing cortex. We do not know whether high doses of estrogen (or estrogen agonists) given perinatally can reverse the cerebral cortical effects of prenatal stress or neonatal gonadectomy in males. Our best evidence that estrogen is involved in cerebral cortical differentiation is based on studies of the ontogeny, location, and distribution of cortical estrogen receptors, rather than from direct studies of estrogen treatment and effects.

Estrogen receptors are present in the cerebral cortex perinatally in many species, including rats, mice, ferrets, and primates (McEwen, 1981). In rats, cortical cytosolic estrogen receptors can be detected prenatally and in the first weeks of postnatal life (MacLusky, Chaptal, and McEwen, 1979; Sandhu, Cook, and Diamond, 1986); their development initially lags a day or two behind that of subcortical estrogen receptors (Lieberburg et al., 1978). A similar pattern is seen in mice (Attardi and Ohno, 1976; Vito and Fox, 1979; Gerlach et al., 1983). In rats, estrogen receptors initially are localized in the deeper layers of the cortex (Toran-Allerand, 1983), as they are in adulthood (Simerly et al., 1990). Estrogen receptors appear several days after the development of cortical neurons (Keefer and Holderegger, 1985). The development of estrogen receptors is an inherent quality of neural tissues and is not dependent on stimulation by gonadal steroid hormones (Paden, Gerlach, and McEwen, 1985).

Although estrogen receptors are present in the developing cortex, little peripherally generated estrogen reaches these receptors (Lieberburg, Wallach, and McEwen, 1977). In 4-day-old female and male castrated rats, no nuclear-bound cerebral cortical or hypothalamic estrogen receptors are detected (Westley and Salaman, 1976), although cytoplasmic estrogen receptors are present (White, Hall, and Lim, 1979), as they are in normal male and female rats in the first weeks postnatally (Barley et al., 1974; Sandhu, Cook and Diamond, 1986). Nuclear translocation of cytoplasmic estrogen receptors can be detected in hypothalamic and limbic regions in normal postnatal males, but less in females or males treated with ATD (MacLusky and Naftolin, 1981). However, treatment of females with an estrogen-receptor antagonist, tamoxifen, reduces still further the size of the SDN-POA (Gorski, 1986). Nuclear translocation of estrogen receptors in the rat cortex has not been detected prior to postnatal day 10 (Dudley, 1981). In male rats, the distribution of nuclear estrogen receptors in subcortical brain regions correlates positively both with serum testosterone levels and with local tissue capacity for aromatization (Krey, Kamel, and McEwen, 1980).

Alpha-fetoprotein (AFP) is present in the neonatal rat and mouse brain in quantities that are sufficient to bind all circulating estradiol and estrone (Soloff, Morrison, and Swartz, 1972; Germain, Campbell, and Anderson, 1978). In general, more AFP is found in those regions of the brain whose development is not steroid-dependent, and less AFP is present in those areas which require estrogen for their differentiation (Toran-Allerand, 1982).

In rats of both sexes, serum levels of estradiol are elevated on the first 2 postnatal days, then decline (Dohler and Wuttke, 1975). These steroids are likely of maternal or placental origin, but may have a prolonged half-life in the neonate because of immaturity of metabolic clearance functions. Another increase in serum estradiol and estrone occurs between postnatal days 9 and 19; estradiol values may reach levels more than twice those of the adult preovulatory phase, and estrone values may be 50 times higher than the highest adult proestrus levels (Dudley, 1981). Although the ovary begins estrogen secretion in the second week of life, much of the estrogen formed during this peak interval is of adrenal origin, and can be eliminated by adrenalectomy (Weisz and Gunsalus, 1973; Ojeda, Kabra, and McCann, 1975).

Administration of exogenous estradiol shortly after birth is associated with a decline in cell division and decreased protein synthesis in the cerebrum and hypothalamus (Vertes, Vertes, and Kovacs, 1973), especially during the first 2 weeks of life. Estradiol given to rats on postnatal days 6 to 10 alters free amino acid levels in rat neocortex compared with oil-injected controls, potentially decreasing inhibitory neurotransmission (Hudson, Vernadakis, and Timiras, 1970); estradiol treatment of adult animals does not duplicate these effects (Timiras, 1971). Neonatal estradiol inhibits the incorporation of ^{14}C lysine into neuroproteins in the cerebral cortex, although it does not appear to inhibit protein syntheses per se (Litteria and Thorner, 1976); estrogen treatment in adulthood has a similar effect (Litteria and Timiras, 1970). Estrogen given to female Long-Evans rats beginning at 45 days of age and continuing until 90 days of age decreases cortical thickness (Pappas, Diamond, and Johnson, 1979).

In explants of amygdaloid tissue from newborn rats maintained in the anterior chamber of adult animals, exogenous estrogen increases dendritic shaft synaptogenesis (Arai et al., 1986). Newborn preoptic tissue, maintained in the third ventricle of adult ovariectomized females, responded to estradiol treatment with increased volume and increased dendritic shaft and spine synapses; explants from parietal cerebral cortex did not (Arai et al., 1986). Hypothalamic, but not cerebral cortical explants maintained in an in vitro tissue culture system show dendritic proliferation and branching in response to estrogen or testosterone (Toran-Allerand, 1978). Kallikreins process kininogens that may be involved in a variety of intracellular processes, including growth; kallikrein activity is present in rat hypothalamus and cerebral cortex. Testosterone increases kallikrein content in castrated male rats, but reduces it in normal females (Chao et al., 1987).

In summary, estrogen receptors are expressed in considerable numbers in the cerebral cortex prenatally and for at least 3 weeks postnatally. Substantial amounts of serum estrogen are present during this interval. Because of AFP, cortical receptors are occupied to a small degree, if at all, by circulating estrogens, and generation of estrogen by cortical aromatization has not been demonstrated in the rat neonatally. Exogenous estrogen causes a number of changes in the developing cortex that may be attributed to rapid maturation and terminal differentiation with loss of cell division. However, the results of administration of estrogen on the cerebral cortex in the adult rats are at present somewhat inconsistent. The results of administration of estrogen on the cerebral cortex vs. the hypothalamus bring about different effects. Often, hypothalamic areas show increases with estrogen administration, whereas cerebral cortical tissue does not: it shows the opposite effect. More work is necessary to clarify the effects of exogenous estrogen on the cerebral cortex.

ARE THE EFFECTS OF TESTOSTERONE MEDIATED BY CEREBRAL CORTICAL ANDROGEN RECEPTORS?

Like estrogen receptors, androgen receptors are present in the developing rat brain (Sheridan, Sar, and Stumpf, 1974; Lieberburg, MacLusky, and McEwen, 1980), mouse (Attardi and Ohno, 1976), and rhesus monkey (Sholl and Kim, 1990). In the neonatal rat brain, androgen receptors are present in smaller quantities than estrogen receptors, and their ontogenesis follows a different pattern (Lieberburg et al., 1978). Androgen receptors are undetectable prenatally, but appear soon after birth, and gradually increase to adult levels over the first 3 to 4 weeks postnatally (Monbon et al., 1974; Meaney and Aitken, 1985). A similar pattern is seen in the mouse brain (Attardi and Ohno, 1976). In fetal rhesus monkey cerebral cortex, androgen receptors are more prevalent than estrogen receptors (Pomerantz et al., 1985), and are lateralized in a sexually dimorphic pattern; sex differences were not seen in 5α-reductase or aromatase activity (Sholl and Kim, 1990).

5α-Reductase activity is present in neural tissue of newborn rats, and the cerebral cortex of both male and female neonatal and adult rats can produce ATD and dihydrotestosterone (DHT) from labeled testosterone. "If ability to form DHT signifies target organ function, then the cortex as well as the hypothalamus contains target organs for testosterone." (Weisz and Philpott, 1971). However, in males, cortical asymmetry is present at birth, before androgen receptors are present, and the effectiveness of ATD in altering cortical asymmetry is evidence for the aromatization hypothesis (see Kaplan and McGinnis, 1989).

IS AROMATASE ACTIVITY PRESENT IN THE CEREBRAL CORTEX DURING THE APPROPRIATE DEVELOPMENTAL PERIOD?

Aromatase activity in general has not been detected in rat neocerebral cortex at any age, although it is present in the hypothalamus (George and Ojeda, 1982; MacLusky et al., 1985), and in hippocampus and cingulate cortex in newborn mice (MacLusky et al., 1987). However, aromatase-containing cells in adult male and female Wistar rats can be demonstrated by immunohistochemistry (Shinoda et al., 1989), and sensitive assay systems show aromatase in adult golden hamster cerebral cortex (Negri-Cesi, Celotti, and Martini, 1989), despite previous reports to the contrary (Callard, Petro, and Ryan, 1979). Apparently, such assays have not been applied to the neonatal rat cerebral cortex. However, in 50-, 80-, and 120-day-old fetal rhesus monkey, aromatase activity is present in the frontal cortex at higher levels than are found in adults, and is sexually differentiated, with greater activity in males (Roselli and Resko, 1986).

Perinatally, hypothalamic aromatase activity peaks are associated with peaks in serum testosterone (Tobet et al., 1985a,b). Adult gonadectomy decreases hypothalamic aromatase activity in rats (Roselli, Ellinwood, and Resko, 1984) and eliminates sex differences in hypothalamic aromatization in rats and doves (Steimer and Hutchison, 1990). In both cases, exogenous androgens restore aromatase activity. Aromatase activity in the hypothalamus is, at least in part, mediated by androgen receptors, since flutamide blocks testosterone-induced increases in aromatization (Roselli and Resko, 1984), and aromatization is deficient in testicular-feminized rats despite their higher circulating androgen levels (Roselli, Salisbury, and Resko, 1987). Prenatal stress decreases hypothalamic aromatase activity in both male and female rats (Weisz, Brown, and Ward, 1982), but intrauterine proximity to male fetuses, which exposes females to increased levels of androgens (Vom Saal and Bronson, 1980), does not (Tobet et al., 1985a). These findings support the contention of Roselli et al. (1987), that both genetic and hormonal factors interact to determine aromatase activity.

The results from the laboratory of Diamond and colleagues reported in this chapter do not address directly the issue of whether aromatization occurs in the developing cerebral cortex. They do, however, demonstrate that ATD, an inhibitor of aromatase, can alter the normal cortical growth pattern (Lewis, 1991), and therefore support a role for aromatization in cerebral cortical differentiation in specific regions. MacLusky et al. (1987) speculate that:

failure to detect aromatization in the rat cerebral cortex might reflect regional or temporal variations in the expression of the enzyme, rather than a complete absence of aromatase activity.... It is conceivable that aromatase activity might change abruptly in different areas of the rodent cortex, during perinatal and early postnatal life. (p. 469)

The increasing sophistication and precision of our investigational tools may well allow us to demonstrate in the near future that the growth and development of a subset of cerebral cortical cells is dependent on aromatization of testosterone.

PREVIOUS EXPERIMENTAL USE OF ATD

Experimentally, compounds that selectively inhibit aromatase are useful in identifying and distinguishing the effects of testosterone and ATD from the effects of their aromatized metabolites, estradiol and estrone, as well as from the effects of testosterone metabolites produced by reductases, especially DHT. ATD has been used in several species prenatally, postnatally, and in adulthood to explore the role of sex steroids in modifying brain morphology, brain chemistry, and reproductive and nonreproductive behavior.

Aromatization is an important process in neonates and adults, both for organization and activation of sexual behavior. ATD is a useful tool to distinguish processes that are directly androgen-dependent from those that depend on androgen-derived estrogen. ATD has been used frequently in behavioral studies, and it seemed that it might prove equally useful in exploring a sexual dimorphism in brain development. The results of the ATD studies are in preparation for publication.

Most of the research on sex differences and asymmetry in the cerebral cortex has been carried out on the rat because rats have a smooth cortex that has no folds. Histological measurements of cortical thickness are relatively easy to determine on the rodent cortex in contrast to cortices of cats, dogs, monkeys, and humans. We have tried several times to obtain cortical thickness data on human brains, but the variation of thickness through the gyri and sulci is too great for reliable results. Therefore, comparable asymmetry data found in rats have not been shown in humans.

Perhaps in the future as the resolution of magnetic resonance imaging (MRI) scans improves, consecutive sections will provide adequate samples to compile average thickness data over considerable areas of human cortex.

SUMMARY AND CONCLUSIONS

Several lines of evidence converge in support of the hypotheses that cerebral cortical asymmetry in Long-Evans rats is largely or entirely hormone-dependent, that testosterone is responsible for sex differences in asymmetry, and that the mechanisms by which testosterone affects the hemisphere differentially is through aromatization to estrogen and interaction with cortical estrogen receptors. Estrogen receptors are present in the developing cortex, and are asymmetrically distributed in a sexually dimorphic pattern. Testosterone is present both before and after birth, at times that coincide with expression of cortical estrogen receptors. Aromatization of testosterone is responsible for sex differences in other sexually dimorphic regions of the brain. Sex differences in testosterone can be demonstrated at specific times during development. Testosterone is present in substantial amounts prenatally, when the cortex expresses estrogen (but not androgen) receptors, and male cortical asymmetry is already present at birth. Interventions that alter circulating testosterone levels in males, including prenatal maternal stress, day 1 gonadectomy, and opioid receptor blockade, also affect male cortical asymmetry.

A corollary of these hypotheses is that mechanisms exist to protect cortical estrogen receptors from peripherally generated estrogen, ensuring that control of sexual differentiation in the cortex depends on local aromatization of testosterone. Fetuses of both sexes are exposed equally to maternal and placental estrogen. However, circulating estrogen is bound with high affinity to AFP, making it unavailable to neural estrogen receptors. In contrast, testosterone binds to circulating proteins with lower affinity, and does gain access to the developing brain. Testosterone is known to serve as a substrate for aromatase and as the source of neural estrogen in other hormone-dependent brain structures.

Undoubtedly, the absolute dimensions of the cortex are due not only to the actions of estrogen but to a wide variety of influences, including the animal's prenatal and postnatal milieu, general metabolic state, nutritional status, maternal sufficiency, and environmental stimulation, as well as the action of other growth-enhancing and growth-inhibiting hormones. However, estrogen may well be substantially responsible for the asymmetry between the cerebral hemispheres, and the development of this asymmetry may also precede the periods of maximal growth and subsequent consolidation. Even if estrogen receptors are only transiently expressed, their effects could be long-lasting.

An alternative hypothesis is that cerebral cortical asymmetry is hormone-dependent, but that both testosterone and ATD act via androgen receptors. Androgen receptors are expressed in the cortex postnatally, and testosterone is present during this time. Since Lewis (1991) gave ATD both prenatally and postnatally, it is possible that ATD modification of normal asymmetry occurred postnatally. Objections to this theory include lack of direct evidence that ATD competes with testosterone for androgen receptors, the effectiveness of prenatal interventions such as maternal stress in altering male cortical asymmetry, and the presence of cortical asymmetry at birth, before androgen receptors are detected in the cerebral cortex.

The most telling objections to applying the aromatase hypothesis to the cerebral cortex are that aromatase activity has not been identified in the developing rat cortex, and neither has nuclear translocation of estrogen-receptor complexes in cortical cells. Both these objections raise technical questions regarding our ability, using current methods, to detect processes that may be quite localized in time and restricted to specific cortical regions.

The timing of expression of cortical estrogen receptors relative to peak periods of cortical growth is another interesting consideration. The period of maximal estrogen receptor expression in the cerebral cortex does not coincide with the period of maximal expansion in cortical thickness during the first postnatal month. In fact it is quite the contrary. The rat cerebral cortex reaches maximal thickness (Diamond et al., 1975) at the same time the estrogen-receptor activity is minimal in the cerebral cortex, approximately 1 month after birth (Sandhu et al., 1986).

One perspective that may help us to understand these complex hormonal systems for sexual differentiation is that every organism requires multiple levels of control over maleness and femaleness. Consider the number of regions in which sex differences exist, each with its own developmental timetable and its own interactions with neighboring and distant tissues. In the central nervous system alone, the differentiation of sexual behaviors involves sexual dimorphism of the hypothalamus, preoptic area, amygdala, pituitary, spinal cord nuclei associated with pelvic musculature, perhaps the cortex, perhaps the hippocampus, perhaps the pineal body; sexual differences in exploratory behavior may involve cerebral cortex, striatum, and hippocampus; sex differences in paternal and maternal behavior involve the hypothalamus, pituitary, and probably additional brain regions as well; sex differences in perception involve differential organization of a variety of sensory processing pathways and associative connections.

It would indeed be remarkable if all these demands for sexual differentiation could be met by modifying the levels of a single hormone during development. To achieve more precise, localized control of growth and differentiation in different tissues at different times during development, a variety of regulatory mechanisms are required. One way an organism can regulate its differentiation as male or female is by control of the production and metabolism of testosterone, another is by differential expression of receptors that respond to testosterone or to its derivative, another is by regulation of the expression of enzymes required to produce active metabolites, and so on. There also is an interplay between these components: estrogen may stimulate formation of estrogen receptors or androgen receptors, sensitizing tissues to future hormone exposure; it may prolong or accelerate the usual timetable of cellular maturation, affecting a tissue's responsiveness to other growth regulators; testosterone can stimulate aromatase activity, leading to greater production of estrogen and amplifying its effects. Any particular tissue may demonstrate some or all of these mechanisms at specific times in its differentiation. Further research on any of the above-mentioned variables will help to clarify, one step at a time, the role of sex steroids in establishing cerebral cortical asymmetry.

REFERENCES

Alba, F., Ramirez, M., Iribar, C., Cantalejo, E., and Oscar, C. (1985). Asymmetrical distribution of aminopeptidase activity in the cortex of rat brain. *Brain Research, 368,* 158–160.

Anderson, R. H., Fleming, D. E., Rhees, R. W., and Kinghorn, E. (1986). Relationships between sexual activity, plasma testosterone and the volume of the sexually dimorphic nucleus of the preoptic area in prenatally stressed and non-stressed rats. *Brain Research, 370,* 1–10.

Arai, Y., Matsumoto, A., Nishizuka, M., and Murakami, S. (1986). Neurotropic action of estrogen on the developing brain—Effect on newborn preoptic and amygdaloid tissues grafted into the brain or into the eye. *Monographs in Neural Science, 12,* 64–68.

Archer, J. E., and Blackman, D. E. (1971). Prenatal psychological stress and offspring behavior in rats and mice. *Developmental Psychobiology, 4*(3), 193–248.

Attardi, B., and Ohno, S. (1976). Androgen and estrogen receptors in the developing mouse brain. *Endocrinology, 99,* 1279–1292.

Barley, J., Ginsburg, M., Greenstein, B. D., MacLusky, N. J., and Thomas, P. J. (1974). A receptor mediating sexual differentiation? *Nature, 252,* 259–260.

Barneoud, P., Neveu, P. J., Vitiello, S., and Le Moal, M. (1987). Functional heterogeneity of the right and left cerebral neocortex in the modulation of the immune system. *Physiology and Behavior, 41,* 525–530.

Bennett, E. L., Rosenzweig, M. R., Diamond, M. C., Morimoto, H., and Hebert, M. (1974). Effects of successive environments on brain measures. *Physiology and Behavior, 12,* 621–631.

Byne, W., and Bleier, R. (1987). Medial preoptic sexual dimorphisms in the guinea pig. I. An investigation of their hormonal dependence. *Journal of Neuroscience, 7*(9), 2688–2702.

Callard, G. V., Petro, Z., and Ryan, K. J. (1979). Conversion of androgen to estrogen and other steroids in the vertebrate brain. *American Zoology, 18,* 511–523.

Chao, J., Chao, L., Swain, C. C., Tsai, J., and Margolius, H. S. (1987). Tissue kallikrein in rat brain and pituitary: Regional distribution and estrogen induction in the anterior pituitary. *Endocrinology, 120,* 475–482.

Christensen, L. W., and Gorski, R. A. (1978). Independent masculinization of neuroendocrine systems by intracerebral implants of testosterone or estradiol in the neonatal female rat. *Brain Research, 146,* 325–340.

Cicero, T. J., Schainker, B. A., and Meyer, E. R. (1979). Endogenous opioids participate in the regulation of the hypothalamic-pituitary-luteinizing hormone axis and testosterone's negative feedback control of luteinizing hormone. *Endocrinology, 104,* 1286–1290.

Cicero, T. J., Wilcox, C. E., Bell, R. D., and Meyer, E. R. (1976). Acute reductions in serum testosterone levels by narcotics in the male rat: Sterospecificity, blockade by naloxone and tolerance. *Journal of Pharmacology and Experimental Therapeutics, 198*(2), 340–346.

Corbier, P., Roffi, J., and Rhoda, J. (1983). Female sexual behavior in male rats: Effect of hour of castration at birth. *Physiology and Behavior, 30,* 613–616.

Denenberg, V. H. (1981). Hemispheric laterality in animals and the effects of early experience. *Behavioral and Brain Sciences, 4,* 1–49.

Diamond, M. C. (1983). New data supporting cortical asymmetry differences in males and females. *Behavioral and Brain Sciences, 3,* 233–234.

Diamond, M. C. (1984). Age, sex and environmental influences. In N. Geschwind and A. M. Galaburda (Eds.), *Cerebral dominance.* Cambridge, MA: Harvard University Press.

Diamond, M. C. (1985). Rat forebrain morphology: right-left, male-female, young-old, enriched-impoverished. In S. Glick (Ed.), *Cerebral lateralization in nonhuman species* (pp 73–88). Orlando, FL: Academic Press.

Diamond, M. C. (1987). Sex differences in the structure of the rat forebrain. *Brain Research Review, 12,* 235–240.

Diamond, M. C. (1988). Enriching heredity: The impact of the environment on the anatomy of the brain. New York, NY: Free Press.

Diamond, M. C., Dowling, G. A., and Johnson, R. E. (1980). Morphologic cerebral cortical asymmetry in male and female rats. *Experimental Neurology, 71,* 261–268.

Diamond, M. C., Greer, E. R., York, A., Lewis, D., Barton, T., and Lin, J. (1987). Rat cortical morphology following crowded-enriched living conditions. *Experimental Neurology, 96,* 241–247.

Diamond, M. C., Johnson, R. E., and Ehlert, J. (1979). A comparison of cortical thickness in male and female rats—normal and gonadectomized, young and adult. *Behavioral and Neural Biology, 26,* 485–491.

Diamond, M. C., Johnson, R. E., and Ingham, C. A. (1975). Morphological changes in the young, adult and aging rat cerebral cortex, hippocampus and diencephalon. *Behavioral Biology, 14,* 163–174.

Diamond, M. C., Johnson, R. E., Young, D., and Sandhu, S. S. (1983). Age-related morphologic differences in the rat cerebral cortex and hippocampus: Male-female, right-left. *Experimental Neurology, 81,* 1–13.

Diamond, M. C., Krech, D., and Rosenzweig, M. R. (1964). The effects of an enriched environment on the histology of the rat cerebral cortex. *Journal of Comparative Neurology, 123,* 111–120.

Dohler, K. D., Coquelin, A., Davis, F., Hines, M., Shryne, J. E., and Gorski, R. A. (1984). Pre- and postnatal influence of testosterone propionate and diethylstilbestrol on differentiation of the sexually dimorphic nucleus of the preoptic area in male and female rats. *Brain Research, 302,* 291–295.

Dohler, K. D., Coquelin, A., Davis, F., Hines, M., Shryne, J. E., Sickmoeller, P. M., Jarzab, B., and Gorski, R. A. (1986). Pre- and postnatal influence of an estrogen antagonist and an androgen antagonist on differentiation of the sexually dimorphic nucleus of the preoptic area in male and female rats. *Neuroendocrinology, 42,* 443–448.

Dohler, K. D., and Wuttke, W. (1975). Changes with age in levels of serum gonadotropins, prolactin and gonadal steroids in prepubertal male and female rats. *Endocrinology, 97,* 898–907.

Dorner, G., and Staudt, J. (1969a). Structural changes in the hypothalamic ventromedial nucleus of the male rat, following neonatal castration and androgen treatment. *Neuroendocrinology, 4,* 278–281.

Dorner, G., and Staudt, J. (1969b). Perinatal structural sex differentiation of the hypothalamus in rats. *Neuroendocrinology, 5,* 103–106.

Dudley, S. D. (1981). Prepubertal ontogeny of responsiveness to estradiol in the female rat central nervous system. *Neuroscience and Biobehavioral Reviews, 5,* 421–435.

Fleming, D. E., Anderson, R. H., Rhees, R. W., Kinghorn, E., and Bakaitis, J. (1986). Effects of prenatal stress on sexually dimorphic asymmetries in the cerebral cortex of the male rat. *Brain Research Bulletin, 16,* 395–398.

George, F. W., and Ojeda, S. R. (1982). Changes in aromatase activity in the rat brain during embryonic, neonatal and infantile development. *Endocrinology, 111,* 522–529.

Gerlach, J. L., McEwen, B. S., Toran-Allerand, C. S., and Friedman, W. J. (1983). Perinatal development of estrogen receptors in mouse brain assessed by radioautography, nuclear isolation and receptor assay. *Developmental Brain Research, 11,* 7–18.

Germain, B. J., Campbell, P. S., and Anderson, J. N. (1978). Role of serum estrogen-binding protein in the control of tissue estradiol levels during postnatal development of the female rat. *Endocrinology, 103,* 1401–1410.

Geshwind, N., and Galaburda, A. M. (1985). Cerebral lateralization—biological mechanisms, associations and pathology: I. A hypothesis and a program for research. *Archives of Neurology, 42,* 428–458.

Gorski, R. A. (1986). Sexual differentiation of the brain: A model for drug-induced alterations of the reproductive system. *Environmental Health Perspectives, 70,* 163–173.

Gorski, R. A., Gordon, J. H., Shryne, J. E., and Southam, A. M. (1978). Evidence for a morphological sex difference within the medial preoptic area of the rat brain. *Brain Research, 148,* 333–346.

Gregory, E. (1975). Comparison of postnatal CNS development between male and female rats. *Brain Research, 99,* 152–156.

Habib, M. (1989). Anatomical asymmetries of the human cerebral cortex. *International Journal of Neuroscience, 47,* 67–79.

Handa, R. J., Hines, M., Schoonmaker, J. N., Shryne, J. E., and Gorski, R. A. (1986). Evidence that serotonin is involved in the sexually dimorphic development of the preoptic area in the rat brain. *Developmental Brain Research, 30,* 278–282.

Heinsbroeck, R. P. W., van Haaren, F., Zantvoord, F., and van de Poll, N. (1987). Sex differences in response rates during random ratio acquisition: Effects of gonadectomy. *Physiology and Behavior, 39,* 269–272.

Hellige, J. B. (1990). Hemispheric asymmetry. *Annual Reviews of Psychology, 41*, 55−80.

Hines, M., and Gorski, R. A. (1985). Hormonal influences on the development of neural asymmetries. In Benson, F. and A. Zaidel (Eds.), *The dual brain* (pp 73−96). New York, NY: Guilford Press.

Hudson, D. B., Vernadakis, A., and Timiras, P. S. (1970). Regional changes in amino acid concentration in the developing brain and the effects of neonatal administration of estradiol. *Brain Research, 23*, 213−222.

Jacobson, C. D., Csernus, V. J., Shryne, J. E., and Gorski, R. A. (1981). The influence of gonadectomy, androgen exposure, or a gonadal graft in the neonatal rat on the volume of the sexually dimorphic nucleus of the preoptic area. *Journal of Neuroscience, 1*(10), 1142−1147.

Jacobson, C. D., Davis, F. C., and Gorski, R. A. (1985). Formation of the sexually dimorphic nucleus of the preoptic area: Neuronal growth, migration and changes in cell number. *Developmental Brain Research, 21*, 7−18.

Juraska, J. M. (1986). Sex differences in developmental plasticity of behavior and the brain. In *Developmental Psychoneurobiology* (pp 409−422). New York, NY: Academic Press.

Kaplan, M. E., and McGinnis, M. Y. (1989). Effects of ATD on male sexual behavior and androgen receptor binding: a reexamination of the aromatization hypothesis. *Hormones and Behavior, 23*, 10−26.

Keefer, D., and Holderegger, C. (1985). The ontogeny of estrogen receptors: Brain and pituitary. *Developmental Brain Research, 19*, 183−194.

Kolb, B., Sutherland, R. J., Nonneman, A. J., and Whishaw, I. Q. (1982). Asymmetry in the cerebral hemispheres of the rat, mouse, rabbit and cat: the right hemisphere is larger. *Experimental Neurology, 78*, 348−359.

Krey, L. C., Kamel, F., and McEwen, B. S. (1980). Parameters of neuroendocrine aromatization and estrogen receptor occupation in the male rat. *Brain Research, 193*, 277−283.

Lewis, D. W. (1991). *Dimensions and asymmetry of the cerebral cortex in Long-Evans rats treated prenatally and postnatally with 1,4,6-androstatriene-3,17-dione, an inhibitor of aromatase.* Thesis, University of California, Berkeley.

Lieberburg, I., MacLusky, N. J., and McEwen, B. S. (1980). Androgen receptors to the perinatal rat brain. *Brain Research, 196*, 125−138.

Lieberburg, I., MacLusky, N. J., Roy, E. J., and McEwen, B. S. (1978). Sex steroid receptors in the perinatal rat brain. *American Zoology, 18*, 539−544.

Lieberburg, I., Wallach, G., and McEwen, B. S. (1977). The effects of an inhibitor of aromatization (1,4,6-androstatriene-3,17-dione) and an anti-estrogen (CI-628) on in vivo formed testosterone metabolites recovered from neonatal rat brain tissues and purified cell nuclei. Implications for sexual differentiation of the rat brain. *Brain Research, 128*, 176−181.

Litteria, M., and Thorner, M. W. (1976). Inhibitory action of neonatal estrogenization on the incorporation of ^{3}H-lysine into cortical neuroproteins. *Brain Research, 103*, 584−587.

Litteria, M., and Timiras, P. S. (1970). In vivo inhibition of protein synthesis in specific hypothalamic nuclei by 17-beta-estradiol. *Endocrinology, 124*, 256−261.

MacLusky, N. J., Chaptal, C., and McEwen B. S. (1979). The development of estrogen receptor systems in the rat brain: Postnatal development. *Brain Research, 178*, 143−160.

MacLusky, N. J., Clark, A. S., Naftolin, F., and Goldman-Rakic, P. S. (1987). Estrogen formation in the mammalian brain: possible role of aromatase in sexual differentiation of the hippocampus and neocortex. *Steroids, 50*(4−6), 459−474.

MacLusky, N. J., and Naftolin, F. (1981). Sexual differentiation of the central nervous system. *Science, 211,* 1294–1303.

MacLusky, N. J., Philip, A., Hurlburt, C., and Naftolin, F. (1985). Estrogen formation in the developing rat brain: Sex differences in aromatase activity during early postnatal life. *Psychoneuroendocrinology, 10*(3), 355–361.

Mayberg, H. S., Moran, T. H., and Robinson, R. G. (1990). Remote lateralized changes in cortical [³H] spiperone binding following focal frontal cortex lesions in the rat. *Brain Research, 516,* 127–131.

McDonald, P. G., and Doughty, C. (1974). Effect of neonatal administration of different androgens in the female rat: Correlation between aromatization and the induction of sterilization. *Journal of Endocrinology, 61,* 95–103.

McEwen, B. S. (1981). Neural gonadal steroid actions. *Science, 211,* 1303–1311.

McEwen, B. S., Lieberburg, I., Chaptal, C., Davis, P. G., Krey, L. C., MacLusky, N. J., and Roy, E. J. (1979). Attenuating the defeminization of the neonatal rat brain: Mechanisms of action of cyproterone acetate, 1,4,6-androstatriene-3,17-dione, and a synthetic progestin, R5020. *Hormones and Behavior, 13,* 269–281.

McEwen, B. S., Lieberburg, I., Chaptal, C., and Krey, L. C. (1977). Aromatization: Important for sexual differentiation of the neonatal rat brain. *Hormones and Behavior, 9,* 249–263.

McEwen, B. S., Plapinger, L., Chaptal, C., Gerlach, J., and Wallach G. (1975). Role of fetoneonatal estrogen binding proteins in the associations of estrogen with neonatal brain cell nuclear receptors." *Brain Research, 96,* 400–406.

McShane, S., Glaser, L., Greer, E. R., Houtz, J., and Diamond, M. C. (1988). Cortical asymmetry —a preliminary study: neurons-glia, female-male. *Experimental Neurology, 99,* 353–361.

Meaney, M. J., and Aitkin, D. H. (1985). [³H]Dexamethasone binding in rat frontal cortex. *Brain Research, 328,* 176–180.

Micevych, P. E., Matt D. W., and Go, V. L. W. (1988). Concentrations of cholecystokinin, substance P, and bombesin in discrete regions of male and female rat brain: Sex differences and estrogen effects. *Experimental Neurology, 100,* 416–425.

Monbon, M., Loras, B., Reboud, J. P., and Bertrand, J. (1974). Binding and metabolism of testosterone in the rat brain during sexual maturation—I. Macromolecular binding of androgens. *Journal of Steroid Biochemistry, 5,* 417–423.

Negri-Cesi, P., Celotti F., and Martini, L. (1989). Androgen metabolism in the male hamster—2. Aromatization of androstenedione in the hypothalamus and in the cerebral cortex; kinetic parameters and effect of exposure to different photoperiods. *Journal of Steroid Biochemistry, 32*(1A), 65–70.

Ojeda, S. R., Kabra, P. S., and McCann, S. M. (1974). Further studies on the maturation of the estrogen negative feedback on gonadotropin release in the female rat. *Neuroendocrinology, 18,* 242–255.

Paden, C. M., Gerlach, J. L., and McEwen B. S. (1985). Estrogen and progestin receptors appear in transplanted fetal hypothalamus-preoptic area independently of the steroid environment. *Journal of Neuroscience, 5,* 2374–2381.

Pappas, C. T. E., Diamond, M. C., and Johnson, R. E. (1978). Effects on ovariectomy and differential experience on rat cerebral cortical morphology. *Brain Research, 154,* 53–60.

Pappas, C. T. E., Diamond, M. C., and Johnson, R. E. (1979). Morphological changes in the cerebral cortex of rats with altered levels of ovarian hormones. *Behavioral and Neural Biology, 26,* 298–310.

Parsons, B., Rainbow, T. C., and McEwen, B. S. (1984). Organizational effects of testosterone via aromatization on feminine reproductive behavior and neural progestin receptors in rat brain. *Endocrinology, 115,* 1412–1417.

Pfaff, D. W. (1966). Morphological changes in the brains of adult male rats after neonatal castration. *Journal of Endocrinology, 36,* 415–416.

Plapinger, L., McEwen, B. S., and Clemens, L. E. (1973). Ontogeny of estradiol-binding sites in rat brain: II. Characteristics of a neonatal binding macromolecule. *Endocrinology, 93,* 1129–1140.

Pomerantz, S. M., Fox, T. O., Sholl, S. A., Vito, C. C., and Goy, R. W. (1985). Androgen and estrogen receptors in fetal rhesus monkey brain and anterior pituitary. *Endocrinology, 116,* 83–89.

Raisman, G., and Field, P. M. (1973). Sexual dimorphism in the neuropil of the preoptic area of the rat and its dependence on neonatal androgen. *Brain Research, 54,* 1–29.

Reddy, V. V. R., Naftolins, F., and Ryan, K. J. (1974). Conversion of androstenedione to estrone by neural tissues from fetal neonatal rats. *Endocrinology, 94,* 117–121.

Renoux, G., Bizier K., Renoux M., Guillaine J. M., and Degenne D. (1983). A balanced brain asymmetry modulates T cell–mediated events. *Journal of Neuroimmunology, 5,* 227–237.

Reyes, J. (1993). The effects of opioid receptor blockade and enriched environment on cortical plasticity. Thesis, University of California, Berkeley.

Rhees, R. W., Shryne, J. E., and Gorski, R. A. (1990). Onset of the hormone-sensitive perinatal period for sexual differentiation of the sexually dimorphic nucleus of the preoptic area in female rats. *Journal of Neurobiology, 21*(5), 781–786.

Robinson, S. M., Fox, T. O., Dikkes, P., and Pearlstein, R. A. (1986). Sex differences in the shape of the sexually dimorphic nucleus of the preoptic area and suprachiasmatic nucleus of the rat: 3D computer reconstructions and morphometrics. *Brain Research, 371,* 380–384.

Roselli, C. E., Ellinwood, W. E., and Resko, J. A. (1984). Regulation of brain aromatase activity in rats. *Endocrinology, 114,* 192–200.

Roselli, C. E., and Resko J. A. (1984). Androgens regulate brain aromatase activity in adult male rats through a receptor mechanism. *Endocrinology, 114,* 2183–2189.

Roselli, C. E., and Resko, J. A. (1986) . Effects of gonadectomy and androgen treatment on aromatase activity in the fetal monkey brain. *Biology of Reproduction, 35,* 106–112.

Roselli, C. E., Salisbury, R. L., and Resko, J. A. (1987). Genetic evidence for androgen-dependent and independent control of aromatase activity in the rat brain. *Endocrinology, 121,* 2205–2210.

Sandhu, S., Cook, P., and Diamond, M. C. (1986). Rat cerebral coritcal estrogen receptors: male-female, right-left. *Experimental Neurology, 92,* 186–196.

Sheridan, P. J., Sar M., and Stumpf, W. E. (1975). Estrogen and androgen distribution in the brain of neonatal rats. In Stumpf, W. E. and Grant, L. D. (Eds.), *Anatomical neuroendocrinology* (pp 134–141). International Conference on Neurobiology of CNS-Hormone Interactions, Chapel Hill, NC.

Sherman, G. F., and Galaburda, A. M. (1985). Asymmetries in anatomy and pathology in the rodent brain. In Glick, S. (Ed.), *Cerebral lateralization in nonhuman species* (pp 89–107). Orlando, FL: Academic Press.

Shinoda, K., Yagi, H., Fujita, H., Osawa, Y., and Shiotani, Y. (1989). Screening of aromatase-containing neurons in the rat forebrain: An immunohistochemical study with antibody against human placental antigen X-P2 (hPAX-P2), *Journal of Comparative Neurology, 290,* 502–515.

Sholl, S. A., and Kim, K. L. (1990). Androgen receptors are differentially distributed between right and left cerebral hemispheres in the fetal male rhesus monkey. *Brain Research, 516*, 122–126.

Simerly, R. B., Chang, C., Muramatsu, M., and Swanson, L. W. (1990). Distribution of androgen and estrogen receptor mRNA-containing cells in the rat brain: An in situ hybridization study. *Journal of Comparative Neurology, 294*, 76–95.

Slob, A. K., Ooms, M. P., and Vreeburg, J. T. M. (1980). Prenatal and early postnatal sex differences in plasma and gonadal testosterone and plasma luteinizing hormone in female and male rats. *Journal of Endocrinology, 87*, 81–87.

Smith, C. G. (1934). The volume of the neocortex of the albino rat and the changes it undergoes with age after birth. *Journal of Comparative Neurology, 60*(2), 319–347.

Soloff, M. S., Morrison, M. J., and Swartz, T. L. (1972). A comparison of the estrone-estradiol-binding proteins in the plasmas of prepubertal and pregnant rats. *Steroids, 20*, 597–608.

Soriero, O., and Ford, D. H. (1971). Age and sex: the effect on the composition of different regions of the neonatal rat brain. In Ford, D. H. (Ed.), *Influence of hormones on the nervous system* (pp 322–333). Proceedings of the International Society for Psychoneuroendocrinology, Brooklyn, NY, 1970.

Steimer, T., and Hutchison, J. B. (1990). Is androgen-dependent aromatase activity sexually differentiated in the rat and dove preoptic area? *Journal of Neurobiology, 21*(5), 787–795.

Stewart, J., and Cygan, D. (1980). Ovarian hormones act early in development to feminize adult open-field behavior in the rat. *Hormones and Behavior, 14*, 20–32.

Stewart, J., and Kolb, B. (1988). The effects of neonatal gonadectomy and prenatal stress on cortical thickness and asymmetry in rats. *Behavioral and Neural Biology, 49*, 344–360.

Tarttelin, M. F., and Gorski, R. A. (1988) . Postnatal influence of diethylstilbestrol on the differentiation of the sexually dimorphic nucleus in the rat is as effective as perinatal treatment. *Brain Research, 456*, 271–274.

Timiras, P. S. (1971). Estrogens as "organizers" of CNS function. In Ford, D. H. (Ed.), *Influence of hormones on the nervous system* (pp 242–254). Proceedings of the International Society for Psychoneuroendocrinology, Brooklyn, NY.

Tobet, S. A., Baum, M. J., Tang, H. B., Shim, J. H., and Canick, J. A. (1985a). Aromatase activity in the perinatal rat forebrain: Effects of age, sex and intrauterine position. *Developmental Brain Research, 23*, 171–178.

Tobet, S. A., Shim, J. H., Osiecki, S. T., Baum, M. J., and Canick, J. A. (1985b). Androgen aromatization and 5-alpha-reduction in ferret brain during perinatal development: Effects of sex and testosterone manipulation. *Endocrinology, 116*, 1869–1877.

Toran-Allerand, C. D. (1978). Gonadal hormones and brain development: Cellular aspects of sexual differentiation. *American Zoology, 18*, 553–565.

Toran-Allerand, C. D. (1982). Regional differences in intraneuronal localization of alpha-fetoprotein in developing mouse brain. *Developmental Brain Research, 5*, 213–217.

Toran-Allerand, C. D. (1983). Cited by Gerlach, J. L., McEwen, B. S., Toran-Allerand, C. S., and Friedman, W. J. Perinatal development of estrogen receptors in mouse brain assessed by radio-autography, nuclear isolation and receptor assay. *Developmental Brain Research, 11*, 7–18.

Van Eden, C. G., Uylings, H. B. M., and Van Pelt, J. (1984). Sex-difference and right-left asymmetries in the prefrontal cortex during postnatal development in the rat. *Developmental Brain Research, 12*, 146–153.

Vertes, Z., Vertes, M., and Kovacs, S. (1973). Effect of postnatal oestradiol treatment on DNA and RNA synthesis in the brain. *Acta Physiologica Academiae Scientiarum Hungaricae, 44,* 428.

Vito, C. C., and Fox, T. O. (1979). Embryonic rodent brain contains estrogen receptors. *Science, 204,* 517–519.

Vom Saal, F. S., and Bronson, F. H. (1980). Sexual characteristics of adult female mice are correlated with their blood testosterone levels during prenatal development. *Science, 208,* 597–599.

Ward, I. L. (1971). Prenatal stress feminizes and demasculinizes the behavior of males. *Science, 175,* 82–84.

Ward, I. L. (1977). Exogenous androgen activated female behavior in noncopulating, prenatally stressed male rat. *Journal of Comparative and Physiological Psychology, 91*(3), 465–471.

Ward, I. L., and Weisz, J. (1980). Maternal stress alters plasma testosterone in fetal males. *Science, 207,* 328–329.

Ward, I. L., and Weisz, J. (1984). Differential effects of maternal stress on circulating levels of corticosterone, progesterone and testosterone in male and female rat fetuses and their mothers. *Endocrinology, 114,* 1635–1644.

Ward, O. B., Monaghan, E. P., and Ward, I. L. (1986). Naltrexone blocks the effects of prenatal stress on sexual behavior differentiation in male rats. *Pharmacology, Biochemistry and Behavior, 251,* 573–576.

Ward, O. B., Orth, J. M., and Weisz, J. (1983). A possible role of opiates in modifying sexual differentiation. *Monographs in Neural Sciences, 9,* 194–200.

Weisz, J., Brown, B. L., and Ward, I. L. (1982). Maternal stress decreases steroid aromatase activity in brains of male and female rat fetuses. *Neuroendocrinology, 35,* 374–379.

Weisz, J., and Gunsalus, P. (1973). Estrogen levels in immature female rats: True or spurious, ovarian or adrenal? *Endocrinology, 93,* 1057–1065.

Weisz, J., and Philpott, J. (1971). Uptake and metabolism of testosterone by the brain of the newborn rat. In Ford, D. H. (Ed.), *Influence of hormones on the nervous system* (pp 282–295). Proceedings of the International Society of Psychoneuroendocrinology, Brooklyn, NY.

Westley, B. R., and Salaman, D. F. (1976). Role of oestrogen receptor in androgen-induced sexual differentiation of the brain. *Nature, 262,* 407–408.

White, J. O., Hall, C., and Lim, L. (1979). Developmental changes in the content of oestrogen receptors in the hypothalamus of the female rat. *Biochemistry Journal, 184,* 465–468.

Yanai, J. (1979a). Strain and sex differences in the rat brain. *Acta Anatomica, 103,* 150–158.

Yanai, J. (1979b). Delayed maturation of the male cerebral cortex in rats. *Acta Anatomica, 104,* 335–339.

Zagon, I. S., and McLaughlin, P. J. (1983a). Increased brain size and cellular content in infant rats treated with an opiate antagonist. *Science, 221,* 1179–1180.

Zagon, I. S., and McLaughlin, P. J. (1983b). Naltrexone modulates growth in infant rats. *Life Sciences, 33,* 2449–2454.

3 Anatomic Basis of Cerebral Dominance

Albert M. Galaburda

The human brain is asymmetric (Galaburda et al., 1978a; Geschwind and Levitsky, 1968; LeMay and Culebras, 1972; Steinmetz et al., 1991; Witelson, 1977a), as are the brains of other animals (Engbretson, Reiner, and Brecha, 1981; Falk, 1978; Sherman, Galaburda, and Geschwind, 1982). The exact relationship between brain asymmetry and side differences in function, however, is not known. In fact, 150 years after the discoveries of Dax and Broca regarding lateralization of language, the neural basis for language is not clearly understood, and as part of this incomplete knowledge the relationship between language lateralization and cerebral asymmetry is at best tentative.

This book deals with cerebral dominance for language and other cognitive functions. Following the tradition of thinking and research in this field, the general emphasis is on the relationship between functions of one hemisphere compared with those of the other. We think of the left hemisphere as doing "this" while the right does "that." On the other hand, as we have learned from the study of brains of persons with developmental dyslexia (Galaburda et al., 1985; Haslam et al., 1981; Hier et al., 1978; Humphreys, Kaufmann, and Galaburda, 1990; Hynd et al., 1990; Larsen et al., 1990; Leonard et al., 1993; Rumsey et al., 1986, 1987; Wood et al., 1991), which is perhaps also the case for other developmental disorders (Andreasen et al., 1982; Brown et al., 1985; Crow et al., 1989; Falkai et al., 1992; Gur et al., 1991; Jernigan et al., 1982; Luchins and Meltzer, 1983; Rossi et al., 1992; Tsai et al., 1983), it is possible to think of asymmetry as compared to lack of asymmetry. The two dichotomies focus, in turn, on directionality of asymmetry—left vs. right—and on magnitude of asymmetry—very asymmetric or not asymmetric at all. The emphasis of this chapter is less on a comparison between left and right hemispheres but rather on the relationship between brain areas that are symmetric compared with those that are asymmetric.

Research on the anatomy of lateralization began in our laboratory 15 years ago with the expectation that we would discover fundamental differences in the ways the left and right hemispheres are organized (architectonic subdivisions and connectivity) and perhaps in the ways chemical characteristics are expressed in the two sides. These types of differences would provide the building blocks for explaining the functional asymmetry between the hemispheres. By and large, however, we have only found side differences in the amount of brain substrate devoted to a particular architectonic area or a particular gross anatomic landmark. In other words, despite the fact that the left hemisphere is significantly different in function from the right, there appears to be no structure or chemical constituent that is present in one hemisphere but not in the other. Therefore, there is a planum temporale both in the right and in the left hemisphere. There are gyri with the same names and general structure on both sides. All architectonic areas are present in both hemispheres. There are no cell types found in one hemisphere but not in the other. There is no known pattern of connections that appears to be specific to the dominant hemisphere. And, as far as has been determined, there are no physiologic properties in neurons of one hemisphere that are not present in the other. This leaves quantitative differences as the only difference between areas present in both hemispheres. The message here is not that quantitative differences are not important and might not even be the whole explanation of cerebral dominance, but it is also likely that quantitative differences lead to qualitative differences by permitting the arrival at thresholds and emergent properties.

On the other hand, we have noted in our work on developmental dyslexia (see Galaburda, 1992, for review), which has been confirmed in neuroimaging studies (Haslam et al., 1981; Hier et al., 1978; Hynd et al., 1990; Larsen et al., 1990; Leonard et al., 1993; Rumsey et al., 1986, 1987; Wood et al., 1991), that one of the features that distinguishes the brains of dyslexic persons from the brains of nondyslexic persons is the degree to which a language area in the brain is asymmetric. It appears therefore that magnitude of asymmetry could be an important issue vis-à-vis specialization of the brain for language function. Therefore, it is useful to compare the anatomic characteristics of brain areas that are symmetric with symmetric homologous areas. This is the focus of the present chapter.

In this chapter I review instances of directional asymmetry, both in the human and animal literature. This is not an exhaustive listing of areas and species in which asymmetries are found, particularly since in the majority of these instances even speculation about the functional correlations of these anatomic asymmetries is risky. I stress instead asymmetries which are understandable from the perspective of the human brain and therefore provide some glimpse of understanding about how asymmetries in human brains could come about and could support the behavioral observations of cerebral dominance. I also review our experiments in which we have tried to understand the differences between asymmetry and symmetry and the relationship between the degree of asymmetry and other more detailed anatomic characteristics. The working hypothesis is that with change in magnitude of asymmetry there is significant change in the circuitry such that at some point the functional capacity of the system changes. This hypothesis would predict, for instance, that a symmetric language system does different things, or does things differently, from an asymmetric one. Hence, in developmental dyslexia lack of asymmetry might be the crucial factor for the demonstrated differences in linguistic capacity. By extension, injury to an asymmetric language system would be associated with a different pattern of functional loss from that seen after injury to a symmetric language system, even though in both of them the same amount of brain tissue is lost. Finally, recovery of function and plasticity surrounding the loss of function would be different in the two types of asymmetric arrangement in that whatever differential developmental pressure leads to the formation of different degrees of asymmetry in different brains could again act during the period following injury, thus leading to a different degree or pattern of reorganization.

ISSUES IN THE DEFINITION OF ASYMMETRY

Three issues appear to be important in a discussion of brain asymmetry: the first is the issue of directionality of asymmetry. In other words, it is important to note whether a brain area is larger on the left side or on the right side. Some areas would be expected to be asymmetric (and functionally dominant) in favor of one hemisphere, whereas other areas are asymmetric (and functionally dominant) in favor of the other hemisphere. In the case of the human brain one could consider that the larger areas are ordinarily in the left hemisphere for most linguistic capacities and in the right hemisphere for many visuospatial skills. Theoretically, the side in which the brain area is larger would presumably correspond to the hemisphere in which a particular function is dominant. This is at present conjecture, because there is no clear-cut evidence that the larger side need be the dominant side. At least it appears plausible that the side with the larger area could be dominant because most of the circuitry (neurons and connections) related to a particular function is located in that hemisphere. Therefore, were there to be damage in that hemisphere, such damage would injure the more substantial portion of the bilateral structure, thus leading to the more substantial deficit. Similar injury in the opposite hemisphere, by virtue of the fact that only a smaller portion of the circuitry is located in that hemisphere, would not take away enough processing capacity and could be compatible with relatively preserved function. This is the concept of cerebral dominance that does not emphasize unique features for the dominant hemisphere but simply a quantitative difference in participation between the two sides in a particular function. In this scenario, it should be possible to demonstrate linguistic anomalies with right hemisphere lesions with tasks that tax the system and require full participation of both the larger left and smaller right side of the assembly. This may in fact be the case for naming objects on confrontation and other tests of semantic processing, whereby right hemisphere lesions do indeed show abnormalities.

Conversely, the quantitative difference between the hemispheres in the partaking of a given anatomically specific structure could confer to the side with the larger portion functions not at all available to the side with the smaller portion. In this scenario a quantitative increase on the dominant side leads to the emergence of new properties on that side. In this case, lesions to the nondominant hemisphere would not produce detectable linguistic loss. On the other hand, the appearance of architectonic areas in the right hemisphere of the human brain differs much less from their left counterparts (other than size differences) than from the brains of apes, e.g., so that some linguistic capacity might be possible on the small side.

The directionality of asymmetry varies in the human population such that a sizable minority exhibits the opposite direction of asymmetry. This makes comparison and testing of the two hypotheses stated above difficult because, in the absence of well-characterized markers of asymmetry in living subjects, it is difficult to determine whether preservation of language function after unilateral injury represents support for one of the hypotheses or reversal of dominance.

In areas related to language, e.g., the planum temporale, approximately two thirds of the brain shows leftward asymmetry, while 10% shows the reverse asymmetry. Why the population is not equally divided between these alternatives is not known, but additional observations on this issue may help in conjecture. For instance, when the planum temporale shows the reverse direction of asymmetry (right larger), the right side now looks like a typical left and the left like a typical right. Similarly, when the architectonic area that contributes most to the planum asymmetry, area Tpt (Galaburda et al., 1978b), is compared in the two cases, those with leftward asymmetry look like mirror images of those with rightward asymmetry. Therefore it would appear that there is nothing special about leftward asymmetry other than that it represents the majority situation. Why is the leftward case more common? It is unlikely that it is because of the greater demise or lesser reproductive capacity of people with the less common rightward case, although explanations such as these have been offered for the related case of left-handedness (Coren and Halpern, 1991). Although early death is possible, in the case of handedness the prevalence of left-handedness has remained stable over many thousands of years, which would argue against something terribly maladaptive about left-handedness. The mirror quality of the comparison between the rightward and leftward planum temporale asymmetries does not suggest that the brains are fundamentally different, and therefore fundamentally unequal to the task of survival. A recent review looks at other possible explanations for a population bias (Bock and Marsh, 1991), but in fact there is no proven explanation. Genetic forces may not play a big role, however, because, as Collins (1981) has shown in his studies of paw preference in rats, it is impossible to breed for direction of preference. On the other hand, a gene locus that appears to control lateralization of somatic organs has been recently identified (Yokoyama et al., 1993).

It is clear that brain areas are not simply leftward- or rightward-asymmetric, but also *very* or *slightly* leftward- or rightward-asymmetric. In some brains, e.g., area Tpt could be five to seven times larger on one side, while in another brain the difference could be asymmetry of only 15%. This is not surprising, because it would be difficult to conceive of a mechanism whereby one side always ends up being a certain number of times larger than the other side. This would imply that there is some way by which the growth of one side can check itself against the growth of the other side, for growth itself is variable and does not lend itself easily to being perfectly coded in the genome. By the same token it would probably be very difficult to design a system by which both sides end up growing exactly to the same degree, since again this would suggest that one side has to know what the other side is doing, and we know of no mechanism by which this communication can take place during development. As it turns out, in all the animals we have looked at and in both the cortex and subcortical structures, it appears that anatomic asymmetry occurs in a continuum whereby all degrees of asymmetry are seen. In this regard, some brain areas are perfectly symmetric, which in our work is defined as less than 10% difference between the two sides, whereas others can be dramatically asymmetric. Moreover, one person can have striking asymmetry in a particular area, say the planum temporale, while another person may show no asymmetry at all in the planum.

NEUROANATOMIC ASYMMETRIES

Asymmetry in the Planum Temporale

In 1968 in the journal *Science*, Norman Geschwind and Walter Levitsky published a paper in which they reported their findings of asymmetry in the planum temporale in 100 autopsied human brains. They found that 65% of the sample showed a longer left planum temporale, whereas the right planum was longer in only 11% and both plana were equal in the remaining 24%. The results were highly significant and were essentially replicated by subsequent studies (Campain and Minckler, 1976; Wada, Clarke, and Hamm, 1975; Witelson and Pallie, 1973). Teszner and colleagues (1972) included brains of newborns and found the left planum larger in 64% and the right larger in 10%. As mentioned above, brains with reversal of planum asymmetry look like mirror images of those with the more common leftward asymmetry. The planum temporale, which contains several auditory association cortices, is thought on the left side to be an important portion of the language network of the left hemisphere. Lesions affecting significant portions of the planum temporale, usually in the left side in right-handed subjects, often lead to Wernicke's aphasia.

Ever since Geschwind and Levitsky (1968) published their paper on asymmetry of the planum temporale there has been growing interest in the potential usefulness of this structure for the understanding of language lateralization in the normal brain and for the study of acquired and developmental disorders of language. From the beginning, however, there has been debate and confusion as to exactly what the planum temporale is. Should it include or exclude a second Heschl's gyrus, if present? What about the posterior branching of the sylvian fissures? Which one of the planes created by such branching constitutes the continuation of the planum temporale? The debate continues to this date and the problem has become more poignant with the realization that it is possible to get an estimate of the shape and size of the planum temporale from the reconstruction of images obtained by magnetic resonance imaging (MRI) in living, behaving subjects and patients.

Review of the recent literature on this topic suggests that a quick resolution of the questions raised about the planum temporale must be reached if we are to compare results obtained by the different investigators in this field. In other words it is important to be sure that what one investigator calls the planum is the same structure that another investigator calls the planum. Of course, I should stress that it is not necessary to study only the planum in this region of brain, since we also know that neighboring areas in the parietal operculum and in the inferior parietal lobule, some of which have fairly predictable sulcal landmarks, participate in language functions as well. Indeed, these regions should be specified and made available to studies of brain-behavior relationships.

When the gross brain is dissected to show the planum on the rear of the superior temporal plane, there can be no doubt as to what the planum is and where its borders lie. However, when working with reconstructions from sections, either histologic or imaging sections, it is easy to reach differing conclusions about the shape, size, and asymmetry of the planum temporale, depending on whether reconstructions are made from sagittal, horizontal, or coronal sections. This problem arises from inherent difficulties in visualization of the planum from any single cross-sectional plane. Sagittal sections present a problem on the lateralmost extent of the planum, as some of the tributaries of the sylvian fissures posteriorly, constituting the parietal operculum dorsally, appear to be a continuation of the plane of the planum. These turn out to be too shallow on deeper cuts and can be excluded, while the true continuation of the planum is better seen in the same deeper cuts. The coronal plane offers a good look at the planum by presenting a direct assessment of the full depth of the sylvian fossa, of which the planum is its floor; it permits easy identification of shallow opercular sulci that do not belong. Its shortcoming, however, is evident when the posterior planum angles upward, as it often does, especially on the right side. Care must be taken in calculating the area of this portion, taking into consideration the mathematical correction needed to fully measure the inclined plane. Failure to do so results in a foreshortened planum on the side of greater inclination. Interestingly, although asymmetries in the planum could be exaggerated by such an error, they are demonstrable even when the error is avoided. The commonly employed horizontal (axial) plane in clinical MRI is particularly unhelpful for the planum temporale because it is too close to the plane of the planum itself, making visualization, if not reconstruction, difficult, even for experienced eyes.

Given today's easily obtained computational support, it is a relatively simple matter to create planum temporale reconstructions from the sagittal and coronal planes and, as an internal check, to compare the resulting frames. It is also possible to mark points along a sulcus on a less advantageous plane and to check its true identity on a more advantageous plane after electronic transposition from one set of images to another. This should allow minimization of error of inclusion of unwanted cortex and exclusion of important parts. Finally, there is the promise of echoplanar MRI, which permits the functional activation of some brain regions by behavioral tasks, as another means for checking the anatomic identity of a region in question. Equal in magnitude to the advances promised and delivered by molecular biology, the ability to probe the mind with better behavioral tests coupled with the capacity to evaluate the living cerebral anatomy should result in great leaps in our understanding of behavior and the brain.

Heschl's gyrus, which represents the anterior border of the planum temporale, and contains the primary auditory cortex, has been reported to be asymmetric as well. There is an asymmetry in the orientation of Heschl's gyrus: the left one is usually more oblique, less transverse than the right one (personal observations). Furthermore, the right Heschl's gyrus tends to be doubled more often than the left (see review in Rademacher et al., 1993). A recent study in a small number of brains (Rademacher et al., 1993), did not confirm the increased doubling on the right side, but Campaign and Minckler (1976) confirmed the asymmetry in 30 brains of adults and children.

The planum temporale is bound laterally by the sylvian fissure, which can be seen on the lateral surface of the brain's convexity. At the end of the nineteenth century this fissure was seen to be asymmetric by Eberstaller, who noted that the left sylvian fissure was longer. Cunningham (1892) noted that the left sylvian fissure was more horizontal than the right. Such asymmetries in the sylvian fissures have been confirmed by Yeni-Komshian and Benson (1976), by Rubens et al., (1976) and by LeMay and colleagues (1976, 1972). Reversal of sylvian asymmetry, as with the planum, illustrates a mirror image of the more standard pattern. Moreover, it appears that the sylvian fissures are asymmetric in roughly the same proportion of brains showing asymmetries in the planum temporale, and until recently the ability to visualize the sylvian fissure in arteriograms could serve as a reasonable indication of asymmetry or lack thereof in the planum temporale. Currently it is possible to assess for planum asymmetry directly with MRI (e.g., see Larsen et al., 1990; Steinmetz et al., 1991).

Absence of asymmetry in the sylvian fissure and planum temporale could potentially be of several types. For instance, the pattern could be that of two left-sided forms or two right-sided forms. Alternatively, the structures could be symmetric but different in shape from either the left or the right configuration. In the planum temporale, e.g., one could find in the symmetric case two large plana similar to the typical left side, two small plana similar to the typical right side, or two plana of some intermediate size. The two sylvian fissures of a symmetric case could be both long and straight, similar to the typical left fissure; both short and curved, similar to the typical right fissure; or of some intermediate configuration. In fact, when the sylvian fissures are symmetric they adopt the configuration of a typical left-sided sylvian fissure, and when the planum temporale is symmetric, both plana look like the typical left-sided planum temporale. Absence of asymmetry, therefore, discloses a brain that appears to have two left hemispheres and none right (cf., Witelson, 1977b). Furthermore, this finding is compatible with the hypothesis that asymmetry is produced by developmental curtailment, rather than developmental enhancement (also, see below).

Asymmetries in the Inferior Frontal Area

The inferior frontal area, composed of the partes opercularis, triangularis, and orbitalis of the inferior frontal gyrus and frontal operculum and the subcentral cortex, is complex, highly folded, and variable among individuals. Likewise the lesion the produces Broca's aphasia varies substantially from patient to patient. In some cases a very small lesion in the left pars opercularis could lead to a severe and unremitting Broca's aphasia, whereas in others a large lesion affecting the pars triangularis, the pars opercularis, and the subcentral region together would be necessary to produce the same degree of aphasia. In yet another patient with the same large lesion, no aphasia may ensue. Explanations for this variability must entail issues of localization of function as well as brain asymmetry. Asymmetries have been demonstrated in this part of the brain, beginning with the time of Eberstaller in the nineteenth century (Eberstaller, 1890).

Eberstaller pointed out that the ascending limb of the sylvian fissure, which separates the pars opercularis posteriorly from the pars triangularis anteriorly, was more often branched on the left side, giving off the diagonal sulcus. Stengel (1930) found the pars opercularis to be more developed on the left in 9 out of 11 cases, and Falzi, Perrone, and Vignolo (1982) found greater surface area on the left side in 9 out of 12 brains from right-handers. Wada and colleagues (1975), on the other hand, measured the surface portion of the pars opercularis and part of the pars triangularis and found it larger on the right. I looked at the photographs of the brains studied by Geschwind and Levitsky (1968) and found a diagonal sulcus on the left in 27 out of 102 brains, on the right in 13 of 102, with the remainder showing either no branching or branching occurring symmetrically (Galaburda, 1980).

Asymmetries in Fetal and Infant Brains

Gross anatomic asymmetries are present in the cerebral cortex before birth. Even though clearly cerebral dominance can be modified after birth (e.g., recovery from early hemispheric injury and ability to switch handedness), the anatomic asymmetries that may underlie functional lateralization are fixed, at least in their gross design, before birth. This is not to say that recovery from early lesions is perfect at any age or that switching handedness leads to equivalent degrees of dexterity with the new hand. We do not know about this, because the control experiment cannot be performed in the individual patient and variability in the population gets in the way of interpreting the results. Thus, we cannot tell in advance how well language would have developed in the ordinary hemisphere before the lesion and how good the right hand would have become before the switch to the left.

The sylvian fissures are visibly asymmetric from about the middle of gestation, demonstrating the pattern usually seen in the adult human (Chi, Dooling, and Gilles, 1977; Fontes, 1944). The planum temporale is also grossly asymmetric before the end of pregnancy (Chi, Dooling, and Gilles, 1977). The study by Witelson and Pallie (1973), which included 14 brains from newborns, found the planum temporale to be larger on the left side in 79% of the cases. Wada and colleagues (1975) made planimetric measurements of 100 adult and 100 newborn and fetal brains and found that the average ratio of the surface area of the right to left planum temporale was 67% in the younger brains and 55% in the adults. (If this difference is significant, did the change indicate that some of the cases with larger right plana do not make it to adulthood?) These authors also noted that the planum temporale asymmetry was visible beginning in the twenty-ninth week of gestation. Chi, Dooling, and Gilles (1977) found that the right Heschl's gyrus was doubled on the right side in 54% of cases and on the left in 18%.

It is important to emphasize here that the gross anatomy of the brain does not change significantly after birth, other than by the appearance of low-order fissuration of the cortex and overall growth. Thus, it would not be expected that the anatomic asymmetries just described would change significantly after birth. This is not to say that the functional expression of these asymmetries could not change by later modulation of the detailed connectivity, synaptic architecture, and other lower-level structural changes that do not change the gross appearance. This hypothesis is consistent with the functional model proposed by Stephen Kosslyn (Kosslyn, 1987, Kosslyn and Koenig, 1992), in which the beginning state of asymmetry in the nervous system can be modified by learning (modification of synaptic weights) so that either more or less functional asymmetry results from that which would have been predicted from the original, innate anatomic pattern. The evidence on the effects of learning on anatomy (Greenough, Black, and Wallace, 1987) indicate that changes would take place at lower levels of structure and would not be reflected in the gross anatomy or even the cytoarchitecture and gross connectivity.

Architectonic Asymmetries

Gross anatomic asymmetry reflects to a great extent asymmetries in underlying architectonic areas,[1] which are subdivisions of cortex with specific cellular architecture, connectivity, and physiology. Cortical folding, however, may also be related to physical forces imposed by the skull during growth, and

Galaburda: Anatomic Basis of Cerebral Dominance

gross anatomic asymmetries may therefore reflect in part bony asymmetries that are unrelated to brain function. It is important, therefore, to ascertain whether asymmetry in the cerebral cortex can be demonstrated at a level that heralds functional differentiation more strictly than the gross anatomic level of lobes, gyri, and sulci—the architectonic level.

Cytoarchitectonics refers to regional cortical differentiation which consists of fluctuations in the thickness (and sometimes numbers) of layers, sizes, and shapes of neurons in the layers, the packing density of these neurons, and local arrangements in clusters and columns. In some cases the transition from one architectonic area to its neighbor is sharp, while in others there is a gradual transition from one to the next. It is possible with experience to draw borders around many cytoarchitectonic areas and to measure their volume in each hemisphere. Having done this we have shown asymmetries in several cortical areas implicated in language function. For instance, area Tpt, which is located on the posterior one third of the superior temporal gyrus extending onto the planum temporale, is larger on the left side in the majority of brains (Galaburda and Sanides, 1980). Asymmetry of area Tpt correlates positively with asymmetry of the planum temporale, and I believe is the cause for the planum asymmetry. In some cases the left planum can be severalfold the size of the right.

The frontal operculum contains predominantly cytoarchitectonic areas 44 and 45, whereby the former covers most of the pars opercularis (the foot of Broca) and the latter covers mainly the pars triangularis (the cape of Broca). Both of these cortices belong to the category of motor association cortex, with area 44 being an inferior premotor cortex and area 45 an inferior prefrontal cortex. The prefrontal cortex would be considered more multimodal (cognitive?) than the premotor cortex, although lesions that result in Broca's aphasia affect area 44 alone more often than area 45 alone, as estimated from descriptions of gyral involvement in the literature. Area 44, which was enhanced by special stains directed at intracellular lipofuscin pigment, was found to be of greater volume in six out of ten brains, nearly symmetric in three, and larger on the right side in one brain from a collection of neurologically normal brains (Galaburda, 1980). There is no information regarding asymmetry of area 45.

We also studied the inferior parietal lobule in ten normal human brains and found predominance of the left area PG in eight of those brains. Area PG (equivalent to Brodmann's area 39) lies mainly on the angular gyrus and is a prototypical, so-called homotypical or high-order association cortex. It is highly multimodal and interposed between cortices dealing respectively with somesthetic, auditory, and visual functions. Lesions on the angular gyrus, which often lead to anomic aphasia, acquired reading and writing disorders, and Gerstmann's syndrome, likely destroy the bulk of area PG.

The same brains with leftward asymmetry of area PG also exhibited predominance of the left planum temporale and of the left area 44. On the other hand, a more dorsal parietal area, area PEG, which by virtue of its architecture and location is less clearly related to language, tended to be larger on the right side and asymmetry in this area did not correlate with asymmetry of the planum temporale or PG (Eidelberg and Galaburda, 1984). This finding could suggest that asymmetries in one region are correlated with asymmetries in another region as long as the two regions are functionally related. In animal studies we found similar correlations of directional asymmetry between adjacent, visually related cortices (Rosen, Sherman, and Galaburda, 1991).

Asymmetries in Other Species

Paradoxically, more is known about asymmetry in brain structures in other species than in the human brain, while cerebral dominance is more obviously evident in humans. Furthermore, particularly in nonhuman primates, the types if not the degree of brain asymmetry are similar to those found in the human brain, which raises questions about what lateralized functions, if any, these structural asymmetries might serve. For instance, Cunningham (1892), who described asymmetries in the sylvian fissures of humans, also found them in other primate brains (see also Falk, 1978; Falk et al., 1990, 1991). If one is permitted to attach significance to the sylvian asymmetry in the human vis à vis linguistic capacity, what then is the meaning of asymmetry in the same structure in the baboon, the orangutan, and the chimpanzee? The planum temporale, on the other hand, is not fully evident in any nonhuman primate. In chimpanzee and orangutan brains, the gyrus of Heschl is prominent enough to suggest a planum temporale posterior to it, but a circumscribed planum temporale emerges for the first time in the human brain. The orangutan and the papions show frontal asymmetries in favor of the left side, a situation that has not been reported in the human brain, where more commonly the right frontal lobe predominates. On the other hand, the baboon shows frontal asymmetry in favor of the right side (LeMay and Geschwind, 1975; Falk, 1978; Cheverud et al., 1990; Falk et al., 1990).

The cerebral cortex emerges for the first time in its six-layered organization in mammals. Asymmetries in structures other than cortex are present, however, in birds, fishes, and amphibians. In the case of birds, the asymmetries are demonstrated mainly in the functional domain and consist of differential effects of neural lesions on the ability of singing birds to sing, with the left predominating (Nottebohm, 1981; Nottebohm and Nottebohm, 1976). Slight left anatomic superiority of one of the song-relevant nuclei (the hypoglossal nucleus) has also been demonstrated (DeVoogd, Pyskaty, and Nottebohm, 1991). Fishes and amphibians often show asymmetries in the habenular nuclei, the functional significance of which is not clear.

In our laboratory we have stressed asymmetries in the cerebral cortex of rodents, which we take to be a useful model for the study of the developmental basis for cortical asymmetries in mammalian species. In the rodent cortex, individual animals are commonly asymmetric but asymmetry at the population level is not striking. Therefore, roughly the same number of animals in a group are right-predominant as left-predominant. Architectonic areas 17 and 18, parts of the visual cortex, are thicker on the right side in male rats (Dowling et al., 1982). Females fail to show this type of asymmetry and instead show predominance on the left side. It has been suggested that this is the consequence of hormonal influences during critical periods of development of cortical asymmetry. Thus, it is possible to convert one asymmetry to the other by diminishing the effect of one sex hormone or increasing the effect of another (Diamond, Dowling, and Johnson, 1981; Dowling et al., 1982). For instance castration in neonatal males leads to the female pattern of cortical asymmetry. One conclusion of this finding would be that critical effects on cortical asymmetry take place after birth. Very little additional research on this interesting area has been carried out, and statements regarding the effects of hormones on asymmetry remain to a large extent speculative.

Asymmetries in Fossils

Occasionally the literature reports a finding of asymmetry in a fossil skull. The best known of these is the asymmetry in the Neanderthal fossil from La Chapelle aux Saints, about 60,000 years old, which showed a sylvian fissure asymmetry similar to that seen in modern humans (LeMay, 1976). There was a suggestion of a comparable asymmetry in the endocast of Peking man, which dates from 500,000 to 600,000 years ago. Asymmetries in perisylvian cortex also appear to exist in australopithecines, *Homo habilis* and *Homo erectus*, which date to up to 3.5 million years (Holloway, 1980). Again, as is the case in nonhuman primates, asymmetries in the sylvian fissure are found in individuals whose language capacity is in question. Whether or not these asymmetries represent linguistic capacities in these early humans, or some preadaptive behavior, is likely to remain unknown. It will help to find out what is it about asymmetry of the modern human brain, if anything, which can explain linguistic capacity.

Asymmetries Demonstrated by Imaging Devices in Living Subjects

Earlier findings of brain asymmetry in living subjects were made with the use of plain skull radiographs, arteriograms, and pneumoencephalograms. Skull films showed petalia, or the erosion of the inner wall of the skull by overgrown brain tissue, and this petalia could be seen in humans and in other primates (Cheverud et al., 1990; LeMay and Kido, 1978). Pneumoencephalograms showed that the left occipital horn of the lateral ventricle is larger in 57% of subjects as compared to 13% showing the opposite asymmetry. Among subjects who are right-handed, the standard asymmetry is found 60% of the time, whereas in those who are left-handed, leftward occipital horn asymmetry is seen only 38% of the time. Symmetric horns are seen in right-handers 40% of the time as compared to 62% of the time in left-handers. These data illustrate that left-handers, no matter how they are classified, do not tend to show the reverse pattern of cerebral asymmetry, but rather a more symmetric pattern. In this regard the left sylvian fissure is found to be longer and straighter than the right in carotid arteriograms in 67% of right-handers as compared to only 29% of left-handed or ambidextrous persons. There is furthermore a correlation between the side of the longer and straighter sylvian fissure and language lateralization as demonstrated by the Wada test. A study found that 66% of subjects having left hemisphere lateralization for the Wada test showed a longer sylvian fissure on the left, whereas only 35% of those having right hemisphere specialization for language had this pattern (Ratcliff et al., 1980). The correlation, however, is not nearly perfect, which suggests that this is the wrong asymmetry to look at or that magnitude, not just directionality, of asymmetry plays a role in the structural-functional correlation.

Computer assisted tomograms of the brain have been used gainfully for the study of brain asymmetry in living subjects. Petalia can easily be seen in this procedure because of the ease with which bone contours can be assessed. The right frontal lobe is often seen to protrude ahead of the left (right frontal petalia) while the left occipital lobe tends to protrude farther toward the back than the right (left occipital petalia). Left occipital petalia is seen in 78% of right-handers, whereas left-handers again are more often symmetric. As a group, left-handers that have a family history of left-handedness are particularly more symmetric than left-handers without such family history, which may suggest a contribution of the environment, either through injury or through learning, to the expression of left-handedness in the latter group. Studies concentrating exclusively on petalia, however, are difficult to interpret because subtle changes in the angle of section can produce significant changes in the appearance of the petalia and the classification of brains into the "wrong" groups. Perhaps this is one explanation for the finding that there is little correlation between occipital petalia and the side of the lesion that results in a language disturbance (Naeser, 1984). Another explanation may relate to the fact that these gross anatomic asymmetries reflect subregions of brain that are asymmetric in opposite directions and that cannot be predicted by the gross anatomic asymmetry alone. Thus, for instance, the right occipital pole may protrude because of growth of visual association cortices, while the left may push out because of growth of temporoparietal cortices just rostral to it.

Mechanisms of Cerebral Asymmetry

Having come to the conclusion that there are no obvious qualitative differences between the two sides of an architectonic area that is asymmetric, the only finding that needs to be explained at present is how the two sides come to be of a different size. Furthermore, we would like to know what determines variability in side differences: for instance, why is it that some areas are severalfold larger on one side than the other, whereas other areas are only a few percentage points different in size between the two sides; and how in some individuals an area is only slightly asymmetric while in another the same area is strikingly asymmetric. Another important question that needs to be answered is whether variability in the directionality and magnitude of asymmetry alters the functional characteristics of the brain.

The phrenologic approach to neuropsychology, which we carry with us for the daily practice of behavioral neurology and neuropsychology, insinuates that the basis for cognitive capacity is large size. For example, our brains are uniquely able to carry out complex cognitive tasks because they are bigger than the brains of other cognitively less gifted primates. Similarly, the left hemisphere is able to support language because some of the perisylvian cortices involved in language are larger than corresponding areas on the right. The phrenologic school in the nineteenth century paid a great deal of attention to local enlargements on the brain (and related skull) surface in order to explain special intellectual gifts. Based on this approach, in the case of cerebral asymmetry one could suppose that a brain grows an area on one side in order to support a special skill or remains small on both sides if the skill does not exist. For example, by comparison with humans, who have language, apes, which do not, would have two small "language areas" while humans would have one small and one large one.

An alternative to the phrenologic concept is provided by the notion that while size may be important for some cognitive functions (e.g., memory) other highly specialized functions may depend more on specificity of organization (e.g., rule learning). Thus, e.g., ants can build complex dwellings with very small brains, but small changes in the brain architecture deal a devastating blow to the task of building those homes. Likewise, building a phonologically competent brain area may require increasing the specificity of the brain substrate by customized reduction rather than enlargement of its components. In this sense, an asymmetric language area would result from the pruning of one side rather than from the enlargement of the other. This is a plausible mechanism in the light of present knowledge about cortical development, since the cerebral cortex, it appears, generates during development more neurons, axons, synapses, and receptors than it finally keeps (for a review, see Cowan et al., 1984). Some of these elements are removed by what seems to be a program of pruning, while others are removed as a result of environmental factors, for instance axonal inputs to neurons, electrical or chemical stimulation, and so forth. The ultimate purpose for overproduction and pruning must be to set up an optimal anatomy to match environmental requirements, which cannot altogether be predicted in advance. An alternative to phrenologic mechanisms for brain asymmetry could therefore be asymmetric pruning, individual variation of which leads to different degrees of asymmetry.

After perusing photographs of the planum temporale from the same brains studied originally by Geschwind and Levitsky (1968), we were impressed to see that strikingly asymmetric plana usually consisted of a large planum and a small planum by comparison to symmetric plana, which usually consisted of two large plana, not two small plana or two medium-sized plana. We then plotted the sum of the areas of the two plana temporale against a coefficient of asymmetry for each brain and found a significant inverse relationship (Galaburda et al., 1987). This meant that as the asymmetry became more pronounced, the total amount of plana temporale, right plus left, was less, and that consequently asymmetric areas were smaller overall than symmetric areas. Furthermore this relationship could not be accounted for by bilateral, albeit asymmetric curtailment, but rather by unilateral curtailment only. In other words, in the asymmetric cases the size of the small side predicted for degree of asymmetry, not the size of both sides. This suggested to us that symmetry was the result of incomplete pruning of one side rather than incomplete unilateral growth. Since this observation on the planum temporale we have confirmed the relationship between total size and asymmetry in rodent brain architectonic areas (Rosen et al., 1989, 1991), which indicates that this may be a general principle governing the relationship of asymmetry and brain space.

The small side of an asymmetric area could have fewer neurons or neurons packed more tightly. Similarly, overall, asymmetric areas could have fewer neurons or neurons packed more tightly than symmetric areas. The number of neurons is by and large controlled during events taking place earlier during development than events controlling the space occupied by neurons and other factors affecting the packing density of neurons. The earlier the event the more likely it is to be governed by genetic rather than environmental factors. Therefore, it appears important to determine which of the two factors (or both) accounts for size differences between architectonic areas in the context of asymmetry.

We measured the volume of cortical area 17 (the primary visual cortex) of the rat and found a negative correlation between the total volume of this area and the degree of asymmetry, as expected. Similarly, asymmetry correlated with the size of the small side, not the size of both sides. We then estimated cell-packing densities in area 17 of each hemisphere and found that, irrespective of the degree of areal asymmetry, there were no asymmetries in this measure. We concluded, therefore, that architectonic asymmetry must result from side differences in neuronal numbers, not side differences in the packing of neurons or a combination of packing and numbers of neurons (Galaburda et al., 1986). That side differences in cell numbers rather than cell packing density relate to areal asymmetry is not surprising, since side differences in packing density large enough to account for the often large areal asymmetries would lead to side differences in architectonic appearance, which are not seen.

Having determined that side differences in neuron numbers account for areal asymmetry and for the difference in size between symmetric and asymmetric architectonic areas, it became important to understand how the number of neurons is determined during cortical development. In the human brain, between the 16th and 24th weeks of gestation, most neurons destined for the cerebral cortex are produced from neuroblasts (mother cells) residing in germinal zones. Prior to that, it is the number of mother cells that is determined, a process that begins very early. A fair amount is known about the production and subsequent migration of neurons from the germinal zones to the cerebral cortex, but very little is known about the production of mother cells. It is known that after neuronal production and migration some of the neurons are eliminated (see above), but it is not known for certain whether mother cells are also overproduced and eliminated. In summary, neuronal numbers in the cerebral cortex depend on the early production (and possible subsequent elimination) of mother cells and the production and subsequent elimination of neurons during development. Neuronal numbers in a particular architectonic area could also depend on assignment of neurons to it, as opposed to a neighboring architectonic area, by shifting borders between the two areas. In this case, while an area in question loses neurons and becomes smaller, its neighbor would gain neurons and become larger.

The same issues that relate to the overall number of neurons in an architectonic area must play a role in determining side differences in the numbers of neurons, which leads to brain asymmetry. As stated above, the number of mother cells in the germinal zones is determined early in gestation, but quantitative assessment of this process has not been possible because of methodologic limitations. It is possible that at that time, when the midline of the neuraxis is established, in some cases this line is not exactly in the middle, leading to asymmetry in the distribution or assignment of neuroblasts to either side of the line. Assuming that mother cells then divide the same number of times on both sides, some cases will end up symmetric while other will end up asymmetric. This mechanism will not explain the fact that the asymmetric cases end up with fewer neurons (see above). There must be, then, an additional difference in the production or elimination of neuroblasts (or both) between the sides. We cannot distinguish between these possibilities.

After the establishment of the midline, neuroblasts may divide the same number of times on both sides or a different number of times to produce a final pool of neuroblasts. After the final pool of mother cells is established in both sides, neuroblasts divide, either symmetrically or asymmetrically, to produce a symmetric or asymmetric number of young neurons. An equivalent scenario may be posed for the elimination of young neurons after completion of neuronal migration: either there is asymmetric destruction after symmetric or asymmetric production, or symmetric reduction. Methodologic advances in this case do permit looking at the possibility of side differences in neuronal production, and to some extent side differences in the elimination of postmigrational neurons, for explaining cortical asymmetries.

Asymmetries in the birth of neurons may reflect side difference in the rates at which mother cells generate young neurons or in the length of time during which they can divide. Likewise, asymmetries in the death of neurons may reflect side difference in the rates at which young neurons die or in the length of time during which neurons die.

As already mentioned, the quantification of neuroblast generation and possibly neuroblast death early in gestation has defied methodologic approaches.

On the other hand, the use of radioactively labeled thymidine, which tags newly produced DNA and signals DNA replication and cell division, has made it possible to date and quantify cell birth at the time when neuroblasts divide for the last time before young neurons migrate to the cerebral cortex. The young neurons, which do not divide, have the highest content of radioactively labeled thymidine in their DNA and can be tracked to their final locations in the emerging cerebral cortex. We used this approach to assess young neuron production in the two sides of asymmetric and symmetric cortical areas in the rat (Rosen et al., 1991). Radioactively labeled thymidine was injected into pregnant rats at several times during the known period of generation of young neurons and the animals were sacrificed in adulthood. We counted heavily labeled neurons in both hemispheres in visual cortex and SM-1 and calculated labeling ratios (proportion of labeled to unlabeled neurons). We argued that if the neuroblasts of one side undergo additional divisions, the label would be more diluted and the labeling ratio lower. We found no differences in label dilution between the two sides irrespective of whether the two sides were symmetric or asymmetric. This indicated to us that there are no substantial differences in the number of neuroblast divisions between the two sides to account for asymmetry in the size of areas represented in both hemispheres. We also looked at overall labeled cell densities to exclude the possibility that the rate of labeling and proliferation (differences in the cell cycle) did not differ between the sides, which it did not.

We have encountered numerous experimental difficulties in assessing the possibility of asymmetric cell death after migration. There are, however, a priori reasons for diminishing the importance of this mechanism. Thus, in order to diminish the size of an architectonic area without changing its appearance, it would be necessary to take away all types of neurons proportionately. In essence, in the layered structure which is the cerebral cortex, this would mean that whole columns of cortex would have to be removed by cell death. Had this happened to a significant extent, it would have been noticed, particularly to explain side differences that are often in the severalfold range; such cell death has not been reported. Furthermore, studies on cell death in the cortex show that some layers are affected more than others and therefore cell death is not proportionate (Finlay and Slattery, 1983; Finlay, Wikler, and Sengelaub, 1987; Sengelaub, Jacobs, and Finlay, 1985; Sengelaub, Dolan, and Finlay, 1986). We, therefore, tentatively attribute the generation of asymmetry to the asymmetric production of neurons, which itself reflects the asymmetric generation or death of neuroblasts early in histogenesis, well before neuronal migration and establishment of cortical connectivity. Such early timing would be consistent with a genetically controlled process rather than with significant environmental influences, and it supports the findings of Robert Collins (1981), which indicate that degree of paw preference in rats, if not direction of asymmetry, appears to be under strong genetic control.

Despite the observations indicating that by and large architecture does not differ between small and large sides of an architectonic area, and that proportions of neurons must be roughly similar on the two sides, we have recently gathered evidence that one neuronal type may differ in the two hemispheres in cerebral asymmetry (unpublished observations under review). We examined cell packing densities of several types of neurons stained by immunohistochemical methods in the rat brain and compared left and right sides vis à vis asymmetry. Again, there was no overall relationship between cell packing density and asymmetry. However, the density of parvalbumin-positive neurons was greater on the larger side in asymmetric cases. Parvalbumin neurons are characterized by having long projections, which would then indicate that the larger (dominant?) side is more connected than the smaller side. This situation would then be compatible with a different functional capacity being possible in the larger side.

Hemispheric differences in connections have not been reported except in the parietal eye of the lizard and other nonmammalian brains. However, most research on connectivity has not specifically compared the two sides. The methodology for studying connections does not lend itself easily to the kind of quantitative comparisons needed for asymmetry work. On the other hand, the findings on parvalbumin-positive neurons suggest subtle connectional hemispheric differences.

In addition, we tried to circumvent the methodologic limitations by sectioning the corpus callosum in the rat and looking at degenerating axonal terminals on the two sides vis à vis asymmetry of targeted architectonic areas (Rosen et al., 1989). We found that, with increasing asymmetry, the proportion of the targeted area receiving callosal connections diminished. In other words, the more asymmetric areas have relatively fewer callosal connections than similar areas that are more symmetric. Cortical areas receive callosal projections in only some locations. Developmentally, a larger complement of callosal connections reach under the cortical plate, but only some of these penetrate it at several sites and establish connectivity with neurons in the cortex (Innocenti, 1981; Innocenti and Frost, 1980; Ivy and Killackey, 1981, 1982). Of those that do not penetrate, some are withdrawn and disappear, while others are rerouted. It appears that in symmetric areas fewer are withdrawn, while in asymmetric areas more are withdrawn. In the latter we do not know specifically whether more are rerouted or simply disappear. If there is more rerouting in the asymmetric cases, this would mean that areas would then connect within the same hemisphere rather than across the hemisphere. Asymmetric areas would be more intrahemispherically connected while symmetric areas would be more interhemispherically connected, which could produce important differences in interhemispheric and intrahemispheric communication.

In summary, asymmetry of cortical areas is associated with changes in the volume of architectonic areas, side differences in overall numbers and densities of some neurons, and variation in the patterns of callosal connections. Indirect evidence suggests, furthermore, that asymmetry is determined early during corticogenesis, probably during the time when the neuroblast pools are being established on the two sides of the midline of the neural tube. The histologic characteristics of symmetric and asymmetric cortical areas do not support the notion that cerebral dominance represents simply a case of storing functional areas in one hemisphere or the other, but rather that there are storage factors as well as factors of network size and detailed connectivity. The implication of this is that cerebral dominance stops being important merely for the understanding of the effects of injury to one hemisphere or the other but also reflects variation in functional properties of symmetric and asymmetric cortical areas, which provides the species with desirable and sometimes problematic individual variation.

For the first time, it is possible to assess the normally functioning human brain with sophisticated methods that can address issues about localization and lateralization of function. With improving anatomic imaging it will be possible to extract individual information rather than sample averages, which will be useful for studies on individual variation of localization and lateralization. This knowledge can then be applied to studies of variability in response to brain injury and of developmental variation in cognitive style and learning disorders.

ACKNOWLEDGMENTS

I am grateful for the collaboration of Drs. Gordon F. Sherman and Glenn D. Rosen. Some of the work described here was supported by NIH grants HD 20806 and NS 27119, grants from the Carl W. Herzog Foundation, the Milton Fund, and the Research Division of the Orton Dyslexia Society.

NOTE

1. When architectonic subdivision of the cortex stresses cellular arrangement, as opposed to the arrangement of fibers, specific molecules, or other cortical features, it is referred to as *cytoarchitectonics*.

REFERENCES

Andreasen, N. C., Dennert, J. W., Olsen, S. A., and Damasio, A. R. (1982). Hemispheric asymmetries and schizophrenia. *American Journal of Psychiatry, 139*, 427–430.

Bock, G. R., and Marsh, J. (1991). *Biological asymmetry and handedness* (p 327). Chichester, England: John Wiley & Sons.

Brown, R., Colter, N., Corsellis, J. A., Crow, T. J., Frith, C. D., Jagoe, R., Johnstone, E. C., and Marsh, L. (1985). Postmortem evidence of structural brain changes in schizophrenia. *Archives of General Psychiatry, 43*, 36–42.

Campain, R., and Minckler, J. (1976). A note on the gross configurations of the human auditory cortex. *Brain and Langguage, 3*, 318–323.

Cheverud, J. M., Falk, D., Hildebolt, C., Moore, A. J., Helmkamp, R. C., and Vannier, M. (1990). Heritability and association of cortical petalias in rhesus macaques (*Macaca-mulatta*). *Brain, Behavior and Evolution, 35*(6), 368–372.

Chi, J. G., Dooling, E. C., and Gilles, F. H. (1977). Gyral development of the human brain. *Annals of Neurology, 1,* 86–93.

Collins, R. L. (1981). A demonstration of an inheritance of the direction of asymmetry that is consistent with the notion that genetic alleles are left-right indifferent. *Behavioral Genetics, 11,* 596–600.

Coren, S., and Halpern, D. F. (1991). Left-handedness: A marker for decreased survival fitness. *Psychological Bulletin, 109*(1), 90–106.

Cowan, W. M., Fawcett, J. W., O'Leary, D. D. M., and Stanfield, B. B. (1984). Regressive events in neurogenesis. *Science, 225,* 1258–1265.

Crow, T. J., Ball, J., Bloom, S. R., Brown, R., Bruton, C. J., Colter, N., Frith, C. D., Johnstone, E. C., Owens, D. G. C., and Roberts, G. W. (1989). Schizophrenia as an anomaly of development of cerebral asymmetry. A postmortem study and a proposal concerning the genetic basis of the disease. *Archives of General Psychiatry, 46,* 1145–1150.

Cunningham, D. J. (1892). *Contribution to the surface anatomy of the cerebral hemispheres.* Dublin: Royal Irish Academy.

DeVoogd, T. J., Pyskaty, D. J., and Nottebohm, F. (1991). Lateral asymmetries and testosterone-induced changes in the gross morphology of the hypoglossal nucleus in adult canaries. *Journal of Comparative Neurology, 307*(1), 65–76.

Diamond, M. C., Dowling, G. A., and Johnson, R. E. (1981). Morphological cerebral cortical asymmetry in male and female rats. *Experimental Neurology, 71,* 261–268.

Dowling, G. A., Diamond, M. C., Murphy, G. M., and Johnson, R. E. (1982). A morphological study of male rat cerebral cortical asymmetry. *Experimental Neurology, 75,* 51–67.

Eberstaller, O. (1890). *Das Stirnhirn. Ein Beitrag zur Anatomie der Oberfläche des Gehirns.* Vienna-Leipzig: Urban & Schwarzenberg.

Eidelberg, D., and Galaburda, A. M. (1984). Inferior parietal lobule. Divergent architectonic asymmetries in the human brain. *Archives of Neurology, 41,* 843–852.

Engbretson, G. A., Reiner, A., and Brecha, N. (1981). Habenular asymmetry and the central connections of the parietal eye of the lizard. *Journal of Comparative Neurology, 198,* 155–165.

Falk, D. (1978). Cerebral asymmetry in old world monkeys. *Acta Anatomica, 101,* 334–339.

Falk, D., Hildebolt, C., Cheverud, J., Kohn, L. A. P., Figiel, G., and Vannier, M. (1991). Human cortical asymmetries determined with 3D-MR technology. *Journal of Neuroscience Methods, 39*(2), 185–191.

Falk, D., Hildebolt, C., Cheverud, J., Vannier, M., Helmkamp, R. C., and Konigsberg, L. (1990). Cortical asymmetries in frontal lobes of Rhesus monkeys (*Macaca-mulatta*). *Brain Research, 512*(1), 40–45.

Falkai, P., Bogerts, B., Greve, B., Pfeiffer, U., Machus, B., Fölsch-Reetz, B., Majtenyi, C., and Ovary, I. (1992). Loss of Sylvian fissure asymmetry in schizophrenia: A quantitative post mortem study. *Schizophrenia Research, 7*(1), 23–32.

Falzi, G., Perrone, P., and Vignolo, L. (1982). Right-left asymmetry in anterior speech region. *Archives of Neurology, 39,* 239–240.

Finlay, B. L., and Slattery, M. (1983). Local differences in the amount of early cell death in neocortex predict adult local specializations. *Science, 219,* 1349–1351.

Finlay, B. L., Wikler, K. C., and Sengelaub, D. R. (1987). Regressive events in brain development and scenarios for vertebrate brain evolution. *Brain, Behavior and Evolution, 30,* 102–117.

Fontes, V. (1944). *Morfologia do cortex cerebral (desenvolvimento)*. Lisbon: Instituto Antonio Aurelio da Costa Ferreirs.

Galaburda, A. M. (1980). La région de Broca: Observations anatomiques faites un siècle après la mort de son découvreur. *Revue de Neurologie (Paris), 136,* 609–616.

Galaburda, A. M. (1992). Neurology of developmental dyslexia. *Current Opinion in Neurology and Neurosurgery, 5,* 71–76.

Galaburda, A. M., Aboitiz, F., Rosen, G. D., and Sherman, G. F. (1986). Histological asymmetry in the primary visual cortex of the rat: Implications for mechanisms of cerebral asymmetry. *Cortex, 22,* 151–160.

Galaburda, A. M., Corsiglia, J., Rosen, G. D., and Sherman, G. F. (1987). Planum temporale asymmetry: Reappraisal since Geschwind and Levitsky. *Neuropsychologia, 25,* 853–868.

Galaburda, A. M., LeMay, M., Kemper, T. L., and Geschwind, N. (1978a). Right-left asymmetries in the brain. *Science, 199,* 852–856.

Galaburda, A. M., and Sanides, F. (1980). Cytoarchitectonic organization of the human auditory cortex. *Journal of Comparative Neurology, 190,* 597–610.

Galaburda, A. M., Sanides, F., and Geschwind, N. (1978b). Human brain: Cytoarchitectonic left-right asymmetries in the temporal speech region. *Archives of Neurology, 35,* 812–817.

Galaburda, A. M., Sherman, G. F., Rosen, G. D., Aboitiz, F., and Geschwind, N. (1985). Developmental dyslexia: Four consecutive cases with cortical anomalies. *Annals of Neurology, 18,* 222–233.

Geschwind, N., and Levitsky, W. (1968). Human brain: Left-right asymmetries in temporal speech region. *Science, 161,* 186–187.

Greenough, W. T., Black, J. E., and Wallace, C. S. (1987). Experience and brain development. *Child Development, 58,* 539–559.

Gur, R. E., Mzoley, P. D., Resnick, S. M., Sahtsel, D., Kohn, M., Zimmerman, R., Herman, G., Atlas, S., Grossman, R., Erwin, R., and Gur, R. C. (1991). Magnetic resonance imaging in schizophrenia. *Archives of General Psychiatry, 48,* 407–412.

Haslam, R. H., Dalby, J. T., Johns, R. D., and Rademaker, A. W. (1981). Cerebral asymmetry in developmental dyslexia. *Archives of Neurology, 38,* 679–682.

Hier, D. B., LeMay, M., Rosenberger, P. B., and Perlo, V. (1978). Developmental dyslexia: Evidence for a sub-group with reversed cerebral asymmetry. *Archives of Neurology, 35,* 90–92.

Holloway, R. L. (1980). Indonesian "solo" (Ngandong) endocranial reconstructions: some preliminary observations and comparisons with neandertal and homo erectus groups. *American Journal of Physical Anthropology, 53,* 285–295.

Humphreys, P., Kaufmann, W. E., and Galaburda, A. M. (1990). Developmental dyslexia in women: Neuropathological findings in three cases. *Annals of Neurology, 28,* 727–738.

Hynd, G., Semrud-Clikeman, M., Lorys, A., Novey, E., and Eliopulos, R. (1990). Brain morphology in developmental dyslexia and attention deficit disorder/hyperactivity. *Archives of Neurology, 47,* 919–926.

Innocenti, G. M. (1981). Growth and reshaping of axons in the establishment of visual callosal connections. *Science, 212,* 824–827.

Innocenti, G. M., and Frost, D. O. (1980). The postnatal development of visual callosal connections in the absence of visual experience or of the eyes. *Experimental Brain Research, 39,* 365–375.

Ivy, G. O., and Killackey, H. P. (1981). The ontogeny of the distribution of callosal projection neurons in the rat parietal cortex. *Journal of Comparative Neurology, 195,* 367–389.

Ivy, G. O., and Killackey, H. P. (1982). Ontogenetic changes in the projections of neocortical neurons. *Journal of Neuroscience, 2,* 735–743.

Jernigan, T. L., Zatz, L. M., Moses, J. A., and Cardellino, J. P. (1982). Computed tomography in schizophrenics and normal volunteers—cranial asymmetries. *Archives of General Psychiatry, 39,* 771–773.

Kosslyn, S. M. (1987). Seeing and imagining in the cerebral hemispheres: A computational approach. *Psychological Review, 94,* 148–175

Kosslyn, S. M., and Koenig, O. (1992). *Wet mind—the new cognitive neuroscience.* New York, NY: Free Press.

Larsen, J., Hoien, T., Lundberg, I., and Odegaard, H. (1990). MRI evaluation of the size and symmetry of the planum temporale in adolescents with developmental dyslexia. *Brain and Language, 39,* 289–301.

LeMay, M. (1976). Morphological cerebral asymmetries of modern man, fossil man, and non-human primate. *Annals of the New York Academy of Sciences, 280,* 349–366.

LeMay, M., and Culebras, A. (1972). Human brain: Morphologic differences in the hemispheres demonstrable by carotid arteriography. *New England Journal of Medicine, 287,* 168–170.

LeMay, M., and Geschwind, N. (1975). Hemispheric differences in the brains of great apes. *Brain, Behavior, and Evolution, 11,* 48–52.

LeMay, M., and Kido, D. K. (1978). Asymmetries of the cerebral hemispheres on computed tomograms. *Journal of Computer Assisted Tomography, 2,* 471–476.

Leonard, C. L., Voeller, K. S., Lombardino, L. J., Morris, M. K., Hynd, G. W., Alexander, A. W., Andersen, H. G., Garofalakis, M., Honeyman, J. C., Mao, J., Agee, O. F., and Staab, E. V. (1993). Anomalous cerebral morphology in dyslexia revealed with MR imaging. *Archives of Neurology, 50,* 461–469.

Luchins, D. J., and Meltzer, H. Y. (1983). A blind, controlled study of occipital cerebral asymmetry in schizophrenia. *Psychiatry Research, 10,* 87–95.

Naeser, M. A. (1984). Relationship between hemispheric asymmetries on computed tomography scan and recovery from aphasia. *Seminars in Neurology, 4,* 136–150.

Nottebohm, F. (1981). Laterality, seasons, and space govern the learning of a motor skill. *Trends in Neurosciences,* 299–301.

Nottebohm, F., and Nottebohm, M. E. (1976). Left hypoglossal dominance in the control of canary and white-crowned sparrow song. *Journal of Comparative Physiology, 108,* 171–192.

Rademacher, J., Galaburda, A. M., Kennedy, D. N., Filipek, P. A. and Caviness, V. S. (1993). Topographic variation of the human primary cortices: Implications for neuroimaging, brain mapping, and neurobiology. *Cerebral Cortex, 3,* 313–329.

Ratcliff, G., Dila, C., Taylor, L., and Milner, B. (1980). The morphological asymmetry of the hemispheres and cerebral dominance for speech: A possible relationship. *Brain and Language, 11,* 87–98.

Rosen, G. D., Sherman, G. F., and Galaburda, A. M. (1989). Interhemispheric connections differ between symmetrical and asymmetrical brain regions. *Neuroscience, 33,* 525–533.

Rosen, G. D., Sherman, G. F., and Galaburda, A. M. (1991). Ontogenesis of neocortical asymmetry: A [^{3}H]thymidine study. *Neuroscience, 41,* 779–790.

Rossi, A., Stratta, P., Mattei, P., Cupillari, M., Bozzao, A., Gallucci, M., and Casacchia, M. (1992). Planum temporale in schizophrenia: A magnetic resonance study. *Schizophrenia Research*, 7(1), 19–22.

Rubens, A. B., Mahowald, M. W., and Hutton, J. T. (1976). Asymmetry of lateral (Sylvian) fissures in man. *Neurology, 26,* 620–624.

Rumsey, J. M., Berman, K. F., Denckla, M. B., Hamburger, S. D., Kruesi, M. J., and Weinberger, D. R. (1987). Regional cerebral blood flow in severe developmental dyslexia. *Archives of Neurology, 44,* 1144–1150.

Rumsey, J. M., Dorwart, R., Vermess, M., Denckla, M. B., Kruesi, M. J. P., and Rapoport, J. L. (1986). Magnetic resonance imaging of brain anatomy in severe developmental dyslexia. *Archives of Neurology, 43,* 1045–1046.

Sengelaub, D., Jacobs, L. F., and Finlay, B. L. (1985). Regional differences in normally occurring cell death in the developing hamster lateral geniculate nuclei. *Neuroscience Letters, 55,* 103–108.

Sengelaub, D. R., Dolan, R. P., and Finlay, B. L. (1986). Cell generation, death, and retinal growth in the development of the hamster retinal ganglion cell layer. *Journal of Comparative Neurology, 246,* 527–543.

Sherman, G. F., Galaburda, A. M., and Geschwind, N. (1982). Neuroanatomical asymmetries in non-human species. *Trends in Neurosciences, 5,* 429–431.

Steinmetz, H., Volkmann, J., Jancke, L., and Freund, H. J. (1991). Anatomical left-right asymmetry of language-related temporal cortex is different in left-handers and right-handers. *Annals of Neurology, 29(3),* 315–319.

Stengel, E. (1930). Morphologische und cytoarchitektonische Studien über den Bau der unteren Frontalwindung bei Normalen und Taubstummen. Ihre individuellen und Seitenunterschiede. *Zeitschrift für die gesamte Neurologie und Psychiatrie, 130,* 631.

Teszner, D., Tzavaras, A., Gruner, J., and Hécaen, H. (1972). L'asymmétrie droite-gauche du planum temporale: À propos de l'étude anatomique de 100 cerveaux. *Revue Neurologique (Paris), 126,* 444–449.

Tsai, L. Y., Nasrallah, H. A., and Jacoby, C. G. (1983). Hemispheric asymmetries on computed tomographic scans in schizophrenia and mania. *Archives of General Psychiatry, 40,* 1286–1289.

Wada, J. A., Clarke, R., and Hamm, A. (1975). Cerebral hemispheric asymmetry in humans. *Archives of Neurology, 32,* 239–246.

Witelson, S. F. (1977a). Anatomic asymmetry in the temporal lobes: Its documentation, phylogenesis and relationship to functional asymmetry. *Annals of the New York Academy of Sciences, 299,* 328–354.

Witelson, S. F. (1977b). Developmental dyslexia: two right hemispheres and none left. *Science, 195,* 309–311.

Witelson, S. F., and Pallie, W. (1973). Left hemisphere specialization for language in the newborn: Neuroanatomical evidence of asymmetry. *Brain, 96,* 641–646.

Wood, F., Flowers, L., Buchsbaum, M., and Tallal, P. (1991). Investigation of abnormal left temporal functioning in dyslexia through rCBF, auditory evoked potentials and positron emission tomography. *Reading and Writing, 4,* 81–95.

Yeni-Komshian, G. H., and Benson, D. A. (1976). Anatomical study of cerebral asymmetry in the temporal lobe of humans, chimpanzees, and rhesus monkeys. *Science, 192,* 387–389.

Yokoyama, T., Copeland, N. G., Jenkins, N. A., Montgomery, C. A., Elder, F. F. B., and Overbeck, P. A. (1993) Reversal of left-right asymmetry: A situs inversus mutation. *Science, 260,* 279–682.

III   Perceptual, Cognitive, and Motor Lateralization

4 Hemispheric Differences in Visual Object Processing: Structural versus Allocation Theories

Halle D. Brown and Stephen M. Kosslyn

John Hughlings Jackson (1874) is usually credited with being the first to argue persuasively that the cerebral hemispheres have different perceptual strengths. Although this general claim is no longer controversial, there is no consensus about how to characterize these differences. In this chapter we adopt a somewhat novel approach toward characterizing the visual abilities of the hemispheres; we ask how they may differ computationally. Specifically, we ask, at which phases of visual form processing and object recognition are the hemispheres likely to be performing different computations on visual input?

Vision, like all other high-level abilities, is not a single process. It is clear that vision is subserved by a host of distinct systems, which compute information about spatial properties of objects, movement, shape, and so forth (e.g., for a review, see chapter 3 of Kosslyn and Koenig, 1992; see also Cavanagh, 1987; Maunsell and Newsome, 1987). We focus here on only one type of visual processing, that which is accomplished by the "ventral" system (computations taking place in the occipitotemporal and inferior temporal cortices). This system has been called the "what" system by Ungerleider and Mishkin (1982), in contrast to the "where" system implemented in the parietal lobe, and is devoted to visual processing for object recognition. We address the question of how the hemispheres operate differently when they encode shapes.

The study of cerebral lateralization is dependent on the more general study of overall brain function in at least two ways. First, until we have a good idea of what the brain does, we cannot even begin to hypothesize about what is lateralized. Fortunately, vision is one of the most advanced areas of study in cognitive neuroscience, in large part because of sophisticated animal models and computer simulations. Hence, we know enough about vision to begin to theorize about what aspects of visual processing may be carried out more effectively in one or the other cerebral hemisphere. Second, the way we characterize what is lateralized depends on how brain function is characterized more generally. Vision is probably the paradigmatic example of a system that is best understood computationally. The system can be decomposed into subsystems, each of which accepts input, operates on it, and produces output (see Kosslyn and Koenig, 1992; Marr, 1982; Rumelhart and McClelland,

1986). Thus, a theory of visual hemispheric specialization should specify differences in the visual computations performed by the two hemispheres. This is the approach we have taken here.

A QUESTION OF SCALE

Marr (1982) argued that many functions of vision would be accomplished most effectively if the system encoded information at multiple levels of scale. For example, one way to distinguish between an edge versus texture (e.g., the edge of a table and the grain on its top) is to determine whether sharp changes in intensity are present at multiple scales: if they are present only with high resolution, they are probably texture variations; if they are present at multiple levels, they are probably edges (see also DeValois and DeValois, 1988). One lesson we have learned from computational models of visual information processing is that when different types of information must be extracted from a single stimulus, it is more efficient to separate the processing into different systems (see Kosslyn and Koenig, 1992). At least in some cases, these different systems may be located in different hemispheres of the brain (cf. Kosslyn et al., 1992; Marsolek, 1992; Rueckl, Cave, and Kosslyn, 1989).

Converging evidence from neuropsychological cases of patients with unilateral brain damage (Delis, Robertson, and Efron, 1986; Robertson and Delis, 1986) and from divided visual field studies with normal subjects (Jonsson and Hellige, 1986; Martin, 1979; Sergent, 1987a,b; Van Kleeck, 1989) indicate that the two hemispheres focus on different types of features of visual stimuli when forming object representations. The left hemisphere appears to focus on smaller parts, higher spatial frequencies, or details (depending on how one chooses to characterize the results); in contrast, the right hemisphere appears to focus on the global form, lower spatial frequencies, or course patterns. Many researchers have advanced theories to explain the basis of these hemispheric differences in visual processing (Palmer and Tzeng, 1990; Robertson and Lamb, 1991; Sergent, 1987b; see also Christman, 1989, and Peterzell, 1991). Indeed, the different "descriptions" of the results are highly theoretically loaded; each implies a different conception of what the hemispheres do.[1]

Global Precedence

Navon (1977) provided evidence that perception proceeds from the global level down to the local level. He described a "global precedence phenomenon," whereby global-level features of a stimulus are apprehended before local-level features. In his Experiment 2, Navon used a clever paradigm in which subjects heard either an H or an S spoken aloud and then produced a manual response with their right hand indicating which of these letters they heard. At the same time, the subjects watched a visual display in which a composite letter was flashed 40 ms before the utterance began on half of the trials. To ensure that the subjects actually monitored the visual display, they had to press a key with their left hand if there had been a flash. The composite stimuli were either a large H, S, or O made up of small versions of each of these letters so that the identity of either the global or local level, both, or neither could conflict with the identity of the auditory stimulus for each trial. Navon found that response time (RT) depended on the relation of the auditory stimulus and the global-level letter. The subjects were fastest when these were the same, and slowest when the auditory stimulus and the global-level letter conflicted. However, there was no difference in RT depending on the relation of the local-level letter to the auditory stimulus. Navon interpreted this selective interference with the global level as evidence that visual processing proceeds from the global to the local level.

Some researchers have administered variants of Navon's task to normal subjects in divided-visual-field experiments in an effort to document a right hemisphere (RH) superiority for processing global-level forms and a left hemisphere (LH) superiority for processing local-level forms (e.g., Boles, 1984; Martin, 1979; Van Kleeck, 1989). The results from these studies have not consistently demonstrated reliable asymmetries. Van Kleeck (1989) noticed that many of the nonsignificant results still had trends in the expected direction, and hence followed up his own experiment with a meta-analysis of his results and those of six additional studies using similar tasks. The meta-analysis did support the LH-local/RH-global distinction, but the effect sizes from individual studies were quite variable.

Thus, we are faced with a puzzle. When many studies are examined, there is evidence for hemispheric specialization, as summarized above. But evidence for such specialization is not robust. Any theory of visual hemispheric specialization must explain not only the findings but the basis of this underlying variability.

Alternative Theories

We can divide accounts for the LH-local/RH-global findings into two classes. *Structural theories* posit that one or more processing subsystems has become specialized in the hemispheres, whereas *allocation theories* posit that the hemispheres tend to employ different strategies that often produce these results— but there are no hard-and-fast structural differences (e.g., see Cohen, 1982). Clearly, at least some linguistic processing involves structural differences, but the issue of structure vs. allocation is open with regard to visual processing. Unlike structural theories, allocation theories lead us to expect different processing in different circumstances. At first glance, the mere fact that the LH-local/RH-global findings are so variable may seem to implicate allocation theories. However, the variability could arise in at least two ways even if the hemispheres differ structurally. First, even subtly different tasks may invoke different component-processing subsystems, which are lateralized differently. Second, there may be widespread individual differences in the way specific subsystems are lateralized, and the different experiments may inadvertently have tested people with different patterns of cerebral lateralization (see Kosslyn, Sokolov, and Chen, 1989). Thus, both classes of theories are viable.

These two classes of theories can be used to generate six alternative hypotheses by considering structural and allocation differences at three levels of processing. Visual processing is typically divided into three phases: "low level," "intermediate," and "high level" (e.g., cf. Marr, 1982), and the hemispheres may differ—structurally or in terms of allocation—at any of these phases. We assume that the subsystems that accomplish each type of processing are duplicated in the two hemispheres, and cerebral lateralization is a matter of degree. Hemispheric asymmetries—in structure or allocation—are not due to the presence or absence of individual subsystems or strategies; rather, the hemispheres differ in the relative efficacy of individual subsystems for particular types of processing (for structural theories) or in their predilection for using certain strategies (for allocation theories).

Low-level Specialization At the lowest level, subsystems organize the input so that distinct "figures" are separated from the "ground." The output of such processing subsystems is represented in something like the structure Kosslyn et al. (1990) called the "visual buffer." This structure includes a group of retinotopically mapped visual areas, including areas V1, V2, V3, V3a, and V4 in the occipital cortex (see Felleman and Van Essen, 1991). Representations in the visual buffer specify edges, regions of common color and texture, and other characteristics that delineate objects from background. This structure is roughly equivalent to that which supports Marr's (1982) "2.5-D Sketch."

The visual buffer contains more information than can be considered in detail, and hence some information must be selected for additional processing. Kosslyn et al. (1990) posit an "attention window" that can be adjusted to a specific size, shape, and location to select a specific region of the visual buffer for further processing (cf. Treisman and Gelade, 1980).

According to structural theories, the hemispheres organize the input in different ways. For example, the RH may more effectively detect large variations in light intensity over space, whereas the LH may more effectively detect small variations in light intensity over space. One way to think of this is that the hemispheres differ in their sensitivity to different spatial frequencies (cf. Sergent, 1987b; Sergent and Hellige, 1986; Jonsson and Hellige, 1986). Jonsson and Hellige (1986) tested this hypothesized hemispheric difference with a physical identity letter-matching task. When letters were very blurred, same/different matching was selectively impaired in the LH relative to the RH, which is consistent with the hypothesis that the LH processes the higher spatial frequency information that was removed by the blurring. It is possible that the LH is sensitive to higher spatial frequencies than the right because of anatomic features, such as the average length of lateral connections in the relevant areas (see Springer and Deutsch, 1989, pp. 315–320). Alternatively, Kosslyn (1987) suggests a "snowball" mechanism that can result in such structural differences via learning; in this mechanism, if a certain kind of information is useful to subsystems downstream, they send feedback that strengthens the relevant processes that send such information (for computer simulations, see Kosslyn et al., 1989).

A strong structural theory that posits differences in the lateralization of low-level vision is probably incorrect: Kitterle, Christman, and Hellige (1990) report no visual-field differences in the ease of detecting gratings that have high or low spatial frequencies. The LH-local/RH-global difference only occurs when subjects must categorize or compare the stimulus in some way.

According to allocation theories, the hemispheres are biased to process the input in different ways. For example, the attention window may be biased to subtend a smaller portion of the LH visual buffer, perhaps because processes downstream have found it useful to receive smaller portions of input in the past. This sort of theory can easily accommodate the fact that the hemispheric differences arise only when the stimulus must be categorized or compared: only then do top-down processes set the attention window appropriately.

Intermediate-level Specialization   Intermediate visual processing organizes the input into perceptual groups that will be useful for later object recognition. In the Kosslyn et al. (1990) model, the contents of the attention window are sent to a "preprocessing" subsystem, instantiated in the occipito-temporal regions. The preprocessing subsystem extracts stimulus features that will be most useful for recognition—the "nonaccidental properties" proposed by Lowe (1985, 1987), texture gradients, and color are good candidates for such features (cf. Biederman, 1987; for further discussion, see chapter 3 in Kosslyn and Koenig, 1992). These features would be present in most views of the object.

The preprocessing subsystem extracts different properties when it operates on different input: if it receives high-resolution information, it can compute small, detailed features of the stimulus; if it receives coarse information, it can compute overall object structure. It is possible that the preprocessing subsystem itself could operate differently in the two hemispheres.

According to structural theories, this subsystem is tuned to extract different kinds of information in the two hemispheres. For example, sometimes we want to look at an overall pattern, such as a face, and other times we want to look at one of its components, such as the eyes of a face. The two kinds of processes are in a sense incompatible: the global process needs to incorporate into a whole the very things that need to be segregated by the local process. Thus, it would be useful if separate processes operate in parallel at the two levels, extracting features that later would be matched to different-sized patterns in memory.

According to allocation theories, the versions of the preprocessing subsystem in the two hemispheres are biased to extract different sorts of information. This bias could arise from bottom-up factors (i.e., the type of information received as input) or by top-down factors (i.e., the computations may become "tuned" by learning which type of information is most useful for subsequent subsystems). The same factors that might result in structural changes could also produce a bias toward encoding features at different levels of scale, but this bias would not be "hard-wired" into the system (cf. Kosslyn, 1987).

High-level Specialization   Finally, high-level vision involves matching input to representations stored in memory. An object is recognized when such a match is successful. In the Kosslyn et al. (1990) model, the output from the preprocessing subsystem serves as the input to the "pattern activation" subsystem, in the inferior temporal lobes. It is here that the perceptual input is compared to stored visual information, and recognition is achieved if a match is made. If the input does not match a previously stored representation well enough, then the new pattern is stored.

Unlike the visual buffer and preprocessing subsystems, size per se is unlikely to be represented at the level of object recognition; neurons in the inferior temporal lobe that are sensitive to high-level visual properties are insensitive to changes in visual angle (for a review, see Plaut and Farah, 1990). Thus, theories that posit hemispheric specialization in the final phases of the recognition sequence cannot explain hemispheric differences that arise when objects subtend different visual angles. Rather, the hemispheres may differ in their preferences for encoding parts vs. wholes, or—a closely related idea—in their preferences for encoding input at different levels of hierarchy in a structural description. A structural description specifies how components are organized to compose a whole; the shape of a person, for example, can be represented by a tree diagram with "body" at the top, "head," "trunk," "arms," and "legs" as branches, "upper arm," "forearm," "hand" as branches from the "arm" branch, and so forth (cf. Marr, 1982; Palmer, 1977).

According to one possible structural theory, one hemisphere could store the (larger) wholes and the other could store the (smaller) parts. Another possible structural theory posits that the hemispheres differ not in the size of the components they store, but in the preferred level of hierarchy: the LH may represent information farther down in a structural hierarchy than the RH. Alternatively, the hemispheres may have different (built-in) matching processes, which are tuned for matching input to stored representations of parts or wholes—or higher or lower levels in the hierarchy.

Finally, according to allocation theories, there is a bias toward matching representations of parts in the LH and wholes in the RH, or a bias toward processing at one or the other relative levels of hierarchy. Allocation theories would posit, however, that the same types of visual information are stored in the two hemispheres.

THREE EXPERIMENTS

We performed three experiments as an initial effort to narrow down the locus of the observed LH specialization for local features and the RH specialization for global features. In the letter stimuli that are typically used in global precedence studies, the features of the global-level object (e.g., two vertical lines and one horizontal line for an H) are determined by the positioning of the local elements. Thus, there is a confounding between size and level of hierarchy: the large letter is composed of smaller letters. We reserve the term "hierarchy" to refer to objects that are composed only of their constituent parts. For example, a human body is hierarchically structured because it is made out of a head, trunk, arms, and so on; nothing remains if these parts are removed. In contrast, patterns on a shirt are not hierarchically related to the shirt; if removed, the shirt would remain intact. In our third experiment, we remove this confounding for letter stimuli. Moreover, in addition to letter stimuli, we use picture stimuli that are not hierarchically arranged, which removes possible contributions of processes that are specialized for reading.

Only a few studies have attempted to test the generality of the global precedence phenomenon by using stimuli other than letters. Antes and Mann (1984) used pictures to investigate the global precedence effect, and found this effect for small scenes that subtended 4 degrees of visual angle, but they found local precedence for large scenes that subtended 16 degrees of visual angle. However, the local-level features were objects within a scene, and the objects themselves defined the nature of the scene (i.e., a global-level description was "farm scene," and local-level features were barn, tractor, etc., thus establishing a semantic relationship between the two levels). The objects were very different at the two levels, which itself is a confounding.

In order to begin to discriminate among the theories, we wanted to determine whether the global precedence effect depends on a hierarchic arrangement (as in the standard letter stimuli) or whether global features are processed faster than local features in general. In most real-world objects, global features provide general information about object identity, whereas local features can be used to distinguish specific exemplars. For example, a shirt can be defined as having two sleeves and a middle portion that covers the body. It may also have a pocket, buttons, or some design on it, or a combination of these. These local-level features are details that distinguish one shirt from another but they exist independently of the features that define the shirt in general.

In our experiments, the pictures used as stimuli were garments with smaller pictures on them; the larger pictures were not composed of the smaller ones, and hence there was no hierarchic relation between the two. The smaller pictures were themselves garments, and hence we had the same types of objects at local and global level without having a hierarchic arrangement.

In addition to using such stimuli, we used a different experimental paradigm from most other studies. We used a divided-attention task rather than a selective-attention task. Most global precedence studies are designed to assess interference effects in a selective-attention task; the subject's attention is focused on one level and responses are compared when the identity of the item at the other level is either the same or different. The logic underlying these studies is that the level that is processed first will selectively interfere with the level that is processed second. For example, in her divided-visual-field study of global precedence, Martin (1979) found that the global level was processed faster than the local level in both hemispheres when the global- and local-level letters were different. However, the global level was processed faster following RH presentation than following LH presentation when subjects attended to the global level. In addition, there was greater interference from the global-level letter when stimuli were presented initially to the RH when the subjects selectively attended to the local level; in this condition, the subjects evaluated the stimuli more quickly when they were presented initially to the LH than to the RH. Boles (1984) was not able to replicate this finding using the same paradigm.

We speculated that hemispheric specialization might be easier to assess in a more challenging task. In a divided-attention task, subjects must search for targets that could appear at either the global or local level. Under such conditions, both levels must be processed simultaneously, and differences in hemispheric specialization for processing global- and local-level features might be more easily detected than in a selective-attention task. Divided-attention tasks are rarely used to investigate the global precedence effect, but Lamb, Robertson, and Knight (1990) did use such a paradigm with unilaterally brain-damaged patients. These researchers used four letters as stimuli, two as targets, and two as distractors, and the subjects were to indicate which target was present on each trial. Only one target was present per trial, and it appeared at the local or global level equally often. We adopted this paradigm for our experiments.

Experiment 1

If the local/global hemispheric specialization is different for hierarchic letters and our nonhierarchic pictures, this result would suggest that the hemispheric difference occurs during high-level visual processing: earlier phases are sensitive to differences in visual angle and size, not hierarchic arrangement. If we obtain such results, we next would want to determine whether the effect was caused by structural or allocation differences between the hemispheres.

Method and Results　We wanted to determine whether the global precedence effect typically found with the standard letter stimuli would also be found with our pictorial stimuli. Hence, the subjects saw two types of stimuli: letters composed of smaller letters and articles of clothing with smaller articles of clothing printed on them as "patterns." Sample stimuli are shown in figure 4.1.

For each stimulus type, we prepared four objects. Two were designated as targets and two were distractors. On each trial, one target and one distractor were paired and the subjects were to indicate (by pressing one of two keys on a computer keyboard) which target object was presented. For example, a stimulus for one trial might be a shirt, which is a target object, with small

Experiment 1

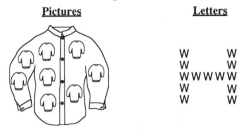

Experiment 2

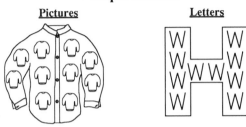

Experiment 3

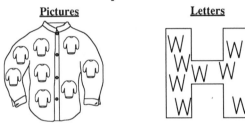

Figure 4.1 Sample picture and letter stimuli used in the three experiments.

sweaters printed on it, so the subject would press the key labeled with a picture of a shirt. The target object for each trial occurred equally often as a large or small object. Stimuli were presented in a pseudorandom order for 100 ms, and were positioned with the near edge 1.4 cm (1.23 degrees of visual angle) to either the left or right of a central fixation point. The order in which stimulus types were seen (pictures first or letters first), and the hand used to respond, were counterbalanced across subjects. The subjects for all three experiments were right-handed men between the ages of 18 and 23.

The pictures in this experiment consisted of six to eight small articles of clothing positioned randomly on larger articles of clothing. Large pictures subtended 4.75 degrees of visual angle, and small pictures subtended 0.88 degree. The letters were hierarchically arranged and contained on average 14 smaller letters. Large letters subtended 2.11 degrees of visual angle, and small letters subtended 0.35 degree. Thirty-three paid subjects were tested.[2]

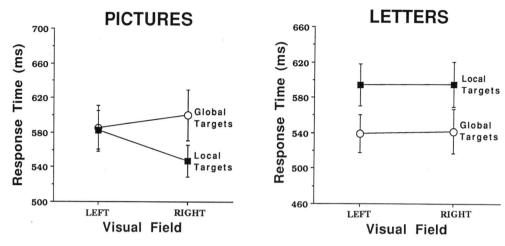

Figure 4.2 Results from Experiment 1.

For all of the experiments reported in this chapter, the data were analyzed with a repeated measures analysis of variance (ANOVA). Visual field and level of target (global or local) were within-subject factors, and the order in which stimulus types were presented and response hand were between-subject factors. Separate ANOVAs were conducted for the picture and letter data. All results discussed met the .05 level of significance.

For the pictures, we found that the subjects did in fact detect targets at the local level faster when the stimuli were shown initially to the LH than the RH, but evaluated targets at the global level equally quickly when they were shown initially to either hemisphere. Thus, local precedence and a trend toward the hypothesized pattern of hemispheric specialization were found for the picture stimuli, as shown in figure 4.2.

In contrast, although we found global precedence for the letter stimuli, this effect was the same when stimuli were presented initially to the RH or to the LH. For letters, the subjects responded faster and made fewer errors when the targets were at the global level than when they were at the local level. But again, this global precedence effect was the same in both hemispheres (see figure 4.2).

These results were unexpected: we failed to find the usual results with the standard type of stimuli, but found evidence that hierarchic organization was not at the root of the hemispheric difference when pictures were used. Although the different results for the two stimulus types would support a high-level theory of hemispheric specialization, we cannot be certain that this alternative is correct. The pictures and letters differed in many ways, so it is unclear why the right and left hemispheres responded differently to global and local levels of pictures but not to letters. In the next experiment, we equated the two stimuli along as many dimensions as possible.

Perceptual, Cognitive, and Motor Lateralization

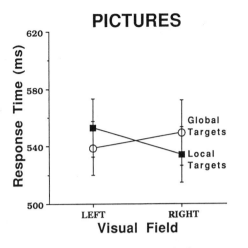

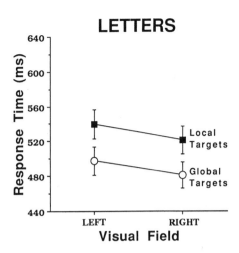

Figure 4.3 Results from Experiment 2.

Experiment 2

We revised the pictures and letters to make them more similar. Both contained ten smaller, local-level forms positioned within an outline that specified the global-level form. In Experiment 1, the smaller pictures were positioned randomly within the global form; in Experiment 2, local forms were positioned more regularly for both pictures and letters. The smaller forms were positioned symmetrically, and consequently appeared more "texture-like." The two stimulus types were also drawn so that they subtended the same visual angle (4.75 degrees); smaller forms also subtended the same (smaller) visual angle (0.88 degree). Thirty-two men who were not tested in Experiment 1 participated as paid subjects.

For the pictures, we did not find strong support for the claim that the hemispheres differ in their ability to encode local and global information, but the trends were in the same direction as in Experiment 1. The subjects detected global targets slightly faster when they were shown initially to the RH, and detected local targets slightly faster when they were shown initially to the LH (figure 4.3). In accordance with our prediction for a divided-attention task, there was a trend toward hemispheric specialization that was equal in magnitude for both global and local targets, without an overall global precedence effect.

For the letters, the pattern of results was similar to Experiment 1. The subjects detected global targets faster overall than local targets, but this effect was the same in both hemispheres. However, we now found that the subjects detected letter targets faster when they were shown initially to the LH (see figure 4.3).

The subjects evaluated the stimuli more quickly overall in this experiment than in the first one, possibly because the larger forms were easier to detect. They were especially fast for the global-level pictures in Experiment 2 compared to Experiment 1. Making the local forms more texturelike for the picture stimuli apparently made the global form more "salient" (possibly due to Gestalt laws of grouping) in Experiment 2 than for the pictures in Experiment 1, where random positioning of few local forms may have made the local level more salient. In both experiments, subjects were faster for the local forms when they were shown initially to the LH than when they were shown initially to the RH. But this specialization was not significant when there were more, regularly positioned local forms in Experiment 2. The subjects evaluated the global forms only slightly faster when they were presented initially to the RH than to the LH in both experiments.

One inference is clear: the results do not support any structural theory of the lateralization of high-level visual processing. However, they can be accommodated by allocation theories. In this case, the attention window may be drawn to inhomogeneities in the visual field (e.g., irregular patterns); in a formal sense, changes in stimulation carry more "information" (see Shannon, 1963). If the relative "saliency" of global- or local-level forms is indeed affecting whether hemispheric specialization emerges, then perhaps the global level of the letter stimuli is always more salient than the local level. This hypothesis was directly investigated in our third experiment.

Experiment 3

This experiment was conducted to determine whether our failure to find evidence for the LH-local/RH-global difference for letter stimuli was caused by a property of letters per se or by the hierarchic arrangement of these stimuli. If we find that the hemispheres encode global and local features differently when the hierarchic arrangement is not present, then we will be encouraged to investigate further the predictions of low-level allocation theories.

Letter stimuli were revised so that smaller letters were positioned randomly inside the outline of a larger letter. In this way, the letters were exactly analogous to the picture stimuli we used in Experiment 1. A new group of 16 subjects was shown the revised letter stimuli along with the picture stimuli from Experiment 1. Both stimulus types now contained six to eight smaller objects, and smaller and larger objects subtended the same visual angles for both letters and pictures.

These subjects detected global-level letters faster than local-level letters overall, but now we now found differences when the stimuli were presented initially to the different hemispheres. Larger letter targets were detected faster than smaller letter targets when they were shown initially to the RH; in contrast, the subjects detected the two types of targets equally fast when they were shown initially to the LH (figure 4.4). For the pictures, this interaction between target and hemisphere was not significant, but the results were similar to the pattern obtained for Experiment 1 in that the subjects detected smaller objects faster overall and also faster than larger objects when they were presented initially to the LH. When pictures were presented initially to

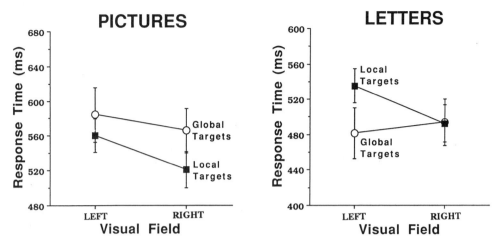

Figure 4.4 Results from Experiment 3.

the RH, the subjects detected smaller and larger targets equally quickly, as in Experiment 1. Also, the subjects responded faster in general when the picture stimuli were presented initially to the LH, as shown in figure 4.4.

Implications of Results

We had trouble obtaining hemispheric differences with the standard letter stimuli, and obtained them only intermittently with picture stimuli. Nevertheless, the findings do bear on the various hypotheses we considered at the outset. First, no structural theory fares well, given the kinds of inconsistencies we observed. One could claim that the inconsistent results with the picture stimuli reflect differences in the subject populations, but all subjects were right-handed male Harvard University undergraduates. Such individual differences may exist, but unless they are specified they can never be disproved— and hence the view is of limited use. The results led us to narrow down the space to the three allocation theories.

Second, given that we found hemispheric specialization with nonhierarchic pictures in Experiment 1, we can rule out the theory that it is caused by processing such representations at the latest phases of visual object recognition. According to that theory, the hemispheres differ in their ability to store or process different levels of hierarchy—and hence hemispheric specialization should not be evident when stimuli are not hierarchically organized. However, this still leaves open the possibility that part/whole relations are stored differently in each hemisphere, even if they are not hierarchic representations.

Third, the fact that the arrangement of the smaller pictures makes a difference suggests that the effect is not due to size per se, as expected if the locus is low-level structural or processing differences in the visual buffer. This inference is consistent with findings reported by Lamb et al. (1990), who studied patients with damage to the left hemisphere superior temporal gyrus (LSTG) or right hemisphere superior temporal gyrus (RSTG). Patients with RSTG damage showed local precedence in a task paradigm similar to ours except that they included many stimulus sizes. They showed local precedence across a range of sizes, except the very smallest (3 degrees), where global precedence was shown. Patients with LSTG damage showed global precedence across all stimulus sizes.

The most plausible account of the present results, along with those in the literature, is that the hemispheres differ in how they preferentially set the attention window. Because the relative saliency of global- or local-level forms affected the magnitude and direction of hemispheric differences, attentional factors must have affected the encoding process.

This interpretation is consistent with strategies that some subjects reported using during our experiments: some subjects claimed that they sought specific features of the pictures, but did not seek such features of the letters; for example, they looked for buttons on the shirt to distinguish it from a sweater. The letters we chose may be sufficiently distinct that subjects did not need to seek specific features to discriminate them, and so any special, hemispheric-specific facility with such attention allocation was not invoked. If this account is correct, then the choice of letters is critical: if letters are highly confusable, we should find strong evidence of LH superiority for local targets.

ATTENTION AND RECEPTIVE FIELDS

Kosslyn and colleagues (1992) offer a specific mechanism that can be used to conceptualize the attention allocation process we envision. They suggest that the RH preferentially monitors outputs from neurons that have relatively large receptive fields, whereas the LH preferentially monitors outputs from neurons that have relatively small receptive fields. In their computer simulation models, they found that when input units had large overlapping receptive fields, the networks could encode the metric location of a dot relative to a bar more effectively than when the input units had small, nonoverlapping receptive fields. The reverse effect (although weaker) was found when the networks categorized whether the dot was above or below the bar. This result is interesting because human subjects evaluate metric location better when stimuli are presented to the RH, and categorize spatial relations better (marginally) when stimuli are presented to the LH (for a review of this literature, see Kosslyn et al., 1992).

Although Kosslyn et al. conceived of their simulations as testing structural theories, their results apply equally well to allocation theories: the hemispheres may differ in their facility at monitoring the outputs from different-sized receptive fields, even if the same outputs are available in both hemispheres.

Jacobs and Kosslyn (in press) extended the computer simulation models of Kosslyn et al. by examining the possible role of differences in receptive field sizes in encoding shapes, in addition to the spatial relations previously examined. They found that networks that received input from units with larger overlapping receptive fields could encode the identity of specific shapes better than networks that received input from units with smaller, nonoverlapping receptive fields. The same network systems could encode metric spatial relations better than those with smaller receptive fields. In contrast, receptive field size had the opposite effect in networks that assigned shapes to categories: smaller receptive fields were more efficient for this computation, as well as encoding categorical spatial relations.

Although Jacobs and Kosslyn did not examine part/whole encoding in their models, we can infer that if shapes are grouped into categories, individual features are likely to be averaged across. In contrast, if individual shapes are encoded, the individual features probably will be preserved.

Jacobs and Kosslyn suggest that the bias to encode outputs from neurons with different-sized receptive fields allows the "ventral" (object properties–encoding) and "dorsal" (spatial properties–encoding) systems to be coordinated. When one is navigating, one not only needs to know precise metric distances of objects (a dorsal function), but also the specific shapes of objects (a ventral function). For example, to avoid hitting a table, one needs to know both its distance and whether it has jutting corners. Hence, the two types of processing need to be linked, and it makes sense that they both are more effective in the same hemisphere, the right (see Kosslyn et al., 1992, and Marsolek, Kosslyn, and Squire, 1992). Similarly, when one is trying to identify objects, one needs to ignore variations in shape among specific examples, and needs only to know the type of spatial relations among parts (such as what is connected to what)—not the specific positions of parts of a given object. For example, to identify a shape as a dog, one would ignore the type of dog and the precise positions of its limbs. The LH appears to have a special role both in generalizing over shapes (Marsolek, 1992) and in categorizing spatial relations (Kosslyn et al., 1989).

Thus, differences in receptive field size could serve to coordinate the encoding of shape and spatial relations, and could conceivably lead the right hemisphere to specialize in computing metric spatial relations and specific shapes and the left hemisphere to specialize in computing categorical spatial relations and categories of shapes.

Some researchers have studied receptive field differences as a possible mechanism underlying global precedence in the center of vision. Hughes et al. (1984) used unique patterns to study global precedence, in which the local-level objects were small lines; the sizes of the lines corresponded to the sizes of receptive field sizes of neurons in primary visual cortex. These lines were arranged into larger, global-level rectangular clusters. The small lines and large rectangle could have different orientations. Thus, local-level components would directly excite individual neurons with small receptive fields while larger clusters of lines would directly excite individual neurons with larger receptive fields. The subject's task was to judge the orientation of either local- or global-level lines. Hughes et al. found a large global precedence effect, which is consistent with the idea that differences in receptive field sizes play a role in this effect.

Spatial Frequencies or Receptive Fields?

We have focused on the idea that the hemispheres differ in how effectively they allocate attention at scales of different size, and have suggested that the underlying mechanism involves sampling outputs from neurons with different-sized receptive fields. However, one could argue that this is nothing more than a restatement of the spatial-frequency hypothesis developed by Sergent and her colleagues. Indeed, the receptive field and spatial-frequency theories predict many of the same results. The two concepts are intimately related: the smaller its receptive field, the higher the spatial frequency a cell will respond to, and the larger the receptive field, the lower the spatial frequency.

Christman (1989) reviewed many studies that address the spatial-frequency hypothesis. In Christman's summary of this literature, he states: "There is evidence that spatial frequency related asymmetries will arise only when some cognitive operation (i.e., identification, discrimination) needs to be performed on the sensory input. Tasks involving simple sensitivity to and detection of a stimulus do not appear to yield reliable asymmetries" (p. 241). Although Jonsson and Hellige (1986), Michimata and Hellige (1987), and Sergent (1987a) blurred stimulus displays to manipulate spatial-frequency content, Christman (1989) notes that blurring affects stimulus perceptibility in addition to spatial frequencies. Only studies involving adaptation to low or high frequency sine wave gratings implicate a direct relationship between spatial-frequency channels and the type of information conveyed in them (e.g., Shulman et al. 1986). Indeed, Peterzell (1991) notes that all of the data from studies of differential hemispheric sensitivity to low or high spatial frequencies can be explained by a total visible information-energy hypothesis or in terms of hemispheric response bias. Thus, he argues that the spatial-frequency hypothesis may not describe the basis of hemispheric differences, and emphasizes, as we have in this chapter, the importance of task parameters that determine the conditions under which hemispheric differences are likely to emerge.

Even though the theories make many similar predictions, this does not imply that they cannot be empirically distinguished. Kosslyn, Anderson, Hamilton, and Hillger (1994) attempted to discriminate between the spatial-frequency hypothesis and the receptive-field hypothesis. They showed subjects small line segments, which were tilted to the left or to the right. The subject had only to classify the orientation, as quickly as possible. The lines were presented sequentially in pairs (with an interstimulus interval long enough that apparent motion did not occur). The logic was that if the outputs from the same neurons were used to represent the orientation of the two lines in a pair, the second line should be "primed." The interesting question was whether such priming would occur when the second line was shifted to a new location, and if so, over what range of locations priming would persist. Thus, the lines were presented either in nearby locations (separated by 1.2 degrees of visual angle) or relatively distant locations (separated by 7.2 degrees of visual angle). The lines that were members of the near and distant pairs appeared equally often in each visual field and in each location.

The receptive-field hypothesis leads us to expect the subjects to require comparable amounts of time for near and distant pairs when they are presented initially to the right hemisphere. The large receptive fields should funnel low-level inputs from a wide range of locations into the same high-level neurons. In contrast, the subjects should require more time for distant pairs than near ones when the lines are presented initially to the LH: the lines in distant pairs should fall into the receptive fields of low-level neurons that do not funnel information into the same high-level neurons, and hence there should be little priming of the second line of a pair. The spatial-frequency hypothesis leads us to expect no difference for the two separations in either hemifield; the lines are presented sequentially, and so each stimulus input has the same spatial-frequency spectrum. The results of this experiment supported the receptive-field hypothesis: the subjects did indeed require more time when the lines appeared at wider separations in the right visual field (and so were seen initially by the LH) than when they appeared in the left visual field. Moreover, as expected, this effect was modulated by attentional variables.

CONCLUSIONS

As is evident in the literature and in the additional experiments we summarize here, the RH does not always compute the global form of an object more effectively than the LH, nor does the LH always compute smaller details more effectively than the RH. In our experiments, the subjects evaluated letter stimuli in the same way when the stimuli were shown initially to the LH or the RH under certain conditions, even when the general features of these stimuli were matched to those of the pictures—which did elicit hemispheric asymmetries in the same conditions. We conclude that structural differences do not underlie the hemispheric differences in visual processing; rather, the hemispheres differ in their predilections for certain types of processing. Moreover, the results suggest that these differences occur because the subjects are led to attend to different characteristics of the stimuli. We hypothesize that the hemispheres differ in their ability to monitor outputs from low-level neurons that have different-sized receptive fields.

In terms of the model of Kosslyn et al. (1990), hemispheric asymmetries in visual processing occur because the hemispheres allocate attention differently, which changes the input to the preprocessing subsystems. The process of allocating attention probably occurs via top-down mechanisms, which seek information that will be useful for performing a task (see Kosslyn et al., 1990; Kosslyn and Koenig, 1992, chapter 3). Thus, task parameters and stimulus characteristics can affect how attention is allocated to outputs from neurons with different-sized receptive fields.

Given this theory, what are the shortcomings of our method of investigating laterality effects? We are using normal subjects with intact brains; trying to tease apart the contributions of each hemisphere to integrated processing is inherently difficult. The divided-visual-field methodology is a poor means by which to try to examine separate hemisphere functions for many reasons: peripheral stimulus presentation for a fraction of a second does not give each hemisphere very high-quality input, response methods may bias one hemisphere over the other, etc. All of these issues have been described and discussed in detail by Sergent and Hellige (1986) and Hellige and Sergent (1986).

A major question still left unanswered is, what determines when attention will be allocated to the global or local level? We have suggested one possibility, namely that attention will be focused on the local level when small details must be discerned to perform the task. But even if this is true, it is unlikely to be the whole story: the same stimuli in a given task sometimes produce laterality effects and sometimes do not. The difficulty in obtaining laterality effects at all, and particularly the failure to replicate findings across studies, should be the focus of future research. Understanding the variability in patterns of hemispheric asymmetry, both within and between individuals, should be explored, as well as the roles of demand characteristics and task parameters.

ACKNOWLEDGMENTS

Preparation of this chapter was supported by NSF grant BNS 90 09619 and NINDS grant 17778-09 awarded to Stephen M. Kosslyn and by an NDSEG Graduate Fellowship awarded to Halle D. Brown.

NOTES

1. For convenience, researchers have typically considered only two levels of information about visual objects. The "global level" contains information about the object as a whole, its general shape, and so forth; the "local level" contains information about parts, texture, or details. From a given vantage point, what we call "global-level features" typically subtend larger visual angles than local-level features. Furthermore, global-level features often define the "lay of the land," the overall structure that organizes local-level features.

2. Additional information about the methodology and results from the three experiments we describe in this chapter are currently being prepared for publication (Brown and Kosslyn, in preparation).

REFERENCES

Antes, J. R., and Mann, S. W. (1984). Global-local precedence in picture processing. *Psychological Research, 46,* 247–259.

Biederman, I. (1987). Recognition by components: A theory of human image understanding. *Psychological Review, 94,* 115–147.

Boles, D. B. (1984). Global versus local processing: Is there a hemispheric dichotomy? *Neuropsychologia, 22,* 445–455.

Brown, H. D., and Kosslyn, S. M. (in preparation). *Hemispheric asymmetry in visual object processing: What underlies the global precedence phenomenon?*

Cavanagh, P. (1987). Reconstructing the third dimension: Interactions between color, texture, motion, binocular disparity, and shape. *Computer Vision, Graphics, and Image Processing, 37,* 171–195.

Christman, S. (1989). Perceptual characteristics in visual laterality research. *Brain and Cognition, 11,* 238–257.

Cohen, G. (1982). Theoretical interpretations of lateral asymmetries. In J. G. Beaumont (Ed.), *Divided visual field studies of cerebral organisation.* New York, NY: Academic Press.

Delis, D. C., Robertson, L. C., and Efron, R. (1986). Hemispheric specialization of memory for visual hierarchical stimuli. *Neuropsychologia, 24,* 205–214.

DeValois, R. L., and DeValois, K. K. (1988). *Spatial vision.* New York, NY: Oxford University Press.

Felleman, D. J., and Van Essen, D. C. (1991). Distributed hierarchical processing in primate cerebral cortex. *Cerebral Cortex, 1,* 1–47.

Hellige, J. B., and Sergent, J. (1986). Role of task factors in visual field asymmetries. *Brain and Cognition, 5,* 200–222.

Hughes, H. C., Layton, W. M., Baird, J. C., and Lester, L. S. (1984). Global precedence in visual pattern recognition. *Perception and Psychophysics, 35,* 361–371.

Jackson, J. H. (1874). On the duality of the brain. In J. Taylor (Ed.), *Selected writings of John Hughlings Jackson.* London: Hodder and Stoughton.

Jacobs, R., and Kosslyn, S. M. (in press). Encoding shape and spatial relations: The role of receptive field size in coordinating complementary representations. *Cognitive Science.*

Jonsson, J. E., and Hellige, J. B. (1986). Lateralized effects of blurring: A test of the visual spatial frequency model of cerebral hemisphere asymmetry. *Neuropsychologia, 24,* 351–362.

Kitterle, F. L., Christman, S., and Hellige, J. B. (1990). Hemispheric differences are found in the identification, but not the detection, of low versus high spatial frequencies. *Perception and Psychophysics, 48,* 297–306.

Kosslyn, S. M. (1987). Seeing and imagining in the cerebral hemispheres: A computational approach. *Psychological Review, 94,* 148–175.

Kosslyn, S. M., Anderson, A. K., Hillger, L. A., and Hamilton, S. E. (1994). Hemispheric difference in sizes of receptive fields or attentional biases? *Neuropsychology, 8,* 139–147.

Kosslyn, S. M., Chabris, C., Marsolek, C. J., and Koenig, O. (1992). Categorical versus coordinate spatial representations: Computational analyses and computer simulations. *Journal of Experimental Psychology: Human Perception and Performance, 18,* 562–577.

Kosslyn, S. M., Flynn, R. A., Amsterdam, J. B., and Wang, G. (1990). Components of high-level vision: A cognitive neuroscience analysis and accounts of neurological syndromes. *Cognition, 34,* 203–277.

Kosslyn, S. M., and Koenig, O. (1992) *Wet mind: The new cognitive neuroscience*. New York, NY: Free Press.

Kosslyn, S. M., Koenig, O., Barrett, A., Cave, C. B., Tang, J., and Gabrieli, J. D. E. (1989). Evidence for two types of spatial representations: Hemispheric specialization for categorical and coordinate relations. *Journal of Experimental Psychology: Human Perception and Performance, 15,* 723–735.

Kosslyn, S. M., Sokolov, M. A., and Chen, J. C. (1989). The lateralization of BRIAN: A computational theory and model of visual hemispheric specialization. In D. Klahr and K. Kotovsky (Eds.), *Complex information processing comes of age*. Hillsdale, NJ: Lawrence Erlbaum Associates.

Lamb, M. R., Robertson, L. C., and Knight, R. T. (1990). Component mechanisms underlying the processing of hierarchically organized patterns: Inferences from patients with unilateral cortical lesions. *Journal of Experimental Psychology: Learning, Memory, and Cognition, 16,* 471–483.

Lowe, D. G. (1985). *Perceptual organization and visual recognition*. Boston, MA: Kluwer.

Lowe, D. G. (1987). The viewpoint consistency constraint. *International Journal of Computer Vision, 1,* 57–72.

Marr, D. (1982). *Vision*. New York, NY: W. H. Freeman & Co.

Marsolek, C. J. (submitted for publication, 1994). Computational incompatibility for processing abstract vs. specific form information.

Marsolek, C. J., Kosslyn, S. M., and Squire, L. R. (1992). Form-specific visual priming in the right cerebral hemisphere. *Journal of Experimental Psychology: Learning, Memory, and Cognition, 18,* 492–508.

Martin, M. (1979). Hemispheric specialization for local and global processing. *Neuropsychologia, 17,* 33–40.

Maunsell, J. H. R., and Newsome, W. T. (1987). Visual processing in monkey extrastriate cortex. *Annual Review of Neuroscience, 10,* 363–401.

Michimata, C., and Hellige, J. (1987). Effects of blurring and stimulus size on the lateralized processing of nonverbal stimuli. *Neuropsychologia, 25,* 397–407.

Navon, D. (1977). Forest before trees: The precedence of global features in visual perception *Cognitive Psychology, 9,* 353–383.

Palmer, S. E. (1977). Hierarchical structure in perceptual representations. *Cognitive Psychology, 9,* 441–474.

Palmer, T., and Tzeng, O. J. L. (1990). Cerebral asymmetry in visual attention. *Brain and Cognition, 13,* 46–58.

Peterzell, D. H. (1991). On the nonrelation between spatial frequency and cerebral hemispheric competence. *Brain and Cognition, 15,* 62–68.

Plaut, D. C., and Farah, M. J. (1990). Visual object representation: Interpreting neurophysiological data within a computational framework. *Journal of Cognitive Neuroscience, 2,* 320–343.

Robertson, L. C., and Delis, D. C. (1986). "Part-whole" processing in unilateral brain-damaged patients: Dysfunction of hierarchical organization. *Neuropsychologia, 24,* 363–370.

Robertson, L. C., and Lamb, M. R. (1991). Neuropsychological contributions to theories of part/whole organization. *Cognitive Psychology, 23,* 299–330.

Robertson, L. C., Lamb, M. R., and Knight, R. T. (1991). Normal global-local analysis in patients with dorsolateral frontal lobe lesions. *Neuropsychologia, 29,* 959–967.

Rueckl, J. G., Cave, K. R., and Kosslyn, S. M. (1989). Why are "what" and "where" processed by separate cortical systems? A computational investigation. *Journal of Cognitive Neuroscience, 1,* 171–186.

Rumelhart, D. E., and J. L. McClelland (Eds.) (1986). *Parallel distributed processing: Explorations in the microstructure of cognition* (pp 77–109). Cambridge, MA: MIT Press.

Sergent, J. (1987a). Failures to confirm the spatial frequency hypothesis: Fatal blow or healthy complication? *Canadian Journal of Psychology, 41,* 412–428.

Sergent, J. (1987b). Information processing and laterality effects for object and face perception. In G. W. Humphreys and M. S. Riddoch (Eds.), *Visual object processing: A cognitive neuropsychological approach* (pp 145–173). Hillsdale, NJ: Lawrence Erlbaum Associates.

Sergent, J., and Hellige, J. B. (1986). Role of input factors in visual-field asymmetries. *Brain and Cognition, 5,* 174–199.

Shannon, C. E. (1963). The mathematical theory of communication. In C. E. Shannon and W. Weaver (Eds.), *The mathematical theory of communication* (pp 29–125). Urbana, IL: University of Illinois Press [Reprinted from *Bell System Technical Journal,* July and October 1948].

Shulman, G. L., Sullivan, M. A., Gish, K., and Sakoda, W. J. (1986). The role of spatial-frequency channels in the perception of local and global structure. *Perception, 15,* 259–273.

Springer, S. P., and Deutsch, G. (1989). *Left brain, right brain.* New York, NY: W. H. Freeman Co.

Treisman, A. M., and Gelade, G. (1980). A feature integration theory of attention. *Cognitive Psychology, 12,* 97–136.

Ungerleider, L. G., and Mishkin, M. (1982). Two cortical visual systems. In D. J. Ingle, M. H. Goodale, and R. J. W. Mansfield (Eds.), *The analysis of visual behavior.* Cambridge, MA: MIT Press.

Van Kleeck, M. H. (1989). Hemispheric differences in global versus local processing of hierarchical visual stimuli by normal subjects: New data and a meta-analysis of previous studies. *Neuropsychologia, 27,* 1165–1178.

Hemispheric Asymmetry for Components of Visual Information Processing

Joseph B. Hellige

The left and right cerebral hemispheres of humans do not handle all aspects of visual information processing with equal ability. Instead, each hemisphere is better able than its partner to handle certain components of processing. Although there continues to be uncertainly surrounding exactly what the relevant components are, it has proved useful to decompose tasks into those processing components that have been hypothesized by contemporary models of perception, cognition, and action. In this chapter, I review some of what this componential approach has revealed about hemispheric asymmetry for visual information processing. In keeping with the general theme of the book, this review considers relationships among various models of visual laterality, the major questions that remain to be answered before we have a truly comprehensive model of hemispheric asymmetry for components of visual processing and the methodologic implications for the study of perceptual asymmetry.

The chapter begins with a brief discussion of what I call a componential approach to the study of hemispheric asymmetry. This is followed by a review of research that demonstrates hemispheric asymmetry for each of three processing distinctions that come from contemporary theories of visual information processing: (1) global vs. local processing, (2) low vs. high visuospatial frequencies, and (3) coordinate vs. categorical spatial relationships. I then discuss how these three processing distinctions may be related to one another and consider the possibility that hemispheric asymmetries of all three types may be different manifestations of the same thing. This is followed by a discussion of certain parallels between hemispheric asymmetry for components of visual processing and hemispheric asymmetry for components of auditory processing and for certain aspects of motor activity. Much of the research presented here involves the study of perceptual asymmetries in neurologically intact persons. This being the case, the chapter ends with a brief discussion of the methodologic implications of the research on hemispheric asymmetry for components of visual processing.

A COMPONENTIAL APPROACH

Cognitive psychology and cognitive neuroscience are characterized by what has come to be known as the information-processing or componential approach.

An important aspect of this approach is the realization that even simple tasks involve a number of information-processing subsystems, modules, or components, and the interactions among those components. It is often impossible to indicate which cerebral hemisphere is superior to the other for an entire task because the direction and magnitude of hemispheric asymmetry is often different for different components of the task (e.g., Allen, 1983; Hellige, 1990, 1993). This being the case, it is necessary to study hemispheric asymmetry in terms of specific processing subsystems or components rather than in terms of larger tasks. This componential approach requires that there be a principled account of the processing components involved in a specific task and some means of distinguishing among the various subsystems empirically. In several domains, it has proved useful to conceptualize various components that have been postulated by contemporary models of perception, cognition, and action and to use experimental manipulations that provide a way of separating the components from one another (for review, see Hellige, 1993). The domain of particular interest here is hemispheric asymmetry for components of visual information processing.

There are several advantages of the componential approach illustrated here. One is that it incorporates the study of hemispheric asymmetry into the larger goal of cognitive neuroscience, to understand how the brain produces cognition. In the past, the study of hemispheric asymmetry has too often been seen as separate from this more general enterprise and has suffered because of the lack of meaningful contact. When viewed from this more general perspective, finding hemispheric asymmetry for specific processing components not only refines our understanding of hemispheric differences but also provides converging evidence that models which decompose tasks into those specific components are on the right track. A second advantage of the componential approach is the possibility that hemispheric asymmetry for a specific processing component will contribute to a wide variety of tasks that require that component, helping us to see interrelationships that might otherwise be overlooked. A third advantage is that an emphasis on processing components rather than tasks is consistent with the observation that both hemispheres are normally involved in one way or another in almost everything we do, even though their contributions may differ. These advantages are illustrated by studies of hemispheric asymmetry for visual processing.

COMPONENTS OF VISUAL PROCESSING

There is a popular view that the right hemisphere of humans is dominant for the processing of nonverbal, visual, and spatial information. The pattern of hemispheric asymmetry for visual processing is actually more complex, with each hemisphere being dominant for processing different types of visual information. The nature of these hemispheric asymmetries has been clarified by using distinctions that have been imported into studies of hemispheric asymmetry from various models of visual information processing. In this section, I review recent studies using three such distinctions: (1) global vs. local aspects of visual stimuli, (2) low vs. high visuospatial frequencies, and (3) coordinate vs. categorical spatial relationships. In each case, the left and right hemispheres seem biased toward efficient processing of different aspects of visual input.

Global vs. Local Aspects of Visual Stimuli

Visual stimuli contain many levels of embedded structure, with smaller (*local*) patterns or parts contained within larger (*global*) patterns or wholes. According to various theories of visual information processing, the same sort of hierarchic organization is contained in the internal representations that are used to represent visual information. A particular pattern can be treated as either global or local depending on the context in which it occurs. For example, a human hand might be considered as a global stimulus, with the thumb being a local element. However, the same hand might be considered a local element in the context of an entire human body. That is, local vs. global patterns are defined by their relative place in what might be considered an entire hierarchy of levels (e.g., Lamb, Robertson, and Knight, 1990; Palmer, 1977; Robertson, 1986).

In this section, I review evidence of hemispheric asymmetry for the processing of global vs. local levels of information in hierarchic visual patterns—evidence that suggests the right hemisphere is superior to the left for the processing of global levels whereas the left hemisphere is superior to the right for the processing of local levels. This pattern of effects sheds light on the nature of hemispheric asymmetry for components of visual processing and also reinforces the notion that hierarchic information is an important aspect of our internal representation of the visual world. The clearest evidence for this particular aspect of hemispheric asymmetry comes from studies of patients with unilateral brain injury, with at least some converging support coming from visual half-field studies with neurologically intact persons.

A number of studies have presented brain-injured patients and neurologically intact persons with hierarchical stimuli similar to those shown in figure 5.1. Note that each of those stimuli consists of small letters (the local elements) arranged in the shape of a large letter (the global pattern). Delis, Robertson and Efron (1986) presented patients with a single pattern of the sort shown in figure 5.1, and asked them to draw the pattern from memory after performing a distractor task for 15 seconds. Patients with unilateral right hemisphere injury often produced the correct local information (e.g., several small *M*'s for figure 5.1a), but did not arrange those elements to produce the correct global pattern. Patients with unilateral left hemisphere injury often drew the correct global pattern (e.g., the large Z in figure 5.1a), but omitted the local detail. This pattern of results suggests that the right hemisphere is necessary for normal processing of global aspects of visual patterns, whereas the left hemisphere is necessary for normal processing of the local aspects of those same patterns.

```
        (a)                    (b)
    M M M M M              E E E E E
            M                      E
          M                      E
        M                      E
      M                      E
    M M M M M              E E E E E

        (c)                    (d)
    M M M M M              E E E E E
          M                      E
          M                      E
          M                      E
          M                      E
```

Figure 5.1 Four examples of hierarchical stimuli composed of small letters (the local elements) arranged into the shape of a large letter (the global pattern).

This pattern of hemispheric asymmetry for processing global vs. local aspects of visual patterns is not restricted to tasks that require patients to draw stimuli. In fact, similar conclusions have been reached in studies of recognition memory for the types of stimuli shown in figure 5.1 (e.g., Delis et al., 1986) and in studies that have patients identify as quickly as possible the letter that appears at either the global level or the local level (e.g., Lamb, Robertson, and Knight, 1989, 1990; Robertson, Lamb, and Knight, 1988, 1991). Based on the entire pattern of results from this series of studies, Lamb et al. (1990) conclude that normal processing of global aspects depends on the posterior superior temporal lobe of the right hemisphere, whereas normal processing of local elements depends on the posterior superior temporal lobe of the left hemisphere. Furthermore, they argue that the relative speed with which the global and local aspects of a pattern can be processed can be modulated by an attentional mechanism associated with the rostral inferior parietal lobe.

Visual half-field studies with neurologically intact persons have also examined hemispheric asymmetry for processing global and local aspects of visual patterns. Some studies have found results consistent with those obtained with patients, but other studies have not. For example, Sergent (1982a) used stimuli similar to those shown in figure 5.1 and found a left visual field (LVF) or right hemisphere advantage for the identification of the large letter, and a right visual field (RVF) or left hemisphere advantage for the identification of the small letters. Martin (1979) and Alwit (1982) also reported a Global/Local × Visual Field interaction, but only the RVF/left hemisphere advantage for the identification of small letters was statistically significant. By way of contrast, neither Alivisatos and Wilding (1982) nor Boles (1984) found any significant visual-field advantages for either large or small letters. Despite including these negative results, Van Kleeck (1989) concludes that there is a Global/Local × Visual-Field interaction in neurologically intact persons based on a meta-analysis of the results from all of these studies.

Some of the inconsistency in the visual half-field studies may reflect noisiness in the paradigm (e.g., Delis et al., 1986) or uncontrolled variation in a host of input and task factors that often vary in an unsystematic way from study to study (e.g., Hellige and Sergent, 1986; Sergent and Hellige, 1986). These aspects of the visual half-field paradigm are discussed in more detail below. It is also possible that, under some viewing conditions, interhemispheric transfer of information is so efficient in the intact brain that hemispheric differences are masked. In any event, taken together, the results from Van Kleeck's meta-analysis (which included studies with negative as well as positive outcomes) and from studies using patients with unilateral brain injury leave little doubt about hemispheric asymmetry for processing global vs. local levels of visual information in hierarchic visual patterns.

Low vs. High Visuospatial Frequency

A number of contemporary theories of visual processing note that each point in the visual field is multiply encoded in the brain by size-tuned filters corresponding to overlapping receptive fields. According to one point of view, the different scales of resolution are determined by outputs from neurons that are tuned to intensity variations over spatial intervals of different sizes—i.e., tuned to different spatial frequencies (e.g., De Valois and De Valois, 1980). A stimulus composed of a single visuospatial frequency consists of a regular sinusoidal variation of luminance across space and looks like alternating dark and light bars with fuzzy borders. Spatial frequency refers to the number of complete dark-light cycles per unit of space. The more cycles per unit of space, the higher the spatial frequency (figure 5.2). The concept of visuospatial frequency has received considerable attention because it is possible, in principle, to decompose any complex image by analyzing which spatial frequencies are present, their orientations, phase relationships, and so forth (e.g., Thomas, 1986). Thus, spatial frequency channels (or something very much like them) could serve as important components of visual information processing.

The concept of visuospatial frequency has proved relevant for thinking about hemispheric asymmetry for processing visual stimuli. Specifically, it has been hypothesized that, at some level of processing beyond the sensory cortex, the left and right hemispheres are biased toward efficient use of higher and lower visuospatial frequencies, respectively (e.g., Sergent, 1982a,b, 1983, 1987a,b). Most tests of this hypothesis have involved divided visual half-field experiments with neurologically intact persons and the results of those experiments have both theoretical and methodologic implications for the study of perceptual asymmetry.

The spatial-frequency hypothesis about hemispheric asymmetry was developed as an attempt to explain various effects of input variables on visual half-field asymmetry. In particular, various forms of perceptual degradation tend to interfere more with performance when stimuli are projected to the RVF/left hemisphere than to the LVF/right hemisphere. The types of perceptual

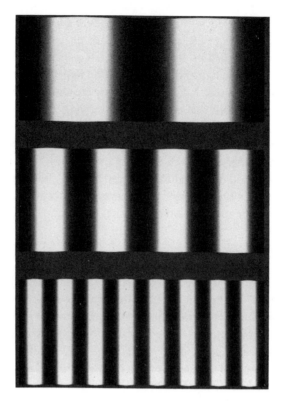

Figure 5.2 Three vertical sine wave gratings. The visuospatial frequency increases from top to bottom. The spatial frequency of the middle grating is twice that of the top grating and the spatial frequency of the bottom grating is twice that of the middle grating.

degradation most often investigated include such things as overlay masks of lines or dots and blurring (e.g., Christman, 1990; Hellige, 1976, 1980; Hellige and Webster, 1979; Jonsson and Hellige, 1986; Michimata and Hellige, 1987; Sergent, 1989; see also Wolcott et al., 1990). Originally, the apparent resistance of the right hemisphere to the detrimental effects of perceptual degradation was discussed in terms of right hemisphere superiority for a variety of visuospatial processes. However, Sergent (1982a, 1983) noted that many effects of this sort could also be explained by the spatial-frequency hypothesis to the extent that the manipulations that had been used to degrade visual input resulted in the selective removal of information carried by higher spatial-frequency channels. One reason that this spatial-frequency hypothesis has generated so much research is that it is, in principle, more amenable to operational definition and empirical test than other explanations that have been proposed.

During the last 10 years, a variety of experiments and literature reviews have attempted to determine the importance of visuospatial frequency for determining visual half-field asymmetry. In general, these experiments and reviews illustrate that spatial frequency is, indeed, important, but they also point to limitations and to modifications of the original spatial-frequency hypothesis. For example, Christman (1989) reviewed the results of those visual half-field studies published between 1965 and 1987 that included manipulations of input parameters that should influence the availability of different ranges of visuospatial frequency. From this review, he concluded that there is moderate support for the spatial-frequency hypothesis. The support seems to be stronger from experiments that involve relatively direct manipulations of spatial frequency than from studies whose manipulations are less direct. For example, blurring (which tends to remove higher relative to lower spatial frequencies) and low-pass filtering of stimuli (which removes higher spatial frequency information from a stimulus in a very precise way) have been found to produce greater impairment of RVF/left hemisphere performance (relative to LVF/right hemisphere performance) in studies that involve a variety of tasks. Such tasks have included letter processing of various sorts (e.g., Jonsson and Hellige, 1986; Sergent, 1989; but see Peterzell, Harvey, and Hardyck, 1989), comparison of nonverbal line figures (Michimata and Hellige, 1987), face processing (Sergent, 1985), and temporal integration (Christman, 1990). Weaker support comes from experiments whose manipulations involve such things as exposure duration, stimulus size, luminance, and retinal eccentricity—which have only indirect effects on the range of spatial frequencies available to be processed. Virtually no support comes from studies using highly linguistic tasks like word identification and lexical decision, which may indicate that hemispheric asymmetries for perceptual processes can be overridden by asymmetry for higher-level cognitive components of a task.

Effects of the range of visuospatial frequencies *contained* in a stimulus are moderated by additional factors. For example, an important factor that also influences visual half-field performance is the range of visuospatial frequencies *required* for optimal performance of whatever experimental task is used. In fact, in developing the spatial-frequency hypothesis, Sergent (1983) suggested that, all other things being equal, a task that demands processing of the high spatial frequencies contained in a complex stimulus will tend to produce a RVF/left hemisphere advantage whereas a task that demands processing of low spatial frequencies contained in the same stimulus will tend to produce a LVF/right hemisphere advantage. Evidence consistent with this prediction has been obtained with studies involving faces (e.g, Sergent, 1985; see also Hellige, Jonsson, and Corwin, 1984) and in studies of temporal integration (e.g., Christman, 1989, 1990).

All of the studies noted so far have used complex visual stimuli (e.g., letters, numbers, faces) and varied perceptual characteristics so as to manipulate the proportion of higher and lower spatial frequencies that are present. The manipulations used in many of these experiments have only indirect effects on the spatial-frequency content of the stimuli, making it difficult to separate the effects of spatial frequency from the effects of other input characteristics such as stimulus perceptibility or the total amount of visible energy (e.g., Jonsson and Hellige, 1986; Michimata and Hellige, 1987; Peterzell, 1991). Even when spatial frequency is manipulated in a direct manner (e.g., by low-pass filtering), it is very difficult in studies with complex stimuli to control exactly which spatial frequencies convey the information needed to perform whatever task is required. One way to circumvent these problems is to use sine wave gratings such as those shown in figure 5.2. A sine wave stimulus consists of only a single spatial frequency, so that we know precisely not only what frequency is present on each trial but what frequency must be processed in order to perform whatever task is being required. With this in mind, Fred Kitterle, Steve Christman and I set out to determine whether visual half-field asymmetries for processing such stimuli varied with spatial frequency in the manner predicted by the spatial-frequency hypothesis of hemispheric asymmetry. What we have found is clear evidence for certain aspects of the hypothesis as well as important qualifications.

In an initial series of experiments, we (Kitterle, Christman, and Hellige, 1990) projected sine wave gratings similar to those shown in figure 5.2, to the LVF/right hemisphere or RVF/left hemisphere of neurologically intact university students, with the gratings varying in spatial frequency (1 vs. 9 cycles/degree of visual angle). Stimulus duration in the various experiments ranged between 20 and 160 ms and the number of experimental trials used in the experiments ranged from 360 to 1680. For some experiments, the task of the observer was to indicate on each trial whether or not a grating stimulus had been presented, without regard for its spatial frequency. In these *stimulus detection* experiments, there was no interaction between Visual Field/ Hemisphere and Spatial Frequency. This replicated earlier experiments using stimulus detection paradigms and indicates that the left and right hemispheres are equally sensitive to both low (1 cycle/degree) and high (9 cycles/degree) spatial frequencies when computational demands are minimal. Such results are consistent with the claim that any hemispheric differences related to spatial frequency must result from processing beyond the sensory level (e.g., Sergent, 1983).

For other experiments, observers were required to identify whether the grating shown on a trial was the "wide" (low frequency) stimulus or the "narrow" (high frequency) stimulus. In these *stimulus identification* experiments there was a LVF/right hemisphere advantage for responding to the low frequency (1 cycle/degree) stimulus but a RVF/left hemisphere advantage for responding to the high frequency (9 cycles/degree) stimulus. This Visual Field/Hemisphere × Spatial Frequency interaction is illustrated in figure 5.3 for two different experiments and is in the direction predicted by the spatial-frequency hypothesis. In still other experiments, we (Christman, Kitterle, and Hellige, 1991) show that the same interaction extends to complex gratings, that are either made up of two low frequency gratings superimposed (0.5 and 1.0 cycle/degree of visual angle) or made up of two higher frequency gratings superimposed (4 and 8 cycles/degree of visual angle). In addition, Kitterle and Selig (1991) have reported the same Visual Field/Hemisphere × Spatial Frequency interaction pattern in a *stimulus discrimination* task that required ob-

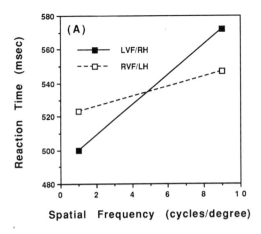

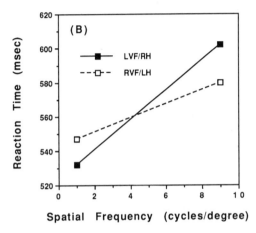

Figure 5.3 Reaction time to identify vertical sine wave gratings of 1 and 9 cycles per degree of visual angle when the gratings were flashed briefly to either the left visual field/right hemisphere (*LVF/RH*) or the right visual field/left hemisphere (*RVF/LH*). The top panel (*A*) shows results from Experiment 4 reported by Kitterle, Christman, and Hellige (1990), with the results averaged across three levels of stimulus contrast. The bottom panel (*B*) shows results from Experiment 5 reported by Kitterle et al. (1990), with the results averaged across three levels of stimulus duration.

servers to indicate whether the second of two successively presented gratings was of higher or lower frequency than the first.

The experiments just reviewed indicate that the spatial frequency contained in the stimulus input is an important determinant of visual half-field asymmetry, but only when the task requires the observer to use information about spatial frequency or stimulus identity. The results of an additional experiment (Kitterle, Hellige, and Christman, 1992) indicate that visual half-field asymmetry for a slightly more complex stimulus also depends on which of the spatial frequencies contained in the stimulus are relevant for performing the task that is required. To examine whether this would be the case, we had

Hellige: Components of Visual Processing

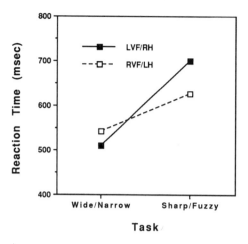

Figure 5.4 Reaction time to respond to square wave stimuli for the Wide/Narrow task and for the Sharp/Fuzzy task when stimuli were flashed briefly to either the left visual field/right hemisphere (*LVF/RH*) or the right visual field/left hemisphere (*RVF/LH*). (After Kitterle, Hellige, and Christman, 1992.)

observers respond to the same four stimuli during two different experimental tasks. Two of the stimuli were sine wave gratings of different spatial frequencies (1 vs. 3 cycles/degree of visual angle). The other two stimuli were square wave gratings that had fundamental frequencies of 1 vs. 3 cycles per degree of visual angle. Note that a square wave stimulus consists of alternating dark and light stripes with sharp edges, in contrast to a sine wave stimulus where there is regular alternation but with no sharp edges. A square wave stimulus consists of several well-defined spatial frequencies. The lowest frequency is the fundamental frequency and corresponds to the width of the bars (i.e., the number of cycles per unit of space). Information about the sharp edge is conveyed by much higher spatial frequencies, the odd higher harmonics of the fundamental frequency. It is these properties that allow us to use different tasks that direct observers' attention to relatively low or high spatial frequencies.

One task required observers to indicate as quickly as possible whether the single stimulus presented on a trial was one of the two wide stimuli (1 cycle/degree) or one of the two narrow stimuli (3 cycles/degree), regardless of whether the bars appeared to have fuzzy or sharp edges. Note that this task requires observers to attend to the relatively low fundamental frequencies. The other task required the observers to indicate as quickly as possible whether the single stimulus presented on a trial was one of the two stimuli with fuzzy edges (the sine wave stimuli) or one of the two stimuli with sharp edges (one of the two square wave stimuli), regardless of the width of the bars. Note that this task requires observers to attend to the relatively high harmonic frequencies. The critical results concern visual half-field asymmetries for processing the square wave stimuli (which contain a wide range of spatial frequencies) during each of the two tasks. As illustrated in figure 5.4, for the wide/narrow (i.e., attend to low frequencies) task there was a LVF/right hemisphere advantage but for the sharp/fuzzy (i.e., attend to high frequencies) task there was a RVF/left hemisphere advantage. Because exactly the same stimuli are used for both tasks, these results cannot be attributed to the range of spatial frequencies contained in the stimuli. Instead, the relevant factor is whether the range of frequencies that was relevant is relatively high or relatively low.

We (Christman et al., 1991) have also found that the visual half-field advantage for processing a particular spatial frequency can depend on the context in which that frequency occurs. For example, a sine wave grating of 2 cycles per degree of visual angle is processed more efficiently on LVF/right hemisphere trials when it is the lowest of three spatial frequencies in a complex stimulus, but the same 2-cycles-per-degree grating is processed more efficiently on RVF/left hemisphere trials when it is the highest of three spatial frequencies in a complex pattern. In this sense, it makes a difference whether the spatial frequency that is critical for performing a task is high or low *relative* to the other frequencies presented in a complex stimulus.

To summarize the findings from these experiments, at least three aspects of spatial frequency influence visual half-field asymmetry: (1) the absolute range of spatial frequencies contained in the input, (2) the range of spatial frequencies that is most relevant for whatever task is being performed, and (3) whether the most relevant frequencies are high or low relative to other frequencies contained in the stimulus. Because different characteristics of a complex stimulus (e.g., a face) are conveyed by different ranges of visuospatial frequency, it is not surprising that visual half-field asymmetry for processing such stimuli are influenced by manipulations of spatial frequency. However, given the complexity of the present findings it is also not surprising that it is difficult to extrapolate to complex stimuli without taking several factors into account.

Coordinate vs. Categorical Spatial Relationships

The two processing distinctions that have been discussed so far both have to do with processing information about the *identity* of a visual stimulus. An equally important aspect of visual information processing is the ability to *localize* a visual stimulus in space. Kosslyn and his colleagues have proposed that the brain computes two different kinds of spatial-relation representations, one which is used to assign a spatial relation to a category such as "on" or "above" and another which preserves location information using a metric coordinate system in which distances are specified with precision (e.g., Kosslyn, 1987; Kosslyn et al., 1989, 1990, 1992). One way to provide converging evidence about the plausibility of this distinction is to show that the two proposed types of spatial-relation representations have different neurologic substrata. It has been hypothesized that the left and right hemispheres make more efficient use of the categorization and coordinate processing subsystems, respectively.

Evidence consistent with this hypothesis about hemispheric asymmetry was first obtained in a series of visual half-field experiments summarized by Kosslyn (1987) and reported in more detail by Kosslyn et al. (1989). In general, there was a significant LVF/right hemisphere advantage for computing coordinate or distance relationships and at least a marginally significant RVF/left hemisphere advantage for computing categorical spatial relationships. For example, in one of their experiments observers saw stimuli consisting of an irregular blob and a dot that was either touching ("on") the blob or separated from ("off") the blob by one of several distances. Their observers performed one of two tasks. For the categorical task, they indicated whether the dot was "on" or "off" the blob. For the coordinate or distance task, they indicated whether the dot was within a distance of 2 mm from the blob. There was a significant Task × Visual Field/Hemisphere interaction, there being a RVF/left hemisphere advantage for the on/off task and a LVF/right hemisphere advantage for the distance judgment task.

Chikashi Michimata and I (Hellige and Michimata, 1989) tested the same hypothesis by having observers either indicate whether a dot was above or below a horizontal line (a categorical task referred to as the Above/Below task) or indicate whether the dot was within 2 cm of the line (a coordinate or distance task referred to as the Near/Far task). Consistent with Kosslyn's hypothesis, there was a Task × Visual Field/Hemisphere interaction, with approximately 85% of the right-handed observers showing an interaction pattern in the predicted direction. For the Above/Below task a RVF/left hemisphere advantage approached statistical significance and for the Near/Far task there was a highly significant LVF/right hemisphere advantage. We have replicated this effect in a new study with right-handed observers and found it to be smaller or absent in left-handed observers (with approximately 60% of left-handed observers showing an interaction pattern in the predicted direction). A similar interaction for right-handed observers has been reported by Sergent (1991), but the interaction disappeared when the luminance of the stimuli was increased well above that used by Hellige and Michimata.

Kosslyn et al. (1989) used their own version of these Above/Below and Near/Far tasks and found a similar Task × Visual Field/Hemisphere interaction on an initial block of trials. However, with their stimuli and viewing parameters, the interaction disappeared quickly with practice. Using these same stimuli, Elizabeth Cowin and I (Cowin and Hellige, 1994) obtained a similar result—as did Koenig, Reiss, and Kosslyn (1990) in a study with children aged 5 and 7 years. A similar pattern of results has also been reported by Rybash and Hoyer (1992). In considering the effects of practice, Kosslyn et al. (1989) suggest that when observers are presented with a coordinate or distance judgment task they may learn to form stimulus categories after sufficient practice, so that coordinate processing becomes unnecessary.

Not all experimental results have been so favorable to the hypothesis about hemispheric asymmetry for processing categorical or coordinate spatial relationships. For example, although Sergent (1991) replicated the results reported by Hellige and Michimata (1989) when the luminance of her stimuli was sufficiently low, the critical Task × Visual Field/Hemisphere interaction disappeared when the luminance increased and the tasks became easier. Sergent also failed to find the critical interaction for a set of additional tasks that are hypothesized to require either categorical or coordinate spatial judgments. What she did find was that the absolute distance between stimuli sometimes influenced performance in tasks that would be regarded as categorical. On this basis, Sergent argued that the distinction between categorical and coordinate types of spatial representation is, at best, unclear. It is obviously important for future experiments to reconcile what seem to be inconsistent empirical results. However, it should also be noted that several neural network simulations presented by Kosslyn et al. (1992) show that models that code only categorical information about whether a dot is above or below a line are still sensitive to the distance between the dot and the line. Thus, the presence of distance effects in a categorical task does not necessarily invalidate the categorical-coordinate distinction. Other simulation models have also been able, to some extent, to mimic the disappearance of the critical Task × Visual Field/Hemisphere interaction with increases in contrast. On this basis, Kosslyn et al. (1992) argue that the disappearance of hemispheric asymmetries at high luminance or contrast does not necessarily invalidate their hypothesis.

RELATIONSHIPS AMONG THE COMPONENTS OF VISUAL PROCESSING

Research on hemispheric asymmetry for the three dimensions of visual information processing discussed in the preceding section developed independently, as if the three dimensions were separable. Although they may be separable in some ways, there is increasing evidence that they are also interrelated in important ways. In this section I consider the nature of those interrelationships and whether the three aspects of hemispheric asymmetry might even be different manifestations of the same thing.

There is a very clear relationship between global and local aspects of a visual stimulus and low vs. high visuospatial frequency. In general, information about the global aspects of a stimulus (e.g., the large Z in figure 5.1a) is carried by a lower range of visuospatial frequencies than is information about the local aspects of the same stimulus (e.g., the small M's in figure 5.1a). This relationship makes it likely that hemispheric asymmetry for processing global vs. local information and for utilizing low vs. high spatial frequencies are manifestations of the same processing difference between the hemispheres. This possibility receives additional support from the fact that hemispheric asymmetry extends to *relatively* high and low spatial frequencies (see the earlier discussion of Christman et al., 1991), because whether a stimulus of a particular size is global or local depends on its relative place in a hierarchy of levels. It is also interesting to note that there is growing evidence that spatial-frequency differences between the global and local levels are particularly important for determining how quickly information at those levels is processed (e.g., Lamb and Yund, 1991). Although there are clearly relationships between the global/local and low/high frequency distinctions, at the present time there is insufficient evidence to decide whether one of the distinctions is more fundamental than the other as a way of describing hemispheric asymmetry for components of visual information processing.

Kosslyn's (1987) original hypothesis about hemispheric asymmetry for processing categorical vs. coordinate spatial relationships argued that this particular asymmetry arose as the result of left hemisphere dominance for the control of speech output and right hemisphere dominance for the control of rapid shifts of attention across space. If this were the case, then hemispheric asymmetry for this dimension would seem to be mostly unrelated to hemispheric asymmetry for the other two dimensions. However, Kosslyn et al. (1992) have presented an alternative account that suggests the possibility of a rather strong relationship. On this view, hemispheric asymmetry for processing spatial relationships is related to the nature of the visual information that is most useful for computing categorical vs. coordinate information. In a set of neural network computer simulations, Kosslyn et al. show that networks with relatively large, overlapping "receptive fields" compute coordinate information (e.g., Is a dot within 3 mm of a line?) better than networks with relatively small, nonoverlapping "receptive fields." Exactly the reverse was found for the computation of categorical information from the same stimuli (e.g., Is a dot above or below a line?). Based on this, and on the findings reviewed earlier about hemispheric asymmetry for processing spatial relationships, Kosslyn et al. suggest that the left hemisphere is biased in favor of information from visual channels with small, nonoverlapping visual fields, whereas the right hemisphere is biased in favor of information from visual channels with large, overlapping visual fields. Consistent with this possibility, they cite Livingstone as having suggested that magnocellular ganglia (which have relatively large, overlapping receptive fields) project preferentially to the right hemisphere. As Kosslyn et al. note, there is similarity between low visuospatial frequency and visual channels with large receptive fields and between high visuospatial frequency and visual channels with small receptive fields, although the two are not completely equivalent.

Some preliminary support for the idea that hemispheric asymmetry for processing categorical vs. coordinate spatial relationships is related to hemispheric asymmetry for processing high vs. low spatial frequencies comes from an experiment reported by Elizabeth Cowin and me (Cowin and Hellige, 1994). Participants in our experiment performed either the Above/Below task or the Near/Far task described earlier for stimuli consisting of a dot and a line on each trial. In addition, the dot and line stimuli were either presented clearly or were blurred by having observers wear distorting lenses. The method of dioptric blurring that we used selectively eliminates information carried primarily by channels tuned to high visuospatial frequencies. Blurring the stimuli consistently disrupted performance of the Above/Below task, suggesting that

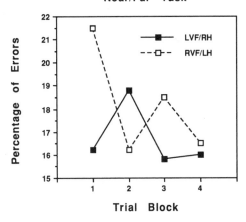

Figure 5.5 Percentage of errors for each of four 24-trial blocks when subjects were performing the Near/Far task involving dots and lines and when stimuli were flashed briefly to either the left visual field/right hemisphere (*LVF/RH*) or the right visual field/left hemisphere (*RVF/LH*). The results shown in the figure are collapsed across Clear and Blurred stimulus conditions because the results were the same for both conditions. (After Cowin and Hellige, 1994.)

high spatial-frequency information is necessary for optimizing the processing of categorical spatial relationships. By way of contrast, blurring the stimuli did not consistently disrupt performance of the Near/Far task, suggesting that the same high spatial-frequency information is not necessary for optimizing the processing of coordinate spatial relationships. Both of these findings are consistent with the hypothesis proposed by Kosslyn et al. (1992). As shown in figure 5.5, we also found significantly fewer errors on LVF/right hemisphere trials than on RVF/left hemisphere trials during the first block of the Near/Far (coordinate) task. Furthermore, this initial LVF/right hemisphere advantage for processing the coordinate relationship between the line and the dot was unaffected by the blurring manipulation, suggesting that the right hemisphere superiority does not depend on information carried by channels tuned to the high spatial frequencies that were eliminated or made difficult to process by our blurring manipulation. Thus, these results are at least consistent with the possibility that hemispheric differences for processing different types of spatial relationships are related to hemispheric differences in utilizing low vs. high visuospatial frequencies.

The possibility considered in this section is that hemispheric asymmetries for at least three dimensions of visual information processing are interrelated. It is important for future research to determine the extent of those interrelationships and whether, in the limiting case, each of these asymmetries is a different manifestation of the same hemispheric difference. Among other things, it will prove interesting to see to what extent individual differences in asymmetry for one dimension (e.g., low vs. high spatial frequency) are correlated with individual differences in asymmetry for the other dimensions (e.g.,

Hellige: Components of Visual Processing

coordinate vs. categorical spatial relationships). To the extent that the different asymmetries are measuring the same thing, significant correlations should be obtained.

It is also interesting to consider how such asymmetries might arise during the course of ontogenetic development. Relative to adults, the visual sensory system of newborns is especially limited in its transmission of information carried by high spatial frequencies (for reviews, see Banks and Dannemiller, 1987; de Schonen and Mathivet, 1989). At the same time, there is evidence that the development of various brain areas is more advanced in the right hemisphere than in the left hemisphere at the time of birth and, perhaps, for a short time thereafter (for discussion of asymmetries in cortical development, see Corballis, 1991; de Schonen and Mathivet, 1989; Geschwind and Galaburda, 1987; Hellige, 1993; Sergent, 1987b; Turkewitz, 1988). A possibility that I have elaborated elsewhere (e.g., Hellige, 1993) is that a certain critical period for being modified by incoming visual input occurs earlier for the right hemisphere than for the left hemisphere, and once modified by highly degraded visual input, the right hemisphere is not only predisposed to become dominant for processing low spatial frequencies but is less able than the left to take full advantage of higher frequencies when they finally appear. The resulting hemispheric differences in visual processing would influence asymmetry for any task that depends on the relevant aspects of visual information, whether the task requires stimulus identification or stimulus localization. Although speculative, this ontogenetic scenario seems sufficiently plausible to merit additional investigation.

PARALLELS IN AUDITORY PROCESSING AND MOTOR PERFORMANCE

Although this chapter deals with hemispheric asymmetry for components of visual processing, it is interesting to consider parallels that do not involve vision. One interesting parallel comes from recent studies of hemispheric asymmetry for processing auditory information. In particular, hemispheric asymmetry for auditory stimuli has been found to be related to temporal frequency. For example, in a pitch discrimination task, Ivry and Lebby (1993) report that persons were faster and more accurate in judging relatively low frequency sounds when they were presented to the left ear (which projects preferentially to the right hemisphere), but were faster and more accurate in judging relatively high frequency sounds when they were presented to the right ear (which projects preferentially to the left hemisphere). This is an interesting parallel to what has been observed in vision, but it is not clear how spatial frequency in vision might be related to temporal frequency in audition. One possibility discussed by Ivry and Lebby is that, in both stimulus modalities, the two hemispheres process information through different asymmetric filters. More specifically, they suggest that the right hemisphere filter is, in some sense, tuned to lower spatial and temporal frequencies than is the left hemisphere filter. This is an interesting possibility in view of visual research reported by Rebai et al. (1986; see also Rebai et al., 1989). They have found that evoked potentials recorded over temporal (but not occipital) leads show opposite hemispheric asymmetries depending on whether a sine wave grating reversed its phase at low (e.g., 4 Hz) or high (e.g., 12 Hz) temporal frequencies. Specifically, the right hemisphere was more responsive than the left at low temporal frequencies, but the left hemisphere was more responsive than the right at high temporal frequencies. Future research that begins to look for a relationship between spatial and temporal frequencies and between vision and audition is likely to prove very interesting.

An interesting parallel to what we have seen in vision is also provided by Guiard (1987; see also Hammond, 1990) in an account of the asymmetric division of labor between the two hands. Guiard proposes that the two hands work together in what is called a kinematic chain, with the nondominant hand performing movements of low temporal and spatial frequency and with the dominant hand building on those movements to perform its own movements of high temporal and spatial frequency. One illustration of this division of labor is what occurs during handwriting, where the nondominant hand arranges and steadies the paper (relatively few large-scale movements) while the dominant hand makes frequent, smaller movements of the writing instrument. Note that each hand is controlled primarily by the contralateral hemisphere, so that in right-handers the direction of this asymmetry is consistent with what has been observed in visual processing. More research is clearly needed to see whether this is more than an interesting coincidence. One possibility is that certain motor areas of the right hemisphere are more fully developed than homologous areas of the left hemisphere at a time in development when only gross movements (and sensory feedback about them) are available to the brain, encouraging the right hemisphere to become dominant for making such movements. This might be followed by a time when the left hemisphere reaches sufficient development to be shaped by the more precise movements (and sensory feedback about those movements) that have become possible.

When a more componential approach has been used to decompose performance, some very interesting parallels have begun to emerge among visual, auditory, and motor asymmetries. Among other things, this illustrates the potential value of what I have called the componential approach to the study of hemispheric asymmetry. It would be premature to argue that there are necessarily strong connections between these various asymmetries. However, we have already seen how certain aspects of visual asymmetry are related in important ways, and parallels such as those just noted suggest the possibility that these relationships go beyond vision.

METHODOLOGIC IMPLICATIONS FOR STUDIES OF PERCEPTUAL ASYMMETRY

Much of what we know about hemispheric asymmetry for components of visual information processing has come from visual half-field studies of perceptual asymmetry. There is little doubt that hemispheric asymmetry is one important determinant of perceptual asymmetry. Very clear evidence of this comes from the results of visual half-field experiments with the so-called split-brain patients, who have had the corpus callosum surgically severed in order to control the spread of epileptic seizures. For example, when a word or picture of a familiar object is flashed briefly to the RVF/left hemisphere, these patients have no trouble naming it. However, when the same stimulus is flashed to the LVF/right hemisphere, the stimulus cannot be named (e.g., Gazzaniga, 1985; Gazzaniga and Le Doux, 1978). These results are clearly caused by the fact that the left hemisphere is typically dominant for a number of linguistic processes and that, in most people, the right hemisphere is virtually unable to generate speech. The fact that similar perceptual asymmetries are found in neurologically intact observers (albeit typically with reduced magnitude) indicates that hemispheric asymmetry influences perceptual asymmetry even when the brain is intact. Thus, visual half-field experiments have become an important tool in the investigation of hemispheric asymmetry.

To be sure, visual half-field differences in neurologically intact persons can be influenced by a number of factors in addition to hemispheric asymmetry. For example, when several stimuli are presented on the same trial, perceptual asymmetry can be influenced by a consistent bias to scan one visual half-field first, especially if some stimuli are in the RVF and others are in the LVF (e.g., Efron, 1990; Hellige, 1991, in press; Hellige and Sergent, 1986). However, the contribution of such effects can be minimized by such things as presenting only a single stimulus on each trial, keeping the stimulus duration sufficiently short to prevent eye movements, presenting the letters in words vertically rather than horizontally, and so forth. In addition to the sources already cited, discussion of various potentially important factors and ways of controlling for their effects can be found in Beaumont (1982), Bryden (1982), and Hellige (1983a), and in a special issue of *Brain and Cognition* (1986, Vol. 5, No. 2).

The studies of visual half-field asymmetry discussed in this chapter were conducted in a way that should minimize the contribution of unwanted factors and maximize the likelihood that the theoretically interesting results reflected information processing differences between the hemispheres. In addition, it is important to note that the critical theoretical predictions have had far less to do with an overall or main effect of visual field than with various Task Variable × Visual Field/Hemisphere interactions. For example, it is the prediction that visual-field differences change in a particular way for low and high spatial-frequency gratings or for global and local aspects of visual stimuli that is important, not an overall visual-field advantage (or even the simple visual-field difference for one particular stimulus). As I have illustrated elsewhere (e.g., Hellige, 1983b; see also Hellige, 1991, in press; Hellige and Sergent, 1986), such Task Variable × Visual Field/Hemisphere interactions are usually more difficult to dismiss as artifacts of nonhemispheric factors than are main effects of visual field or the simple effects of visual field at any one level of some task variable. In fact, a perceptual asymmetry in one condition considered completely in isolation is almost impossible to interpret (e.g., Efron, 1990; Hellige, 1991). Therefore, an additional benefit of the componential approach to the study of hemispheric asymmetry is that the important predictions almost always are about the form of one or more Task Variable × Visual Field/Hemisphere interactions.

The fact that the two hemispheres are asymmetric in their processing of visual information is of obvious theoretical importance. In fact, the theoretical implications are the main focus of this chapter. However, the existence of such effects is also of considerable methodologic importance in the design and interpretation of visual half-field studies, especially when the purpose of the studies is to examine hemispheric asymmetry for something other than visual processing per se (e.g., semantic categorization or some other equally abstract, nonvisual aspect of cognition). In any visual experiment, relevant stimuli must be presented very briefly and to off-center areas of the retina that are not the most well adapted for identifying visual stimuli. In this sense, the entire paradigm may be particularly susceptible to hemispheric asymmetries that occur relatively early in visual processing, and this might tend to obscure asymmetry for more abstract aspects of processing. In addition, in any visual half-field experiment, the stimuli must be presented at some specific size, location from the center of the fovea, duration, luminance, contrast, and so forth. The results reviewed here indicate that many of these input factors can influence the direction and magnitude of visual half-field asymmetry. This is almost certainly one reason for variation in the results of experiments that differ in the values of input parameters but that are otherwise very similar. This being the case, it is critical that input parameters be held constant across all conditions in visual half-field experiments that are not, themselves, designed to manipulate input parameters. It is equally important that the possible effects of different input parameters be considered in comparing what seem to be similar experiments reported by different authors or conducted in different laboratories.

CONCLUDING COMMENTS

I began the chapter by noting that the left and right hemispheres of humans do not handle all aspects of visual information processing with equal ability. My purpose has been to review what I see as the most promising approaches for understanding exactly what the critical differences are. It is interesting that some of these hemispheric asymmetries can be described by three processing distinctions that come from contemporary theories of visual information processing: (1) global vs. local processing, (2) low vs. high visuospatial frequencies, and (3) coordinate vs. categorical spatial relationships. It is even more interesting that these three processing distinctions seem interrelated in a variety of ways, so that the three aspects of hemispheric asymmetry may be different manifestations of the same underlying mechanisms. I have speculated about what those mechanisms could be and how the asymmetries might emerge during the course of ontogenetic development. Although I suspect that many of the speculations will be proved wrong, at least in terms of their particulars, they point toward a number of fruitful research directions for the future.

ACKNOWLEDGMENTS

The preparation of this chapter and much of the author's own research reviewed therein was supported in part by grant DBS-9209534 from the National Science Foundation.

REFERENCES

Alivisatos, B., and Wilding, J. (1982). Hemispheric differences in matching Stroop-type letter stimuli. *Cortex, 18*, 5–21.

Allen, M. (1983). Models of hemispheric specialization. *Psychological Bulletin, 93*, 73–104.

Alwitt, L. F. (1982). Two neural mechanisms related to modes of selective attention. *Journal of Experimental Psychology: Human Perception and Performance, 8*, 253–272.

Banks, M. S., and Dannemiller, J. L. (1987). Infant visual psychophysics. In P. Salapatek and L. Cohen (Eds.), *Handbook of infant perception*, Vol. 1 (pp 115–184). Orlando, FL: Academic Press.

Beaumont, J. G. (Ed.) (1982). *Divided visual field studies of cerebral organization.* New York, NY: Academic Press.

Boles, D. B. (1984). Global versus local processing: Is there a hemispheric dichotomy? *Neuropsychologia, 22*, 445–455.

Bryden, M. P. (1982). *Laterality: Functional asymmetry in the intact brain.* New York, NY: Academic Press.

Christman, S. (1989). Perceptual characteristics in visual laterality research. *Brain and Cognition, 11*, 238–257.

Christman, S. (1990). Effects of luminance and blur on hemispheric asymmetries in temporal integration. *Neuropsychologia, 28*, 361–374.

Christman, S., Kitterle, F. L., and Hellige, J. B. (1991). Hemispheric asymmetry in the processing of absolute versus relative spatial frequency. *Brain and Cognition, 16*, 62–73.

Corballis, M. C. (1991). *The lopsided ape: Evolution of the generative mind.* Oxford, England: Oxford University Press.

Cowin, E. L., and Hellige, J. B. (1994). Effects of blurring on hemispheric asymmetry for processing spatial information. *Journal of Cognitive Neuroscience, 6*, 156–164.

Delis, D. C., Robertson, L. C., and Efron, R. (1986). Hemispheric sepcialization of memory for visual hierarchical stimuli. *Neuropsychologia, 24*, 205–214.

de Schonen, S., and Mathivet, E. (1989). First come first served: A scenario about the development of hemispheric specialization in face recognition during infancy. *European Bulletin of Cognitive Psychology (CPC), 9*, 3–44.

De Valois, R. L., and De Valois, K. K. (1980). Spatial vision. *Annual Review of Psychology, 31*, 117–153.

Efron, R. (1990). *The decline and fall of hemispheric specialization*. Hillsdale, NJ: Lawrence Erlbaum Associates.

Gazzaniga, M. S. (1985). *The social brain*. New York, NY: Basic Books.

Gazzaniga, M. S., and Le Doux, J. (1978). *The integrated mind*. New York, NY: Plenum Press.

Geschwind, N., and Galaburda, A. M. (1987). *Cerebral lateralization: Biological mechanisms, associations, and pathology*. Cambridge, MA: MIT Press.

Guiard, Y. (1987). Asymmetric division of labor in human skilled bimanual action: The kinematic chain as a model. *Journal of Motor Behavior, 19,* 486–517.

Hammond, G. R. (1990). Manual performance asymmetries. In G. R. Hammond (Ed.), *Cerebral control of speech and limb movements* (pp 59–78). Amsterdam: North-Holland.

Hellige, J. B. (1976). Changes in same-different laterality patterns as a function of practice and stimulus quality. *Perception and Psychophysics, 20,* 267–273.

Hellige, J. B. (1980). Effects of perceptual quality and visual field of probe stimulus presentation on memory search for letters. *Journal of Experimental Psychology: Human Perception and Performance, 6,* 639–651.

Hellige, J. B. (1983a). *Cerebral hemisphere asymmetry: Method, theory and application*. New York: Praeger.

Hellige, J. B. (1983b). Hemisphere by task interaction and the study of laterality. In J. B. Hellige (Ed.), *Cerebral hemisphere asymmetry: Method, theory and application* (pp 411–443). New York: Praeger.

Hellige, J. B. (1990). Hemispheric asymmetry. *Annual Review of Psychology, 41,* 55–80.

Hellige, J. B. (1991). Book review of *Hemispheric specialization and psychological function* and *The decline and fall of hemispheric specialization*. *American Journal of Psychology, 104,* 447–474.

Hellige, J. B. (1993). *Hemispheric asymmetry: What's right and what's left*. Cambridge, MA: Harvard University Press.

Hellige, J. B. (in press). Divided visual field technique. In *The Blackwell dictionary of neuropsychology*. Oxford, England: Basil Blackwell.

Hellige, J. B., Jonsson, J. E., and Corwin, W. H. (1984). Effects of perceptual quality on the processing of human faces presented to the left and right cerebral hemispheres. *Journal of Experimental Psychology: Human Perception and Performance, 10,* 90–107.

Hellige, J. B., and Michimata, C. (1989). Categorization versus distance: Hemispheric differences for processing spatial information. *Memory and Cognition, 17,* 770–776.

Hellige, J. B., and Sergent, J. (1986). Role of task factors in visual field asymmetries. *Brain and Cognition, 5,* 200–222.

Hellige, J. B., and Webster, R. (1979). Right hemisphere superiority for initial stages of letter processing. *Neuropsychologia, 17,* 653–660.

Ivry, R. B., and Lebby, P. (1993). Hemispheric differences in auditory perception are similar to those found in visual perception. *Psychological Science, 4,* 41–45.

Jonsson, J. E., and Hellige, J. B. (1986). Lateralized effects of blurring: A test of the visual spatial frequency model of cerebral hemisphere asymmetry. *Neuropsychologia, 24,* 351–362.

Kitterle, F. L., Christman, S., and Hellige, J. B. (1990). Hemispheric differences are found in the identification, but not the detection, of low vs. high spatial frequencies. *Perception and Psychophysics, 48,* 297–306.

Kitterle, F. L., Hellige, J. B., and Christman, S. (1992). Visual hemispheric asymmetries depend on which spatial frequencies are task relevant. *Brain and Cognition, 20,* 308–314.

Kitterle, F. L., and Selig, L. M. (1991). Visual field effects in the discrimination of sine-wave gratings. *Perception and Psychophysics, 50,* 15–18.

Koenig, O., Reiss, L. P., and Kosslyn, S. M. (1990). The development of spatial relation representations: Evidence from studies of cerebral lateralization. *Journal of Experimental Child Psychology, 50,* 119–130.

Kosslyn, S. M. (1987). Seeing and imagining in the cerebral hemispheres: A computational approach. *Psychological Review, 94,* 148–175.

Kosslyn, S. M., Chabris, C. F., Marsolek, C. J., and Koenig, O. (1992). Categorical versus coordinate spatial relations: Computational analyses and computer simulations. *Journal of Experimental Psychology: Human Perception and Performance, 18,* 562–577.

Kosslyn, S. M., Flynn, R. A., Amsterdam, J. B., and Wang, G. (1990). Components of high-level vision: A cognitive neuroscience analysis and accounts of neurological syndromes. *Cognition, 34,* 203–277.

Kosslyn, S. M., Koenig, O., Barrett, A., Cave, C. B., Tang, J., and Gabrieli, J. D. E. (1989). Evidence for two types of spatial representations: Hemispheric specialization for categorical and coordinate relations. *Journal of Experimental Psychology: Human Perception and Performance, 15,* 723–735.

Lamb, M. R., Robertson, L. C., and Knight, R. T. (1989). Attention and interference in the processing of hierarchical patterns: Inferences from patients with right and left temporal-parietal lesions. *Neuropsychologia, 27,* 471–483.

Lamb, M. R., Robertson, L. C., and Knight, R. T. (1990). Component mechanisms underlying the processing of hierarchically organized patterns: Inferences from patients with unilateral cortical lesions. *Journal of Experimental Psychology: Learning, Memory, and Cognition, 16,* 471–483.

Lamb, M. R., and Yund, E. W. (1991). Effects of hierarchical structure and spatial frequency on Global/Local analysis. Paper presented at the Annual Convention of the Psychonomic Society, San Francisco, CA, November 1991.

Martin, M. (1979). Hemispheric specialization for local and global processing. *Neuropsychologia, 17,* 33–40.

Michimata, C., and Hellige, J. B. (1987). Effects of blurring and stimulus size on the lateralized processing of nonverbal stimuli. *Neuropsychologia, 25,* 397–407.

Palmer, S. E. (1977). Hierarchical structure in perceptual representation. *Cognitive Psychology, 9,* 441–474.

Peterzell, D. H. (1991). On the nonrelation between spatial frequency and cerebral hemispheric competence. *Brain and Cognition, 15,* 62–68.

Peterzell, D. H., Harvey, L. O., and Hardyck, C. (1989). Spatial frequencies and the cerebral hemispheres: Contrast sensitivity, visible persistence, and letter classification. *Perception and Psychophysics, 46,* 443–455.

Rebai, M., Mecacci, L., Bagot, J., and Bonnet, C. (1986). Hemispheric asymmetries in the visual evoked potentials to temporal frequency: Preliminary evidence. *Perception, 15,* 589–594.

Rebai, M., Mecacci, L., Bagot, J., and Bonnet, C. (1989). Influence of spatial frequency and handedness on hemispheric asymmetry in visually steady-state evoked potentials. *Neuropsychologia, 27,* 315–324.

Robertson, L. C. (1986). From gestalt to neo-gestalt. In T. J. Knapp and L. C. Robertson (Eds.), *Approaches to cognition: Contrasts and controversies* (pp 159–188). Hillsdale, NJ: Lawrence Erlbaum Associates.

Robertson, L. C., Lamb, M. R., and Knight, R. T. (1988). Effects of lesions of temporal-parietal junction on perceptual and attentional processing in humans. *Journal of Neuroscience, 8,* 3757–3769.

Robertson, L. C., Lamb, M. R., and Knight, R. T. (1991). Normal global-local analysis in patients with dorsolateral frontal lobe lesions. *Neuropsychologia, 29, 959–968.*

Rybash, J. M., and Hoyer, W. J. (1992). Hemispheric specialization for categorical and coordinate spatial representations: A reappraisal. *Memory and Cognition, 20, 271–276.*

Sergent, J. (1982a). The cerebral balance of power: Confrontation or cooperation? *Journal of Experimental Psychology: Human Perception and Performance, 8, 253–272.*

Sergent, J. (1982b). About face: Left-hemisphere involvement in processing of physiognomies. *Journal of Experimental Psychology: Human Perception and Performance, 8, 253–272.*

Sergent, J. (1983). The role of the input in visual hemispheric asymmetries. *Psychological Bulletin, 93, 481–514.*

Sergent, J. (1985). Influence of task and input factors on hemispheric involvement in face processing. *Journal of Experimental Psychology: Human Perception and Performance, 11, 846–861.*

Sergent, J. (1987a). Information processing and laterality effects for object and face perception. In G. W. Humphreys and M. J. Riddoch (Eds.), *Visual object processing: A cognitive neuropsychological approach* (pp 145–173). Hillsdale, NJ: Lawrence Erbaum Associates.

Sergent, J. (1987b). Failures to confirm the spatial-frequency hypothesis: Fatal blow or healthy complication? *Canadian Journal of Psychology, 41, 412–428.*

Sergent, J. (1989). Image generation and processing of generated images in the cerebral hemispheres. *Journal of Experimental Psychology: Human Perception and Performance, 15, 170–178.*

Sergent, J. (1991). Judgments of relative position and distance on representations of spatial relations. *Journal of Experimental Psychology: Human Perception and Performance, 17, 762–780.*

Sergent, J. and Hellige, J. B. (1986). Role of input factors in visual-field asymmetries. *Brain and Cognition, 5, 174–199.*

Thomas, J. (1986). Seeing spatial patterns. In K. R. Boff, L. Kaufman, and J. P. Thomas (Eds.), *Handbook of perception and human performance,* Vol 1. New York, NY: John Wiley & Sons.

Turkewitz, G. (1988). A prenatal source for the development of hemispheric specialization. In D. L. Molfese and S. J. Segalowitz (Eds.), *Brain lateralization in children: Developmental implications* (pp 73–81). New York: Guilford Press.

Van Kleeck, M. H. (1989). Hemispheric differences in global versus local processing of hierarchical visual stimuli by normal subjects: New data and a meta-analysis of previous data. *Neuropsychologia, 27, 1165–1178.*

Wolcott, C. L., Saul, R. E., Hellige, J. B., and Kumar, S. (1990) Effects of stimulus degradation on letter-matching performance of left and right hemispheric stroke patients. *Journal of Clinical and Experimental Neuropsychology, 2, 222–234.*

6 Dichotic Listening: Probing Temporal Lobe Functional Integrity

Kenneth Hugdahl

Dichotic listening (DL) is a behavioral technique used to study a broad range of cognitive and emotional processes related to brain laterality and hemispheric asymmetry (Kimura, 1961; Bryden, 1988; Hugdahl, 1992a); attention (Broadbent, 1954; Näätänen, 1982; Hillyard et al., 1973), conditioning and learning (Corteen and Wood, 1972; Dawson and Schell, 1982; Hugdahl and Brobeck, 1986); memory (Christianson, Nilsson, and Silfvenius, 1986; Hugdahl, Asbjørnsen, and Wester, 1993); and psycholinguistics (Repp, 1977; Lauter, 1982). In neuropsychological practice, DL is typically used to index language function (Studdert-Kennedy and Shankweiler, 1970; Tartter, 1988). The view taken in this chapter is that the DL technique has a much broader field of application than the identification of a left hemisphere phonetic speech processor related to rapidly changing acoustical events (cf. Schwartz and Tallal, 1980). Dichotic listening is a measure of temporal lobe function (Spreen and Strauss, 1991), attention, and stimulus processing speed, in addition to being a measure of hemispheric language asymmetry (cf. Hugdahl, 1992a). Auditory lateralization is probably not related to a single mechanism (cf. Jäncke, Steinmetz, and Volkmann, 1992), but is related to several mechanisms involving both perceptual and other cognitive components. This means that it should not be a surprise when DL shows low intercorrelations with other laterality tasks, like the visual half-field technique, since these tasks probably index different laterality modules. There is no such thing as *the* laterality function that can be assessed with whatever laterality task or test. Each hemisphere subserves multiple functions that need not correlate with one another. What should correlate, however, are measures of general activation of a hemisphere and tasks that tap specific functions within that hemisphere. This was exemplified in recent data collected by Richard Davidson in Madison, Wisconsin (personal communication, April 1993). Davidson showed that the magnitude of the right ear advantage (REA) in the DL task significantly correlated with resting electroencephalographic (EEG) asymmetry. Subjects with larger-left-than-right EEG resting activation also had better recall from the right as compared to the left ear in DL. This is an important study, showing how DL performance is linked to individual differences in traitlike hemisphere asymmetry.

The basic feature of the dichotic situation is to provide more elements to be processed at any moment in time than the brain is capable of processing. That is to say, more stimulus components are presented at the same time than can be consciously analyzed. The question then becomes which elements or components of the stimulus input will be selected, or attended to (cf. Holender, 1986). The dichotic situation thus not only allows for analysis of structural effects of laterality differences between the hemispheres of the brain but also for analysis of dynamic cognitive effects. A typical task in conscious selection involves monitoring and shadowing the message in one ear while ignoring the message presented to the other ear (Cherry, 1953). Several studies have shown that subjects may still process what is presented in the unnoticed ear to a certain degree (e.g., Moray, 1959; Treisman, 1964). However, critics have argued that most of these studies did not adequately control for rapid shifts of attention to the ignored ear when the critical stimulus components were presented (see Holender, 1986, for a review). The issue of unconscious selection is therefore still an open question.

Although the DL technique has its broadest applications in neuropsychology, DL procedures are frequently also used in other type of studies, e.g., in selective attention, particularly when looking for brain potential correlates of attentional behavior (e.g., Hillyard et al., 1973; Näätänen, 1990). A typical task for the study of brain potentials in selective attention is to have trains of dichotic stimulus presentations at a fast rate. The subject is instructed to attend to one ear, and to discriminate between two tones varying in pitch, while at the same time ignoring a similar input presented to the unattended ear. This task thus involves active monitoring of the message in one channel and simultaneously suppressing input from the other channel. Event-related potentials (ERPs) typically differ when recorded to the attended and unattended stimuli, with the so-called processing negativity component (Näätänen, 1990) as an early gatekeeper for admitting a stimulus to further processing after initial selection and memory comparison have occurred. Although a dichotic situation, the tone-monitoring paradigms have not resulted in laterality differences depending on which ear is the active monitored channel and which ear is the passive, unattended channel. As mentioned above, a critical methodologic issue related to the use of dichotic stimulus presentations to unravel hemisphere differences in unconscious processing is the possibility that subjects may rapidly shift attention to the nonattended channel when the critical test stimuli are presented (see Dawson and Schell, 1982; Holender, 1986). Hugdahl and L. Andersson (1986) showed that the standard dichotic procedure is sensitive to attentional influences, where a hemisphere-specific ear advantage may be shifted if attention is focused to the ipsilateral ear (see also Hugdahl, 1992b).

It was Broadbent (1954) who originally developed the DL technique to simulate the attentional load experienced by air traffic controllers when simultaneously receiving multiple flight information. However, it was Kimura (1961) who developed the present-day version of the DL technique for the study of hemisphere function in normal persons and brain-lesioned patients (see Bryden, 1988, for a historical review). As a tool for probing of brain laterality, DL has been used in literally thousands of research and clinical reports related to: language processing (Tartter, 1988; Blumstein and Cooper, 1974); emotional arousal (Bryden, 1988); hypnosis and altered states of consciousness (Frumkin, Ripley, and Cox, 1978; Crawford, Crawford, and Koperski, 1983); stroke patients (Hugdahl, Wester, and Asbjørnsen, 1990); psychiatric disorders (Nachshon, 1980; Wexler,1986; Bruder, 1983); child disorders, including dyslexia (Bakker and Kappers, 1988; Obrzut and Boliek, 1988; Cohen, Hynd, and Hugdahl, 1992), congenital hemiplegia (Carlsson et al., 1992); and autism (Blackstock, 1978), to mention a few examples. Although DL is frequently used as a behavioral test of brain function, and particularly frontotemporal functional integrity, the field is surprisingly neglected with respect to more general reviews, with the exception perhaps of the 1988 *Handbook of Dichotic Listening* (Hugdahl, 1988).

This chapter is focused on the use of consonant-vowel (CV) syllables as stimuli in the dichotic situation, with a few exceptions to be specified in later sections. Among the variety of tasks and situations used with the DL test, recall or monitoring of dichotically presented CV syllables has, on the whole, given the most robust ear advantages across subjects and experimental conditions (e.g., see Bradshaw, Burden, and Nettleton, 1986; Springer and Deutsch, 1989; Hugdahl, 1992a).

THE RIGHT EAR ADVANTAGE

A common finding in DL is the right ear advantage (REA): superior reports from the right ear, compared with the left ear, under divided-attention conditions. Focused-attention conditions are discussed separately. According to Kimura (1967), the REA is a consequence of the anatomy of the auditory projections from the cochlear nucleus in the ear to the primary auditory cortex in the temporal lobe, and of a left hemisphere superiority for the processing of language-related materials. The auditory system may conveniently be divided into five separate relay stations (Brodal, 1981; Nerad, 1992). An auditory stimulus activates neurons in the cochlear nucleus (CN) at the level of the vestibulocochlear nerve. Among the subdivisions of the cochlear nucleus, the ventral acoustic stria (VAS) enters the second level, the superior olivary complex (SOC). From here, both inhibitory and excitatory impulses are projected within the lateral lemniscus (LL) to the dorsal and ventral nuclei of the LL, which make up the third-level relay station. Up to the level of the nuclei of the LL, the auditory system projects bilaterally. However, from the nuclei of the LL, projections are mainly contralateral, projecting to the fourth relay station, the inferior colliculus (IC) in the tectum. The contralateral fibers then innervate the medial geniculate body (MGB) in the pulvinar thalamus, which is the fifth relay station, sending its axons to neurons in the auditory cortex in the posterior superior temporal gyrus (Price et al., 1992; Brugge and Reale,

1985). Thus, although auditory signals from one ear reach both auditory cortices in the temporal lobes, the contralateral projections are stronger and preponderant. Furthermore, although the input to the inferior colliculus is both ipsi- and contralateral, the projections *from* the inferior colliculus are greater from the contralateral ear. This will, in the end, favor representation of the contralateral ear in the auditory cortex (cf. Brodal, 1981).

The Classic Model

The "classic" model (e.g., Kimura, 1967; Sparks and Geschwind, 1968; Sidtis, 1988) argues that the REA is caused by several interacting factors. First of all, as mentioned above, the auditory input to the contralateral hemisphere is more strongly represented in the brain. Second, the left hemisphere (for right-handers) is specialized for language processing. Third, auditory information that is sent along the ipsilateral pathways is suppressed, or blocked, by the contralateral information. Fourth, information that reaches the ipsilateral right hemisphere has to be transferred across the corpus callosum to the left hemisphere language-processing areas.

Taking all of these steps together, the REA will thus reflect a left hemisphere language-dominant hemisphere. The classic model was supported by the papers of Sparks and Geschwind, (1968), and Milner, Taylor, and Sperry (1968). These authors reported a complete, or near-complete extinction in the left ear channel in commissurotomized patients after dichotic presentations. The argument was that in order to report from the left ear, the signal had to travel from the right auditory cortex, via the corpus callosum, to the language-dominant left region. Damage to the pathway anywhere along this route should consequently yield extinction of the left ear input. A similar argument was made that lesions in the left auditory region would produce a left ear extinction effect. By the same token, a left ear advantage (LEA) would typically indicate a right hemisphere processing dominance, and a no ear advantage (NEA) would indicate a bilateral, or mixed, processing dominance. Unpublished data from our laboratory have shown that persons with crossed laterality, i.e., crossed hand and eye preference, fail to demonstrate a significant REA in DL compared with persons with noncrossed eye-hand laterality.

A nice demonstration of how dichotic stimuli are lateralized in the brain, probably involving a "hard-wired" anatomic basis, may be seen in figure 6.1. The data in figure 6.1 are from a study by Heikki Lyytinen and his colleagues at the University of Jyvaeskylae, Finland. Using ERPs from the scalp, time-locked to the presentation of each dichotic CV stimulus pair, these researchers compared the electrophysiologic "answers" from the brain whenever a dichotic stimulus was presented. Lyytinen compared a group of stable REA subjects with a group of LEA subjects. In order to be classified as an REA or LEA subject, each subject had to show a 10% or larger ear advantage in the same direction on three consecutive DL tests. Interestingly, as can be seen in figure 6.1, during the nonforced recall condition, the REA subjects showed

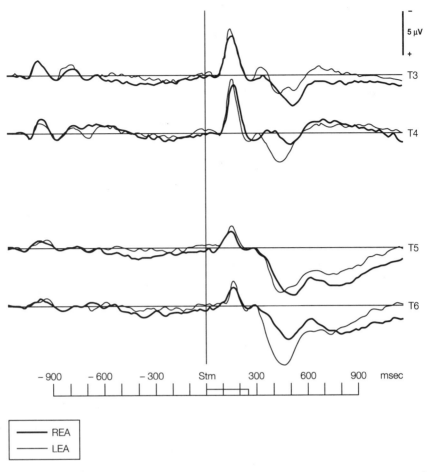

Figure 6.1 Event-related potentials (ERPs) from the left (T3/T5) and right (T4/T6) temporal leads after presentation of dichotic CV syllables. REA, subjects with a consistent right ear advantage; LEA, subjects with a consistent left ear advantage. Negativity up. Vertical line marks presentation of the stimulus. Averaged across 10 subjects. (Data from Heikki Lyytinen, Department of Psychology, University of Jyvaeskylae, Finland.)

enhancement of the P3 component over the *left* auditory cortex (T3/T5), whereas the LEA subjects showed enhanced P3 amplitudes over the homologous *right* hemisphere (T4/T6). These data are the first demonstration, as far as I know, of a direct relationship between performance scores on the DL test and activation of specific brain areas in the two cortical hemispheres.

The Attention Model

Several studies have reported a right ear preference for monaurally presented verbal stimuli (Palmer, 1964; Blackstock, 1978). Furthermore, Bakker (e.g., 1969, 1970) found that children showed better recall from the right compared with the left ear input under monaural presentation. Such results would pose a problem for the classic model of ear asymmetries in DL since monaural input should not suppress the ipsilateral left ear signal; thus an REA should not occur during monaural stimulation. For this reason, Bradshaw and Nettleton (1988) argued that a DL situation is not necessary in order to generate ear asymmetries. Instead, they suggested that it is the perceived position of a sound source rather than ear of entry that determines behavioral asymmetries (see also Bertelson, 1982). Bradshaw and his colleagues showed an REA by arranging loudspeakers in the room that were unknown to the listener (Pierson, Bradshaw, and Nettleton, 1983). A similar view was advocated by Geffen and Quinn (1984; see also Clark, Geffen, and Geffen, 1988), who concluded that there were was strong support for the view that sounds in one half of space are quantitatively better processed in the contralateral hemisphere. This was supported by voluntary direction of attention, showing that the inherent perceptual asymmetry may be overcome.

A more elaborate attentional explanation for the ear advantage in DL was provided by Kinsbourne (e.g., 1970, 1974). Kinsbourne's main argument was that anticipation of a verbal stimulus "primes" the left hemisphere, which increases arousal in the (left) language-specialized hemisphere. It also directs attention to the stimulus source contralateral to the language hemisphere (i.e., to the right ear).Thus, there are two major explanatory models for the REA effect in DL, one that refers to the anatomy and physiology of the auditory system, and another that refers to attentional and other cognitive or emotional influences. This is addressed at length later in this chapter. For now it may suffice to say that looking at the structural vs. attentional controversy in DL, comparing DL results against more "structural" techniques would provide some tentative answers. The most frequently used method of validating DL performance and brain function is the administration of amobarbital sodium (Sodium Amytal) to the left or right hemisphere, and recording how speech function is suppressed when amobarbital is injected into one hemisphere at a time (Strauss, 1988). Although this probably is the most reliable method for observing brain asymmetry for language, the amobarbital technique mainly measures expressive speech function, while DL, in addition, picks up functions related to language reception.

Another way of looking at the structural vs. attentional explanation for the REA is to study patients with unilateral lesions restricted to one hemisphere. Several studies have reported a lesion effect such that unilateral damage to areas involving auditory pathways may lead to reduced frequency of correctly reported items from the contralateral ear (e.g., Sparks, Goodglass, and Nickel, 1970). Furthermore, Roberts and colleagues (1990) showed that patients with complex partial seizures improved their DL performance after anticonvulsant medication. This is what may be expected from a structural explanation for the REA effect. However, from an attentional explanation, unilateral left temporal lobe damage should not necessarily lead to a drastic reduction in the contralateral right ear report; the decrease may as well be manifested in a reduction of correct reports from the ipsilateral ear. A third way of studying the influence of modulatory factors, like attention, in DL is to add specific instructions to the subject to attend either to the left or right ear (cf. Bryden, Munhall, and Allard, 1983), or to orient to the left or right in space (Bradshaw and Nettleton, 1988). This is addressed below.

STIMULUS MATERIALS

In all of the studies from our laboratory reviewed below, the stimuli were paired presentations of the six stop consonants /b,d,g,p,t,k/ together with the vowel /a/ to form CV syllable pairs of the type /ba-ga/, /ta-ka/, etc. The syllables were paired with one another for all possible combinations, thus yielding 36 dichotic pairs, including the homonymic pairs. The homonymic pairs were included as test trials, and were not included in the statistical analyses. Each CV pair was recorded three times on the tape, with three different randomizations of the 36 basic pairs. Thus, the total number of trials on the tape was 108. The 108 trials were divided into three trial blocks, each of 36 pairs, one trial block for each instructional condition, nonforced attention (NF), forced right (FR), and forced left (FL) (see below for details). In some studies only the NF condition was used. For each condition, the analysis was based on 30 trials. Each subject was given a standardized set of instructions prior to the test. The instructions were of the format: "You should listen to the six different sounds which are given on this page [show the six syllables on a page of paper]. After each presentation, you should repeat whatever sound you hear. Say the sound loud and clear directly after it has been presented. Sometimes it will seem as if you hear two different sounds at the same time. Don't worry about this, but say the sound you seemed to hear best or most clearly. Don't spend time thinking, but just repeat the sound as soon as it has been presented." In some instances, e.g., when testing patients with expressive language difficulties, the experimenter asked the patient to point to a sheet of paper on which the syllables were written in capital letters (e.g., Hugdahl et al., 1990).

The syllables were read by a male voice with constant intonation and intensity. Mean duration was approximately 350 ms, and the intertrial interval was about 4 seconds. The syllables were read through a microphone and digitized for computer editing on an IBM-compatible 486-PC, equipped with a DT 2801 A/D and D/A board. After digitization, each CV pair was displayed on the screen and synchronized for simultaneous onset and offset between the right and left channels. The synchronization was performed on the 486-PC computer with a specially developed software (SWELL) running as an application under MS-Windows 3.1.

After computer editing, the CV pairs were taken from the computer (over the D/A board) and recorded on a Revox B-77 stereo reel-to-reel tape recorder. The reel-to-reel tape was then copied onto a chrome dioxide cassette and played to the subject from a SONY Walkman WM DDII stereo minicassette player. The output from the minicassette player was calibrated between channels, and the mean output intensity was 75 dB sound pressure level when measured with a Bruel and Kjaer 2204 sound level meter equipped with a Bruel and Kjaer 4521 "artificial ear." The CV syllables were presented to the subject with the help of miniature plug-in-type earphones.

In most of the studies, the subjects were tested for differences between the ears in hearing acuity. Hearing thresholds were determined for each ear for the frequencies 500, 1000, 2000, 3000, and 5000 Hz. Subjects with threshold differences between the ears larger than 5 dB on any of the frequencies tested were excluded from the study. The range of 500 to 5000 Hz was chosen because most of the spectral energy in the CV syllables is in this range.

Procedure

The data presented were all collected with a common procedure, involving three different attentional instructions labeled NF, FR, and FL, respectively.

The Nonforced Condition   In this condition, which always was presented first for reasons of not confusing the subject, the subject was told that he or she would hear repeated presentations of the six CV syllables /ba, da, ga, pa, ta, ka/, and that he or she should report which syllable was heard after each trial. The subjects were further told that "on some occasions there seems to be two sounds coming simultaneously." They were told that they should not bother about this, and just report the one they heard first, or best. Subjects were instructed not to think about the syllables but to give the answer that spontaneously came to mind after each presentation. They were usually shown a cardboard sheet with all six syllables written on it before the experiment started. In our laboratory, we have shifted to the use of only single-correct trials, which are scored, or alternatively, the subject is instructed always only to report *one* item on each trial irrespective of whether he or she perceived one or both items (see Bryden, 1988, for a discussion of single vs. double answers).

The Forced-Right and Forced-Left Conditions   When subjects are left free to report the items as in the NF situation, they may choose the order in which they report. They may also differentially attend to the right and left ear inputs (see Bryden et al., 1983; Hugdahl and L. Andersson, 1986). It may even be the case that right-handed subjects find it easier to focus attention on items from the right ear, rather than from the left. Thus, in order to control for strategy effects, subjects were requested to "only listen to, and report from the right ear" on the following one third of the trials. Using a focused-attention condition makes it possible to simultaneously study structural and dynamic laterality effects within the same paradigm. The NF condition basically taps a structural laterality component, while the FR and FL conditions tap the modification of structural laterality by dynamic cognitive factors, like attention. This is discussed in detail below. In the forced-attention situations, subjects were required to report only the *right* ear input in one third of the trials, and to attend to and report only the *left* ear input in another third of the trials (see Bryden et al., 1983; Hugdahl and L. Andersson, 1986). The presentation order of the FR and FL conditions was counterbalanced across subjects.

NORMATIVE DATA

In the following, data from a large number of normal subjects, both children and adults, are presented. The sample consists of 488 right-handed persons for the NF condition and 303 right-handed persons for the FR and FL conditions. A smaller sample of 139 left-handers have also been studied in our laboratory. Data on the left-handers are restricted to the NF recall condition, owing to lack of an adequate sample size for the other two recall conditions. The age span of the subjects ranged from 8 to 70 years. Thus both children and adults are included in the tables. However, separate analyses, split for age groups (children, adolescents, adults, older persons) showed similar trends in the data for the NF condition, although the children showed a specific pattern of responding for the forced-attention conditions, which is discussed in detail later.

Table 6.1 shows descriptive statistics for the entire sample of right-handers for all three attentional instructions. As can be seen in the table, there was an overall mean of 46.08% correct reports from the right ear and 35.83% from the left ear during the NF condition. Thus the mean REA was 10.25%. This was highly significant ($P < .001$). The distribution was also reasonably normalized, as can be seen from the skewness and kurtosis values in table 6.1. During the FR condition, the REA increased to 23.99% ($P < .001$). However, during the FL condition, there was an LEA of 7.13% ($P < .05$). Thus, when instructed to focus attention on the left ear, and only report from that ear, subjects can overcome a hard-wired REA and switch to an LEA (see also Hugdahl and L. Andersson, 1986). This means that dynamic temporary factors influence and change the ear advantage observed in DL.

Turning to the left-handed group (n = 139), the mean of right ear correct reports was 45.41% and of left ear correct reports, 42.19% (not significant). Thus, the left-handed group did not show a significant REA during the NF recall condition. However, in a more recent study, adult left-handers also showed a significant REA. A more detailed description of the left-handed group is seen in table 6.2 for the NF attentional condition.

Looking at the number of subjects with either an REA, LEA, or NEA, figure 6.2 shows distributions of the right- and left-handed subjects for the NF condition. The 45-degree symmetry line means that a subject falling on this line has an NEA. Subjects falling below the 45-degree line show an REA, and subjects falling above the 45-degree line show an LEA. Corresponding data for the right-handers for the FR and FL attentional conditions are seen in figure 6.3. The ellipse in each panel shows a confidence interval encompassing

Table 6.1 Normative data for right-handers expressed as percent correct reports from the left and right ear across the three major attentional instructions (See text for further details)

	Mean	Median	SD	Kurtosis	Skewness	+95% CI	−95% CI	Index
				Nonforced (N=488)				
RE	46.08	46.67	10.70	0.522	0.007	47.04	45.13	
LE	35.83	36.67	10.23	0.421	0.257	36.75	34.93	12.65

Percentiles	2th	16th	50th	84th	98th			
Z-scores	−2	−1	0.0	+1	+2			
RE	23.33	36.11	46.67	56.67	66.67			
LE	16.67	25.60	36.67	44.44	61.11			

	Mean	Median	SD	Kurtosis	Skewness	+95% CI	−95% CI	Index
				Forced-Right (N=303)				
RE	51.33	50.00	14.24	−0.213	0.277	52.93	49.71	
LE	27.43	26.67	9.98	0.493	0.409	28.56	26.30	29.36

Percentiles	2th	16th	50th	84th	98th			
Z-scores	−2	−1	0.0	+1	+2			
RE	23.33	36.67	50.00	66.67	83.33			
LE	7.69	16.67	26.67	36.67	50.00			

	Mean	Median	SD	Kurtosis	Skewness	+95% CI	−95% CI	Index
				Forced-Left (N=303)				
RE	34.75	33.33	12.54	−0.309	0.187	36.17	33.33	
LE	41.88	38.89	15.62	−0.353	0.511	43.65	40.11	−7.98

Percentiles	2th	16th	50th	84th	98th			
Z-scores	−2	−1	0.0	+1	+2			
RE	12.50	22.22	33.33	47.22	60.00			
LE	16.67	26.67	38.89	60.00	76.67			

RE = right ear; LE = left ear.

Table 6.2 Normative data for left-handers (see table 6.1 for further explanation)

	Mean	Median	SD	Kurtosis	Skewness	+95% CI	−95% CI	Index
				Nonforced (N=139)				
RE	45.41	46.9	9.14	0.402	−0.174	43.88	46.95	
LE	42.20	42.7	9.55	0.177	−0.144	40.59	43.80	3.80

Percentiles	2th	16th	50th	84th	98th			
Z-scores	−2	−1	0.0	+1	+2			
RE	23.33	36.67	46.90	54.00	66.00			
LE	19.00	33.00	42.70	51.01	63.00			

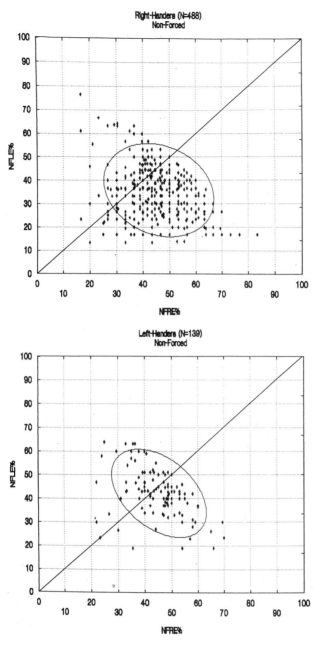

Figure 6.2 Percent correct reports from the left and right ears in 488 right-handers and 139 left-handers. Each dot = one subject. Non-forced, NF (divided-attention condition); LE, left ear; RE, right ear.

Hugdahl: Dichotic Listening

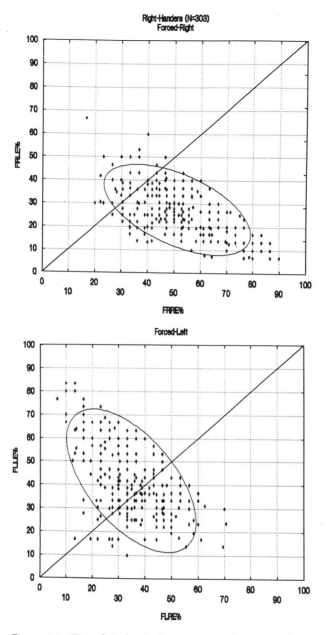

Figure 6.3 Data plotted as in figure 6.2, but only for right-handers during forced attention to the right (FR) or left (FL) ear.

95% of the subjects. For the right-handers, 77% had an REA, 17% an LEA, and 6% an NEA during the NF condition. The corresponding numbers for the left-handers were 64% REA, 26% LEA, and 10% NEA. During the FR condition, 88% of the right-handers showed an REA, 10% an LEA and 2% an NEA. During the FL condition the corresponding figures were 41% REA, 55% LEA, and 5% NEA.

Taken together, the data clearly show a majority of the subjects with an REA in the right-handed sample. During the forced-attention conditions, this pattern is either enhanced or reduced depending on the direction of the attentional instruction, focusing on the right or left ear input.

Correlations between Ear Scores

Correlating the right and left ear scores for both the right- and left-handed subjects showed a weak negative correlation for the right-handers during the NF condition ($r = -.205$, $P < .05$). The correlation becomes somewhat stronger during the FR ($r = -.550$, $P < .05$) and FL conditions ($r = -.580$, $P < .05$). The correlation for the left-handers during the NF condition was $r = -.439$, $P < .05$. Thus, although showing a significant correlation coefficient, although only $-.205$ owing to the large number of subjects, the left and right ear scores are actually weakly correlated during the standard NF recall condition in right-handers.

The lack of a strong correlation between the left and right ear scores during a divided-attention condition suggests a parallel processing model of DL, with the left ear input being initially processed in the right hemisphere. The classic model of DL (e.g., Kimura, 1967; see also Eslinger and Damasio, 1988) assumed that the major auditory pathways involved the contralateral, uncrossed, fibers from the cochlea to the auditory cortex. Ipsilateral input is thus inhibited, or blocked, by the contralateral pathways. An ear advantage emerges because the contralateral pathways from that ear would have direct access to the dominant hemisphere, which for a clear majority of all people is the left hemisphere. The classic model would therefore predict a strong negative correlation between the right and left ear scores. That is, the left ear stimulus would have to be transferred across the corpus callosum in order to be processed, and the more items that are processed from the right ear, the fewer resources would be left for processing of the left ear stimulus. Thus, the better the recall from the right ear, the worse the recall from the left ear. A negative correlation would also be predicted under forced-attention conditions, since allocation of dynamic cognitive resources, like selective attention, would add to the unique processing of the contralateral stimulus. A weak, or nonexistent, correlation, on the other hand, would indicate a kind of parallel processing in the two hemispheres, with the right hemisphere possibly performing an initial processing of the left ear input that is independent of the left hemisphere (right ear) processing.

Table 6.3 Percentage of subjects with a right ear advantage (REA), left ear advantage (LEA), or no ear advantage (NEA) across three consecutive measures (M1, M2, M3) (N = 35)

	M1	M2	M3
REA	25 (71%)	25 (71%)	26 (74%)
NEA	2 (3%)	8 (23%)	8 (23%)
LEA	8 (26%)	2 (6%)	2 (3%)
Total	35 (100%)	35 (100%)	36* (100%)

*Disparity is the result of rounding to the nearest whole number.

RELIABILITY AND VALIDITY

Looking at ear stability across measures, a small sample of 35 adult subjects were measured three times with only a couple of days between measurements. The percentage of subjects with REA, LEA, OR NEA are seen in table 6.3. As can be seen in the table, the data were quite consistent across measures for each of the three ear advantages.

A study by B. Andersson and Hugdahl (1987) showed that 28 of 32 subjects (87.5%) maintained an REA when retested after a year. Since invasive tests for language laterality typically show that more than 95% of right-handed adults have left hemisphere language representation (Rasmussen and Milner, 1977; Strauss, Gaddes, and Wada, 1987), one should therefore expect the DL task to yield an REA in at least 95% of the right-handed population. Most DL studies report proportions that vary from 65% to about 90% (depending on the type of test given and the type of scoring procedure used) (Bryden and Allard, 1978; Hiscock and Kinsbourne, 1977). A majority of the studies have not taken into account differences in the magnitude of the REA between individuals. Two studies may show equal REA proportions, although the distribution of individuals across the magnitude spectrum may vary substantially between the same studies. Measures of reliability of DL scores in children vary in general between .70 and .90. Bakker, Van der Flugt, and Claushuis (1978) studied children up to fifth grade, and found correlations to vary between .70 and .87. Harper and Kraft (1986) reported figures between .78 and .87, and between .88 and .93. The variation in figures usually stems from differences in the index scores used, the kind of stimuli, and the age levels of subjects.

Looking at left-handers, Hugdahl and B. Andersson (1989) found that 65% of left-handed children showed an REA, 25.4% an LEA, and 9.6% an NEA. These figures should be compared with amobarbital data from 122 epileptic patients reported by Rasmussen and Milner (1977), who found 70% left hemisphere language dominance in the left-handers, 15% right hemisphere dominance, and 15% mixed. Thus, DL identified 5% fewer left-handed persons with left hemisphere language dominance than did the invasive technique. Considering the random error always attached to a noninvasive behavioral technique, the 65% hit rate is quite impressive.

MODULATORY FACTORS

Attention

The first modulatory factor to be considered when discussing DL data is focusing of attention to the left or right ear, or to the left or right side in space. Since there may be a variety of factors influencing the ear advantage, some authors have claimed that there may be an attentional bias to attend to the right ear which may confound the REA (e.g., Mondor and Bryden, 1991). Thus, attentional factors in DL should be investigated separately from a laterality factor. In our laboratory we have devoted considerable effort to this issue over the years (see, e.g., Hugdahl and L. Andersson, 1986; Hugdahl, 1992b). Our basic strategy has been to have subjects perform the focused-attention tasks (FR,FL), and to compare their performance with the divided-attention (NF) task. The general findings are that the REA is enhanced during the FR condition, and attenuated and sometimes even reversed to an LEA during the FL condition. In particular, adults seem to be able to attenuate, and even reverse the REA during the FL condition. However, children cannot do this. In the study by Hugdahl and L. Andersson (1986) 8- to 9-year-old children and adults were compared during both NF and forced-attention instructions. The children still showed an REA during the FL attentional condition, particularly the boys. Interestingly, when the data were split for 8- and 9-year olds, there was a clear difference in the data. Whereas the 8-year olds could not modify their REA with attention to the left side, 9-year olds could. This is seen in figure 6.4.

The change in ability to affect the ear advantage by focusing attention to the left ear between the ages of 8 and 9 years may be linked to literacy and the development of reading skills. Hugdahl and B. Andersson (1987) showed that the ability of attentional shifts away from the right ear was increased as the child advanced in reading ability. The effect was also more pronounced for boys than for girls. These findings may be linked to an interaction between development of literacy and attentional capacity, on the one hand, and hemisphere asymmetry, on the other. The results in figure 6.5 and reported by Hugdahl and B. Andersson (1987) indicate that while the ability to switch attention in a DL task is related to both age and reading acquisition, hemisphere asymmetry obviously is not. This is reinforced by other studies (e.g., Witelson and Pallie, 1973; Molfese and Molfese, 1979) which have demonstrated functional differences between the hemispheres of the brain already at the infant level.

Other authors have also investigated the extent to which attention may bias the frequency of correct reports to either the left or right ear. Hiscock and Stewart (1984) showed that if subjects are required to focus attention to one ear first, and are then given an NF divided-attention instruction, their ear advantage during the NF second task seemed to have been "primed" by the focused-attention instruction. Moreover, Mondor and Bryden (1991)

NF

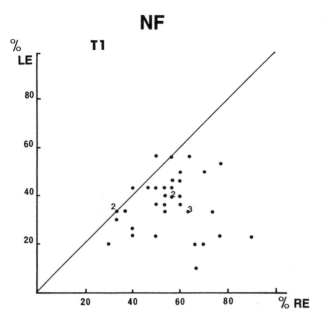

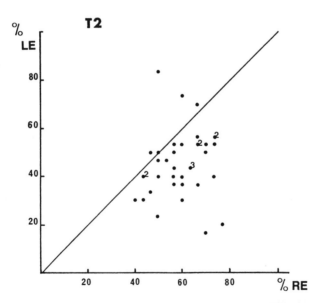

Figure 6.4 Data plotted as in figures 6.2 and 6.3. NF, nonforced, divided-attention condition; T1, test at the age of 8 years; T2, test at the age of 9 years. *Left hand panels,* boys; *right hand panels,* girls. LE, left ear; RE, right ear. (Data from Hugdahl and B. Andersson, 1987.)

NF

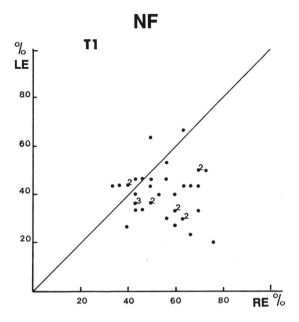

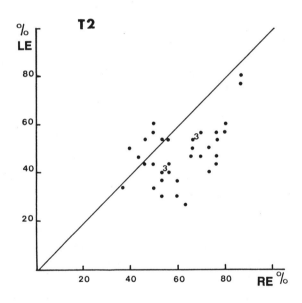

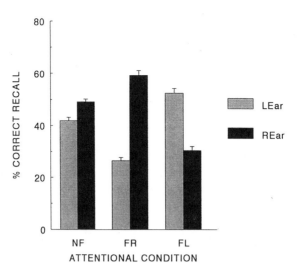

Figure 6.5 Mean percent correct recall from the left and right ear during the three attentional conditions; NF, nonforced; FR, forced-right; FL, forced-left focused attention.

presented a tone to one ear just before the presentation of a dichotic stimulus to indicate which ear to report from. In one condition the tone cue appeared 150 ms before the dichotic stimuli. In another condition it appeared 750 ms before the stimuli. The interval between the cue and the dichotic stimuli is called stimulus onset asynchrony (SOA). If attention contributes to the ear advantage, then the effect should be larger for the longer SOA since the subject would have time to orient attention to the cued ear. The results showed that as SOA grew longer, the more the ear advantage was affected, particularly the REA when the subject was cued to report from the left ear. It should therefore be clear that attention may modify the ear advantage observed in a typical DL task. However, attention usually affects the magnitude rather than the direction of the ear advantage. The view taken here is that any laterality task may tap both a hard-wired bias for one hemisphere to perform a particular task, and modulatory processes that may either enhance or attenuate the obtained ear advantage depending on whether it acts in an additive or subtractive way with regard to the built-in laterality for that task. Thus, factors other than functional laterality influence perceptual asymmetries (cf. Speaks, Niccum, and Carney, 1982).

Although most researchers would agree that attentional factors play a role in DL, and may modify a structurally based ear advantage, there is no generally accepted model of the causes for the attentional effect. As argued by Asbjørnsen and Hugdahl (1993), attention can affect the ear advantage either through enhancing reports from the attended ear, or suppressing reports from the nonattended ear. If attention acts to suppress correct reports from the nonattended ear there should be decreased overall performance compared to a divided-attention NF condition. On the other hand, if attention acts through facilitation of scores at the attended ear, then the result should show a better overall performance during a forced-attention compared to an NF condition. From a strict structural point of view, Kimura's (1967) theoretical model would predict that attention to one side in space should either have no effect at all on the ear advantage, or it should facilitate correct reports from the attended ear, particularly from the attended right ear. On the other hand, if attention acts to reduce the number of correctly reported items from the nonattended ear, this would imply an active role for callosal transfer. Alternatively, it may point toward parallel processing in the left and right hemispheres, even for phonetic stimuli such as CV syllables. These issues were addressed in a study by Asbjørnsen and Hugdahl (1993) of 62 normal right-handed adults during NF, FR, and FL attentional instructions. The results are shown in figure 6.5.

As can be seen in figure 6.5, there was a clear change in ear advantage as a consequence of attentional instruction. This was primarily caused by suppression of correct reports from the nonattended ear. Although the major finding was reduction of correct reports from the nonattended ear, there was also a small but significant increase in correctly reported items from the attended ear. These results point toward a more complex model of DL performance than the structural model would acknowledge. The overall picture is of parallel processing of the right and left ear items in the standard DL situation. Thus, the left ear item is not uncritically transferred to the left hemisphere for processing, with the right hemisphere acting as a passive "slave" whose only role is to shuffle the stimulus over to the other side. Quite the contrary, DL performance with CV syllables actually reflects the action of both the left and right hemispheres, with a hard-wired predominance for the left hemisphere. This predominance can, however, be overcome by activating dynamic processes, like attention, to increase the activation level of the right hemisphere. Such a model could then explain not only interindividual differences in DL but also intraindividual differences over time. For example, Morton and Kershner (1991) found that normal-achieving children differed from reading-disabled children on a DL task, when tested in the morning but not in the afternoon. The normal children were more strongly lateralized compared to the reading-disabled children when instructed to selectively attend to the right ear input. This may indicate a lack of control of attentional resources in the morning for reading-disabled children. It also shows temporary and dynamic modulations of a supposedly structural laterality pattern. Thus, ear advantages in DL reflect a structural hard-wiring of lateralized cognitive functions that are put under modulatory influences by dynamic processes, being switched in and out depending on the general level of activation, attentional focus, and emotional saliency.

Arousal

Although the REA is a robust empirical phenomenon, we have seen that it is affected by attention. Another possible modulator of DL performance may be motivational effort, or arousal. Level of arousal has been shown to exert considerable effects on complex cognitive tasks (see, e.g., Hockey, 1979). In spite of this, little is known of how arousal and activation may affect the scores in DL. This was studied by Asbjørnsen, Hugdahl, and Bryden (1992). An LEA has often been reported for the identification of emotional stimuli (e.g., Haggard and Parkinson, 1971; Carmon and Nachson, 1973; Ley and Bryden, 1982; Bryden and MacRae, 1988). In these studies, subjects are typically asked to identify emotional sounds or words. The LEA in such a task can arise for two reasons. Firstly, the processing of affect may be separable from the processing of content, so that the affective value of the specific stimulus may activate right hemisphere mechanisms. Secondly, the presentation of an emotional stimulus and the instruction to attend to and identify the emotional properties of the stimulus may make the *task* an emotional one, thereby leading to increased arousal and a generalized activation of the right hemisphere (cf. Kinsbourne, 1974; Tucker, 1981). As mentioned previously, this kind of explanation is supported by the argument that asymmetries of hemispheric arousal may explain not only interindividual differences but also intraindividual differences, when the same person is measured on several different occasions (Levy et al., 1983). Contrary to this, Wexler and colleagues (1986) found that highly anxious subjects showed an increase in REA to dichotically presented positively valued words. While this might appear to suggest a left hemisphere locus for positive affect, it is also possible that the positive valence of the material reduced the otherwise high level of right hemisphere arousal in such subjects.

In the study by Asbjørnsen et al. (1992), arousal was manipulated independently of the specific task being used. Thus, subjects were either threatened with an aversive event (electric shock or loud noise) for incorrect answers, or promised a positive event (monetary reward) for correct answers. In addition, a neutral or baseline condition was included, so that each subject was tested under three different conditions. Furthermore, half of the subjects were tested under high-arousal conditions, in which the positive incentive was a substantial amount of money and the aversive stimulus the threat of electric shock to the hand, and half were tested under low-arousal conditions, in which the positive incentive was a small monetary reward, and the aversive stimulus the threat of an irritating noise.

A majority of studies on DL and affect have been concerned with *perception* of affect, or emotionality. However, it might be argued that stimulus-dependent changes in magnitude or direction of ear advantage are not caused by superior right hemisphere perception, but rather because there is a generalized superior right hemisphere capacity to perform under increased stress or arousal (cf. Kinsbourne, 1974; Tucker, 1981; Heilman and Van den Abell, 1979). If an LEA is observed it might be because the right hemisphere perceived and processed the stimulus more accurately, or because the stimulus activated a generalized right hemisphere affective state. If a perceptual explanation is the most likely, then manipulating the affective state in the subject

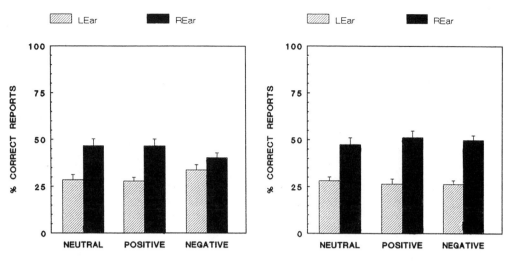

Figure 6.6 Mean percent correct reports during different arousal conditions. See text for further explanation. (Data from Asbjørnsen, Hugdahl, and Bryden, 1992.)

while presenting a nonaffective stimulus should not result in a reduced REA or a shift to an LEA. In a similar way, it could be predicted that positive arousal manipulations, e.g., a promise of monetary rewards for correct answers, should increase the REA (cf. Wexler et al., 1986; Reuter-Lorentz and Davidson, 1981).

Thirty-six females participated in the study. Heart rate was recorded as an independent measure of change in level of arousal as a function of the experimental instructions. The results are seen in figure 6.6, and basically show that the high negative condition abolished the REA effect, with a nonsignificant difference between ears. This was caused by both an increase in correct left ear reports and a decrease in correct right ear reports. The other arousal conditions had no effect on the REA.

On the basis of these results it could be argued that threat of shock not only differentially activated or primed the processing capacity of the right hemisphere (cf. Ley and Bryden, 1982), but it also facilitated callosal transfer of the left ear signal. The reduction in correct right ear reports would then be explained as due to left ear signal interference, competing for the same processing resources as the right ear signal. The left ear signal would normally, in a nonactivated right hemisphere state, not be processed to the same extent as the right ear signal owing to callosal delay. However, an activated or aroused state causes callosal facilitation, with the left ear signal arriving at the left hemisphere at about the same time as the right ear signal. An important aspect of the findings is that they do not support the view that the ear advantage in DL is independent of state shifts in arousal. The same could be said regarding the question whether all changes in arousal, irrespective of valence, will affect the REA because of increased right hemisphere activation (cf. Heilman and

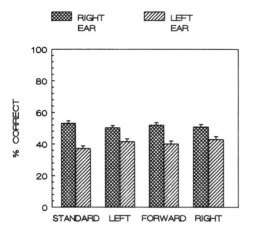
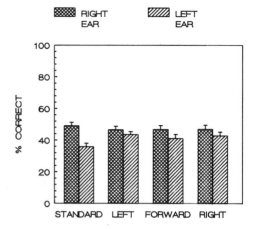

Figure 6.7 Mean percent correct reports from the left and right ears for subjects instructed to move their eyes or head to the left or right side in space. See text for further explanation. (Data from Asbjørnsen, Hugdahl, and Hynd, 1990.)

Van den Abell, 1979). The results are, however, not absolutely clear regarding this matter. Anyway, it is argued that aversive, but not positive arousal, yielded suppression of the REA, pointing toward a unique role for the right hemisphere in aversive affect.

Head and Eye Movements

As reviewed above, in their critique of the classic structural model, Bradshaw and Nettleton (1988) advocated a "functional" model of DL performance, stressing the source of stimulation in three-dimensional space, rather than the ear of entry, as the critical determinant of an ear advantage. The argument, therefore, is that sounds presented in half of space are more easily processed in the contralateral hemisphere. The notion that spatial orientation (either through head or eye turns) may affect the ear advantage was tested in a study by Asbjørnsen, Hugdahl, and Hynd (1990). Subjects were instructed to actively attend to either the right or left side by either turning their head or their eyes to the left or right in space during the dichotic task. The study involved two groups, one instructed to move their head, the other to move their eyes. There were four conditions for each group: the standard NF condition as baseline, and turning the head (or eyes) to the right, to the left, and looking straight ahead. The results are presented in figure 6.7, and show basically that the REA was preserved during all four conditions.

Thus, the REA seems to be unaffected by spatial orientation through eye gaze or head turn. However, as can be seen in figure 6.7, the REA was larger during the standard NF condition compared to the three other conditions. This indicates that spatial orientation had an effect on the REA. A closer analysis showed that fewer subjects showed an REA during spatial orientation, although the magnitude of the REA of those remaining was enough to yield a significant difference. The fact that fewer subjects showed an REA during spatial orientation may represent interference between allocation of motor responses and attention. Thus, rather than facilitating the REA, which may be predicted from lateral priming theory (e.g., Kinsbourne, 1970), the result was an inhibition of the REA in some subjects. However, the overall results showed that ear of entry seems to be a far more powerful determinant of the ear advantage in DL than the perceived sound source in space. This has consequences for models of DL, supporting the structural model of ipsilateral suppression and contralateral gating of the auditory signal. The ipsilateral suppression furthermore seems to be peripheral rather than central. If the suppression was centrally mediated, then turning one's head to the right or left should have had a greater impact on the ear advantage than what was observed in the Asbjørnsen et al. (1990) study.

CLINICAL APPLICATIONS: CASE STUDIES

In this section, a series of clinical case studies from our laboratory are presented, to which we have applied the DL technique. A more comprehensive review of clinical applications in neuropsychology of the DL technique may be found in Eslinger and Damasio (1988), and in Hugdahl and Wester (1992). Because of its simplicity, the DL technique should be an ideal vehicle for an understanding of brain dysfunction, and of language asymmetry dysfunction in particular. Similarly, because a structurally located brain lesion would be an ideal vehicle for validating different theoretical models of dichotic performance, testing DL on brain-lesioned patients is important for its own purpose.

Case 1
The patient was a young left-handed woman who had suffered a severe head injury in a traffic accident a few years before. She had virtually no remaining left hemisphere tissue owing to surgery (figure 6.8). She showed no signs of speech or language disturbance despite an almost nonexistent left hemisphere. Thus, her right hemisphere had to be the site of language. It was therefore predicted that she should demonstrate a drastic reduction in *right ear* performance in the DL test, while left ear performance should remain intact, or even be enhanced. According to the structural model, there should furthermore be no major changes in performance when the patient was instructed to attend to either side. An attentional explanation would, however, mean that although the *contralateral* right ear signal would be blocked because of tissue loss in the left hemisphere, the *ipsilateral* pathway would be intact, with the result that *attending* to the right ear should increase right ear performance. Figure 6.8 shows a CT image revealing the substantial tissue loss in the left hemisphere. The patient had normal hearing thresholds on both ears when tested with screening audiometry. The DL results are seen in figure 6.9, compared to a group of normal left-handed young women for the NF condition.

As can be seen in figure 6.9, the patient's performance was quite anomalous compared to the group as a whole. Her right ear score approached zero,

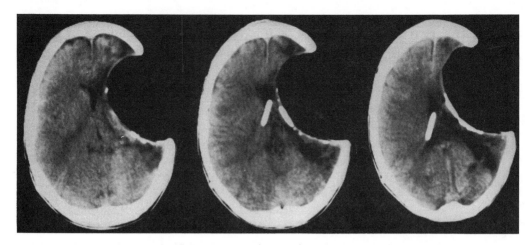

Figure 6.8 Three CT scans from patient 1 showing removal of large portions of the left hemisphere. The right side of the CT scan is the left side of the brain according to standard neuroradiologic conventions. (From Hugdahl and Wester, 1992.)

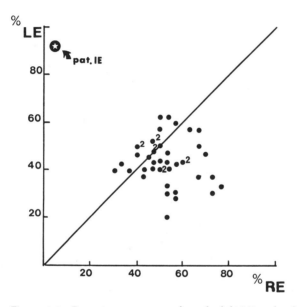

Figure 6.9 Percent correct reports from the left (LE) and right (RE) ears in patient 1 (star, patient I.E.) compared with a group of healthy left-handed women. (Data from Hugdahl and Wester, 1992.)

whereas she actually increased the left ear correct reports compared to the group. Instructing her to attend to either the left or right ear had no effect whatsoever. There are two arguments why she may be considered right hemisphere–dominant for language before the accident: (1) she was left-handed, with an increased probability of right hemisphere language dominance (Fennell, 1986); (2) her language functions were intact after near-complete destruction of the left hemisphere. The data favor a structural rather than an attentional explanation of DL performance. The zero report from the right ear must be attributed to the fact that the contralateral right ear signal was not transferred after reaching the (remaining) left temporal areas. Attending to either ear did not affect the right ear scores. The number of correctly reported items were zero in both the forced-attention conditions. It is therefore unlikely that an attentional model, which attributes the ear advantage to a biased priming effect of attending to a particular ear of input, can alone explain DL performance (cf. Kinsbourne, 1970).

Case 2
The second patient had a subarachnoid hemorrhage involving an aneurysm of the left medial cerebral artery. He had a manifest motor aphasia when admitted to the hospital, which gradually improved during the next 3 weeks. He was treated conservatively for the hemorrhage with bed rest for 3 weeks at the hospital. He was tested with DL a first time 2 days before he was released from the hospital, i.e., about 3 weeks after the acute illness. He was retested after 3.5 months. The results are shown in figure 6.10.

As can be seen in figure 6.10, the patient had reduced correct right ear reports (down to the order of 10%). This was furthermore independent of attentional instruction. Thus, instructing the patient to attend to the right ear did not affect his right ear scores. Left ear performance was in the normal 60% to 70% region, with a slight decrease during the FR condition, and an increase during the FL condition. Thus, correctly reported items from the left ear were affected by the attentional conditions. Right ear performance was, however, *not* affected by the attentional instructions. It therefore seems that the hemorrhage in the language area in the left hemisphere suppressed processing of the contralateral right ear signal, and this cannot be counteracted by focusing attention on the right ear. Thus, the attentional model for explanation of DL performance was not supported in the data from this patient.

Case 3
The third case study involves a patient with an arachnoid cyst in the left temporal lobe that was drained after craniotomy. He showed no overt signs of language disturbance in the neurologic examination. The patient was a right-handed 23-year-old man. He was tested the first time the day before the craniotomy operation, and again on the day after the operation. He was then followed up in a third test 6 weeks after the operation. The results are shown in figure 6.11 (only data from the NF attentional condition are shown).

The most conspicuous finding in this patient was the absence of an REA preoperatively. This is probably explained as a result of increased force of brain tissue in the temporal lobe critically involved in auditory processing. The absence of the REA indicates that the right ear signal was suppressed because of displacement of tissue in this region of the brain. Looking at the results from the two postoperative tests (the middle and right-hand panels), the REA appeared immediately the day after operation, and it was still present

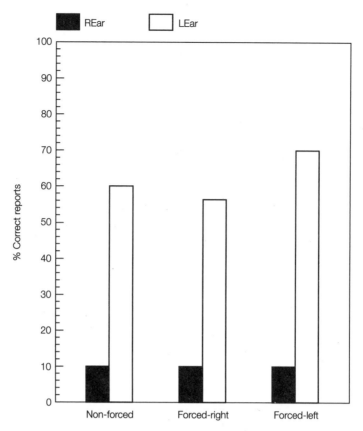

Figure 6.10 Percent correct reports from the left and right ears in patient 2 during the three attentional conditions. (Data from Hugdahl and Wester, 1992.)

at the 6 weeks' follow-up test (the right hand panel). Another important aspect of the data shown is that not only did the REA appear already on the day after the operation but that overall right ear performance also increased into the normal range. A final aspect of the results is that the REA during the two postoperative tests was caused by an *increase* in right ear performance. Since right ear performance in DL is both anatomically (Kimura, 1967; Eslinger and Damasio, 1988), and physiologically (Strauss, 1988) linked to left temporal lobe functioning, it is difficult to escape from the conclusion that DL may be a sensitive measure of functional brain recovery after neurosurgery, especially temporal lobe functioning.

We recently had the opportunity to collect data on five other patients undergoing surgery for subarachnoid cysts. All patients had the cyst located in the left sylvian fissure, growing from under the fissure. As a consequence, a large portion of the left temporal lobe was compressed in these patients. Interestingly, most cysts seem to be located in the left side of the brain, affecting mainly males (Wester, 1992). There seems to be no apparent explanation for this asymmetry in localization of the cyst. All five patients were operated on under local anesthesia with a shunt procedure that did not in-

Perceptual, Cognitive, and Motor Lateralization

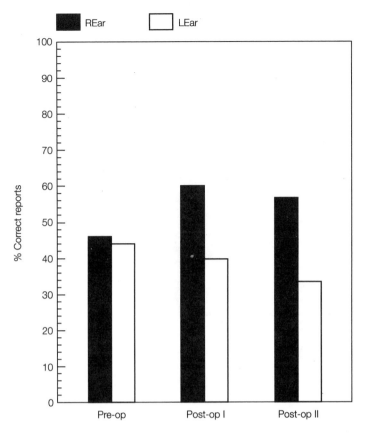

Figure 6.11 Percent correct reports from the left and right ears in patient 3 preoperatively and at two postoperative tests. (Data from Hugdahl and Wester, 1992.)

volve opening the skull. This made it possible to retest the patients much earlier after the operation than is the case with patients post craniotomy. Retesting some of the patients as early as 4 hours after the operation showed that the preoperative LEA already had switched to an REA. The REA then remained at retesting 24 hours, 1 week, and at 3 to 6 months after the operation. It thus seems as if the removal of the pressure exerted on the brain tissue in the left temporal lobe immediately restitutes the functional integrity of that area of the brain, even after long-standing compression, since most of these patients have had their cysts for years, perhaps since birth.

SUMMARY AND CONCLUSIONS

The DL technique can be looked at as a fine-tuned instrument for probing *hemisphere-specific* functions in the temporal areas of the brain that is not so easily done with other standardized neuropsychological tests. A similar view was taken by Darley in 1972 who argued that DL scores might be used to reflect uniquely lateralized changes in the function of the cerebral hemispheres.

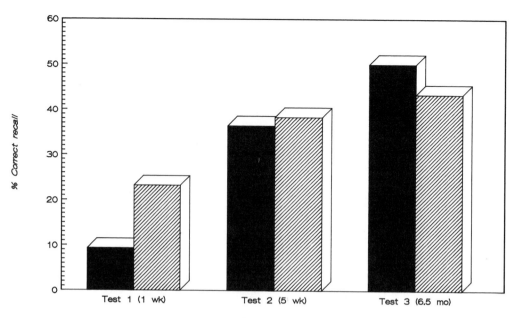

Figure 6.12 Percent correct recall from the left and right ears in a patient with a left-sided hemorrhage due to an arteriovenous malformation (*AVM*) resulting in motor aphasia. The patient was tested on three occasions. (Data from Hugdahl, Wester, and Asbjørnsen, 1990.)

Thus, recovery of, e.g., language function after stroke would then correlate with a shift from an LEA to an REA as recovery progresses. Such a relationship was found by Niccum and colleagues (1986) who studied aphasic patients. However, extent of language recovery was not related to changes in ear scores. Niccum et al. (1986) stressed the importance of the dichotic test in picking up changes occurring in the superior temporal lobe. Following up on this, we recently had the opportunity to repeatedly test a male aphasic patient from the acute phase to recovery after 6.5 months (Hugdahl et al., 1990). He was tested with the DL CV test on three occasions during his clinical recovery. The patient, a young man, was acutely admitted to the hospital for an intracerebral hemorrhage caused by an arteriovenous malformation (AVM) underlying Broca's area. At the first DL test (after 1 week) he could not speak, but understood well. He was therefore required to point at a large paperboard to indicate which syllable he heard on each trial. At the second test (after 5 weeks) he uttered one-syllable words, and could answer yes and no to questions. At the third test he could speak whole sentences, although slowly and stutteringly. His results on the DL test are shown in figure 6.12, and they closely parallel his clinical recovery. Note that the patient pointed at the syllable he heard on each trial at all three test occasions.

On the first test, the patient showed an LEA and his overall performance was reduced compared to what might be expected from someone his age. On the second test, his overall performance increased, particularly his right ear scores, and he showed about an equal percentage of correct reports from the right and left ears, i.e., an NEA. On the third test his overall performance was in the normal range for his age group, and he showed an REA, with about a 10% difference between the ears. Thus, this patient clearly demonstrated a parallel in the development of DL performance and language recovery after left-sided stroke.

In this chapter I have presented data on DL performance on CV syllables from a large number of subjects (N > 400). In general, the results showed an REA in about 80% of subjects, and in 65% of left-handers. The magnitude of the REA is usually in the region of 10% to 15%, while overall performance is between 80% and 95% correct reports. Children usually have lower scores compared to adults, although the REA is a robust finding among children down to the age of 5 years. Thus, the REA to CV syllables seems to be a genuine empirical phenomenon, easily replicated in almost any population studied. Although the REA is related to the anatomic structure of the auditory system, and to the structural organization of the two cerebral hemispheres of the brain, there is no doubt that dynamic cognitive and emotional factors can influence the magnitude of the ear advantage. This is probably best seen in the so-called forced-attention paradigm (Hugdahl and Andersson, 1986) in which adults can switch to an LEA by focusing on the left ear input and only reporting from that ear. Children, though, have difficulties performing this attentional switch, especially before the age of 9, which may be related to the acquisition of reading and writing skills.

In addition to attention, transient changes in activation and arousal also influences the ear advantage, particularly the threat of aversive events. This may reflect a right hemisphere saliency for negative affect which changes the balance between the hemispheres in activation level for processing of dichotic stimuli.

The study of patients with specified lesions in the left or right side of the brain may yield valuable insights into the functional basis of ear advantages in DL. The data presented from a series of case studies provide an empirical underpinning for the theoretical argument made in this chapter, that ear advantages in DL are founded on a hard-wired difference between the left and right hemisphere in processing capacity. This hard-wiring can, however, be modulated by such factors as attention, arousal, spatial orientation, and the nature of the stimulus to be processed. It is also argued here that the right hemisphere is not a passive "slave," acting only as a relay station for the left ear signal. As data from both normals and brain-lesioned patients have shown, the right hemisphere does process the left ear stimulus to some degree, even when the stimulus is a CV syllable. The DL technique is therefore a simple, but reliable, method for precise probing of the functional status of both the left and right temporal cortex.

ACKNOWLEDGMENTS

The present study was supported financially by the Norwegian Council for Research in the Social Sciences (NAVF-RSF) and by Nansenfondet. Special thanks to the neurosurgery department at the Hankelund University Hospital.

REFERENCES

Andersson, B., and Hugdahl, K. (1987). Effects of sex, age, and forced attention on dichotic listening in children: A longitudinal study. *Developmental Neuropsychology, 3,* 191–206.

Asbjørnsen, A., and Hugdahl, K. (submitted for publication, 1993). Attentional effects in dichotic listening.

Asbjørnsen, A., Hugdahl, K., and Bryden, M.P. (1992). Manipulations of subjects' level of arousal in dichotic listening. *Brain and Cognition, 19,* 183–194.

Asbjørnsen, A., Hugdahl, K., and Hynd, G. (1990). The effects of head and eye turns on the right ear advantage in dichotic listening. *Brain and Language, 39,* 447–458.

Bakker, D. J. (1969). Ear asymmetry with monaural stimulation: Task influences. *Cortex, 5,* 36–42.

Bakker, D. J. (1970). Ear-asymmetry with monaural stimulation: Relations to lateral dominance and lateral awareness. *Neuropsychologia, 8,* 103–117.

Bakker, D. J., and Kappers, E. J. (1988). Dichotic listening and reading (dis)ability. In K. Hugdahl (Ed.), *Handbook of dichotic listening: Method, theory, and research* (pp 513–526). Chichester, England: John Wiley & Sons.

Bakker, D. J., Van der Flugt, H., and Claushuis, M. (1978). The reliability of dichotic ear asymmetry in normal children. *Neuropsychologia, 16,* 753–757.

Bertelson, P. (1982). Lateral differences in normal man and lateralization of brain function. *International Journal of Psychology, 17,* 173–210.

Blackstock, E. G. (1978). Cerebral asymmetry and the development of early infantile autism. *Journal of Autism and Childhood Schizophrenia, 8,* 339–353.

Blumstein, S., and Cooper, W. E. (1974). Hemispheric processing of intonation contours. *Cortex, 10,* 146–158.

Bradshaw, J. L., Burden, V., and Nettleton, N. C. (1986). Dichotic and dichaptic techniques. *Neuropsychologia, 24,* 79–90.

Bradshaw, J. L., and Nettleton, N. C. (1988). Monaural asymmetries. In K. Hugdahl (Ed.), *Handbook of dichotic listening: Theory, methods and research.* Chichester, England: John Wiley & Sons.

Broadbent, D. E. (1954). The role of auditory localization in attention and memory span. *Journal of Experimental Psychology, 47,* 191–196.

Brodal, A. (1981). *Neurological anatomy in relation to clinical medicine,* (ed 3). New York, NY: Oxford University Press.

Bruder, G. E. (1983). Cerebral laterality and psychopathology: A review of dichotic listening studies. *Schizophrenia Bulletin, 9,* 134–151

Brugge, J. F., and Reale, R. A. (1985). Auditory cortex. In A. Peters and E. G. Jones (Eds.), *Cerebral cortex,* New York, NY: Plenum Press.

Bryden, M. P. (1988). Dichotic studies of the lateralization of affect in normal subjects. In K. Hugdahl (Ed.), *Handbook of dichotic listening: Theory, methods, and research*. Chichester, England: John Wiley & Sons.

Bryden, M. P., and Allard, F. A. (1978). Dichotic listening and the development of linguistic processes. In M. Kinsbourne (Ed.), *Asymmetrical function of the brain* (pp 392–404). New York, NY: Cambridge University Press.

Bryden, M. P., and MacRae, L. (1988). Dichotic laterality effects obtained with emotional words. *Neuropsychiatry, Neuropsychology, and Behavioral Neurology, 1*, 171–176.

Bryden, M. P., Munhall, K., and Allard, F. (1983). Attentional biases and the right-ear effect in dichotic listening. *Brain and Language, 18*, 236–248.

Carlsson, G., Hugdahl, K., Uvebrant, P., Wiklund, L.-M., and von Wendt, L. (1992). Pathological left-handedness revisited: Dichotic listening in children with left vs. right congenital hemiplegia. *Neuropsychologia, 30*, 471–481.

Carmon, A., and Nachshon, I. (1973). Ear asymmetry in perception of emotional non-verbal stimuli. *Acta Psychologica, 37*, 351–357.

Cherry, E. C. (1953). Some experiments on the recognition of speech with one and two ears. *Journal of the Acoustical Society of America, 25*, 975–979.

Christianson, S.-Å., Nilsson, L.-G., and Silfvenius, H. (1986). Initial memory deficits and subsequent recovery in two cases of head trauma. *Scandinavian Journal of Psychology, 28*, 267–280.

Clark, C. R., Geffen, L. B., and Geffen, G. (1988). Invariant properties of auditory perceptual asymmetry assessed by dichotic listening. In K. Hugdahl (Ed.), *Handbook of dichotic listening: Theory, methods and research*. Chichester, England: John Wiley & Sons.

Cohen, M., Hynd, G., and Hugdahl, L. (1992). Dichotic listening performance in subtypes of developmental dyslexia and a left temporal lobe tumour contrast group. *Brain and Language, 42*, 187–202.

Corteen, R. S., and Wood, B. (1972). Autonomic responses to shock-associated words in an unattended channel. *Journal of Experimental Psychology, 94*, 308–313.

Crawford, H. J., Crawford, K., and Koperski, B. J. (1983). Hypnosis and lateral cerebral function as assessed by dichotic listening. *Biological Psychiatry, 18*, 415–427.

Darley, D. L. (1972). The efficacy of language rehabilitation in aphasia. *Journal of Speech and Hearing Research, 37*, 3–21.

Dawson, M.E., and Schell, A. M. (1982). Electrodermal responses to attended and nonattended significant stimuli during dichotic listening. *Journal of Experimental Psychology: Human Perception and Performance, 8*, 82–86.

Eslinger, P. J., and Damasio, H. (1988). Anatomical correlates of paradoxic ear extinction. In K. Hugdahl (Ed.), *Handbook of dichotic listening: Theory, methods, and research*. Chichester, England: John Wiley & Sons.

Fennell, E. B. (1986). Handedness in neuropsychological research. In J. Hannay (Ed.), *Experimental techniques in human neuropsychology* (pp 15–44). New York, NY: Oxford University Press.

Frumkin, L. R., Ripley, H. S., and Cox, G. B. (1978). Changes in cerebral hemispheric lateralization with hypnosis. *Biological Psychiatry, 13*, 741–750.

Geffen, G., and Quinn, K. (1984). Hemispheric specialization and ear advantages in processing speech. *Psychological Bulletin, 96*, 273–291.

Haggard, M., and Parkinson, A. M. (1971). Stimulus and task factors as determinants of ear advantages. *Quarterly Journal of Experimental Psychology, 23,* 168–177.

Harper, L. V., and Kraft, R. H. (1986). Lateralization of receptive language in preschoolers: Test-retest reliability in a dichotic listening task. *Developmental Psychology, 22,* 553–556.

Heilman, K. M., and Van Den Abell, T. (1979). Right hemisphere dominance for mediating cerebral activation. *Neuropsychologia, 17,* 315–321.

Hillyard, S. A., Hink, R. F., Schwent, V. L., and Picton, T. W. (1973). Electrical signs of selective attention in the human brain. *Science, 182,* 177–180.

Hiscock, M., and Kinsbourne, M. (1977). Selective listening asymmetry in preschool children. *Developmental Psychology, 13,* 217–224.

Hiscock, M., and Stewart, C. (1984). The effect of asymmetrically focused attention upon subsequent ear differences in dichotic listening. *Neuropsychologia, 22,* 337–351.

Hockey, R. (1979). Stress and the cognitive components of skilled performance. In V. Hamilton and D. M. Warburton (Eds.), *Human stress and cognition: An information processing perspective.* Chichester, England: John Wiley & Sons.

Holender, D. (1986). Semantic activation without conscious identification in dichotic listening, parafoveal vision, and visual masking: A survey and appraisal. *Behavioral and Brain Sciences, 9,* 1–66.

Hugdahl, K. (1988). (Ed.). *Handbook of dichotic listening: Theory, methods, and research.* Chichester, England: John Wiley & Sons.

Hugdahl. K. (1992a). Brain lateralization: Dichotic listening studies. In B. Smith and G. Adelman (Eds), *Encyclopedia of neuroscience: Neuroscience year 2.* Boston, MA: Birkhauser.

Hugdahl, K. (1992b). A practical guide to dichotic listening in children. In M. Tramontana and R. Hooper (Eds.). *Advances in child neuropsychology,* Vol. 1. New York, NY: Springer-Verlag.

Hugdahl, K., and Andersson, B. (1987). Dichotic listening and reading acquisition in children: A one-year follow-up. *Journal of Clinical and Experimental Neuropsychology, 9,* 631–649.

Hugdahl, K., and Andersson, B. (1989). Dichotic listening in 126 left-handed children: Ear advantages, familial sinistrality, and sex differences. *Neuropsychologia, 27,* 999–1006.

Hugdahl, K., and Andersson, L. (1986). The "forced-attention paradigm" in dichotic listening to CV-syllables: A comparison between adults and children. *Cortex, 22,* 417–432.

Hugdahl, K., Asbjørnsen, A., and Wester, K. (1993). Memory performance in Parkinson's disease. *Neuropsychiatry, Neuropsychology, and Behavioral Neurology, 6,* 170–176.

Hugdahl, K., and Brobeck, C. G. (1986). Hemispheric asymmetry and human electrodermal conditioning: The dichotic extinction paradigm. *Psychophysiology, 23,* 491–499.

Hugdahl, K., and Wester, K. (1992). Dichotic listening studies of hemispheric asymmetries in brain damaged patients. *International Journal of Neuroscience, 63,* 17–29.

Hugdahl, K., Wester, K., and Asbjørnsen, A. (1990). Dichotic listening in aphasic male patient after a subcortical hemorrhage in the left fronto-parietal region. *International Journal of Neuroscience, 54,* 139–146.

Jäncke, L., Steinmetz, H., and Volkmann, J. (1992). Dichotic listening: What does it measure? *Neuropsychologia, 30,* 941–950.

Kimura, D. (1961). Cerebral dominance and the perception of verbal stimuli. *Canadian Journal of Psychology, 15,* 166–171.

Kimura, D. (1967). Functional asymmetry of the brain in dichotic listening. *Cortex, 3,* 163–168.

Kinsbourne, M. (1970). The cerebral basis of lateral asymmetries in attention. *Acta Psychologica, 33,* 193–201.

Kinsbourne, M. (1974). Mechanisms of hemispheric interaction in man. In M. Kinsbourne and W. L. Smith (Eds.), *Hemispheric disconnection and cerebral function.* Springfield, IL.: Charles C Thomas.

Lauter, J. (1982). Dichotic identification of complex sounds: Absolute and relative ear advantage. *Journal of the Acoustical Society of America, 71,* 701–707.

Levy, J. Heller, W., Banich, M. T., and Burton, L. A. (1983). Are variations among right-handed individuals in perceptual asymmetries caused by characteristic arousal differences between hemispheres? *Journal of Experimental Psychology: Human Perception and Performance, 9,* 329–359.

Ley, R. G., and Bryden, M. P. (1982). A dissociation of right and left hemispheric effects for recognizing emotional tone and verbal content. *Brain and Cognition, 1,* 3–9.

Milner, B., Taylor, L., and Sperry, R.W. (1968). Lateralized suppression of dichotically presented digits after commissural section in man. *Science, 161,* 184–186.

Molfese, D. L., and Molfese, V. J. (1979). Hemisphere and stimulus differences as reflected in the cortical responses of newborn infants to speech stimuli. *Developmental Psychology, 15,* 505–511.

Mondor, T. A., and Bryden, M. P. (1991). The influence of attention on the dichotic REA. *Neuropsychologia, 29,* 1179–1190.

Moray, N. (1959). Attention in dichotic listening: Affect cues and the influence of instructions. *Quarterly Journal of Experimental Psychology, 9,* 56–60.

Morton, L. L., and Kershner, J. R. (1991). Effects of time-of-day on neuropsychological testing as measured by dichotic listening. *International Journal of Neuroscience, 59,* 241–251.

Näätänen, R. (1982). Processing negativity: An evoked potential reflection of selective attention. *Psychological Bulletin, 92,* 605–640.

Näätänen, R. (1990). The role of attention in auditory information processing as revealed by event-related potentials and other brain measures of cognitive function. *Behavioral and Brain Sciences, 13,* 201–288.

Nachshon, I. (1980). Hemispheric dysfunctioning in schizophrenia. *Journal of Nervous and Mental Disease, 168,* 241–242.

Nerad, L. (1992). *Dichotic listening* dissertation, Czechoslovak Academy of Sciences, Prague.

Niccum, N., Selnes, O. A., Speaks, C., Risse, G. L., and Rubens, A. B. (1986). Longitudinal dichotic listening patterns for aphasic patients III. *Brain and Language, 28,* 303–317.

Obrzut, J. E., and Boliek, C. A. (1988). Dichotic listening: Evidence from learning and reading disabled children. In K. Hugdahl (Ed.), *Handbook of dichotic listening: Theory, methods, and research* (pp 475–512). Chichester, England: John Wiley & Sons.

Palmer, R. D. (1964). Cerebral dominance and auditory asymmetry. *Journal of Psychology, 58,* 157–167.

Pierson, J. M., Bradshaw, J. L., and Nettleton, N. C. (1983). Head and body space to left and right, front and rear—1. Unidirectional competitive auditory stimulation. *Neuropsychologia, 21,* 463–473.

Price, C., Wise, R., Ramsay, S., Friston, K., Howard, D., Patterson, K., and Frackowiak, R. (1992). Regional response differences within the human auditory cortex when listening to words. *Neuroscience Letters, 146,* 179–182.

Rasmussen, T., and Milner, B. (1977). The role of early left-brain injury in determining lateralization of cerebral speech function. In S. J. Dimond and D. A. Blizzard (Eds.), Evolution and lateralization of the brain. *Annals of the New York Academy of Sciences, 229*, 355–369.

Repp, B. (1977). Measuring laterality effects in dichotic listening. *Journal of the Acoustical Society of America, 42*, 720–737.

Reuter-Lorentz, P., and Davidson, R. J. (1981). Differential contribution of the two cerebral hemispheres to the perception of happy and sad faces. *Neuropsychologia, 19*, 609–613.

Roberts, R. J., Varney, N. R., Paulsen, J. S., and Richardson, E. D. (1990). Dichotic listening and complex partial seizures. *Journal of Clinical and Experimental Neuropsychology, 12*, 448–458.

Schwartz, J., and Tallal, P. (1980). Rate of acoustic change may underlie hemispheric specialization for speech perception. *Science, 207*, 1380–1381.

Sidtïs, J. J. (1988). Dichotic listening after commissurotomy. In K. Hugdahl (Ed.), *Dichotic listening: Theory, methods, and research*. Chichester, England: John Wiley & Sons.

Sparks, R., and Geschwind, N. (1968). Dichotic listening in man after section of neocortical commissure. *Cortex, 4*, 3–16.

Sparks, R., Goodglass, H., and Nickel, B. (1970). Ipsilateral versus contralateral extinction in dichotic listening resulting from hemispheric lesions. *Cortex, 6*, 249–260.

Speaks, C., Niccum, N., and Carney, E. (1982). Statistical properties of responses to dichotic listening with CV nonsense syllables. *Journal of the Acoustical Society of America, 72*, 1185–1194.

Spreen, O., and Strauss, E. (1991). *A compendium of neuropsychological tests*. New York, NY: Oxford University Press.

Springer, S., and Deutsch, G. (1989). *Left brain, right brain*. San Francisco: W. H. Freeman & Co.

Strauss, E. (1988). Dichotic listening and Sodium-Amytal: Functional and morphological aspects of hemispheric asymmetry. In K. Hugdahl (Ed.), *Handbook of dichotic listening: Theory, methods and research*. Chichester, England: John Wiley & Sons.

Strauss, E., Gaddes, W. H., and Wada, J. (1987). Performance on a free-recall verbal dichotic listening task and cerebral speech dominance determined by the carotid amytal test. *Neuropsychologia, 25*, 747–755.

Studdert-Kennedy, M., and Shankweiler, D. P. (1970). Hemispheric specialization for speech perception. *Journal of the Acoustical Society of America, 48*, 579–594.

Tartter, V. C. (1988). Acoustic and phonetic feature effects in dichotic listening. In K. Hugdahl (Ed.), *Handbook of dichotic listening: Theory, methods, and research* (pp 283–321). Chichester, England: John Wiley & Sons.

Treisman, A. M. (1964). Selective attention in man. *British Medical Bulletin, 20*, 12–16.

Tucker, D. M. (1981). Lateral brain function, emotion and conceptualization. *Psychological Bulletin, 89*, 19–46.

Wester, K. (1992). Gender distribution and sidedness of middle fossa arachnoid cysts: A review of cases diagnosed with computed imaging. *Neurosurgery, 31*, 940–944.

Wexler, B. E. (1986). Alterations in cerebral laterality during acute psychotic illness. *British Journal of Psychiatry, 149*, 202–209.

Wexler, B. E., Schwartz, G., Warrenburg, S., Servis, M., and Tarlatzis, I. (1986). Effects of emotion on perceptual asymmetry: Interactions with personality. *Neuropsychologia, 24*, 699–710.

Witelson, S. F., and Pallie, W. (1973). Left-hemisphere specialization for language in the human newborn: Neuroanatomic evidence of asymmetry. *Brain, 96*, 641–646.

7 Hemispheric Contribution to Face Processing: Patterns of Convergence and Divergence

Justine Sergent

The idea that the brain is organized into distinct areas of relative functional autonomy and specialization is a basic principle of cognitive neuroscience. This principle is supported and illustrated by the selectivity of behavioral and mental deficits that result from focal cerebral injury, and it governs the research aimed at understanding brain-behavior relationships. It implies that the brain realizes its functions by the conjoint activation of several of its component structures, each performing specific operations, and one of the goals of cognitive neuroscience is to uncover *what* operations are performed by each of these structures and *how* these operations are coordinated and related to one another to produce adapted behavior. Because the logic of the underlying processes cannot be operationalized at a neurophysiologic level, the understanding of brain-behavior relationships must rely on a clear and exhaustive description of the processes at a psychological level. Psychological and cognitive functions are no longer viewed as made of unitary processes (e.g., reading, writing, object recognition) but rather as being composed of several subprocesses (e.g., featural analysis, structural encoding, activation of biographic memories) organized in specific ways (e.g., in parallel or in succession, independently or interactively), and the cognitive architecture of mental functions is best characterized by a compartmented organization of interactive components. It is therefore through a decomposition of a given function into its component operations, thus providing a theoretical framework specifying the nature, the goals, the logical order, and the interactive relations of the processing steps to be performed for the realization of the function under study, that a better specification of the functional organization of the cerebral cortex can be achieved. The understanding of brain-behavior relationships can then be conceived of as an enterprise that aims at mapping a fractionated set of interrelated mental operations underlying cognitive functions onto their corresponding interconnected cerebral structures.

Such an enterprise is confronted with a variety of theoretical and methodologic problems. First and foremost, there is no guarantee that the brain divides its functions according to the psychological principles we apply to describe the component subprocesses that make up mental functions. A conceptual decomposition of a cognitive function does not necessarily correspond to the cerebral fractionation of its realization. What is considered as a single mental operation may in fact be implemented in the brain by the interactive recruitment of several structures. For instance, what can be described, at a psychological level, under the unitary concept of spatial function is not necessarily performed by a single processing structure, located in one hemisphere, at an anatomic level. In addition, even if there is evidence supporting a structural and functional *modular* organization of the brain, as indicated by the selectivity of cognitive impairments following focal brain damage, there is also considerable evidence pointing to the close interdependence of cerebral structures (e.g., Mesulam, 1990; Felleman and Van Essen, 1991), and the modularity of the brain is embedded within a highly *interactive* nervous system (Sergent, 1984b). Yet, in spite of the current state of knowledge of structures and connections of the primate brain underlying visual cognition—for example, 32 distinct visual areas have been identified in the monkey's brain, with more than 300 connecting pathways among these areas (Felleman and Van Essen, 1991)—the methods currently available for uncovering human brain-behavior relationships impose limitations on the level of sophistication that can be achieved, especially when dealing with higher-order cognitive processes.

The understanding of the neurofunctional organization of cerebral structures is further complicated by the asymmetric distribution of functions in the brain and by the fact that the two cerebral hemispheres are simultaneously active in the realization of any higher-order cognitive function. Whereas it is firmly established that the hemispheres are not functionally equivalent and are endowed with processing abilities unique to each one, there is no simple way of uncovering how they join their respective resources and conjointly contribute to the performance of a given task. The large variety, if not inconsistency, of findings related to cerebral lateralization of functions attests to the complexity of the phenomenon and illustrates the involvement of many factors in determining the particular contribution of each hemisphere to the realization of specific cognitive activities. The purpose of this chapter is to address some questions related to the study of cerebral lateralization by focusing on one particular area of research, that of face processing, and by examining what different approaches, and different subject populations, tell us about the functional organization of the brain.

It is important to note that the issue of the functional asymmetry of the hemispheres is only one aspect of the larger problem of the neurofunctional organization of cerebral structures. Although it is often convenient to speak of the left and the right hemispheres as single entities with their specific and unique processing abilities, this is of little help for the understanding of the actual role played by each hemisphere and of the distribution of competences between the two hemispheres. There probably is more similarity in processing ability between two homotopic areas of the two hemispheres than between two distinct areas of the same hemisphere. Therefore, attributing a "processing style" to one hemisphere in the realization of a given function cannot inform us much about the underlying organization of the cerebral hemispheres, unless one specifies the actual operations performed by that hemisphere, how this processing style influences the respective operations carried out by each hemisphere, and how the implementation of each hemisphere's operations is coordinated.

In this chapter, I first briefly describe diverse approaches to which different populations can be subjected in order to obtain relevant information about functional hemispheric asymmetry, and I then present a general model of face processing that will guide the various questions to be asked when examining the neurofunctional organization of cerebral structures. Subsequently, I briefly review the main findings bearing on hemispheric asymmetry in face processing and finally I discuss areas of convergence and divergence from different techniques and populations.

DIFFERENT TECHNIQUES AND POPULATIONS

Research on hemispheric asymmetry has benefited from a large variety of techniques that can be used to make inferences about the role of each cerebral hemisphere in the control of behavior. Some techniques are highly democratic, such as dichhaptic tests for somatosensory functions or lateral tachistoscopic presentations for visual functions, as they are inexpensive, easy to apply, and, therefore, available to any researcher interested in this issue. On the other hand, other techniques are restricted to a few privileged centers, such as event-related potentials (ERPs), magnetoencephalography, or positron emission tomography (PET), and they allow correlations to be made between neurophysiologic activity and behavioral manifestation of cerebral processing. This variety of techniques can be seen as a blessing, because, despite the diversity and contradictions that sometimes result from their application, each provides a unique sample of brain functioning, tapping different levels of processing, and together they may offer a broader, yet better constrained, picture of the functional organization of the brain. The same applies to the diversity of populations that can be subjected to the study of hemispheric asymmetry, and the different conclusions that would sometimes impose themselves from the pattern of results of normal and neurologic subjects in fact contain in themselves information about the dynamic effects of brain damage on processing. In this sense, divergences of findings are as important and revealing as convergences and need not necessarily be dismissed as nuisance. Inasmuch as a study is properly controlled, its findings constitute a faithful manifestation of cerebral activity associated to specific mental operations and may therefore lend themselves to valid inferences about brain-behavior relationships.

Studies of Brain-damaged Patients

The main source of information about the neurobiological substrates of cognition in humans has, for a long time, come from the study of brain-damaged patients, and it is essentially obtained through two distinct but complementary approaches. One is the anatomicoclinical method that seeks to establish correlations between the site of a lesion and the patterns of successes and failures on behavioral tasks, in an attempt to identify the contribution of the damaged cerebral area to cognition (e.g., Hécaen and Albert, 1978; McCarthy and Warrington, 1990). This approach generally involves group studies and it focuses primarily on the locus of the lesion responsible for specific impairments in broadly defined functions rather than on the nature and properties of the processes normally underlying the defective function. It is thus concerned with averages or general trends, and by so doing runs the risk of arriving at conclusions that do not necessarily reflect the true nature of the deficit. For instance, if performance by a group of brain-damaged patients on a given task is bimodal, then the "average" performance used to characterize the group may not be a genuine description of the actual capacities of any of these patients. Nonetheless, when the purpose of a study is to uncover the contribution of a specific cerebral area to cognitive functions, studying patients with damage in this particular area and examining their performance provide a straightforward manner of determining which functions this area may be participating in. In addition, group study does not preclude examination of individual data, and as long as interpretations take full account of its limitations, this type of study can offer valuable information.

The other approach is computationally oriented, relies essentially on single-case studies, and uses the examination of brain-damaged patients to infer the functional architecture of cognition from the pattern of disruption that characterizes the cognitive breakdown, generally irrespective of the actual site and nature of the cerebral lesion (e.g., Shallice, 1988; Caramazza and Badecker, 1989). Such an approach imposes an in-depth examination of the patient so as to achieve a detailed description of the pattern of spared and defective functions. On the other hand, this approach runs the risk of giving undue importance to idiosyncrasies, makes generalizations across patients more difficult to achieve, and may lead to the creation of as many ad hoc models as there are single patients examined, because no two patients are ever exactly alike. In spite of the current debate over the respective merits of these two approaches (e.g., Caramazza vs. Zurif, in successive issues of *Brain and Cognition*, 1989–1992), and notwithstanding their inherent limitations, both have the potential to yield relevant and complementary information, and together may contribute to achieve a more exhaustive and comprehensive specification of the mapping of mental functions onto cerebral structures.

Two special categories of patients have been of particular importance in the study of hemispheric asymmetry. One category consists of those epileptic patients whose neocommissures have been severed for the relief of intractable epilepsy and whose cerebral hemispheres have thus become disconnected ("split brain"). Such patients may appear as ideal for examining the respective competence of each cerebral hemisphere and, indeed, early experiments by Sperry and his collaborators (1969) launched the modern study of hemispheric specialization. One may add, however, that the split-brain model has often been transposed uncritically to the normal brain which has been conceived of as if its two hemispheres engaged as little as possible in interhemispheric communication. Such a split-brain model has contributed strongly to examining the question of hemispheric asymmetry from a *specialization* point of view, at the expense of the equally important aspect of interhemispheric *communication*. There would be no functional "specialization" if the two hemispheres could not communicate between one another, and there would be no need for communication if the two hemispheres were not functionally specialized.

The second category of patients concerns hemispherectomized subjects in whom one hemisphere has been ablated as a result of massive damage that disturbed the functioning of the intact hemisphere. When such an ablation is performed at a young age, some subjects later exhibit relatively few sequelae at the higher-order cognitive level. The fact that a single hemisphere, in some patients, can sustain nearly all major cognitive functions at a level of efficiency comparable to that of normal subjects with two intact hemispheres (Smith and Sugar, 1975) is a clear illustration that the cerebral lateralization of functions is a developmental process during which the two hemispheres normally interact in distributing and acquiring their respective competences (see Sergent, 1989b). On the other hand, hemispherectomy at the adult age results in severe deficits not easily compensated for by the remaining intact hemisphere (Villemure and Sergent, in press). These two categories of patients offer relevant information about the competence of one hemisphere taken in isolation, but there is no guarantee that the mode of operation of an isolated hemisphere corresponds to how it would operate if it were to work in conjunction with the other hemisphere (cf. Sergent, 1990).

Studies of Normal Subjects

The study of brain-behavior relationships has also relied on techniques derived from experimental psychology to examine the respective contribution of the *intact* cerebral hemispheres to cognitive functions. In the visual modality, this approach takes advantage of the anatomic arrangement of the visual pathways whereby information appearing in one half of the visual field is initially, and entirely, projected to the contralateral hemisphere. By restricting stimulus presentation to the retinal lateral periphery, and by observing the manner in which the speed and accuracy of responses to various types of stimuli and task requirements differ as a function of field of presentation, it is possible to make inferences about the functional asymmetry of the cerebral hemispheres (e.g., Sergent, 1983; Hellige, 1993). Although such a technique is necessarily coarse with respect to the cerebral localization of functions, the manipulation of stimulus and task variables and the examination of the resulting interactions in the patterns of performance provide information regarding hemispheric specialization and cooperation and how the brain organizes and distributes its resources at a hemispheric level. The difficulties associated with this approach are multifold (e.g., Hellige and Sergent, 1986; Sergent and Hellige, 1986), and they lie at the procedural, experimental, theoretical, and interpretative levels. Thus, performance may vary as a function of apparently trivial factors like exposure duration or retinal eccentricity, so that a given finding is dependent on a specific set of procedural parameters, and patterns of interaction rather than main effects of hemispheric superiority have to be considered. In addition, there is, at present, very little understanding of the distribution and unfolding, within cerebral structures, of the information to be processed after unilateral stimulation, and despite interesting suggestions to disentangle alternative interpretations (e.g., Zaidel, 1983; Hellige, 1993), it remains unclear what actually accounts for visual-field asymmetries and what the relation is between hemispheric processing superiority and visual-field advantage. Yet, as will be discussed later, this approach provides pertinent data about dynamic factors of brain processing and hemispheric interactions that are not as easily obtainable with other approaches.

A more recent approach to uncovering the functional organization of the *normal* human brain consists in PET measurements of local changes in cerebral blood flow (CBF) during the performance of behavioral or mental tasks. With the advance in activation techniques (Raichle et al., 1983), data analyses (Mintun, Fox, and Raichle, 1989), and stereotactic mapping of physiologic changes (Fox, Perlmutter, and Raichle, 1985; Evans et al., 1988), local CBF increases underlying sensory and motor processing can be detected reliably and translated into images of the activated cerebral structures highlighting the areas participating in the realization of a given function (e.g., Lueck et al., 1989). The introduction of paired-image subtraction and intersubject averaging (Fox et al., 1988) has enhanced the sensitivity of PET measurements of regional CBF (rCBF) and has further opened the way to the study of anatomic-functional correlations of higher-order cognitive processing whose neural substrates are more broadly distributed and less intensively activated than are primary sensory and motor cerebral areas. The use of short-lived isotopes (such as ^{15}O) allowing successive tasks in the same subjects, and the application of the subtraction method whereby measurements made in a control task are subtracted from those made in a functionally activated state (Raichle, 1990) in order to "isolate" the cerebral areas concerned with the operations that differentiate the two tasks, have given the opportunity to map the functional organization of the brain underlying cognition in neurologically intact subjects (e.g., Petersen et al., 1989; Posner et al., 1988).

This approach is not immune to methodologic and theoretical difficulties, however, and there are a large number of problems that have to be surmounted to obtain reliable data that lend themselves to unequivocal interpretations. Among such problems, some are worth mentioning, such as (1) the morphologic variability of cerebral structures across subjects, which makes the averaging procedure of activation data questionable, although normalization can be achieved through stereotactic mapping (Evans et al., 1989); (2) because of the low temporal resolution of the technique, the required scanning time (about 40–60 seconds) implies that the actual data are an accumulation of neural activity over time during which *all* mental operations performed by the subject contribute to the total activation in each scanned area, whether or not these operations were relevant to the task; (3) the assumptions that underlie the use of the subtraction method to isolate the cerebral structures specifically involved in the component operations that differentiate two tasks violate some basic properties of cerebral processing (Sergent et al., 1992b); (4) the choice of "control" tasks whose activation is subtracted from that of the "experimental" task is of utmost importance in the design of cognitive PET studies, because the pattern of blood flow changes resulting from the subtraction (and, therefore, considered as reflecting the involvement of the activated areas in the operations specific to the experimental task) is dependent on the activation associated with the control task (see Sergent et al., 1992b). More critically with respect to the study of cerebral lateralization, one still does not know how hemispheric *superiority* manifests itself in terms of changes in CBF. For instance, one could assume that the higher the CBF in a given area, the more involved this area is in the process under study, and, therefore, one may infer that it is specialized for this particular process; alternatively, it is conceivable that the higher the CBF in a given area, the less competent this area is, as the larger activation may reflect the greater difficulty of this area in performing the operations inherent in the task (see Sergent, 1990, for further discussion). Each of these potential problems needs to be further examined and resolved in order to ensure that cognitive PET studies produce reliable findings. As it currently stands, the probability is high that many failures to replicate will emerge as a result of a lack of control and understanding of many parameters that have a nontrivial influence on cognitive processing and its measurement and monitoring.

Nonetheless, when considered within the aforementioned theoretical framework and experimental approaches, the study of the structural and functional organization of cognition and its asymmetric disposition in the cerebral hemispheres may proceed with fewer degrees of freedom as findings from different sources provide converging evidence and constrain one another for their interpretation. In addition, this multidisciplinary procedure offers the possibility to better identify the strengths and weaknesses of each approach by comparing areas of convergence and divergence between these different sources. The remainder of this chapter is devoted to describing such a research strategy in the study of face processing in an attempt to (1) uncover the cerebral structures underlying these functions, the specific roles of these structures, and the interrelationships among them, and (2) identify and better understand the respective merits and limits of different experimental approaches to the understanding of the neurobiological substrates of cognition.

PROCESSING OF FACES

Inquiry into the processes underlying the perception and recognition of faces has led to the development of computational models that describe the various

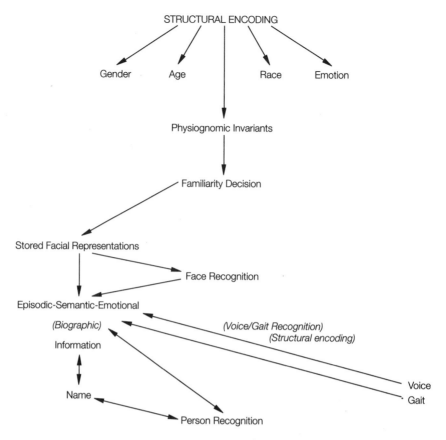

Figure 7.1 Schematic description of some of the steps leading from the perception of a face to the recognition of the person. (From Sergent, J. (1993). In B. Gylyás, D. Ottoson, and P. Roland (Eds.), *The functional organization of the human visual cortex.* Oxford, England: Pergamon Press.)

operations that must be implemented for a face to become meaningful and be identified. Faces convey a variety of information about individuals. Some of this information is *visually derived* in the sense that it can be accessed on the sole basis of the physical attributes of the physiognomy irrespective of the identity of the individual (e.g., gender, age, emotion, etc.), whereas other information is *semantically derived* in the sense that it can be accessed only after the perceived representation of the face "makes contact" with a corresponding stored representation from which biographic information about the individual can then be reactivated (Bruce and Young, 1986; Young and Bruce, 1991; Sergent, 1989a).

Functional Decomposition of Face Processing

The foregoing considerations suggest the existence of a hierarchic organization of the processes underlying face recognition, which is schematically described in figure 7.1. A first necessary step is a structural encoding of the physical facial information so as to achieve as veridical a description as possible of the attributes and properties of a perceived face. Such a description provides the basis on which all face-related processes begin, and the representations thus derived can highlight different featural or configurational properties of the face depending on the nature of the information the perceiver seeks to obtain from that face. For instance, different combinations of facial features convey the pertinent information about the gender, the age, or the identity of a face (Sergent, 1989a), such that different operations must be performed to have access to the different information contained in a facial description. That is, we do not process the same facial features when determining the gender or the age of a face, and different processes, on different combinations of features, are required to have access to these two types of information.

Access to the identity of the face further requires that the physiognomic invariants that specifically describe a face be recovered from the structural description, as the appearance of faces, their emotion, viewpoints, lighting conditions, and so on, are ever changing and complicate the perceptual operations necessary to uncover what is unique to a face and makes it that of a specific individual. Only if such invariants are detected can a face be perceived as being familiar, which implies the reactivation of stored facial representations. Such a reactivation may then spread to pertinent memories related to the bearer of the face, which includes episodic, semantic, emotional, and other biographic information. From this information also, the name of the person can be accessed, but the name itself is not directly "connected" to the representation of the face, such that a face can be recognized even if the name cannot be recalled. On the other hand, the biographic information accessible from a face can also be accessed from the name, or from other attributes that uniquely discriminate an individual from all others (e.g., voice, gait). Thus, the face is only one among several means by which stored knowledge about an individual can be accessed, and the breakdown of face processing results in prosopagnosia but does not preclude person recognition through other means.

This description of some of the steps inherent in the processing of faces, and its schematic representation in figure 7.1, provide a general outline for the study of the neurobiological bases of face processing. Such a model is obviously meant to be improved, modified, or even disproved, but it has nonetheless received some confirmation in the study of brain-damaged subjects, particularly those rare prosopagnosic patients who find themselves unable to recognize persons they know through the visual inspection of their faces (Sergent and Villemure, 1989; Sergent and Poncet, 1990; Sergent and Signoret, 1992a,b; Young and Bruce, 1991). What the study of these patients has shown is that prosopagnosia, though a functionally well-delineated impairment (i.e., an inability to experience a feeling of familiarity at the view of faces of known persons and, consequently, to identify these faces), may manifest itself differently across patients. Some patients display a complete inability to perform any operation on faces, even to tell men apart from women, and one may therefore assume that their underlying disturbance affects the *structural encoding* stage (see figure 7.1); others, in contrast, have no difficulty in processing the gender, age, or emotion of faces, and even in recognizing different views of the same face as representing the same person, but they are deficient as soon as the identity of the face is a critical factor, suggesting a deficit beyond the *physiognomic invariant* stage but before that calling for a *familiarity decision*. In addition, the deficit in face recognition can be highly selective in most patients, and it does not extend to the recognition of objects, although some, but not all, patients have difficulty in identifying objects of the same category when they are physically similar (e.g., feline animals) and in recognizing objects presented from an unusual viewpoint (Landis et al., 1988).

Although the location of the cerebral lesion varies considerably across these patients, it has been suggested that prosopagnosia is the result of a bilateral posterior damage, involving principally the mesial occipitotemporal junction (Damasio, 1985). Yet the pattern of damage does not conform to this general rule in all patients, and there are cases in which the lesion is unilateral (e.g., Michel, Poncet, and Signoret, 1989) or does not invade the posterior cortex (e.g., Sergent and Poncet, 1990). There are, therefore, variations both in the cognitive stage at which the processing of faces breaks down and the location of the lesion responsible for the prosopagnosic deficit, and these variations cannot easily be accounted for on the sole basis of data from brain-damaged patients, as there may be no two patients showing the same pattern of face-processing impairments, associated deficits, and spared functions. This is further complicated by additional contingencies. For instance, in most patients, the lesion is extensive, such that more cortical tissue than would theoretically be necessary to produce prosopagnosia may be destroyed, which makes it difficult to precisely identify the cortical regions specifically involved in face recognition. Moreover, because structural integrity, as identified from radiologic images such as magnetic resonance imaging (MRI), does not guarantee functional normality, as a result of distant detrimental effects of brain damage, it cannot be unequivocally determined whether the damaged areas are those that normally underlie the processing of faces or whether the lesion also disturbs the processing of adjacent intact regions which normally contribute to face processing (see Sergent, 1984b). A clear example of such a possibility comes from patient P.C. (Sergent and Signoret, 1992b), a long-standing prosopagnosic patient with damage in the white matter surrounding the right lingual and fusiform gyri. MRI of this patient's brain indicated no damage to the cortex of the right fusiform and parahippocampal gyri, yet a fluodeoxyglucose F18 (^{18}FDG) PET study revealed that, metabolically, the posterior ventromedial region of the right hemisphere, including the fusiform and parahippocampal gyri, was totally inactive (Michel et al., 1989), suggesting that, functionally, the cerebral damage was much more extensive than one would have inferred on the basis of the structural (MRI) radiologic data.

The foregoing findings illustrate some of the difficulties inherent in inferring brain-behavior relationships from patterns of functional disturbances and structural damage, and, by the same token, raise a series of questions to which the study of neurologically intact subjects may bring some elements of answers. These questions are concerned with the respective role of the cerebral hemispheres in face processing, the organization of the component operations underlying face recognition, and the nature and properties of the processes performed at each stage. The study of normal subjects through laboratory behavioral experiments is particularly well suited to examining these questions, and research in this area has been especially useful in delineating the various operations inherent in face processing and in producing cognitive models of face recognition (Bruce, 1988; Bruce and Young, 1986; Bruyer, 1989; A. Ellis, 1992; H. Ellis, 1992; Sergent, 1989a; Young and Bruce, 1991). On the other hand, questions bearing on the actual cerebral structures engaged in the processing of faces, the participation of these structures depending on the particular operations to be performed on the facial representations, the extent to which these structures are involved specifically in the processing of faces, contributing to other operations, or to the processing of other categories of objects, all lend themselves to cognitive studies based on the PET methodology, and the next sections describe relevant findings obtained with each of these techniques.

Divided-Visual-Field Studies of Face Processing

As noted earlier, there are considerable inconsistencies across results of divided-visual-field studies, and the investigation of face processing with this technique is no exception. A good deal of progress has been made in uncovering some of the reasons for these inconsistencies (e.g., Hellige and Sergent, 1986; Sergent and Hellige, 1986; Hellige, 1990), and they are worth pointing out.

Some Problems Inherent in Divided-Visual-Field Studies One major reason for these inconsistencies came from the absence until the early 1980s of a cognitive model of face processing. Before then, face processing was considered as a single, monolithic process, and any task involving faces was thought to be well suited to make inferences about the role of the cerebral hemispheres in their processing. In particular, no distinction was made between familiar and unfamiliar faces, and, in fact, most studies involved the presentation of unfamiliar faces. Yet, evidence from brain-damaged patients should have warned researchers that such an approach was inappropriate, as Warrington and James (1967) had shown that there was no correlation between the discrimination of unfamiliar faces and the recognition of familiar faces, and that impairment of these two tasks resulted from lesions in different parts of the cortex. Moreover, Benton and Van Allen (1972) had presented evidence that some prosopagnosic patients, who are no longer able to recognize familiar faces, performed within the normal range on a test requiring the discrimination of unfamiliar faces. As will be discussed later, this distinction between the processing of familiar and unfamiliar faces has received support from PET studies, as different cortical areas are activated depending on the category of faces which are presented.

Related to the distinction between familiar and unfamiliar faces is the variation in processing demands across studies. Faces convey a large variety of information about individuals, and they can be subjected to different operations each of which makes different and specific processing demands. Whereas familiar faces can be subjected to any such operations, a smaller range of operations can be performed on unfamiliar faces which, by definition, have no stored representations in the subjects' memory. Figure 7.1 illustrates some of these variations, and it also makes it clear that even unfamiliar faces lend themselves to different types of operation. That is, age estimation, gender categorization, and emotion recognition each call for a specific set of operations which do not make the same processing requirements and are not necessarily carried out in the same regions of the brain. Different tasks on facial representations may therefore entail the recruitment of different brain regions, and one should expect different patterns of results depending on the type of information being accessed from a face.

Still another set of reasons contributing to inconsistencies across studies is the influence of procedural variables inherent in the design of divided-visual-field experiments. A large number of variables have to be manipulated in such experiments (e.g., exposure duration, luminance, contrast, retinal eccentricity, and so forth), and each of these variables influences performance in a significant, but still incompletely understood way (Sergent, 1983). Because any procedural variable must have some positive value, each contributes, in a very intricate manner, to the final outcome, such that this outcome is a complex interactive function of the particular set of variables under which the experiment was conducted. Although studies have been carried out in an attempt to disentangle the respective contributions of these variables, it is nearly impossible to determine the extent of the contribution of each variable to an observed pattern of results, which makes it necessary to conduct a series of closely related experiments and to focus on interactions between the manipulated variables. Unfortunately, few such studies have been carried out, and it remains difficult to tell unequivocally what accounts for a particular pattern of results in divided-visual-field studies.

Also of importance is the choice of the dependent variable. There is, at present, no clear rationale that would allow a clear justification for opting for latency or accuracy as the main dependent variable. However, the setup of experiments that use one or the other dependent variable may in itself have a nontrivial influence on the outcome. For instance, if latency is the main dependent variable, a small number of errors must be made by the subjects to guarantee a large sample of reaction times which are inherently a highly "noisy" measure of performance (e.g., Takane and Sergent, 1983). Such a high level of accuracy requires high-quality stimulus presentation, which can be accommodated by long exposure, high contrast, and small retinal eccentricity, and these characteristics have been found to bias performance toward a relatively more efficient processing of the left hemisphere (e.g., Sergent, 1983). Conversely, the use of accuracy as the dependent variable requires an experimental design leading to a sufficiently high number of errors for reliable statistical analysis, which in turn imposes experimental conditions that entail less-than-optimal performance. These conditions are obviously different from, and sometimes opposite to, those prevailing in reaction-time experiments, and different patterns of results may thus prevail for reasons that have little to do with the processing demands of the particular task as such.

Hemispheric Contribution to Face Processing   On the basis of the results of divided-visual-field studies of face processing, and assuming that a visual-field advantage implies a processing superiority of the contralateral hemisphere, it would seem justified to conclude that both cerebral hemispheres are equipped with the necessary structures to carry out the discrimination and recognition of faces, as well as the processing of visually derived semantic properties of faces (e.g., age, gender, race). Such a conclusion relies on the fact that one can always find at least one study showing that the left or the right hemisphere is the more competent at any of the operations that have been examined, with one exception. There is, to my knowledge, no lateral tachistoscopic study indicating that the left hemisphere is better than the right at performing delayed matching of faces, whereas there are several studies showing better left hemisphere ability to identify famous or well-known faces (e.g., Marzi and Berlucchi, 1977). This might suggest a special role for the right hemisphere in the initial storage of facial information, but an equal ability of the cerebral hemispheres to access permanently stored facial information.

Most experiments using accuracy as the main dependent variable have yielded a right hemisphere superiority. On the other hand, much of the evidence suggesting a role of the left hemisphere in the processing of faces has been obtained in experiments using latency as the main dependent variable, although not all reaction-time experiments produced a left hemisphere advantage. This makes it difficult to draw definitive conclusions from these studies. Were they the only source of information about the neural bases of face processing, a thorough and systematic examination of the current literature would be necessary. However, because of the complexities and poorly understood intricacies inherent in these studies, such an examination would benefit from findings obtained through other approaches and populations, and more will be said about it toward the end of this chapter.

Studies of Face Processing in Brain-damaged Patients

The study of nonprosopagnosic, unilaterally brain-damaged patients has produced essentially unequivocal evidence of a critical, if not exclusive, role of the right hemisphere in the processing of faces. Group studies by Hécaen (1972), De Renzi, Faglioni, and Spinnler (1968), Benton et al. (1983), and others have shown that a lesion in the posterior region of the right hemisphere disrupts the discrimination and recognition of faces, whereas a similar lesion in the posterior left hemisphere leaves the processing of faces essentially unaffected. There are exceptions to these general findings (e.g., Hamsher, Levin, and Benton, 1979), and they indicate that damage to the posterior left hemisphere that produces aphasia may result in defective discrimination of faces (left hemisphere damage that does not produce aphasia is not associated with such a face-processing deficit). However, the actual and respective contributions of the hemispheres to the processes underlying face recognition have not been clarified on the basis of these studies. It must also be noted that these group studies are performed on patients that do not complain of face-recognition impairments, and the observed differences depending on lesion site are brought to the fore in experiments that compare optimal performance between groups. From these findings, it seems to be clear that the posterior right hemisphere plays a critical role in the processing of faces, irrespective of the types of operations that are performed on faces. However, as noted earlier, further examination of this issue indicates dissociations between these different operations, as the deficits displayed by the patients on different tasks are not correlated (e.g., DeKosky et al., 1980), and lesions in different regions of the posterior right hemisphere result in qualitatively different deficits (e.g., Warrington and James, 1967).

In contrast, different conclusions would be drawn from the studies of select groups of brain-damaged patients: prosopagnosic, hemispherectomized, and split-brain patients. It was long believed that a bilateral lesion was necessary to produce a complete inability to recognize faces (prosopagnosia), as pointed out by Meadows (1974). Indeed, among the 14 cases that came to autopsy, all but two had a bilateral lesion, and, as noted by Damasio (1985), this could not be a coincidence. However, the bilaterality of the lesion did not always include both posterior hemispheres, and in some cases the lesion in the left hemisphere was very small and in a region that had little involvement in visual processes, whereas the right hemisphere damage always included the posterior region. More important, with the advances in brain imaging techniques during the last few years, particularly in magnetic resonance, it has become possible to obtain reliable information on localization of lesions in damaged brains. The results of such imaging have revealed a large number of cases of prosopagnosia with cerebral injury restricted to the right hemisphere (e.g., Landis et al., 1986; Michel et al., 1989). The fact that prosopagnosia can result from unilateral right hemisphere damage strongly suggests a crucial role for the right hemisphere in the processing of faces, and may even indicate that this hemisphere is both necessary and sufficient to sustain face-recognition abilities. It is therefore unclear, on the basis of data from prosopagnosic patients, what the respective roles of the cerebral hemispheres are with respect to the processing of faces.

The examination of hemispherectomized patients had, for a long time, suggested a functional equivalence of the hemispheres in processing faces, as no case of face-processing deficit had been reported in these patients (Damasio, 1985). However, Sergent and Villemure (1989) presented the case of a 33-year-old woman (B.M.), hemispherectomized at age 13, who was totally unable to recognize faces and was not even aware that she was lacking a particular skill (i.e., she did not complain of her deficit, and, because of her rather restricted social life, did not appear to be inconvenienced by it). This particular patient, who had been examined by neuropsychologists on several earlier occasions without their noticing her impairment, suggests that prosopagnosia might be more prevalent among hemispherectomized patients than is commonly thought, and that a systematic examination of face-processing abilities could reveal similar cases. Nonetheless, even if new cases are reported, prosopagnosia does not seem to be a necessary consequence of right hemisphere ablation is these patients, and there may be specific conditions that contribute to the emergence of such a deficit in hemispherectomized patients. Therefore, findings from hemispherectomized patients tend to contradict those from prosopagnosic patients and could support the view of a functional equivalence of the cerebral hemispheres in face processing.

Such a hemisphere equivalence is also suggested by research on split-brain patients which has strongly contributed to the idea that both hemispheres are competent at processing faces. Levy, Trevarthen, and Sperry (1972) showed that both the right and the left hemispheres were capable of recognizing faces and associating a name with a face, and that each could do so without the contribution of the other.

The study of brain-damaged patients thus appears to yield conflicting findings with respect to the contribution of the cerebral hemispheres to the processing of faces. Whereas unilateral brain damage produces face-processing impairment nearly exclusively after right hemisphere lesion, evidence from split-brain and hemispherectomized patients suggests that there may be functional equivalence of the two hemispheres with respect to the processing of faces or, at least, that destruction of areas in both hemispheres is necessary to produce a complete inability to process faces. However, these findings cannot be considered independently of the particular neurologic conditions of the patients, and, examining the site of the lesion responsible for impairment in face processing does not necessarily lead to the same answer as asking which cerebral areas *normally* underlie the processing of faces.

Positron Emission Tomography Studies of Face Processing

The foregoing discussions illustrate the difficulties in obtaining a clear picture of the neurofunctional anatomy of face processing. Several factors contributing to this state of affairs have already been pointed out. An additional factor is concerned with the large diversity of tasks that have been used in different populations and with different techniques, and the observed inconsistencies may partly reflect the fact that the results of these experiments do not tap the same functional level of processing because they are derived from different tasks. Cognitive PET studies are much more recent, and they could therefore benefit from the lessons learned from all the difficulties encountered in earlier research. In particular, to ensure valid comparisons across studies, it would make sense to subject the diverse populations to the same experiments carried out under the same procedural conditions. This was attempted by conducting the same experimental tasks in the laboratory and under PET measurement with normal subjects, as well as in the laboratory with prosopagnosic patients for whom detailed information about the site of their lesion was available. The main aspects of the PET study will first be described, and its results will then be compared to those obtained in the laboratory in normal and prosopagnosic subjects (Sergent et al., 1992a).

The approach used in the PET experiment introduced some new controls and variables so as to enhance the validity of the findings. The speed and accuracy of responses were recorded in order to obtain information about the pattern of reaction times and errors and to ensure that the subjects were effectively performing what they were asked to do. In addition, because face recognition necessarily involves the presentation of familiar faces and because subjects vary with respect to the faces they actually know, the selected faces were drawn from a pool of faces individually established earlier for each of the subjects. As a result, the rate of response accuracy was above 85% in all subjects compared to about 70% in most experiments on face recognition. Moreover, as noted earlier, each of the tasks performed by the subjects was later carried out by the same subjects in the laboratory, using lateral tachisto-scopic presentation so that the pattern of functional hemisphere asymmetry that can be inferred from the divided-visual-field technique could be compared to the actual respective engagement of the cerebral hemispheres of the same subjects performing the same task as derived from the PET study.

In this experiment (Sergent et al., 1992a), the main control condition was a grating discrimination task in which subjects had to judge whether the orientation of the centrally presented grating was vertical or horizontal. The spatial frequency bandwidths of the gratings varied from 0.5 to 16 cycles per degree of visual angle, so that they encompassed most of the spatial frequencies of the face and object stimuli. The three main experimental tasks constituted a face gender categorization (Is the face that of a man or a woman?), a face professional categorization (Is the face that of an actor or a politician?), and an object semantic categorization (Is the object natural or man-made?). Each of these tasks had been validated earlier on normal subjects and had also been tested on prosopagnosic patients (Sergent and Signoret, 1992b). The results (Sergent et al., 1992a) can be summarized as follows: (1) the gender categorization task engaged the right lingual gyrus and the posterior part of the fusiform gyrus, along with the lateral occipital cortex of the left hemisphere, in an area that was also activated during the object recognition task; (2) the face recognition task produced activation of both fusiform gyri, of the right parahippocampal gyrus, and of the anterior cortex of the temporal lobe of both hemispheres; (3) the object recognition task resulted in activation of the left fusiform gyrus and of the lateral occipitotemporal cortex, as well as of the left middle temporal gyrus; (4) when the activation state associated with the object task was subtracted from the face-categorization task, the previously significant rCBF change in the left fusiform gyrus during face recognition was no longer significant, whereas all the areas of the right hemisphere that were significant in the previous comparison were still significant. This suggests, on the one hand, that the participation of the left fusiform gyrus in face recognition may not be specific to the processing of faces as such and may reflect the operation of perceptual analysis common to the processing of both objects and faces; on the other hand, the absence of overlap of right hemisphere activation in the processing of faces and objects suggests a dissociation between these two functions.

Together, these findings indicate a bilateral, yet asymmetric, involvement of the cerebral hemispheres in the normal processing of faces. The right hemisphere seems to play a crucial role in the perceptual aspects of face processing and in reactivating the biographic information necessary for a face to become meaningful and be identified. The left hemisphere does not seem to be a "silent partner" in these processes, but its involvement did not appear to be specific to the processing of faces.

Comparisons of Findings from Different Populations

A comparison of these findings with the radiologic data of prosopagnosic patients (figure 7.2) may offer a better understanding of the actual involvement of cerebral structures in the processing of faces. Such a comparison indicates that at least one of the areas of the *right* hemisphere activated during the PET face identification task is found to be destroyed or disconnected in prosopagnosic patients, suggesting that the integrity of each of these areas is required for the normal recognition of faces (Sergent and Signoret, 1992a). This may explain the large variability in the location of the lesion responsible for prosopagnosia across patients. Such a variability reflects the large neural network underlying the processing of faces, located essentially in the right hemisphere and composed of locally specialized structures that perform the specific operations through which facial representations have to be subjected to achieve face recognition.

The comparison of PET and other radiologic data also allows a specification of the contribution of each of these areas to face recognition on the basis of the patients' patterns of successes and failures (table 7.1) as a function of the location of their lesion. Among the cortical areas involved in the processes leading to the recognition of faces, the right lingual and fusiform gyri are

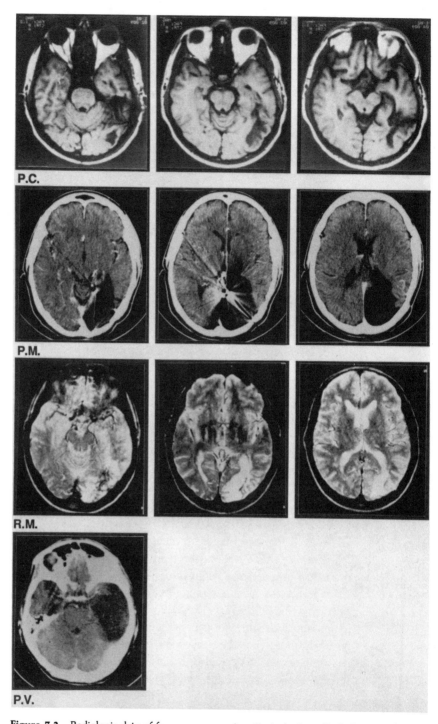

Figure 7.2 Radiologic data of four prosopagnosic patients (patients P. C., P. M., and R. M. have unilateral right hemisphere lesions; patient P. V. has a bilateral lesion, with involvement of the pole of the left temporal lobe along with the right anterior temporal lobe).

Table 7.1 Summary data of neuropsychological tests performed on three prosopagnosic patients

	P.C.	P.M.	R.M.	Controls (range)
WAIS Verbal	114	108	103	
WAIS Performance	101	97	102	
Weschler Memory Quotient	109	111	112	
Objects/canonical	52/54	54/54	52/54	49–54
Objects/noncanonical	24/54*	18/54*	23/54*	36–54
Benton's tests[a]	34/54* (6, 19, 9)	38/54 (6, 13, 19)	19/54* (4, 7, 8)	42–54
Mooney (gender)	19/40*	27/40	16/40*	28–40
Age estimation	17/20	16/20*	4/20*	17–20
Face matching, simultaneous[b]	20/20	18/20*	12/20*	20–20
Face matching, simultaneous, different[c]	15/20*	12/20*	8/20*	19–20
Face matching immediate[d]	9/20	6/20	6/20	14–20
Face matching immediate, different[e]	10/20*	11/20*	7/20*	13–20
Face matching delayed[f]	11/20*	8/20*	3/20*	12–20
Face emotion, recognition	12/24	8/24*	6/24*	18–24
Face emotion, matching	11/24*	13/24*	6/24*	19–24

* Indicates that performance time was slower than the slowest of the control subjects.
[a] The 3 numbers between brackets correspond to scores in 3 categories of face matching: 1: First 6 plates, with same views of test and target faces; 2: 24 comparisons of faces viewed from different angles but same lighting; 3: 24 comparisons of faces viewed from same angle but different lighting.
[b] Matching of 2 simultaneously presented same views of faces.
[c] Matching of 2 simultaneously presented different views of faces.
[d] Presentation of 20 front-view target faces, immediately followed by the presentation of 40 front-view faces including the 20 targets.
[e] Presentation of the same 20 front-view target faces as in test 4, immediately followed by the presentation of 40 faces seen from a different angle, including the 20 targets.
[f] Presentation, one hour after test 5, of 40 front-view faces, including the 20 targets presented in tests 4 to 5.

engaged in the perceptual operations inherent in the structural encoding and the extraction of a configuration that uniquely describes a face. Destruction of these areas results in an inability to perform elementary operations on faces (e.g., patients R.M. and P.M.), whereas sparing of these areas leaves essentially unaffected the ability to extract the physiognomic invariants of faces (e.g., patients P.C. and P.V.). The right parahippocampal gyrus appears to be involved in establishing a link between a facial representation and its related memories, and it thus plays a crucial role in reactivating the relevant biographic information without which a facial representation cannot be perceived as that of a specific individual. Finally, the anterior temporal lobes seem to contain the relevant biographic information related to individual entities.

Whether the two hemispheres differ in their functions at this level cannot be determined on the sole basis of the aforementioned studies, but is suggested by findings from brain-damaged patients (e.g., Ellis, Young, and Critchley, 1989; Damasio et al., 1991). Thus, damage to the right temporal lobe may prevent access to any biographic information, whether it be accessed through a face or a name, whereas proper name–finding difficulties seem to be restricted to damage to the left anterior temporal lobe. The latter finding has recently been confirmed in a PET study (Sergent et al., 1992b) in which activation of the pole of the temporal lobe was detected when normal subjects processed proper names of known persons, but not their faces.

 On the other hand, the finding of a left hemisphere contribution to object processing, as observed in the PET study, and of a dissociation between face and object processing, as observed in prosopagnosic patients, indicate that different neural substrates are involved in processing faces and objects. An examination of the radiologic data and patterns of associated deficits of patients described in the literature (e.g., Kertesz, 1979; Sergent and Signoret, 1992a) shows that the conjoint disruption of face and object processing is observed only in patients with a bilateral posterior lesion, whereas a unilateral right posterior lesion systematically spared the processing of objects (as long as they are seen from an unusual viewpoint, e.g., Landis et al., 1988).

Whereas the foregoing discussion indicates a fair amount of convergence across findings, other results exhibit some serious divergence. When the subjects that participated in the PET study were also tested in the divided-visual-field study, their results were at odds with those of the PET study and of the prosopagnosic patients. That is, the pattern of visual-field asymmetry suggested a significantly better performance of the left hemisphere in the face-recognition task, and one would therefore conclude from such results that the left hemisphere is more adept at recognizing faces than the right hemisphere. It thus seems that the conclusion that can be drawn from the divided-visual-field experiment does not correspond to the pattern of cerebral activation observed in the PET study for the same subjects. Yet, as noted earlier, such a left hemisphere superiority in face recognition is not an isolated finding in normal subjects, and there is also evidence that split-brain patients are able to recognize faces projected to their left hemisphere, suggesting that they are equipped with the necessary structures to perform all the operations required, from face perception to recognition. On the basis of the PET findings, this would suggest that the activation found in the left fusiform gyrus may be responsible for this outcome. However, if this were the case, why do not prosopagnosic patients, who have an intact left hemisphere, make use of this area to perform the recognition task?

To examine this question, an experiment was carried out on the three patients whose lesions were clearly unilateral (P.C., P.M., and R.M. in figure 7.1; Sergent and Signoret, 1992b). They were presented with 12 faces of familiar individuals whom they could not identify, and the corresponding names were then placed below each face. They were requested to learn the association of each face with its name and they were given as many trials as were necessary to correctly associate each name with its face on five consecutive trials. All three patients eventually succeeded in learning the 12 face-name associations. This task was performed at the end of a testing session. The following day, they were again presented with the 12 names, and they were asked to place the 12 faces above their corresponding names. The patients performed perfectly, indicating that they had been able to discriminate among the 12 faces some facial characteristics uniquely associated with each one and to establish a connection between each face and its respective name—all this, presumably, through operations performed by the left hemisphere. One may therefore conclude that the left hemisphere is not without capacity to process faces, and that it can learn to recognize faces not only within a short experimental time but also that it can store the relevant information and recall it the next day. This would then be consistent with the results obtained with the normal and commissurotomized subjects.

However, if the left hemisphere were capable of such a true face recognition, why are these patients still prosopagnosic? For instance, patient P.M., who had an occipital ablation and has been prosopagnosic for 20 years, still fails to recognize her husband when she does not expect to see him. Clearly, the way the prosopagnosic patients performed this learning task does not correspond to the processes one normally uses to recognize faces, and perhaps this is what usually happens in laboratory experiments with normal and split-brain subjects displaying a left hemisphere competence at recognizing faces. To examine this possibility, the prosopagnosic patients, right after the recall task performed in the morning, were presented with the faces of the same 12 persons, but different versions of the faces were used. The results indicated that each patient performed at chance, suggesting an inability to transfer the stored knowledge associated with the first version of a face to the new version. In other words, their left hemisphere is not equipped to extract the configuration of a face that contains the physiognomic invariants, and it treats different views of the same faces as different faces. What the patients had learned, therefore, presumably with their left hemisphere, was a specific view of a face which was useless as soon as a new version had to be recognized, and this cannot be of much help in compensating for their disturbance.

Now, if we consider how experiments with normal subjects are carried out, especially those reaction-time experiments that frequently yield a left hemisphere superiority, it is important to note that they involve few faces appearing under the same format and viewpoint, and comprise many trials with several repetitions of the same faces. Under such conditions, the left hemisphere may achieve a significant level of efficiency, as the performance of the patients suggests, which does not necessarily reflect the true processes that normally underlie the recognition of an unexpected face. This explanation may also account for the performance of the split-brain patients on a face-recognition task. In the well-known study by Levy et al. (1972), the patients were shown four faces, from a single viewpoint, repeated many times, and they were given a long practice to learn to associate each face with a name. Under such circumstances, the left hemisphere may very well have learned to recognize faces, but the operations underlying this recognition may have little in common with the processes that are normally involved in recognizing faces.

CONCLUSIONS

An exhaustive description and explanation of functional cerebral asymmetry is a far-fetched goal which encounters a large variety of obstacles on its path. It is now clear that the search for a single, bipolar principle that would encompass the functional properties of the two hemispheres would be futile, but even a characterization of the functional organization of the cerebral structures underlying face processing, which should be a more modest and simple achievement, is still elusive. The information presented in this chapter illustrates some of the difficulties inherent in making inferences about the respective contributions of the cerebral hemispheres to a well-delineated cognitive function, and it also suggests that the roles played by the hemispheres in this function cannot be described in simple terms restricted to a localization of the cerebral regions involved. In addition to specifying the neurofunctional anatomy of a given function, which is concerned with rather static aspects of cerebral processing, the understanding of functional asymmetry must take into consideration the dynamic aspects of cerebral lateralization, which manifest themselves at all levels of processing, whatever the type of technique being used to investigate this phenomenon (Sergent, 1990).

None of the techniques appear to be self-sufficient, their reliability cannot be perfect, and they produce results that may sometimes contradict one another. There is probably much to learn from these inconsistencies, both within and between techniques, and deciphering what underlies the various patterns of convergence and divergence of findings across studies and experimental approaches may yield some of the more important information about the dynamic aspects of cerebral processing.

REFERENCES

Benton, A. R., Hamsher, K. D. S., Varney, N., and Spreen, O. (1983). *Contributions to neuropsychological assessment: A clinical manual.* New York, NY: Oxford University Press.

Benton, A. R., and Van Allen, M. W. (1972). Prosopagnosia and facial discrimination. *Journal of Neurological Sciences, 15,* 167–172.

Bruce, V. (1988). *Recognising faces.* London: Erlbaum.

Bruce, V., and Young, A. W. (1986). Understanding face recognition. *British Journal of Psychology, 77,* 305–327.

Bruyer, R. (1989). Disorders of face processing. In A. W. Young and H. D. Ellis (Eds.), *Handbook of research on face processing* (pp. 437–473). Amsterdam: North Holland.

Burton, A. M., Young, A. W., Bruce, V., Johnston, R. A., and Ellis, A. W. (1991). Understanding covert recognition. *Cognition, 39,* 129–166.

Caramazza, A., and Badecker, W. (1989). Patient classification in neuropsychological research. *Brain and Cognition, 10,* 256–295.

Damasio, A. R. (1985). Prosopagnosia. *Trends in Neuroscience, 8,* 132–135.

Damasio, A. R., Damasio, H., Tranel, D., and Brandt, J. P. (1991). The neural regionalization of knowledge access: Preliminary evidence. *Cold Spring Harbor Symposium of Quantitative Biology, 55,* 1039–1047.

DeKosky, S. T., Heilman, K. M., Bowers, D., and Valenstein, E. (1980). Recognition and discrimination of emotional faces and pictures. *Brain and Language, 9,* 206–214.

De Renzi, E., Faglioni, P., and Spinnler, H. (1968). The performance of patients with unilateral brain damage on face recognition tasks. *Cortex, 4,* 17–34.

Ellis, A. W. (1992). Cognitive mechanisms of face processing. *Philosophical Transactions of the Royal Society, London, Series B, 335,* 113–119.

Ellis, A. W., Young, A. W., and Critchley, E. M. R. (1989). Loss of memory for people following temporal lobe damage. *Brain, 112,* 1469–1483.

Ellis, H. D. (1992). The development of face processing skills. *Philosophical Transactions of the Royal Society, London, Series B, 335,* 105–111.

Evans, A., Marrett, S., Collins, L., and Peters, T. M. (1989). Anatomical-functional correlative analysis of the human brain using three-dimensional imaging systems. *Proceedings of the Society of Photographic and Optical Instrumentation and Engineering, 1092,* 264–274.

Felleman, D. J., and Van Essen, D. C. (1991). Distributed hierarchical processing in the primate cerebral cortex. *Cerebral Cortex, 1,* 1–47.

Fox, P. T., Perlmutter, J. S., and Raichle, M. E. (1985). A stereotactic method of anatomical localization for positron emission tomography. *Journal of Computer Assisted Tomography, 9,* 141–153.

Fox, P. T., Mintun, M. A., Reinman, E. M., and Raichle, M. E. (1988). Enhanced detection of focal brain responses using intersubject averaging and change-distribution analysis of subtracted PET images. *Journal of Cerebral Blood Flow and Metabolism, 8,* 642–653.

Hamsher, K., Levin, H. S., and Benton, A. L. (1979). Facial recognition in patients with focal brain lesions. *Archives of Neurology, 36,* 837–839.

Hécaen, H. (1972). *La neuropsychologie humaine.* Paris: Masson.

Hécaen, H., and Albert, M. (1978). *Human neuropsychology.* New York, NY: John Wiley & Sons.

Hellige, J. B. (1990). Hemispheric asymmetry. *Annual Review of Psychology, 41,* 55–80.

Hellige, J. B. (1993). *Hemispheric asymmetry. What is left and what is right.* Cambridge, MA: Harvard University Press.

Hellige, J. B., and Sergent, J. (1986). Role of task factors in visual-field asymmetries. *Brain and Cognition, 5,* 200–223.

Kertesz, A. (1979). Visual agnosia. The dual deficit of perception and recognition. *Cortex, 15,* 403–419.

Landis, T., Cunnings, J. L., Christen, L., Bogen, J., and Imhof, H.-G. (1986). Are unilateral right posterior cerebral lesions sufficient to cause prosopagnosia? Clinical and radiological findings in six additional patients. *Cortex, 22,* 243–252.

Landis, T., Regard, M., Bliestle, A., and Kleihues, P. (1988). Prosopagnosia and agnosia for noncanonical views. An autopsied case. *Brain, 111,* 1287–1298.

Levy, J., Trevarthen, C., and Sperry, R. W. (1972). Perception of bilateral chimeric figures following hemisphere disconnexion. *Brain, 95,* 61–78.

Lueck, C. J., Zeki, S., Friston, K. J., Deiber, M.-P., Cope, P., Cunningham, V. J., Lammertsma, A. A., Kennard, C., and Frackowiak, R. S. J. (1989). The colour center in the cerebral cortex of man. *Nature, 340,* 386–389.

Marzi, C., and Berlucchi, G. (1977). Right visual field superiority for accuracy of recognition of famous faces in normals. *Neuropsychologia, 15,* 751–756.

McCarthy, R. A., and Warrington, E. K. (1990). *Cognitive neuropsychology. A clinical introduction.* London: Academic Press.

Meadows, J. C. (1974). The anatomical basis of prosopagnosia. *Journal of Neurology, Neurosurgery and Psychiatry, 37,* 489–501.

Mesulam, M.-M. (1990). Large-scale neurcognitive networks and distributed processing for attention, language, and memory. *Annals of Neurology, 28,* 597–613.

Michel, F., Poncet, M., and Signoret, J.-L. (1989). Les lésions responsables de la prosopagnosie sont-elles toujours bilatérales? *Revue Neurologique, 145,* 764–770.

Mintun, M., Fox, P. T., and Raichle, M. E. (1989). A highly accurate method of localizing neuronal activity in the human brain with positron emission tomography. *Journal of Cerebral Blood Flow and Metabolism, 9,* 96–103.

Petersen, S. E., Fox, P. T., Posner, M. I., Mintun, M., and Raichle, M. E. (1989). Positron emission tomography studies of the processing of single words. *Journal of Cognitive Neuroscience, 1,* 153–170.

Posner, M. I., Petersen, S. E., Fox, P. T., and Raichle, M. E. (1988). Localization of cognitive functions in the brain. *Science, 240,* 1627–1631.

Raichle, M. E. (1990). Images of the functioning human brain. In H. Barlow, C. Blakemore, and M. Weston-Smith (Eds), *Images and understanding* (pp 284–296). Cambridge, UK: Cambridge University Press.

Raichle, M. E., Martin, W. R. W., Herscovitch, P., Mintun, M. A., and Marham, J. (1983). Brain blood flow measured with intraveinous $H_2^{15}O$. II. Implementation and validation. *Journal of Nuclear Medicine, 24,* 790–798.

Sergent, J. (1983). The role of the input in visual hemispheric asymmetries. *Psychological Bulletin, 93,* 481–512.

Sergent, J. (1984b). Inferences from unilateral brain damage about normal hemispheric functions in visual pattern recognition. *Psychological Bulletin, 96,* 99–115.

Sergent, J. (1989a). Structural processing of faces. In A. W. Young and H. D. Ellis (Eds.), *Handbook of face processing.* Amsterdam: Elsevier.

Sergent, J. (1989b). Ontogenesis and microgenesis of face perception. *The European Bulletin of Cognitive Psychology, 5,* 123–128.

Sergent, J. (1990). Les dilemmes de la gauche et de la droite: Confrontation, cohabitation ou coopération? In X. Seron (Ed.), *Psychologie et cerveau.* Paris: Presses Universitaires de France.

Sergent, J., and Hellige, J. B. (1986). Role of input factors in visual field asymmetry. *Brain and Cognition, 5,* 174–199.

Sergent, J., Ohta, S., and MacDonald, B. (1992a). Functional neuroanatomy of face and object processing: A PET study. *Brain, 115,* 15−29.

Sergent, J., and Poncet, M. (1990). From covert to overt recognition of faces in a prosopagnosic patient. *Brain, 113,* 989−1004.

Sergent, J., and Signoret, J.-L. (1992a). Functional and anatomical decomposition of face processing: Evidence from prosopagnosia and PET study of normal subjects. *Philosophical Transactions of the Royal Society of London. Series B: Biological Sciences, 335,* 55−62.

Sergent, J., and Signoret, J.-L. (1992b). Varieties of functional deficits in prosopagnosia. *Cerebral Cortex, 2,* 375−388.

Sergent, J., and Villemure, J.-G. (1989). Prosopagnosia in a right hemispherectomized patient. *Brain, 112,* 975−995.

Sergent, J., Zuck, E., Lévesque, M., and MacDonald, B. (1992b). Positron emission tomography study of letter and object processing: Empirical findings and methodological considerations. *Cerebral Cortex, 2,* 68−80.

Shallice, T. (1988). *From neuropsychology to mental structures.* Cambridge, England: Cambridge University Press.

Smith, A., and Sugar, O. (1975). Development of above normal language and intelligence 21 years after left hemispherectomy. *Neurology, 25,* 813−818.

Sperry, R. W., Gazzaniga, M. S., and Bogen, J. E. (1969). Interhemispheric relationships: The neocortical commissures, syndromes of hemispheric disconnection. In P. J. Vinken and G. W. Bruyn (Eds.), *Handbook of clinical neurology,* Vol. 4: *Disorders of speech, perception and symbolic behavior.* Amsterdam: Elsevier.

Takane, Y., and Sergent, J. (1983). Multidimensional scaling models for reaction-time and same-different judgments. *Psychometrika, 48,* 393−423.

Villemure, J.-G., and Sergent, J. (in press). Hemispherectomy. In J. G. Beaumont and J. Sergent (Eds.), *Dictionary of neuropsychology.* Oxford: Basil Blackwell.

Warrington, E. K., and James, M. (1967). An experimental investigation of facial recognition in patients with unilateral cerebral lesions. *Cortex, 3,* 317−326.

Zaidel, E. (1983). Disconnection syndrome as a model of laterality effect in the normal brain. In J. B. Hellige (Ed.), *Cerebral hemisphere asymmetry.* New York, NY: Praeger.

Editor's Note

We note with regret the death of Justine Sergent during the production of this book.

8 Handedness and Its Relation to Other Indices of Cerebral Lateralization

Michael Peters

Nevertheless, though I think the superiority of the right hand is acquired and is a result of its more frequent use, the tendency to use it, in preference to the left, is so universal that it would seem rather natural. I am driven, therefore, to the rather nice distinction, that, though the superiority is acquired, the tendency to acquire the superiority is natural.

Humphrey, 1861 (p. 202)

Handedness is the most easily observed expression of cerebral lateralization. Because of its seemingly dichotomous nature, the phenomenon of handedness should be very amenable to neuropsychological research. This expectation has not been met. Handedness has proved to be a complex and multifaceted manifestation of lateral preferences that has so far resisted any unified explanation. In particular, a general theory of handedness that does justice to the observed preference and performance patterns is lacking. Much of the research on handedness tracks isolated problems, and tends not to allow generalizations beyond specific tasks and methods. As a result, any general review of the current state of handedness research will not allow broad insights. Instead, this chapter provides an account of the specific remaining difficulties in the study of handedness, and some areas where progress has been made.

PREVALENCE AND CLASSIFICATION

What Is the Proportion of Left- and Right-handers in the Population?

The first, and most obvious question to be asked is: How many left-handers and right-handers are there in the population? To answer this question in a satisfactory way presumes that there is some agreement about handedness classification. There is not, and because the association of handedness with other indices of cerebral lateralization can only be explored fully if problems of classification and measurement are solved, the current status of these will have to be discussed in some detail. The question of classification and prevalence interacts with theory. After all, how can one determine the prevalence of left-handedness if one does not know what exactly it is that is to be classified? I shall sidestep that issue for the moment, and begin with a very loose and commonly shared understanding of handedness as a preference of one hand over the other if a choice is possible. This understanding will only serve as a point of departure and its labile status will become immediately obvious.

The first obstacle to understanding the demographics of handedness lies in the interference of cultural values with the expression of hand preferences. Pressures against left hand use may take a general form that is well illustrated by Suetonius' observation: "Claudius never behaved less informally than at these picnics—exposing his left hand in the Plebeian fashion when he distributed prizes, instead of keeping it decently covered by the toga." (Suetonius, 1979; section 21, p. 199). In addition, the general form of disapproval of the left hand finds reflection in specific exclusions, such as discouragement of writing with the left hand. The strength of pressures against the use of the left hand varies, and is reflected by the fact that the prevalence of left-handed writers in contemporary societies varies from less than 1% in countries such as Korea (Kang and Harris, 1993) to some 12% or more in North America (Gilbert and Wisocki, 1992). Such cultural effects make it difficult to estimate the prevalence of left-handedness if one has the ambition to do this across cultures and across time. However, it is reasonable to accept the basic proposition that in countries like the United States and Canada there is no longer a uniform systematic pressure against the use of the left hand as the writing hand. For this reason, U.S. population estimates of people writing with the left hand, such as the 10.5% reported for females and 13% reported for males of the current generation (Gilbert and Wisocki, 1992), can be accepted as valid minimal estimates, minimal because there continue to be, in ethnic and religious subpopulations of the United States, pressures against the left hand as the writing hand. Gilbert and Wisocki's data also show that there are more left-handed men than women. McManus (1991) thought it necessary to modify his genetic model to account for this factor, by invoking a modifier gene. However, it is premature to assume that genetic factors must underlie the male-female difference. In a recent study of over 600 left-handers (Peters, in preparation), females stated significantly more often than males that they had been pressured to change handedness. In addition, the same study showed that in North American samples a significantly higher portion of left-handed females write with the noninverted position and this, too, is attributed to greater pressures on females to conform. Perhaps the existence of population data in which no sex differences in the prevalence of left-handedness in males and females are found (Seddon and McManus, in preparation) can be interpreted in terms of the possibility that cultural pressures rather than modifier genes are responsible for sex differences in prevalence of left-handedness.

These figures provide the most conservative estimate of the prevalence of left-handers. It is assumed here that in other countries, where the prevalence of left-handed writing is lower, a similar proportion of left-handed writers to that in the United States would be observed in the absence of cultural pressures. The question is, What other factors enter the classification of handedness, and are there more satisfactory classification schemes than those based on single indicators such as writing hand?

The Question of Subclassification

Writing Position In the absence of a theory of handedness, various attempts at subclassification have been made on the basis of observations of phenotype, or association of handedness with some other condition or event. A powerful and imaginative attempt of subclassification was made by Levy (e.g., Levy and Reid, 1978). Levy suggested that left-handers may be subdivided in terms of fundamental differences in the organization of the neural machinery that guides the hands. Left-handers who write with the inverted, hooked position are said to have ipsilateral control of the digits, as opposed to left-handers who write much like right-handers, but with the left hand. However, Levy's speculation has not found wide acceptance (Weber and Bradshaw, 1981), and few researchers in the field would now subscribe to the idea that writing position in left-handers or right-handers is related to some fundamental differences in neuromotor organization. Instead, there is a conviction that writing position can be modified quite readily by sociocultural factors and that the inverted writing position confers some technical advantages for the left-handed writer who writes in cursive style. Evidence for environmental influences derives from the finding that in a sample of left-handers, the prevalence of the inverted writing position differs significantly for the older and younger generations (Peters, in preparation). In the sample, among 242 left-handed persons younger than 40 years of age, 52% wrote with the inverted position and 116 wrote with the noninverted position. Among 165 persons older than 40, only 32% ($\chi^2 = 15.8$, $P < .0001$) did so. There was also a marked effect of sex. Of 206 males, 58% wrote with the inverted position, while of 263 females, only 25% wrote with the inverted position ($\chi^2 = 51.6$, $P < .00001$). These data suggest that use of the writing position in left-handers to infer neurologic organization of the hand motor system is questionable. There remains the problem of how to account for those studies in which a positive association between handwriting position and some other index of cerebral lateralization was found (e.g., Moscovitch and Smith, 1979). Part of the answer may lie in the findings of Guiard and Millerat (1984), who showed that the relation between hand movement and visual half-field in inverted writers is influenced by their habit of crossing hands during writing. If this is an important factor, the positive findings in the literature may be explained in terms of acquired differences in the way in which the visual half-fields relate to fine motor control in inverted writers—not because of underlying neurologic differences, but because of differential experience in guiding movement relative to a given visual half-field.

Familial vs. Nonfamilial Left-handedness Another subclassification, and one that has significant implications for any theory of handedness, focuses on familial handedness. That is, some researchers distinguish between persons who have left-handedness in their family background and those who do not. In principle, this would allow a distinction between left-handedness as an inherited rather than an "acquired" trait. A considerable number of papers have reported significant differences between "familial" and "nonfamilial" left-handers on the basis of their performance on various neuropsychological tests. The contradictory nature of results, combined with the uncertainties of assessing familial handedness, are a source of some concern. Of particular interest is Bishop's (1990a) doubt about the usefulness of familial sinistrality in the subclassification, especially of right-handers. Her argument goes as follows. If familial sinistrality information were useful, the presence of familial sinistrality in an individual should allow the prediction that this individual has a significantly higher probability of having a genotype associated with left-handedness than an individual without familial sinistrality. Using Annett's (1985) genetic model, Bishop shows that the probabilities are not sufficiently different to use familial sinistrality as a useful subclassification tool and that manifest handedness of the individuals in question allows a significantly better prediction of genotype than familial handedness. Similar conclusions would be reached if McManus' (1991) genetic model were used as basis for the probability calculations.

Bishop's argument should temper any undue enthusiasm in the acceptance of positive findings associated with the familial sinistrality variable, especially for small subject samples.

Hormones and the Ontogeny of Cerebral Differentiation Geschwind and Galaburda's (1985) influential theory suggests that differential rates of left and right hemisphere maturation that are subject to finely timed effects of hormones play a major role in the development of hand preferences. An extensive discussion of this theory has been provided by McManus and Bryden (1991) who have transformed an amorphous mass of intriguing speculations and associations into a theoretical framework that allows falsification. It now remains to be seen whether the mechanisms suggested by Geschwind and Galaburda to determine the development of handedness will in fact be shown to have such an effect.

Pathology Unhappily, the "pathology" model itself is subject to some form of subclassification (Harris and Carlson, 1988). While the unifying feature of the pathology model is that left-handers are at increased risk, the question of how the pathology enters the picture is rarely put in an intelligible way. Perhaps the clearest statement is made by those (e.g., Bakan, Dibbs, and Reed, 1973) who believe that the normal human condition is right-handedness, and that all left-handedness is due to some form of insult, most likely incurred during the birth process. This does not, however, exclude the possibility of a genetic element because it may also be suggested that left-handedness is a marker for various problems (Geschwind and Behan, 1982; Geschwind and Galaburda, 1985; Kinsbourne, 1988). This, then, is the second variant of the pathology model in which left-handedness as such is not pathologic but may indicate the risk for difficulties. A third variant would distinguish between "normal" left-handedness and pathologic left-handedness (Satz, 1972; Satz et al., 1985), and this variant suggests that some left-handers come to be left-handers through whatever mechanism determines handedness and some come to be left-handers because something went wrong. Yet a further variation suggests that a sizable proportion of left-handed children are "subclinical" pathologic left-handers. In this group, underlying neurologic disturbances of varying etiology are not sufficiently strong to lead to overt paralysis of the nonpreferred hand but cause a shift of hand preference from the (normally chosen) right hand to the left hand (Bishop, 1984). Bishop (1990b), in her excellent book on handedness and developmental disorders, estimates that about 1 in 20 left-handers might be a pathologic left-hander.

In one of the more dramatic developments in this area, Coren and Halpern (1991) have suggested that not only is there pathology involved in left-handedness but that it has major implications for the life expectancy of left-handers. For full measure, they add two additional risk factors for left-handers. First, they invoke the Geschwind and Galaburda (1985) hypothesis, which has as one of its predictions that left-handers should suffer disproportionately more from autoimmune disorders. Second, they speculate that left-handers are at a greater risk in terms of accidents because they live in a world which is designed to meet the needs of right-handers. Coren and Halpern (1991) believe that direct evidence for the greater mortality rates of left-handers lies in population prevalence figures for left-handedness. Because such prevalence data are of general interest not only with regard to the pathology model of handedness and its interaction with classification but also with regard to the model of inheritance, a closer look at prevalence data is desirable. The best set of data on the prevalence of left-handedness is that published by Gilbert and Wisocki (1992). Their data are extremely useful because the questionnaire on which it is based was not directed at left-handers and therefore reduces bias in the sample due to self-selection. In addition, the sample is by an order of magnitude the largest collected so far. Of the various questions, two were related to handedness: Which hand do you write with? And, Which hand do you throw with? Figure 8.1A and B shows the proportion of left-handed males and females according to age groupings. It can be seen that the proportion of left-handers in the population is fairly stable up into the forties, with a decline thereafter. Specifically, left-handers become rare in the older age cohorts. Coren and Halpern interpret this in terms of greater mortality rates for left-handers. To do so, they have to discount the so-called modification hypothesis. This hypothesis is based on the broad understanding that older left-handed people will have encountered pressures to change the writing hand to the right hand in their youth. As a result, they will show up as right-handed

A
Males

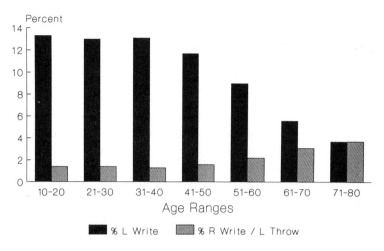

B
Females

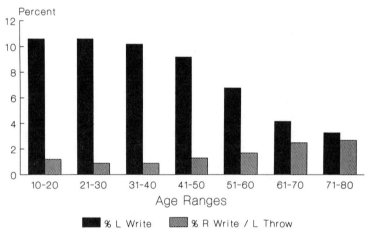

Figure 8.1 Proportion of left-handed writers in various age groups, and proportion of persons who write with the right hand and throw with the left hand. (Computed from numerical data provided by Gilbert and Wisocki, 1992, for 665,223 females and 509,552 males.)

writers when sampled now (Hugdahl et al., 1993). The data in figure 8.1 give indirect evidence of social pressures. Shown in addition to left-handed writers are persons who write with the right hand and who throw with the left hand. These are twice as prevalent in the older generation than in the current generation. Applying Coren and Halpern's logic one would have to argue that these persons enjoy a selective advantage in longevity over all other groups. Applying the modification hypothesis, a different interpretation offers itself: there were direct environmental pressures against left-handed writing in the older generation but not against left-handed throwing. Because of this, there will be proportionately more people with the "right write—left throw" pattern than in the current generation.

While the thesis that left-handers die younger has some heuristic appeal because of the multitude of possible reasons why that should be the case, the actual evidence is disappointingly weak. That applies to *all* of the evidence that has been marshaled to bolster the idea of the vulnerable left-hander; not a single domain of evidence, ranging from mortality data to birth difficulties, provides clear and incontrovertible support (for an extended discussion of the nature of the evidence, see Harris, 1993). A cautious interpretation would be that while some persons might die earlier because they are left-handed, the proportion would be so low as to question continued preoccupation with this topic. For this reason, we exclude the pathologic left-hander from further consideration.

Quantitative Approaches to Classification   In the above analysis of the Gilbert and Wisocki data, it was stated that some 10.5% of females and 13% of males in the United States write with the left hand. Few would argue with classifying these people as left-handers. However, an appreciable number of people are rather more difficult to classify by any simple criteria. For instance, in the Gilbert and Wisocki data, there are individuals who write with the right and throw with the left hand, and individuals who write with the left and throw with the right hand. Should these be classified as left-handers, too? A rather simple solution to this dilemma has been provided by those who give a list of preference questions to subjects, and classify all those who answer exclusively "right" as right-handers and the remainder as "non-right-handers". This may suit the purposes of individual researchers but changes the distributions drastically. With increasing length of the questionnaire, fewer and fewer persons answer "right" to all alternatives. Taking this to a ludicrous extent, when a 60-item questionnaire is used, some 92 out of 100 persons are non-right-handers. Even with a more conservative 14-item questionnaire, non-right-handers become a rather large proportion. Consider the dilemma of a scientist who attempts to develop a genetic model to account for handedness: What has to be explained? Should the model account for the existence of approximately 12% left-handed writers in the population, or should it account for 17% of the population who do a number of important activities with the left hand, or should it, let us say, account for 35% non-right-handers and 65%

Table 8.1 Prevalence of left-handedness as function of classification criteria

Criteria	Right-handers (%)	Non-right-handers (%)
A. Righthander if 100% "always rights" choices on 5-point scale	13.3	86.7
B. Righthander if 90% "always right" choices on 5-point scale	52.1	47.9
C. Righthander if 100% "right" choices on "right/left" option	64.5	35.5
D. Righthander if to the right of mid-point zero on continuous scale	90.6	9.4

right-handers, both proportions being quite arbitrary. There are some weighty implications behind such classification procedures. While in the case of classification by writing hand only, left-handers are a definite minority, classifications that recognize right-handers only on the basis of exclusive right-handed choices can lead to right-handers being the minority and non-right-handers being in the majority—depending on the number of questionnaire items. In either case, the classification procedure selects out individuals who represent, in many ways, the extreme of a spectrum of possible hand preferences. Some examples from Peters (1992a) make the point.

In table 8.1, percentages of right-handers and non-right-handers are given as a function of classification criteria for a single questionnaire that was given to 576 college students twice, once with a forced choice and once with a graded procedure. The items used were: write, throw, hammer, use knife to cut bread, hold toothbrush, hold match while striking, open jar lid, hold racquet, use scissors, draw, use spoon, hold needle while mending something. In criterion A, subjects answered on a five-point scale (1 = always left, 2 = mostly left, 3 = either hand, 4 = mostly right, 5 = always right). Only those who chose "always right" for all questions were considered right-handers. In B, a slightly relaxed criterion was applied; subjects who had 90% of a perfect "always right" maximum were considered right-handers. In C, subjects were answering either "left" or "right," and only those who chose only "right" were considered right-handers. In D, subjects were classified according to the midpoint between perfect "always left" and "always right" extremes.

Depending on classification procedures, then, the percentage of non-right-handers varies from 9.4% to 86.7% for the same subjects and the same questionnaire items. The influence of item selection is illustrated by the fact that when the item "open jar lid" is dropped from the questionnaire the prevalence of right-handers in C increases by almost 20%. It should be noted that if the classification procedure used for D is adopted (individuals with scores below the midpoint of scores classed as "left-handers" and those above classed as "right-handers"), very stable prevalence estimates can be obtained. For instance, using the Waterloo 60-item questionnaire (Steenhuis and Bryden,

1989) with a 1 to 5 graded answer scheme, a 30-item selection from this questionnaire with a 1 to 5 graded answer scheme, the above 12-item questionnaire with graded or forced left/right choices, and 8- and 4-item questionnaires with forced and graded choices each, the average prevalence figure for left-handedness across all 8 questionnaires is 9.4%, with an SD of 0.98. Unhappily, reliability does not indicate validity, as will be seen in the discussion of functionally defined subgroups below. However, it is clear that the discovery of important relations between handedness and other neuropsychological variables, as based on the "right-hander"/"non-right-hander" classification procedure must be viewed with reservation.

Some investigators have tried to put the classification on a more formal basis—procedurally, if not conceptually—by trying to find some method by which handedness questionnaire items can be selected systematically. One such method would be to perform a factor analysis on a large number of items, with the aim of grouping items that load under a common factor (e.g., Healey, Liederman, and Geschwind, 1986; Steenhuis and Bryden, 1989; Williams, 1986). Unfortunately, such an approach suffers from a major flaw. In all of the existing work, the data from left-handers and right-handers have been combined; a procedure that goes against the principle that data from subgroups of the population that are known, a priori, to be heterogeneous, should not be pooled. The resulting factor structure tells us nothing we do not know beforehand: items that load very highly on the first factor (the one that accounts for most of the variance) are the items for which left-handers choose the left hand and right-handers choose the right hand. Thus, one can expect to find the items "write" and "draw" loading under the first factor. If the factor analysis is done only for right-handers, the factor structure becomes unintelligible and "write" and "draw" no longer load under the first factor. Instead, factors that show some variability for right-handers (activities that "do not matter," such as the hand chosen to pick up a marble) show up under the first factor (Peters and Murphy, 1993). A similar situation can be seen in the sample of native Amazonians studied by Bryden, Ardila, and Ardila (1993). Although their sample was too small to sustain a credible factor analysis, the pattern of essentially meaningless factor loadings observed with deliberate selection of right-handers only can also be seen; their sample consisted almost entirely of phenotypic right-handers.

In left-handed writers, some items that show no variability for right-handed writers, such as "throwing," still load under the first factor. One possibility is that left-handers can be classified into subgroups according to this item. When a cluster analysis is performed on *individuals* rather than *items*, the latter possibility becomes quite attractive. When a relatively large number of persons are subjected to a cluster analysis, a 14-item questionnaire yields three handedness groups: one group of right-handers, one group of left-handers characterized most succinctly by congruence of writing and throwing hand, and one group of left-handers who write with the left hand and who throw with the right hand. A discriminant function analysis shows that people can be assigned to these three groups with a very high degree of accuracy and very little overlap (Peters and Murphy, 1992).

Functionally Defined Subgroups   The identification of a group of left-handers who throw with the right and write with the left hand is of more than passing interest. According to the data provided by Gilbert and Wisocki (1992), they represent 30% of all left-handed writers when averaged over age groups. In persons younger than 40 years old, the proportion approaches 40%. In the case of the small group of persons who write with the right hand and throw with the left hand it could be argued that these are originally left-handed persons who have been forced to change the writing hand but resisted changing the throwing hand, but no such argument can be found for the existence of the left-handed writers who throw with the right. The combination of subgroups is likely responsible for many of the statements in the literature that left-handers, as a group, show much smaller differences between hands than right-handers. For example, when hand strength is compared for the left and right hand of left-handers, no systematic group difference is found and this has been considered one of the defining features of left-handers. Right-handers, in contrast, show a convincing right-hand superiority in hand strength. However, it turns out that left-handers who throw with the left and write with the left have a convincingly stronger left hand whereas left-handers who throw with the right and write with the left have a convincingly stronger right hand. When left-handers as a group are compared on hand strength, the marked asymmetry favoring the right hand in the latter group is sufficient to reduce or even eliminate the asymmetry in hand strength favoring the left hand in the former group (Peters, 1992b). This is only one illustration of how subgrouping of left-handers or handedness groups in general can have important implications for how one looks at handedness and leads into a general discussion of the implications of subgrouping.

IMPLICATIONS OF DEFINING SUBGROUPS OF LEFT-HANDERS IN NEUROPSYCHOLOGY

The Relation of Handedness to Other Behavioral Asymmetries

Next to hand preference, foot preference is the most salient behavioral asymmetry. The relation between handedness and footedness is of practical and theoretical interest. Historically, the relation between footedness and handedness has been recognized because they are not mutually independent (Humphrey, 1861). A clear indication of how foot and hand preference are interrelated comes from Virgil's *Aeneid* "... Lucagus ... now took up position for combat, his left foot advanced: as he did so, Aeneas' spear passed through the rim of his shining shield, at the bottom, then penetrated the left groin ..." (Virgil, 1962, p. 240, lines 563–593). Here, foot movement is dictated by the fact that the shield is held in the left, and the sword in the right hand. The warrior leads with the left foot, and so do armies when marching (Peters, 1988a). But the relation between hand and foot preference is not quite as simple as it seems. While right-handers as a group show a marked preference for the right foot in kicking (over 90% of right-handed writers), the situation for left-handers is reminiscent of strength comparisons between the two hands. Thus, left-handers as a group do not seem to prefer the left foot as clearly as right-handers seem to prefer the right foot (Annett and Turner, 1974; Peters and Durding, 1979). Annett and Turner (1974) already suggested that the foot preference of left-handers depends on the consistency of their hand preference choices. This was narrowed down to a relation between lateral preference for throwing and foot chosen for kicking by Peters (in preparation): some 82% of left-handers who preferred the left arm for throwing preferred the left foot for kicking, while 78% of left-handers who preferred the right arm for throwing preferred the right foot for kicking. From a functional point of view it makes sense that there should be a meaningful correlation between choice of arm for strength and ballistic activities and choice of leg for kicking. Because right-handers have such a consistent right-side preference, this relation emerges clearly only when left-handers are examined.

In the case of foot preference, the logic of search for its association with hand preference lies in the functional dynamics of hand and foot use in humans and the question of whether it is the musculature of a whole body half that is involved in motor preference. Attempts have also been made to investigate the congruence of other eyedness and handedness (Porac and Coren, 1981) and ear dominance and handedness. Lateral preference for the eyes and the ears especially is less clearly expressed than hand preference. Right-side congruence is the norm for eye and hand use, but ear and hand association is counfounded, a priori, by the fact that the majority of left-handers have left hemisphere language and speech dominance.

Handedness in the Context of Selected Brain Structures and Functions

Motor Tracts   Because handedness is such a clearly observed asymmetry, at least in right-handers, considerable efforts have been made to relate this variable to a number of structural variables in the brain (Harris and Carlson, 1988, p. 321). The best known asymmetry is the tendency of pyramidal tract fibers from the left hemisphere to cross over at a higher level than the fibers from the right side (Yakovlev and Rakic, 1966). The intriguing fact is that these researchers reported an asymmetry favoring higher crossover from the left side in 87% of the brains, a figure that is very close to the prevalence figures for left-handedness in the Gilbert and Wisocki (1992) study. Unhappily, even the very limited number of left-handers studied by Kertesz and Geschwind (1971) allows the conclusion that there is no simple relation between crossover patterns and handedness. Complicating the situation even further is the observation that the uncrossed anterior corticospinal tract is *larger* on the right side in the great majority of cases (Nathan, Smith, and Deacon, 1990). This arrangement suggests that while the crossing arrangements of the dorsal corticospinal tract favor the left brain half, the descending fibers of the uncrossed anterior (ventral) corticospinal tract reveal an asymmetry favoring the right brain half. The former tract controls the musculature of the digits and is identified with skilled manual movements. The latter controls the more proximal portions of the limbs and the trunk. If the structural asymmetries are even weakly related to hand preference, there is an asymmetry favoring the left hemisphere for fine manual movements and an asymmetry favoring the right hemisphere for limb and trunk movements. The possibility of different lateral specializations of the distal and proximal musculature has been mentioned by Healey et al. (1986). A direct test of this possibility was carried out by Peters and Pang (1992). Beginning with the observation that some left-handed writers prefer the right arm for throwing, they speculated that this group might have fine motor control lateralized for the left hand, and arm movement control lateralized for the right arm. However, while this group was very clearly specialized for throwing in the right hand, arm-tapping speed favored the left arm. It was concluded that the type of movement, rather than musculature (distal vs. proximal), was the crucial variable in lateral specialization.

Speculations about the relation between structure of the descending motor tracts and handedness must await a great deal more detailed information than is available now. Such information would have to include:

• The nature of termination patterns of the dorsolateral corticospinal tracts on alpha motor neurons serving the digits and toes on the left and right side

• The relationship between crossover patterns and the termination patterns on alpha motor neurons serving hands and feet

• The overall relation between tract size and fiber composition of the corticospinal tracts, especially in relation to the anterior corticospinal tract

• The relation of termination patterns of the direct and indirect corticospinal tracts

• The degree to which preferential use interacts with structural asymmetries in these tracts

The Cerebellum   In the literature on handedness, the cerebellum does not normally enter the discussion. However, there are good reasons to focus some attention on this structure. The lateral portions of the cerebellar hemispheres are implicated in movement of the digits by a number of indicators. First, the evolution of the lateral portions of the cerebellum parallels the degree to which animals can make use of the distal portions of their limbs. For instance, in birds, there is very little lateral development of the cerebellum. In animals that have no independent function of the digits, the intermediate portion of the cerebellum is well developed, but not the lateral portion. That the role of the lateral cerebellum lies in higher-order aspects of motor control is indirectly suggested by the fact that the enormous flow of information that reaches the cerebellum from the cortex via the pons and the middle cerebellar peduncle comes not only from the motor and sensory areas of the cortex but also from many other areas of the cortex.

The outflow from the intermediate regions of the cerebellum is directed at the motor machinery involved with the distal portion of the limbs, and the outflow of the lateral regions of the cerebellum is directed at those regions of the cortex (and other basal ganglia) that are involved with the planning and organization of movement. There is an especially close relationship between the outflow nuclei of the lateral cerebellum, the dentate nuclei, and the premotor and supplementary cortices, which are directly implicated in the organization, planning, and modification of motor activities (Allen, Gilbert, and Yin, 1978; Halsband et al., 1993). The point made here is that (a) the lateral neocerebellum is likely to play a very important role in skilled movements of the hands and (b) the role played in skilled movement of the hands is likely to be at the level of organization, planning, and learning, as well as execution of skilled motor patterns. Unfortunately, the study of the sequelae of cerebellar lesions has been abandoned prematurely in favor of the technically more challenging work on microstructure and neurophysiology of the cerebellum. As a result, the knowledge in these latter areas far outstrips our knowledge of how cerebellar lesions and especially lesions of the cerebellar cortex affect behavior (Eccles, 1982; Ghez, 1992). Neuropsychological work on cerebellar lesions is especially important because when neocortical lesions are examined with conventional neurologic methods, no or only minimal impairments are noted (Growdon, Chambers, and Liu, 1967; Keller, Roy, and Chase, 1937; Peters and Filter, 1973; Russell, 1970). The lack of clear signs is yet another indicator that higher-order motor mechanisms are involved, and their study demands sophisticated behavioral approaches such as those developed in neuropsychology.

The focus on cerebellar involvement in hand movement is particularly pertinent in view of the fact that there has been an evolutionary shift between primate and nonprimate mammalian orders that implicates a highly developed neocerebellar role in the control of the distal musculature for the former (Ito, 1984). Nowhere is this clearer than in the original descriptions of patients with cerebellar lesions by Holmes (1917) "The slowness, awkwardness and irregularity of the finger movements in handling objects and the difficulty in bringing each finger of the affected hand separately and accurately to the tip of the thumb have been described above, but these effects are even more apparent when the patient attempts to use simple and familiar tools" (p. 490). For the development of our argument it is important to realize that these observed effects are not only due to problems in execution but also to those aspects of movement that require timing and assembly of the component acts into a meaningful whole. Holmes comments specifically that, "In writing, too, these disturbances are very obvious when the wound involves the right half of the cerebellum" (p. 490). The point made here is that cerebellar involvement in hand movement will interact with hand preferences at levels close to motor execution *and* at levels that are closer to planning and organization of movement. For instance, in fine skilled movements, the timing of component movements that are assembled in the course of a voluntary movement is crucial in execution (Ivry and Keele, 1989; Ivry, Keele, and Diener, 1988). To the extent that the timing involves proper sequencing, such a function involves both the actual provision of timing as the movement process progresses and the "syntax" of timing specific elements which involves at a very minimum the premotor cortex and the supplementary motor areas (Halsband et al., 1993). It is unthinkable that hand preference, which to a very large extent involves the development of expertise for certain movements, does not involve cerebellar functions.

The question is, Does cerebellar involvement develop with the expression of hand preferences, determined elsewhere, or is it part and parcel of the determining factors of hand preference? The question remains open. There is one aspect of cerebellar involvement that directly touches on handedness. In Levy and Reid's (1978) original model, left-handers with the inverted writing position were said to have a motor organization that favored ipsilateral corticospinal pathways. If this were the case, there would have to be a massive rearrangement of cerebrocerebellar relations. The cerebellar hemispheres exert their influence on the ipsilateral musculature of the body. That is, the outflow from the left cerebral hemisphere reaches the right neocerebellar hemisphere and, conversely, a complex system of double crossovers from the neocerebellum to the red nucleus ensures that the ascending and descending communications of the cerebellum meet up with the motor control processes of the contralateral cerebral hemisphere.

The Corpus Callosum   Witelson (1985) reported that the corpus callosum of non-right-handers is significantly larger than that of "consistent right-handers." This statement applies to males only; no significant relation between these variables was observed for females. Subsequent discussion about the validity of this claim (e.g., Habib et al., 1991; Kertesz et al., 1987; Witelson, 1989) has largely revolved around replicability of the results, and about method. As in all other such situations, the question of classification is all-important. Witelson (1985) distinguishes between those persons who in a given questionnaire prefer the right hand for all activities and calls them "consistent right-handers." Those who do not show such consistent differences are called "inconsistent right-handers." By means of this classification, Witelson includes persons who write with the right hand and those who write with the left hand under the same category of "non-right-handers." Bryden and Steenhuis (1991) suggested that one of the dangers of using this procedure is that the term "non-right-handers" becomes "left-handers," even though it denotes nothing of the sort. Their concern is justified; although Witelson's (1985) classification was strictly concerned with the identification of non-right-handers, the title of her paper is "The Brain Connection: The Corpus Callosum is Larger in Left-Handers." In addition, the frequencies of right-handers and non-right-handers defined by Witelson's classification are entirely a function of the length of the questionnaire, as pointed out above. However, it is not necessary to engage in lengthy discussions about classification in this context. A recent paper by Steinmetz et al. (1992) used the same classification methods described by Witelson to define non-right-handers, and methods that are not subject to criticism that might be leveled at other work in the literature. Steinmetz et al. failed to find any significant differences related to handedness.

From a functional perspective, behavioral data do not reveal any significant differences in information transfer across the corpus callosum between right-handers and left-handers (e.g., Piccirilli, Finali, and Sciarma, 1989). However, there is some evidence from the animal literature that the corpus callosum plays a role in the development of paw preference. What this role is remains unclear. In the work of Gruber et al. (1991), male mice with a congenitally absent corpus callosum show weaker paw preferences, while in the work of Schmidt, Manhaes, and DeMoraes (1991), animals with corpus callosum malformations show a greater asymmetry favoring the left than do animals of the same strain without such malformations.

Three significant problems prevent any conclusive statements about the role of the corpus callosum in relation to handedness. First, the role of the corpus callosum in central nervous system function is still very much a subject of speculation. In particular, there is little acknowledgment in the literature of the fact that the very large majority of fibers in the corpus callosum are unmyelinated and very slow. If there is any relation between the corpus callosum and handedness, would only the large and fast fibers be involved, and if so, how? What possible role could there be for the huge proportion of very slowly conducting unmyelinated fibers in hand preference? It *is* known that the corpus callosum is important in the integration of bimanual movement, an aspect of hand movement that figures largely in hand preference, but it is quite unclear how this could be a factor in hand preference asymmetries.

Second, the anatomic data on callosum size, especially for humans, are too meager at this point to permit extensive speculation. What is the relationship between overall size of the callosum or its parts and the number and composition of its fibers? What is the significance of the very marked interindividual differences in callosal size and shape of parts (i.e., shape of the splenium in particular)? Third, the documentation of significant handedness differences seems to rest on a handedness classification that is very arbitrary. How will different ways of classifying handedness affect the relation between handedness and callosal parameters? If it is degree rather than direction of lateralization that matters in handedness-callosal interrelations, why do the Steinmetz et al. data not show such a relation?

The conclusion to be drawn is that the speculations relating handedness to callosal parameters outstrip by far the body of reliable data that is available on this question. The approach taken by Witelson and others may yet prove very useful in the classification of handedness. In particular, there is a conceptual link between handedness and callosal function, however weakly developed. Kinsbourne (1973) and Levy (1985) have stressed the possibility of a crucial role of the corpus callosum in directing attention, and Peters (1988b), suggesting multiple callosal roles, also believes that the allocation of attention was one of its major functions. These speculations assume some significance in view of the argument, developed later in this chapter, that hand preference is more directly related to asymmetries in the allocation of attention than to structural asymmetries at the executing level of the motor system.

Speech and Language Lateralization in Relation to Handedness   One of the more frustrating aspects of relating handedness to other aspects of cerebral lateralization concerns the relation between handedness and lateralization for speech and language. For the purposes of this discussion it is necessary to separate lateralization for speech from lateralization for language. By "speech" we refer to the specialized motor mechanisms that translate language into vocal productions. By "language" we refer to all the linguistic processes that occur prior to the provision of motor output specifications. On a conceptual level, it is easy to see that while there might be a need for lateral specialization in language processes, this specialization is likely to be flexible and allow for interhemispheric interactions, as in the interplay of the left and right hemispheres in the integration of syntax, semantics, and general context within which the communication occurs. At the level of thought, there is likely great flexibility in terms of where and how hemispheric processes contribute and interact. However, in the process of translating thought into motor specifications for speech production, the necessity to produce a very finely timed and modulated movement of the bilateral speech apparatus does not permit great flexibility; motor instructions have to be precisely sequenced and formulated. Elsewhere (Peters, 1990a) an account has been given of how the operation of the bilateral musculature of the speech apparatus requires unilateral specialization. There is no claim that speech and language lateralization is independent because as linguistic processes evolve toward articulation of thought there is a distinct advantage in having the final path from linguistic processes to articulation commands in a congruent hemisphere. However, the argument made here is that speech production will be more sharply localized to only one hemisphere (in principle, it can be either one) at a time, while language processes may show more flexibility in terms of lateral specialization (Vallar, 1990).

This distinction is important because the means by which language and speech lateralization are assessed traditionally differ in the degree to which speech and language are addressed. For instance, when tachistoscopic and dichotic methods are used to assess language lateralization in normal subjects, the final lateralization for the speech outflow path is not accessible. In the amobarbital sodium (Amytal Sodium) technique, both speech and language processes are affected and confounded as is the case in the examination of aphasia after brain insult. In this latter situation, a dissociation between speech and language processes can be achieved by distinguishing between Broca's aphasia from other aphasias, with the emphasis that this is only a relative dissociation because Broca's aphasia very rarely occurs in the complete absence of disorders of comprehension or other aphasic disturbances.

This lengthy preamble to the discussion of lateralization of speech and language relative to handedness is necessary because it flavors the interpretation of existing evidence. There is little disagreement that the overwhelming majority of right-handers have left hemisphere lateralization for speech and language. However, a majority of left-handers—albeit not as large a proportion as left-speech right-handers—also show left hemisphere specialization for language. In addition, there have also been claims that left-handers show a greater prevalence of bilateral involvement in language functions (Segalowitz and Bryden, 1983), as based on a review of the literature that largely concerns amobarbital tests and the sequalae of unilateral lesions. However, the data on language lateralization of left-handers are not at all comparable in volume and quality to the evidence available for right-handers, and there is some reason for caution. Basso et al. (1990) did not find significant differences between recovery rates for right-handers and non-right-handers, and Borod, Carper, and Naeser (1990) could not find any convincing differences between recovery rates of left-handers and right-handers after unilateral left lesions. While it is true that these last two papers themselves are not without methodologic problems, it is prudent to reserve judgment on this issue until larger samples of left-handed patients have been studied.

Dichotic listening studies also suggest that the majority of left-handers (a smaller majority than is the case for right-handers) are left hemisphere–dominant for language. It should also be noted that a strong attentional component of the dichotic listening task (e.g., Bryden, Munhall, and Allard, 1983) cautions researchers to use dichotic data to draw hard-and-fast conclusions about the lateralization of speech mechanisms.

Perhaps it has been a mistake to focus too much on the data which suggest that speech and language lateralization in left-handers is more often on the right hemisphere than it is in right-handers. The status of right hemisphere speech and language, or bilateral speech and language in left-handers, is not securely established and it might very well be the case that instances of relatively pure Broca's aphasia after *right* hemisphere lesions in left-handers are extremely rare. What is securely established is that the majority of left-handers share with right-handers a left hemisphere specialization for this domain. Thus, there is a clear dissociation between lateralization for preferred hand and lateralization for speech and language in left-handers. Recently, it has been pointed out that all persons, whether right- or left-handed, share a common asymmetry in one of the most important neural pathways underlying speech. The recurrent branches of the vagus nerve form the final motor control outflow to the muscles of the larynx and in all persons, the left branch of the recurrent nerve has a significantly longer access path to its target musculature than the right branch (Walker, 1987, 1988). In order to achieve synchronous activation of the larynx, this asymmetry imposes common restraints as to laterality on all persons (Peters, 1992b).

The conclusion drawn from this is that the underlying asymmetry, especially for motor speech control, favors the same side in right- and left-handers. Why and under what circumstances the pattern in left-handers would differ from that of right-handers is considered below.

Handedness and Abilities

There is a rather interesting body of literature that attempts to relate verbal and spatial abilities to handedness. The evidence used to make the case has been either indirect or direct. Indirect evidence, for instance, would be derived from associations between hand preference and certain professions. We disregard here the associations between handedness and footedness and sports such as tennis, soccer, cricket, and baseball, because in some sports there are selective advantages for particular handedness profiles and disproportionately high prevalence figures for left-handers do not mean that left-handers excel in these sports. More to the point are widely quoted claims that there is a significant excess of left-handers among architects (Peterson and Lansky, 1977). If valid, this would support claims about differing patterns of strengths in certain cognitive domains between left-handers and right-handers. However, there is sufficient doubt about this particular relation (Shettel-Neuber and O'Reilly, 1983; Wood and Aggleton, 1991) to question the claim of a high prevalence of left-handedness among architects.

Annett and Kilshaw (1982) suggested a link between mathematical ability and left-handedness, a link which was subsequently also claimed for students who were mathematically gifted (Benbow, 1988). Bishop's (1990b, pp. 158–161) discussion of the literature indicates that the link is by no means well established. The same can be said for the speculation (Levy, 1969) that left-handers might be superior in verbal abilities and right-handers in visuospatial abilities. Since that time, numerous claims have been made that focus on verbal and visuospatial abilities relative to handedness (e.g., see the reviews by Bishop, 1990b, and McKeever, 1991). Of all the work in which handedness is to be related to some other variable, this presents the most variable results and it is our judgment that the area is not ready for an interpretative review at this point. The reluctance of researchers to attempt straight replications of reported findings, together with the failure to report effect sizes and the power of significance tests makes assessment of reports especially difficult when many of the significant findings are based on higher-order interactions or idiosyncratic handedness groupings, or both (e.g., Casey, Pezaris, and Nuttall, 1992; Harshman, Hampson, and Berenbaum, 1987).

At present, the most interesting postulate concerning handedness and abilities is that by Annett (cf. Annett and Manning, 1989). Annett seems to have abandoned the position that left-handers are specifically favored in mathematical ability and suggests that strong right-handers are generally at a disadvantage across the entire range of the intellectual spectrum. Some caution is advised because of the way in which "strong right-handers" are selected. First, the selection is made on the basis of the peg-moving task, and this is a rather narrow base from which to proceed. More important, because it is the performance differential between the left and right hand that is looked at, there is a real danger that the selection for "strong right-handers" accumulates persons who are bound to have very poor left-hand performance in the presence of average right-hand performance. Indeed, Annett's classification procedure may select for the right-handed counterparts of Bishop's (1984) "subclinical pathology" left-handers.

In summary, the literature on the relation between handedness and intellectual abilities does not inspire confidence, in spite of the fact that some promising indications of some relation do exist. However, neuropsychologists would be served well to be extremely conservative in asserting the existence of simple relations when the evidence relies very substantially on uncertain handedness classification and notoriously fickle interactions.

SPECULATIONS ABOUT NEUROPHYSIOLOGIC MECHANISMS THAT UNDERLIE HANDEDNESS

What Is It that Is Lateralized in Handedness?

In order to address the question of lateral specialization, one first has to establish what it is that one thinks is lateralized. In voluntary bimanual movement, three conceptually separate levels can be recognized.

Level 1 This is the level at which the goal is formulated, and where the component contributions of the two hands to the goal are established in terms of which hand does what and where attention is directed in the control of hand movement. The most important functional aspect of hand use is that the hands can act in a complementary fashion. In naturally occurring activities, complementarity implies role specialization (Guiard, 1987; Peters, 1985). The most fundamental way in which such role specialization can be characterized is that one hand acts on something which the other hand holds and positions. It has been pointed out (Peters, 1991, 1992b, 1994) that because attention cannot be divided in the concurrent guidance of two different motor activities —although the illusion that this is so might arise—focal attention can only be directed at one hand at a time. When the actual movements of the two hands are identical in terms of complexity but differ in terms of temporal demands in their concurrent control, attention is asymmetrically distributed in right-handers, favoring the right hand when both hands compete for attention (Guiard, 1989; Peters, 1981, 1985). Here, it is argued that not only is attention asymmetrically distributed to the two hands but that this is the essential prerequisite for skilled bimanual activity. Naturally, attentional biases will also affect the use of hands in unimanual activities in the sense that the hand that is more directly associated with the goal of the movement and which requires most directly the generative capacities of the left cerebral hemisphere (Corballis, 1989; Oldfield, 1969) will also be the hand chosen in skilled voluntary unimanual activities. However, the focusing of attention must be flexible because attention must be capable of being switched between the hands (Peters and Schwartz, 1988), and for this reason lateral bias will not be driven in any powerful way for unimanual movements. In contrast, role selection for bimanual movements implies a double specialization in the sense that it is not only the preferred hand that specializes for its role, but the nonpreferred hand that specializes for its own component role. As a result, the commitment to adopt the use of a hand for a particular role in bimanual activities has greater consequences in terms of skill acquisition than for unimanual activities. As an example, in mastering throwing with both hands, little is expected of the nonthrowing hand, but in changing hand roles in playing a string instrument, not only does the right hand have to learn a complex new role but the left hand has to do so as well.

All this accounts for lateralization but does not address the issue of why in the majority of the population it should be the left hemisphere that is associated with generativity in action and, by association, with the selective focusing of attention to the right hand. Directionally consistent lateralization arises because several action domains such as motor speech control, manipulation of food and objects with lips, tongue, and jaw movements (Peters, 1988c), in addition to bimanual hand control, all demand a unilateral source of control. Lateral congruence of a superordinate system by which action is generated and components assembled for all of these systems would seem a much more efficient design than having independently lateralized systems that all provide the same kind of higher-order control processes for these action domains. By far the most efficient way of ensuring congruence is to have lateral specialization of a generative (Corballis, 1989) mechanism that is one order removed from the actual machinery that operates jaws, larynx, intrathoracic musculature, and the hand, rather than having a separate mechanism that performs the same sort of task for each of these domains.

Level 2 This is the level where the precisely timed commands for the initiation and termination of the movement trajectories of the two hands are issued. Once an attentional bias is lateralized, the lateral specialization of control at level 2 is also determined. The timing of onset and offset of the complementary movements of the two hands would be extremely inefficient if it had to be arranged by back-and-forth communication between the hemispheres. Instead, it is reasonable from a functional design perspective to have the initiation and termination commands for the two hands issued from one side, and in right-handers this will be the left side. Confirmation of this speculation comes from the predominance of left hemisphere lesions in the production of apraxia *in the left hand* in right-handers (Liepmann, 1905), and the disruption of the timing of component movement sequences, especially after premotor cortex lesions of the left hemisphere, in the absence of problems in movement execution (Halsband et al., 1993).

Level 3   This is the level that governs the final outflow of control for the particular hand that allows the hand to perform the movement as required. In the consideration of corticospinal pathways, some asymmetries of the final motor outflow paths have been described, together with the observation that such asymmetries as have been documented do not map well onto known handedness prevalence figures. Two additional considerations mitigate against considering such peripheral asymmetries as important players in the determination of hand preferences. First and foremost, in human skilled bimanual activities, both hands have to perform very complex and delicate activities. It would be extremely limiting if structural constraints were to make one or the other hand less capable of performing certain movements. Second, when social and environmental circumstances or the nature of artifacts require that the nonpreferred hand perform complex movements, this can be done without problems. For instance, the left hand of the right-hander copes well with fingering movements in the playing of string instruments, although these can hardly be considered less demanding than the movements performed by the right hand (Peters, 1986). In typing, both hands perform equivalent and highly complex movements. Finally, in countries like Korea, virtually all left-handers write with the right hand (Kang and Harris, 1993).

In summary, it is suggested that the fundamental underlying and directionally biased asymmetry lies with the processes that take place at level 1. This suggestion is not novel; Kinsbourne (1973) speculated about the asymmetry of higher-order processes and came to similar conclusions, but not in reference to handedness. This underlying asymmetry will then lead to functional asymmetries at level 2, and structural asymmetries at level 3, such as between-hand differences in strength (Peters, 1990b).

Implications of "Attentional Bias" as Causal Agent in Hand Preference

The Locus of Underlying Asymmetries for Level 1 Processes   Several important practical implications follow from the assumption that attentional asymmetries are the causal agent for hand preference. In terms of neural underpinnings, the emphasis on attention shifts the locus of structural asymmetries from the executing motor machinery to a far more complex neural system. From an evolutionary point of view, attentional processes are likely related to sleep mechanisms because the most rudimentary form of directing global attention is provided by the brainstem mechanisms that regulate sleep and wakefulness. From such a diffuse process, differentiated paths of directing attention evolve through a process that is analogous to the parcellation process advanced by Ebbeson (1984) to explain how "new" functional circuits can arise in the central nervous system. Indeed, it is suggested that the activational processes by which some circuits are kept active within a collective of possible circuits is a prototypical attentional process that directs the selectivity by which the parcellation process carves out new pathways out of a preexisting amorphous network of connections. Seen in this way, the asymmetries observed in the location of transmitters that by virtue of their characteristics are far more suitable to the distribution of attention than to the hard-and-fast business of analyzing sensory events or controlling movement (Bracha et al., 1987; Glick and Shapiro, 1984) are not only supportive of the argument developed here but essential to its validity. Their location in the thalamus is also predictable. If fundamental attentional asymmetries underlie cortical activation, the source must be sought at the level of the ascending portions of the reticular activating system, and in the mechanisms by which meaningful action is initiated and terminated (both basal ganglia and limbic system structures are implicated here). Indeed, to the extent that the profound asymmetry of the recurrent nerve of the vagus is implicated in speech, the autonomic nervous system enters the picture as well.

How Attentional Asymmetries Confound the Degree of Manifest Handedness   Any initial asymmetry, however slight, will have a cumulative interaction with the mechanisms at levels 2 and 3. As a given hand comes to be preferred for certain activities, expertise develops in terms of efficiency of timing for certain activities and the degree to which movement intent is reliably translated into action. The relation between a subtle attentional bias and the subsequent sharpening of asymmetry through practice can hardly be put more succinctly than Humphrey did well over 100 years ago: "I am driven, therefore, to the rather nice distinction, that, though the superiority is acquired, the tendency to acquire the superiority is natural" (Humphrey, 1861, p. 202). The implications of this line of reasoning for the classification of handedness are immediately obvious. Because performance superiority of one hand over the other is stated to be the outcome of extensive asymmetric motor experience, it follows that the degree to which hand performance differs, one from the other, is a measure that is determined by the idiosyncratic motor and life experience of an individual. This view does not coincide with the idea that the degree of between-hand performance differences (skill differences) rather than the directionality of such differences is the important variable in the measurement of handedness (Annett, 1985; Bryden, 1982).

If magnitude of between-hand differences is a fundamental characteristic of handedness that is somehow related to underlying genetic mechanisms, a simple prediction follows. For different skilled activities that do *not* involve topographically similar skills (because these involve strong transfer of practice effects; cf. Annett, 1992), strong correlations should be found between the magnitude of between-hand differences of the different skills. In contrast, if it is simply a directional bias that is the fundamental determinant of handedness, there is no reason to expect strong correlations between different skilled tasks.

For instance, the latter position, which is held here, would suggest that there will be only a low or nonsignificant correlation between hand differences on Annett's (1985) peg-placing task and Peters and Durding's (1979) finger-tapping task. A different way of putting this is to emphasize that it is not skill that is heritable but direction of preference (McManus et al., 1992).

It is not suggested that the measurement of the degree of between-hand differences for certain motor skills is not useful. For instance, knowledge of the normal range of between-hand performance differences for relatively experience-neutral activities such as finger-tapping and peg-placing allows identification of disturbances in motor function that are manifested by unusually large between-hand performance differences (e.g., Bishop, 1984). In addition, there is much to be learned from the normal range of between-hand performance differences on certain tasks in terms of the design of man-machine interfaces in ergonomics. However, it is asserted here that the degree of between-hand differences will be so contaminated by motor experience that it is of questionable use in the construction of handedness theories.

All of these statements are made mostly with right-handers in mind. What about left-handers? In terms of the two major genetic models (those of Annett and McManus), two rather different predictions emerge. Beginning with the present position, that the underlying factor in hand preference is attentional in nature, Annett's model would state that left-handers (L) lack the inherent attentional bias (i.e., lack the "right-shift" gene) that is present in right-handers (R). Their hand performance asymmetries would be brought about by the dynamics that impose lateral specialization in skilled bimanual and unimanual activities. McManus' model differs in its predictions. Although McManus' states that a population that is homozygous for the "chance" (C) gene will not show any directional bias, *individuals* within that population will show a consistent lateral bias, which may be toward the right or the left. This phenomenon is termed *fluctuating asymmetry*. Left-handed writers would, in Annett's model, belong to either to a group lacking the right-shift gene in Annett's model, or possibly to a group that is heterozygous for the right-shift gene, but not very likely to the group that is homozygous for the right-shift gene. In McManus' model, left-handers would either be homozygous for the chance allele of the handedness gene, or represent a heterozygous genotype with chance in one allele and "dextral" (D) in the other.

Unfortunately, these predictions are difficult to falsify because existing phenotypes, exemplified by persons who write with the left but throw with the right hand, or those who show persistent lateral biases for the left hand, can be accounted for in terms of both Annett's and McManus' models, albeit with different arguments. This weakness of testing handedness models has been acknowledged by McManus and Bryden (1993). Preliminary work with dual tasks that stress allocation of attention rather than motor skill as such suggest (Peters, 1987) that left-handers do differ from right-handers in their allocation of attention, but it is rather difficult to assert that motor experience plays no role in this.

SUMMARY AND CONCLUSIONS

How to Classify Handedness for Practical Purposes

The alpha and omega of relating handedness to other neuropsychological variables or indices of lateral specialization lies in the classification of handedness. It has been shown that especially with a classification scheme that involves the "right-handers" and "non-right-handers," the proportions of these two groups are extremely sensitive to relatively small differences in scoring procedures, item composition, and number of items. As a result, any claims of associations between the handedness thus defined and some other neuropsychological variable must be viewed with caution. What, then, is a conservative and practical measure of handedness for researchers in neuropsychology? Here, the answer is based on the argument that the underlying variable in hand preference is attentional in nature and that direction of lateral bias is a more fundamental variable than skill differences. In countries (e.g., Australia, Canada, New Zealand, United States) where pressures against use of the left hand as the writing hand are restricted to religious and ethnic minorities, the choice of writing hand will provide the single most stable indicator of a bias toward the left hand. Thus, if only a single question were possible, it should concern the writing hand.

When it is feasible to collect additional information, short questionnaires (8–14 items) that contain references to major classes of skilled manual and arm activities (cf. Kronenberg and Beukelaar, 1983) should be used in industrialized societies:

• *Fine manual skill*, e.g., writing, drawing, using tweezers, holding a needle when sewing, holding a tool when repairing something

• *Hand-wrist skill*, e.g., using a razor, combing hair, cutting bread

• *Hand-wrist-arm skill*, e.g., throwing a ball, holding a racquet in sports, using a hammer

• *Strength*, e.g., which hand or arm is stronger

• *Activity that reflects preference, but not necessarily skill*, e.g., picking up a book, or a small object

In calculating handedness scores from such questionnaires, the most stable results will be obtained when handedness is defined in terms of "below and above midpoint" criteria. This procedure will underestimate the prevalence of left-handedness in cultures in which there is no pressure against using the left hand for writing because there will be left-handed writers who do many things with the right hand. However, in cultures in which there is pressure against use of the left hand as the writing hand, this procedure will yield prevalence figures of left-handedness that are much closer to those obtained by the "writing hand" criterion (Kang and Harris, 1993; Maehara et al., 1988). The least stable results will be obtained if a categorization into "right-handers" and "non-right-handers" is made on the basis of exclusive "right" answers. Slightly more stable is a classification that is based on "right-handers," "mixed preference handers," and "left-handers," based on extreme choices in either direction and intermediate choices. This classification method may be of value if right- and left-handed persons are to be identified who are extremely rigid in their preferences.

If possible, subjects should be given the same questionnaire twice, first with forced choices (left/right) and second, with graded choices (always left, mostly left, either side, mostly right, always right). For short questionnaires this should take little time. The choice of a few representative questions will allow flexibility in defining handedness in case advances are made in the theory of handedness. Thus, retroactive analysis of data can be performed, with different criteria of handedness. From the point of multivariate analyses it is not desirable to include too many items that ask similar questions. For example, multiple questions of the type "pick up small object, pick up marble, pick up paper clip" will lead to distortions of factor structure in factor-analytic studies.

Promising New (and Revival of Old) Avenues of Investigation

Cross-cultural Studies   In keeping with the general theme of this chapter, promising new directions lie in the accumulation of detailed handedness data from a variety of different industrial and nonindustrial cultures (e.g., Bryden et al., 1993; Connolly and Bishop, 1992; Dellatolas et al., 1991; Kang and Harris, 1993; Maehara et al., 1988). Careful examination of highly detailed handedness studies from different cultures will permit identification of handedness activities that are subject to different degrees of social pressure in terms of hand use. In addition, by careful examination of the patterns of items that are less directly influenced, some meaningful cross-cultural comparisons can be made. Work in this area can also give a clearer perspective on the sex differences in the prevalence of left-handedness. The new decade might well bring evidence that explanations for this difference are to be sought at the cultural-environmental rather than the biological level.

Work in the Kinesiology of Handedness   Research in this area will provide information about the exact motor requirements of different classes of movements that are used to define handedness. This information can be used to evaluate the possibility that, contrary to my position, neuromuscular specializations that are not simply the result of differential practice underlie hand preference.

Research on Nonhuman Lateral Motor Preferences   Work in this area has been given new impetus (Fagot and Vauclair, 1991; Harris, 1989; MacNeilage, Studdert-Kennedy, and Lindblom (1987), and will allow a broader interpretation of the dynamics underlying handedness.

Positron Emission Tomography Studies of Unimanual and Bimanual Hand Use with Groups of Left-handers and Right-handers This technology will help in answering the question of the different hemispheric localization of higher-order motor mechanisms in right- and left-handers. Specifically, persons with clearly defined handedness can be asked to imagine execution of a simple movement with one hand, to execute a simple movement requiring strength with one hand, to execute a complex unimanual sequence of movements, to execute a complex bimanual sequence of movements, and to imagine carrying out these movements without actually performing them. Of especial interest will be the pattern of cerebral activity in the premotor cortex and the supplementary motor cortex of both hemispheres and the intra- and interhemispheric pattern of activity in complex bimanual activities in right- and left-handers. Such work can answer the question of the lateralization of the higher-order motor corteces, especially in left-handers.

Genetic Models Both models have weaknesses in terms of their differential predictions for the phenotypic distinctions between the heterozygous and homozygous conditions that increase the probability of left-handedness. In Annett's (1985) case, this involves the distinction between the phenotypic expectations for R+/R− vs. R−/R−, and in McManus' (1991), the expectations for D/C vs. C/C. A most exciting direction of future research would lie in the identification of putative loci for a handedness gene, with initial speculations by McManus (1991) that a locus might lie in the pseudoautosomal region of the X chromosome. Also in the area of genetic models, work that will inform about the degree to which skill differences between the hands correlate across different skilled activities will allow an evaluation of the different predictions made by the two handedness theories.

Neuroanatomy of Corticospinal Tracts The functional significance of the asymmetry in crossing corticospinal fibers at the level of the pyramids remains to be resolved, as does the question of the functional significance of differences in size of descending dorsolateral and anterior corticospinal tracts. Ideally, work would deal with postmortem studies in persons for whom handedness information is complete, with sufficient numbers of cases to evaluate classification of left-handedness relative to anatomic structure. Work on the functional neurophysiology of spinal reflexes, such as the research by Tan (1989), will complement the neuroanatomic data.

ACKNOWLEDGMENT

The support of the Natural Sciences and Engineering Research Council of Canada grant No. A7054 is gratefully acknowledged.

REFERENCES

Allen, G. I., Gilbert, P. F. C., and Yin, T. C. T. (1978). Convergence of cerebral inputs onto dentate neurons in monkey. *Experimental Brain Research, 32,* 337–341.

Annett, M. (1985). *Left, right, hand and brain: the right shift theory.* Hillsdale, NJ: Lawrence Erlbaum Associates.

Annett, M. (1992). Five tests of hand skill. *Cortex, 28,* 583–600.

Annett, M., and Kilshaw, D. (1982). Mathematical ability and lateral asymmetry. *Cortex, 18,* 547–568.

Annett, M., and Manning, M. (1989). The disadvantages of dextrality for intelligence. *British Journal of Psychology, 80,* 213–226.

Annett, M., and Turner, A. (1974). Laterality and the growth of intellectual abilities. *British Journal of Educational Psychology, 44,* 37–46.

Bakan, P., Dibbs, G., and Reed, P. (1973). Handedness and birth stress. *Neuropsychologia, 11,* 363–366.

Basso, A., Farabola, M., Grassi, M. P., Laiacona, M., and Zanobia, M. E. (1990). Comparison of aphasia profiles and language recovery in non-right-handed and matched right-handed patients. *Brain and Language, 38,* 233–252.

Benbow, C. P. (1988). Sex differences in mathematical reasoning ability in intellectually talented preadolescents: their nature, effects, and possible causes. *Brain and Behavioral Sciences, 11,* 169–232.

Bishop, D. V. M. (1984). Using non-preferred hand skill to investigate pathological left-handedness in an unselected population. *Developmental Medicine and Child Neurology, 26,* 214–226.

Bishop, D. V. M. (1990a). On the futility of using familial sinistrality to subclassify handedness groups. *Cortex, 26,* 153–155.

Bishop, D. V. M. (1990b). *Handedness and developmental disorder.* Hove, England: Lawrence Erlbaum Associates.

Borod, J. C., Carper, J. M., and Naeser, M. (1990). Long-term language recovery in left-handed aphasic patients. *Aphasiology, 4,* 561–572.

Bracha, H. I., Seitz, D. J., Otemaa, D. J., and Glick, S. D. (1987). Rotational movement (circling) in normal humans: Sex differences and relationship to hand, foot and eye preference. *Brain Research, 411,* 231–235.

Bryden, M. P. (1982). *Laterality: functional asymmetry in the intact brain.* New York, NY: Academic Press.

Bryden, M. P., Ardila, A., and Ardila, O. (1993). Handedness in native Amazonians. *Neuropsychologia, 31,* 301–308.

Bryden, M. P., Munhall, K., and Allard, F. (1983). Attentional biases and the right-ear effect in dichotic listening. *Brain and Language, 18,* 236–248.

Bryden, M. P. and Steenhuis, R. E. (1991). Issues in the assessment of handedness. In F. L. Kitterle (Ed.), *Cerebral laterality: theory and research* (pp 35–51). Hillsdale, NJ: Lawrence Erlbaum Associates.

Casey, M. B., Pezaris, E., and Nuttall, R. L. (1992). Spatial ability as predictor of math achievement: the importance of sex and handedness patterns. *Neuropsychologia, 30,* 34–45.

Connolly, K., J., and Bishop, D. V. M. (1992). The measurement of handedness: a cross-cultural comparison of samples from England and Papua New Guinea. *Neuropsychologia, 30*, 27—34.

Corballis, M. C. (1989). Laterality and human evolution. *Psychological Review, 96*, 492—505.

Coren, S., and Halpern, D. F. (1991). Left-handedness: a marker for decreased survival fitness? *Psychological Bulletin, 109*, 90—106.

Dellatolas, G., Tubert, P., Castresana, A., Mesbah, M., Giallonardo, T., Lazaratou, H., and Lelouch, J. (1991). Age and cohort effects in adult handedness. *Neuropsychologia, 29*, 225—261.

Ebbeson, S. O. (1984). Evolution and ontogeny of neural circuits. *The Behavioral and Brain Sciences, 7*, 321—331.

Eccles, J. C. (1982). The future of studies on the cerebellum. In S. L. Palay and V. Chan-Palay (Eds.), *The cerebellum—new vistas* (pp 607—620). Heidelberg: Springer-Verlag.

Fagot, J., and Vauclair, J. (1991). Manual laterality in nonhuman species: a distinction between handedness and manual specialization. *Psychological Bulletin, 109*, 76—89.

Geschwind, N., and Behan, P. (1982). Left-handedness: Association with immune disease, migraine, and developmental disorder. *Proceedings of the National Academy of Sciences of the United States of America, 79*, 5097—5100.

Geschwind, N., and Galaburda, A. M. (1985). Cerebral lateralization. Biological mechanisms, associations and pathology: II. A hypothesis and a program for research. *Archives of Neurology, 42*, 521—552.

Ghez, C. (1992). The cerebellum. In E. R. Kandel, J. H. Schwartz, and T. M. Jessell (Eds.), *Principles of neural science* (pp 626—646). New York, NY: Elsevier.

Gilbert, A. N., and Wisocki, C. J. (1992). Hand preference and age in the United States. *Neuropsychologia, 30*, 601—608.

Glick, S. D., and Shapiro, R. M. (1984). Functional and neurochemical asymmetries. In N. Geschwind and A. M. Galaburda (Eds.), *Cerebral dominance: the biological foundations* (pp 147—166). Cambridge, MA: Harvard University Press.

Growdon, J. H., Chambers, W. W., and Liu, C. N. (1967). An experimental study of cerebellar dyskinesia in the rhesus monkey. *Brain, 90*, 603—632.

Gruber, D., Waanders, R., Collins, R. L., Wolfer, D. P., and Lipp, H. P. (1991). Weak or missing paw lateralization in a mouse strain (I/LnJ) with congenital absence of the corpus callosum. *Behavioral Brain Research, 46*, 9—16.

Guiard, Y. (1987). Asymmetric division of labor in human skilled bimanual action: the cinematic chain as a model. *Journal of Motor Behaviour, 19*, 486—517.

Guiard, Y. (1989). Failure to sing the left-hand part of the score during piano performance: loss of the pitch and stroop vocalizations. *Music Perception, 6*, 299—314.

Guiard, Y., and Millerat, F. (1984). Writing posture in lefthanders: inverters are hand crossers. *Neuropsychologia, 22*, 535—538.

Habib, M., Gayraud, D., Oliva, A., Regis, J., Salamon, G., and Khalil, R. (1991). Effects of handedness and sex on the morphology of the corpus callosum: a study with brain magnetic resonance imaging. *Brain and Cognition, 16*, 41—61.

Halsband, U., Ito, N., Tanji, J., and Freund, H. J. (1993). The role of premotor cortex and the supplementary motor area in the temporal control of movement in man. *Brain, 116*, 243—266.

Harris, L. J. (1989). Footedness in parrots: three centuries of research, theory and mere surmise. *Canadian Journal of Psychology, 43*, 369—396.

Harris, L. J. (1993). Do left-handers die sooner than right-handers? Commentary on Coren and Halpern's "Left-handedness: a marker for decreased survival fitness." *Psychological Bulletin, 114,* 203–234.

Harris, L. J., and Carlson, D. F. (1988). Pathological left-handedness: An analysis of theories and evidence. In D. Molfese and S. J. Segalowitz (Eds.), *Brain lateralization in children* (pp 289–372). New York, NY: Guilford Press.

Harshman, R. A., Hampson, E., and Berenbaum, S. A. (1987). Normal variation in human brain organization: relation to handedness, sex and handedness differences in ability. *Canadian Journal of Psychology, 37,* 144–192.

Healey, J. M., Liederman, J., and Geschwind, N. (1986). Handedness is not a unidimensional trait. *Cortex, 22,* 33–53.

Holmes, G. (1917). The symptoms of acute cerebellar injuries due to gunshot injuries. *Brain, 40,* 461–535.

Hugdahl, K., Satz, P., Mitrushina, M., and Miller, N. E. (1993). Left-handedness and old age: do left-handers die earlier? *Neuropsychologia, 31,* 325–333.

Humphrey, G. M. (1861). The human foot and the human hand. Cambridge, England: Macmillan.

Ito, M. (1984). *The cerebellum and neural control.* New York, NY: Raven Press.

Ivry, R. B., and Keele, S. W. (1989). Timing functions of the cerebellum. *Journal of Cognitive Neuroscience, 1,* 136–152.

Ivry, R. B., Keele, S. W., and Diener, H. C. (1988). Timing functions of the cerebellum. *Experimental Brain Research, 73,* 167–180.

Kang, Y., and Harris, L. (1993). *Social-cultural influences on handedness: a cross-cultural study of Koreans and Americans.* Paper presented at the TENNET (Theoretical and Experimental Neuropsychology) Meeting, Montral, May 1993.

Keller, A. D., Roy, R. S., and Chase, W. P. (1937). Extirpation of the neocerebellar cortex without eliciting so-called cerebellar signs. *American Journal of Physiology, 118,* 720–733.

Kertesz, A., and Geschwind, N. (1971). Patterns of pyramidal decussation and their relationship to handedness. *Archives of Neurology, 24,* 326–332.

Kertesz, A., Polk, M., Howell, J., and Black, S. E. (1987). Cerebral dominance, sex and callosal size. *Neurology, 37,* 1385–1388.

Kinsbourne, M. (1973). Lateral interactions in the brain. In Kinsbourne, M., and Smyth, L. W. (Eds.), *Hemispheric disconnection and cerebral function* (pp 239–259). Springfield, IL: Charles C Thomas.

Kinsbourne, M. (1988). Sinistrality, brain organization, and cognitive deficits. In D. Molfese and S. J. Segalowitz (Eds.), *The developmental implications of brain lateralization* (pp 259–280). New York, NY: Guilford Press.

Kronenberg, L. J., and Beukelaar, P. M. (1983). Towards a conceptualization of hand preference. *British Journal of Psychology, 74,* 33–45.

Liepmann, H. (1905). Die linke Hemisphäre und das Handeln. *Münchener medizinische Wochenschrift, Nov. 28,* 2322–2326, 2375–2378.

Levy, J. (1969). Possible basis for the evolution of lateral specialization in the human brain. *Nature, 224,* 614–615.

Levy, J. (1985). Interhemispheric collaboration: Single mindedness in the asymmetric brain. In C. T. Best (Ed.), *Hemispheric function and collaboration in the child* (pp 11–31). New York, NY: Academic Press.

Levy, J., and Reid, M. (1978). Variations in cerebral organization as a function of handedness, hand posture in writing, and sex. *Journal of Experimental Psychology: General, 107,* 109–144.

MacNeilage, P. F., Studdert-Kennedy, M. G., and Lindblom, B. (1987). Primate handedness reconsidered. *Behavioral and Brain Sciences, 10,* 247–301.

Maehara, K., Negishi, N., Tsai, A., Iizuka, R, Otsuki, N., Suzuki, S., Takahashi, T., and Sumiyoshi, Y. (1988). Handedness in the Japanese. *Developmental Neuropsychology, 4,* 117–127.

McKeever, W. F. (1991). Handedness, language laterality and spatial ability. In F. L. Kitterle (Ed.), *Cerebral laterality: theory and research* (pp 53–70). Hillsdale, NJ: Lawrence Erlbaum Associates.

McManus, I. C. (1991). The inheritance of left-handedness. In J. Marsh (Ed.), *Biological asymmetry and handedness (CIBA Symposium 162)* (pp 251–267). London: John Wiley & Sons.

McManus, I. C., Murray, B., Doyle, K., and Baron-Cohen, S. (1992). Handedness in childhood autism shows a dissociation between skill and preference. *Cortex, 28,* 373–381.

McManus, I. C., and Bryden, M. P. (1991). Geschwind's theory of cerebral lateralization: developing a formal causal model. *Psychological Bulletin, 110,* 237–253.

McManus, I. C., and Bryden, M. P. (1993). The neurobiology of handedness, language, and cerebral dominance: a model for the molecular genetics of behavior. In M. H. Johnson (Ed.), *Brain development and cognition* (pp 679–702). Cambridge, England: Basic Blackwell.

Moscovitch, M., and Smith, L. C. (1979). Differences in neural organization between individuals with inverted and noninverted handwriting postures. *Science, 205,* 710–713.

Nathan, P. W., Smith, M. C., and Deacon, P. (1990). The spinocortical tracts in man. *Brain, 113,* 303–324.

Oldfield, R. C. (1969). Handedness in musicians. *British Journal of Psychology, 60,* 91–99.

Peters, M. (1981). Attentional asymmetries during concurrent bimanual performance. *Quarterly Journal of Experimental Psychology, 33,* 95–103.

Peters, M. (1985). Constraints in the coordination of bimanual movements and their expression in skilled and unskilled subjects. *Quarterly Journal of Experimental Psychology. 37A,* 171–196.

Peters, M. (1986). Hand roles and handedness in music. *Psychomusicology, 6,* 29–34.

Peters, M. (1987). A nontrivial motor performance difference between right-handers and left-handers: Attention as intervening variable in the expression of handedness. *Canadian Journal of Psychology, 41,* 91–99.

Peters, M. (1988a). Footedness: Asymmetries in foot preference and skill and neuropsychological assessment of foot movement. *Psychological Bulletin, 103,* 179–192.

Peters, M. (1988b). The size of the corpus callosum in males and females: Implications of a lack of allometry. *Canadian Journal of Psychology, 42,* 313–324.

Peters, M. (1988c). The primate mouth as agent of manipulation and its relation to human handedness. *Behavioral and Brain Sciences, 11,* 729.

Peters, M. (1990a). Interaction of vocal and manual movements. In G. Hammond (Ed.), *Cerebral control of speech and limb movement. Advances in Psychology* (pp 535–574). Amsterdam: North-Holland

Peters, M. (1990b). Subclassification of lefthanders poses problems for theories of handedness. *Neuropsychologia, 28,* 279–289.

Peters, M. (1991). Laterality and motor control. In J. Marsh (Ed.), *Biological asymmetry and handedness (CIBA Symposium 162)* (pp 300–311). London: John Wiley & Sons.

Peters, M. (1992a). How sensitive are handedness prevalence figures to differences in handedness classification procedures? *Brain and Cognition, 18,* 208–215.

Peters, M. (1992b). Cerebral asymmetry for speech and the asymmetry in path lengths for the right and left recurrent nerves. *Brain and Language, 43,* 349–352.

Peters, M. (in preparation). Preference profiles of lefthanders.

Peters, M. (1994). When attention can absolutely not be divided. *Journal of Motor Behavior, 26,* 196–199.

Peters, M. and Durding, B. (1979). Footedness of left-and right-handers. *American Journal of Psychology, 92,* 133–142.

Peters, M., and Filter, P. M. (1973). Performance of a motor task after cerebellar cortical lesions in rats. *Physiology and Behavior, 11,* 13–16.

Peters, M., and Murphy, K. (1992). Cluster analysis reveals at least three, and possibly five distinct handedness groups. *Neuropsychologia, 30,* 373–380.

Peters, M., and Murphy, K. (1993). Factor analysis of pooled handedness questionnaire data is of questionable value. *Cortex, 29,* 305–413.

Peters, M., and Pang, J. (1992). Do "right-armed" lefthanders have different lateralization of motor control for the proximal and distal musculature? *Cortex, 28,* 391–399.

Peters, M., and Schwartz, S. (1988). Coordination of the two hands and effects of attentional manipulation in the production of a bimanual 2 : 3 polyrhythm. *Australian Journal of Psychology, 41,* 215–224.

Peterson, J. M., and Lansky, L. M. (1977). Left-handedness among architects: partial replication and some new data. *Perceptual and Motor Skills, 45,* 1216–1218.

Piccirilli, M., Finali, G., and Sciarma, T. (1989). Negative evidence of difference between right- and lefthanders in interhemispheric transfer of information. *Neuropsychologia, 27,* 1023–1026.

Porac, C., and Coren, S. (1981). *Lateral preferences and human behavior.* New York, NY: Springer-Verlag.

Russell, G. (1970). Discussion. In W. S. Fields and W. D. Willis, *The cerebellum in health and disease* (p 409). St. Louis MO: Warren H. Green.

Satz, P. (1972). Pathological Left-handedness: An explanatory model. *Cortex, 8,* 121–137.

Satz, P., Orsini, D. L., Saslow, E., and Henry, R. R. (1985). The pathological lefthandedness syndrome. *Brain and Cognition, 4,* 27–46.

Schmidt, S. L., Manhaes, A. C., and DeMoraes, V. Z. (1991). The effects of total and partial callosal agenesis on the development of paw preference performance in the BALB/cCF mouse. *Brain Research, 545,* 175–182.

Seddon, B. M., and McManus, I. C. (in preparation). The incidence of left-handedness: a meta-analysis.

Segalowitz, S. J., and Bryden, M. P. (1983). Individual differences in hemispheric representation of language. In S. J. Segalowitz (Ed.), *Language functions and brain organization* (pp 341–372). New York, NY: Academic Press.

Shettel-Neuber, J., and O'Reilly, J. (1983). Handedness and career choice: another look at supposed left/right differences. *Perceptual and Motor Skills, 57,* 391–397.

Steenhuis, R. E., and Bryden, M. P. (1989). Different dimensions of hand preference that relate to skilled and unskilled activities. *Cortex, 25,* 289–304.

Steinmetz, H., Jäncke, L., Kleinschmidt, A., Schlaug, G., Volkmann, J., and Huang, Y. (1992). Sex but no hand difference in the isthmus of the corpus callosum. *Neurology, 42,* 749–752.

Suetonius (1979). *The twelve caesars.* R. Graves (Trans.). London: Penguin.

Tan, Ü. (1989). The H-reflex recovery curve from the wrist flexors: lateralization of motoneuronal excitability in relation to handedness in normal subjects. *International Journal of Neuroscience, 48,* 271–284.

Thach, W. T., Kane, S. A., Mink, J. W., and Goodkin, H. P. (1992). Cerebellar output: multiple maps and modes of control in movement coordination. In R. Llinas and C. Sotelo (Eds.), *The cerebellum revisited* (pp 283–300). New York, NY: Springer-Verlag.

Vallar, G. (1990). Hemispheric control of articulatory speech output in aphasia. In G. Hammond (Ed.) *Cerebral control of speech and limb movement. Advances in Psychology* (pp. 388–416). Amsterdam: North-Holland.

Virgil (1962). *The Aeneid.* C. D. Lewis (Trans.). London: New English Library.

Walker, S. F. (1987). Or in the hand, or in the heart? Alternative routes to lateralization. *Behavioral and Brain Sciences, 10,* 288.

Walker, S. F. (1988). Language, handedness and the larynx. *Behavioral and Brain Sciences, 11,* 731–732.

Weber, A. M., and Bradshaw, J. L. (1981). Levy and Reid's neuropsychological model in relation to writing/hand posture: an evaluation. *Psychological Bulletin, 90,* 74–88.

Williams, S. M. (1986). Factor analysis of the Edingurgh handedness inventory. *Cortex, 22,* 325–326.

Witelson, S. F. (1985). The brain connection: the corpus callosum is larger in left-handers. *Science, 229,* 665–668.

Witelson, S. F. (1989). Hand and sex differences in the isthmus and genu of the human corpus callosum. *Brain, 112,* 700–835.

Wood, C. J., and Aggleton, J. P. (1991). Occupation and handedness: An examination of architects and mail survey biases. *Canadian Journal of Psychology, 45,* 395–404.

Yakovlev, P. I., and Rakic, P. (1966). Patterns of decussation of bulbar pyramids and distribution of pyramidal tracts on two sides of the spinal cord. *Transactions of the American Neurological Association, 91,* 366–367.

IV Attention and Learning

9 Attentional Asymmetries

Kenneth M. Heilman

The purpose of this chapter is to discuss attentional asymmetries. Before we can discuss functional asymmetries we need to define terms. Unfortunately, terms such as *attention* and *intention* are notoriously difficult to define because they are processes rather than objects or actions. The brain receives more simultaneous sensory input than it can possibly process. Therefore, the brain makes priorities based on goals and needs. Based on these priorities, the brain selects a subset of stimuli to process fully (attended stimuli) and a subset of stimuli that will not be fully processed (unattended stimuli). The brain also decides when to continue attending to stimuli or a portion of space while waiting for stimuli (viligance) and when to discontinue attending to stimuli (extinction and habituation).

In regard to intention, there are at least two major premotor systems that influence motor acts. The production or praxis system (see Heilman and Rothi, 1993) is critical for programming the spatial trajectory, the timing, and the sequencing of motor acts. Unlike these praxic or "how" systems, the intentional or "when" systems provide instructions to the motor system in relation to goals and needs. Intentional instructions parallel attentional instructions. There are, in general, four types of intentional instructions: "when" to initiate a motor act; "when" not to initiate a motor act; "when" to continue a motor act; and "when" to stop a motor act.

There is increasing evidence that the neuronal systems that mediate attentional and intentional instructions are asymmetrically organized in the brain. Much of this evidence originally came from neurobehavioral studies of brain-impaired subjects. More recently, studies of normal subjects using behavioral and physiologic paradigms have not only confirmed impressions gained from observations of brain-damaged subjects but have also added to our knowledge of the neuronal basis of these attentional asymmetries. Therefore, in this chapter I not only discuss the attentional asymmetries seen in brain-impaired subjects but also the studies on normal subjects. Based on these studies, I attempt to develop neuropsychological models that account for these attentional asymmetries. Because we have recently reviewed intentional asymmetries (see Heilman and Watson, 1991), they are not discussed here.

ASYMMETRIES OF ATTENTIONAL DISORDERS

Inattention

Visual Inattention (Visual Neglect or Pseudohemianopsia)   Visual inattention or visual neglect refers to the unawareness of contralesional visual stimuli in patients with central nervous system lesions in locations other than the primary visual area of the visual projection systems. Patients with visual inattention may be distinguished from patients with hemianopsia because they can detect stimuli when aided by instructional cues, novel stimuli, or stimuli with strong motivational value. In other patients, hemianopia can be distinguished from body-centered inattention by having the patient gaze toward the ipsilesional side. Patients with body-centered inattention may fail to detect contralesional stimuli when they look straight ahead or look toward contralateral hemispace, but when their gaze is directed to ipsilesional hemispace, placing the contralateral visual field within the ipsilesional head or body hemispace, they may be able to detect visual stimuli even in the contralesional retinal field (Kooistra and Heilman, 1989; Nadeau and Heilman, 1991). In some patients, inattention cannot be behaviorally distinguished from hemianopsia, and therefore one may rely on evoked potentials (Vallar et al., 1991b) or one can rely on knowledge that the lesion did not ablate the primary visual cortex or projections to this cortex.

Because visual attention is often difficult to distinguish from hemianopsia, there have not been systematic studies that attempted to learn if there are hemispheric asymmetries. However, the five cases of pseudohemianopsia reported by Kooistra and Heilman (1989), Nadeau and Heilman (1991), and Vallar et al. (1991b) all had right hemisphere lesions. As we discuss in subsequent sections, there are patients without hemianopsia or pseudohemianopsia that have hemispatial or unilateral spatial neglect and fail to cancel contralesional targets, fail to copy contralesional sides of figures, and fail to correctly bisect lines deviating to the ipsilesional sides. Even though hemispatial neglect can be explained by intentional disorders, these patients can also have attentional disorders. Multiple studies have demonstrated that hemispatial neglect is more commonly associated and is more severe with right than with left hemisphere lesions.

Tactile Inattention (Pseudohemianesthesia)   Vallar et al. (1991a) reported a patient who appeared to have contralateral hemianesthesia from a large right hemisphere cerebral infarction. Although this patient did not report being stimulated on the left side, tactile stimulation did produce psychophysiologic responses as determined by electrodermal skin conductance. Vallar et al. (1991b) reported three patients who had left hemianesthesia from right hemisphere lesions and normal evoked potentials to left-sided stimuli.

Many of the symptoms associated with the neglect syndrome may be temporarily improved by stimulating the contralateral ear with cold water

(Rubens, 1985). Vallar and co-workers (1990) report three patients who appeared to have hemianesthesia that was reduced with caloric stimulation. All of the cases had left hemianesthesia from right hemisphere lesions.

Using selective hemispheric anesthesia or Wada testing in 18 epileptic patients, Meador et al. (1988) found that contralateral tactile inattention was present in 8 patients after right hemisphere injections but in only two subjects after left-sided injections.

Extinction to Simultaneous Stimulation

As patients with inattention improve, they may develop extinction to simultaneous stimuli. Whereas patients with inattention are unaware of stimuli presented to the side opposite their lesion (pseudohemianopsia and pseudohemianesthesia), patients with extinction are aware of contralesional stimuli, but when given bilateral simultaneous stimuli, they fail to report the stimulus presented to the contralesional side.

Schwartz and co-workers (1979) studied patients with hemispheric lesions for extinction and noted that extinction was more frequent for stimuli presented to the left than the right hand. However, in this study a verbal response was required and Schwartz et al. attributed this asymmetry in part to the exclusion of aphasic patients and the possibility that extinction in some cases may be related to a right hemisphere disconnection such that lesions prevented stimuli that were perceived on the left side, by the right hemisphere, from reaching language cortex in the left hemisphere.

Meador et al. (1988) studied extinction in 18 epileptic patients who were undergoing Wada testing for preoperative evaluation. They found that contralateral extinction was more commonly associated with selective anesthesia of the right hemisphere than of the left hemisphere.

Although tactile and visual extinction are most commonly reported when the simultaneous stimuli are presented to opposite sides of the body or visual field, extinction can be seen when both stimuli are presented to the same side of the body or the same visual field, including the side ipsilateral to the lesion (Rapscak, Watson, and Heilman, 1987; Feinberg, Habor, and Stacy, 1990). In all these cases of ipsilateral extinction, the patients had right hemisphere lesions.

Hemispatial Neglect (Unilateral Spatial Neglect)

Patients with hemispheric lesions may fail to perform normally on spatial tasks that require both detection and action. For example, they may not eat off of one side of their trays or plates. When requested to copy a picture, they may only copy the ipsilesional half of the picture. When asked to bisect horizontally oriented lines they may deviate their bisection toward the ipsilesional side, and when requested to cancel stimuli randomly distributed over a page they may fail to cancel the contralesional stimuli. Contralesional hemispace may be defined by (1) the viewer's body such that stimuli to the left of the body are neglected more than those to the right of the body (Heilman and Valenstein, 1979), (2) by the environment such that even when the patient lies on his or her side the left half of the environment is neglected (Ladavas, 1987), or (3) by the object such that they neglect the contralesional side of the target (Rapcsak et al., 1989).

Spatial neglect is a complex disorder, and at least three neuropsychological mechanisms have been proposed to account for it: (1) attentional disorders, (2) intentional or motor activation disorders, and (3) representational disorders. Coslett et al. (1990) and Bisiach et al. (1990) performed studies on patients with hemispatial neglect to determine if the defect was being caused by a sensory attentional disorder or an action intentional disorder. Although they used different techniques, both attempted to dissociate the side or direction of action from the side or direction to which attention was directed. Both investigators demonstrated that there were patients with primary action intentional deficits and others with primary attentional deficits. In this section we discuss only the attentional deficits.

There are four attentional hypotheses that may explain the attentional disorder associated with hemispatial neglect: (1) contralateral spatial inattention, (2) ipsilesional attentional bias, (3) inability to disengage, and (4) reduced sequential attentional capacity or premature habituation. These hypotheses are not mutually exclusive.

According to the attentional hypothesis (Heilman and Watson, 1977), patients with left hemispatial neglect fail to act in or toward left hemispace because they are unaware of stimuli in left hemispace. Support for the attentional hypothesis of hemispatial neglect comes from several studies. The severity of neglect may be decreased by providing attentional cues (Riddoch and Humphreys, 1983). These cues may modify the distribution of attention in a "top-down" manner. Unlike cues, novelty may influence attention in a "bottom-up" manner. Butter, Kirsch, and Reeves (1990) showed that novel stimuli presented on the contralesional side also reduced spatial neglect.

Many patients with hemispatial neglect do not demonstrate inattention or pseudohemianopsia. Rather than suffering with almost total unawareness, as seen with inattention or pseudohemianopsia, patients with hemispatial neglect may be less aware of stimuli on the left than on the right. This may cause an ipsilesional attentional bias. Support for this bias comes from the observation that when patients with hemispatial neglect perform either line bisection or cancellation tasks, they initiate the search from the ipsilesional side. Also, support for the bias hypothesis comes from the observation that right hemisphere—damaged patients with hemispatial neglect have more rapid reaction times to ipsilateral (right) than contralesional (left) stimuli (Ladavas, Petronio, and Umicta, 1990). Mark, Kooistra, and Heilman (1988) gave patients a cancellation task wherein the subjects would either mark or erase stimuli. The subjects performed better in the erase condition than they did in the mark condition. Erasing a stimulus removes stimuli from the display, and one cannot be biased toward a stimulus that is not present. Therefore, the erase procedure may reduce attentional bias.

However, removing the attentional bias as Mark et al. did in their study did not entirely eliminate all the patients' neglect. It is possible that other environmental objects in ipsilateral space drew their attention, and the bias was so strong that subjects could not disengage their attention from these objects (Posner et al., 1984). Alternatively, it is possible that the bias was primarily a top-down process. Therefore, ipsilesional stimuli are more likely to capture attention than are contralesional stimuli, but even in the absence of ipsilesional stimuli, the attentional bias persists. Although the Ladavas et al. (1990) reaction times study produced support for this top-down bias hypothesis, a recent report by Chatterjee, Mennemeier, and Heilman (1992) raises some important questions about the bias hypothesis.

Chatterjee et al. (1992) studied a woman who had left-sided hemispatial neglect on standard cancellation tasks. When requested to alternatively cancel targets on the right and left side of an array, the patient was partially able to overcome her right-sided bias. However, when using this technique she did not cancel more targets than when she performed the cancellation tasks in the traditional manner. However, now she neglected targets in the center rather than on the left. These results cannot be explained by left-sided inattention, right-sided bias, or inability to disengage. These findings suggest that whereas bias or inattention may determine where stimuli are neglected, a limited sequential capacity or inappropriate habituation may also lead to hemispatial neglect.

Many neurologists thought that hemispatial neglect was more frequently associated with right than left hemisphere lesions (Brain, 1941; Critchley, 1966). However, Battersby, Bender, and Pollack (1956) thought that the association between neglect and right hemisphere lesions was induced by a sampling bias. They believed that patients with left hemisphere lesions were often severely aphasic and therefore were excluded from study. However, subsequent studies that accounted for possible subject selection bias continued to demonstrate that hemispatial neglect was more frequently associated with right hemisphere lesions (Gainotti, Messerli, and Tissot, 1972; Costa et al., 1969), and when the hemispatial neglect is seen with left hemisphere lesions in general it is not as severe as that seen with right hemisphere lesions (Albert, 1973). In addition, several investigators note that, whereas spatial neglect induced by right hemisphere lesions is most severe for stimuli in contralateral left space, even stimuli placed in ipsilateral right space may be neglected (Albert, 1973; Heilman and Valenstein, 1979; Weintraub and Mesulam, 1987).

When normal subjects are asked to bisect lines, they are overall more likely to displace their bisection toward the left than toward the right (Bowers and Heilman, 1980; Bradshaw et al., 1985). Geldmacher, Doty, and Heilman (1991) performed cancellation tasks on a large population of normal subjects. These investigators also found that normal subjects were more likely to be unaware of targets on the right than on the left, suggesting that a normal subject's attention is either slightly biased toward the left part of space or stimuli that fall in the left visual field (and hence directed the right hemisphere) are attended to more than those that fall in the right visual field.

Arousal and Vigilance Asymmetries

Arousal Arousal is both a behavioral and physiologic construct. An aroused organism is alert. It is prepared to process incoming stimuli. An unaroused organism is comatose. It is not prepared to process stimuli and is unaware of stimuli. Physiologically, arousal also refers to the excitatory state or the propensity of neurons to discharge when appropriately activated (neuronal preparation).

Changes in the level of activity of the peripheral autonomic nervous system often mirror arousal changes in the central nervous system. Using the galvanic skin response (which reflects changes in hand sweating) as a measure of arousal, several investigators have demonstrated that patients with right hemisphere lesions have a reduced response when compared to normals and left hemisphere–damaged controls (Heilman, Schwartz, and Watson, 1978; Schrandt, Tranel, and Domasio, 1989). Compared with normal controls, patients with left hemisphere lesions appear to have greater autonomic response (Heilman et al., 1978; Schrandt et al., 1989). Using changes in heart rate as a peripheral measure of arousal, Yokoyama et al. (1987) obtained similar results to those obtained using galvanic skin response. Using electroencephalography (EEG) as a measure of central arousal, it has also been demonstrated that patients with right hemisphere lesions have more delta and theta activity over their nonlesioned (left) hemisphere than patients with left hemisphere lesions have over their right hemisphere (Heilman, 1979).

Vigilance The ability to sustain attention is termed *vigilance*. Arousal and vigilance are closely linked so that when arousal wanes, vigilance diminishes, and vice versa. Using a monotonous single-detection task Wilkens, Shallice, and McCarthy (1987) demonstrated that, when compared with left hemisphere–damaged controls, patients with right hemisphere lesions had impaired sustained attention. Dimond (1979) studied patients with callosal disconnection and noted that the right hemisphere was more vigilant than the left. Whitehead (1991) studied the ability of normal subjects to sustain attention and found a right hemisphere superiority for sustained visual attention. Lastly, Deutsch et al. (1987) studied blood flow during a sustained attention task and found a greater increase of blood flow to the right than to the left hemisphere.

THE NEURAL SUBSTRATE OF ATTENTIONAL BEHAVIOR

Since this chapter is primarily directed at discussing attentional asymmetries, we will only briefly discuss the neural system that mediates attention. For a full discussion of this topic, the reader is referred to Heilman, Valenstein, and Watson (1993b).

In humans, lesions of the inferior parietal lobe are most often associated with disorders of attention (Critchley, 1966; Heilman, Valenstein, and Watson, 1983). Temporoparietal ablations in monkeys also induce contralesional attentional disorders, primarily extinction (Heilman, Pandya, and Geschwind, 1970; Lynch, 1980).

Physiologic studies employing recordings from cells in the parietal lobes of monkeys appear to support the postulate that the parietal lobe is important in directing attention. Unlike cells in visual cortex, the rate of firing of these "attentional" cells appears to be associated with the importance of the stimulus to the monkey such that important stimuli are associated with a higher firing rate than unimportant stimuli (see Bushnell, Goldberg, and Robinson, 1981; Lynch, 1980; Motter and Mountcastle, 1981).

Some of these cells are most active when the monkey fixes its gaze on an important object ("fixation neurons"), other cells discharge when the animal is visually tracking a moving object that is important to the monkey ("tracking neurons"), and still other neurons become active before a visual saccade to a significant stimulus ("saccade neurons"). Lastly, there are neurons that become active when important stimuli come into peripheral vision ("light-sensitive neurons").

Ungerleider and Mishkin (1982) posited that visual and visual association areas are organized into two cortical visual pathways. The ventral pathway consists of a multisynaptic occipitotemporal project system that interconnects the striate, prestriate, and inferior temporal areas. This pathway is critical for the visual identification of objects and faces. The dorsal pathway consists of a multisynaptic occipitoparietal projection system interconnecting the striate, prestriate, and inferior parietal areas. This dorsal pathway is crucial for the localization of objects in space.

The spatial loci of important stimuli are often different from the spatial loci of irrelevant stimuli, and when an organism is confronted with more stimuli than it can simultaneously process, it selectively processes the important stimuli by focusing attention on their spatial location. In addition to the optical focusing or foveation brought about by eye movements, there is physiologic focusing such that stimuli in attended locations have a processing advantage over stimuli in unattended locations (Desimone et al., 1990).

Goldberg and Robinson (1977) and Robinson, Goldberg, and Stanton (1978) demonstrated that the activity of some parietal attentional neurons are spatially selective. The parietal lobe also receives input from other sensory modalities, and the coding of spatial location is probably multimodal. Because cells in the parietal lobe code the spatial location of important stimuli and show increased activity when important stimuli are presented in specific spatial locations, it appears that the parietal lobe is crucial for spatial attention.

Primary sensory cortices project only to their association cortex. Each of these unimodal association areas converges upon polymodal association areas, including, in the monkey, the frontal cortex (periarcuate, prearcuate, and orbitofrontal), and both banks of the superior temporal sulcus (Pandya and Kuypers, 1969). Polymodal conversion areas may be important for sensory synthesis and cross-modal association. Polymodal convergence areas project to the supramodal inferior parietal lobe (Mesulam et al., 1977).

Whereas the determination as to whether the stimulus is novel may be mediated by sensory association cortex, stimulus significance requires knowledge as to both the meaning of the stimulus and the motivational state (needs and goals) of the organism.

The limbic system monitors the internal milieu, and limbic input into regions important in determining stimulus significance may provide information about immediate biological needs. In contrast, the frontal lobe may play a role in goal-directed behavior. Ablation studies have revealed that the frontal lobes play a critical role in goal-directed behavior and in developing sets (see Damasio, 1985; Stuss and Benson, 1986). Therefore, unlike limbic system input, the frontal input into the attentional systems may provide information about goals that are not motivated by an immediate biological need. The temporoparietal region that we have discussed has strong connections with both the limbic system, such as the cingulate gyrus, and the prefrontal cortex.

Support for the postulate that these frontal and limbic (cingulate) connections with the parietal lobe may be the anatomic substrate by which motivational states influence attentional systems comes from the observation that unilateral neglect in humans and monkeys can be induced by dorsolateral frontal (Heilman and Valenstein, 1972; Welch and Stuteville, 1958) and cingulate lesions (Heilman and Valenstein, 1972; Watson et al., 1973).

In cats and monkeys, profound sensory neglect also results from lesions of the mesencephalic reticular formation (Reeves and Hagaman, 1971; Watson et al., 1974). As discussed above, arousal is a physiologic state that prepares the organism for sensory processing by increasing neuronal sensitivity and the signal-to-noise ratio. Stimulation of the mesencephalic reticular formation (MRF) in animals induces behavioral arousal (increased alertness) and is associated with desynchronization of the EEG, a physiologic measure of central arousal (Moruzzi and Magoun, 1949). However, unilateral MRF stimulation causes more desynchronization in the ipsilateral than in the contralateral hemisphere (Moruzzi and Magoun, 1949), and unilateral lesions of the MRF result in contralateral neglect (Watson et al., 1974).

There are three means by which the MRF may influence cortical processing (i.e., make cortical neurons more responsive to sensory input). Shute and Lewis (1967) posited an ascending cholinergic reticular formation. Acetylcholine increases neuronal responsivity and the signal-to-noise ratio (McCormick, 1989). The nucleus basalis has cholinergic projections to the cortex, and these cholinergic projections appear important for increasing neuronal responsivity (Sato et al., 1987).

The MRF may influence the cortex through its projections to the thalamus. Steriade and Glenn (1982) demonstrated that the centralis lateralis and paracentralis thalamic nuclei project to widespread cortical regions. Thirteen percent of neurons with cortical or caudate projections could be activated by stimulation of the mesencephalic reticular system. The third possible mechanism to account for arousal involves the nucleus reticularis, which envelops the thalamus, projects to the sensory thalamic relay nuclei, and may inhibit thalamic relay of sensory information to the cortex (Scheibel and Scheibel, 1966). When a stimulus is important to the organism, corticofugal projects may inhibit the nucleus reticularis and allow the thalamus to relay sensory input to the cortex.

NEUROPSYCHOLOGICAL MECHANISMS THAT MAY ACCOUNT FOR ATTENTIONAL AND AROUSAL ASYMMETRIES

The monkey parietal lobe "attentional" neurons discussed above have predominantly contralateral fields (e.g., important stimuli activate cells when presented in the contralateral visual field). However, some of the neurons also had bilateral receptive fields such that when meaningful stimuli were presented to either the contralateral or ipsilateral visual field, these neurons had increased activity. To account for the asymmetries of attention seen in humans, Heilman and Van Den Abell (1980) proposed that each hemisphere of the human brain has attentional systems that direct attention in and toward the contralateral space. However, for most humans the right hemisphere is more likely to have systems that cannot only direct attention in and toward contralateral space but also direct attention in and toward the ipsilateral space. Rather than a sharp midsagittal spatial demarcation that separates contralateral and ipsilateral space, there may be attentional spatial gradients, the left hemisphere gradient being greater as it approaches ipsilateral space than the right hemisphere gradient. This graded attentional asymmetry hypothesis not only explains why contralateral inattention is more often associated with right than with left hemisphere lesions, it also explains why ipsilateral inattention is more common with right than with left hemisphere lesions. If the left hemisphere is injured, severe neglect would be unlikely because the right hemisphere can attend ipsilaterally. However, because the left hemisphere cannot attend ipsilaterally when the right hemisphere is injured, severe neglect is common. Since the right hemisphere plays a more important role in attending to ipsilateral stimuli when the right hemisphere is injured, ipsilateral inattention is more likely to be seen than when the left hemisphere is injured. Lastly, the gradient hypothesis also explains why it is the leftmost stimulus that is neglected in an extinction paradigm even when both stimuli are in the ipsilateral hemifield (Rapcsak et al., 1987).

To test the hemispheric asymmetry hypothesis, visual warning stimuli were presented to the left or right visual field. These warning stimuli were followed by an imperative reaction time stimulus. During the time the subjects were performing this task, their EEG was being recorded. If activation of attentional networks in the parietal lobe induces local EEG desynchronization and the right hemisphere attends bilaterally but the left hemisphere contralaterally, the right hemisphere should desynchronize to stimuli on either side of space, but the left hemisphere should desynchronize primarily to right-sided stimuli. Heilman and Van Den Abell (1980) found that whereas the left hemisphere desynchronized primarily to the right-sided stimuli, the right hemisphere desynchronized to stimuli on either side. Pardo, Fox, and Raichle (1991) demonstrated a similar phenomenon using positron emission tomography (PET) scanning. Neville and Lawson (1987) found larger evoked potentials over the right than over the left hemisphere and suggested that the special role of the right hemisphere in spatial attention may be limited to an analysis of information of visual periphery. Although these physiologic studies provide support for the postulate that the right hemisphere plays a dominant role in spatially directed attention, the gradient hypothesis has not been fully tested. However, as mentioned, clinical observations also provide support for this hypothesis.

Patients with hemispatial neglect and extinction have an attentional bias. For example, when performing cancellation tasks, they will start from the far ipsilateral part of the page and when given simultaneous stimuli in the ipsilateral visual field, they are more often unaware of the stimulus that is more contralesional. To explain this attentional bias, Kinsbourne (1970) posited that each hemisphere directs attention toward the contralateral space and that normally attentional systems of one hemisphere inhibit those of the opposite hemisphere. Therefore, when one hemisphere is injured, the other becomes attentionally hyperactive, and attention is biased to the side of space opposite the normal hemisphere.

Heilman and Watson (1977) agree with Kinsbourne's (1970) hypothesis that each hemisphere orients attention toward contralateral space and that after a right hemisphere lesion there is an ipsilesional attentional bias. However, Heilman and Watson (1977) believe that this bias is not being induced by a hyperactive hemisphere but rather by a hypoactive hemisphere. The mechanisms of this hypoactivity have been discussed above. If each hemisphere orients attention in the contralateral direction and one hemisphere is hypoactive, this will also produce an ipsilateral attentional bias. There is both behavioral and physiologic support for the hypoactive vs. hyperactive hemisphere attentional bias hypothesis. For example, Ladavas et al. (1990) reported that attentional shifts between vertically aligned stimuli were slower when stimuli were in contralesional hemispace than when they were in ipsilesional hemispace. There is also EEG slowing of the nonlesioned (left) hemisphere of patients with neglect (Heilman, 1979), and evidence from PET studies also show the lower energy metabolism in the hemisphere contralateral to the lesion inducing neglect (Fiorelli et al., 1991).

Although this ipsilesional bias hypothesis may explain why attention is biased in the ipsilesional direction, it cannot by itself explain why there is more ipsilesional attentional bias after right than after left hemisphere lesions. There are at least two explanations for the preponderance of rightward bias.

One of these has already been partially discussed. Each hemisphere may not only be important for attending to contralateral stimuli, it may also be important for moving attention in a contralateral direction. Whereas the left hemisphere moves attention rightward, the right hemisphere can move attention in either direction. Therefore, with left hemisphere leisons, there would be no or minimal bias, but with right hemisphere lesions, there would be a strong rightward bias. The second hypothesis used to explain the rightward bias is that of language activation as proposed by Kinsbourne (1970). Behavioral and psychophysiologic studies of normal subjects have demonstrated that language may induce left hemisphere activation with a rightward attentional bias (Kinsbourne, 1974; Bowers and Heilman, 1976). When being tested for neglect, patients are given verbal instructions, and during the task the patient may be using verbal strategies. Kinsbourne (1970) proposed that language-induced activation of the left hemisphere may make neglect associated with right hemisphere lesions more severe because it would increase the ipsilateral bias. Language-induced left hemisphere activation may make neglect from left hemisphere lesions less severe because it would decrease the ipsilesional bias. Heilman and Watson (1978) tested patients that had left-sided neglect with cancellation tasks that were either verbal or nonverbal. Patients appeared to have more severe neglect on the verbal than on the nonverbal tasks. Joanette et al. (1986) and Halligan and Marshall (1989) tested patients for neglect using their right or left hands and found that left-sided neglect was less severe when subjects used their left hands than when they used their right hands. Both verbal stimuli and use of the right hand may activate the left hemisphere and using visuospatial stimuli or using the left hand may activate the right hemisphere. Even though these findings are consistent with Kinsbourne's hypothesis, there are alternative explanations. In Heilman and Watson's (1978) study, the verbal stimuli may have placed more demands on focused attention. Rapcsak et al. (1989) demonstrated that patients with neglect perform more poorly on tasks that require focused attention. In regard to the study of Joanette et al. and the Halligan and Marshall study, it has been demonstrated that use of the right hand induces a rightward movement or intentional bias and use of the left hand induces a leftward bias (Heilman, Bowers, and Watson, 1984). Unfortunately, to date there has been no clinical experiment that distinguishes between the hemispheric asymmetry hypothesis and the verbal activation hypothesis. In addition, these hypotheses are not mutually contradictory.

The brain mechanisms underlying the reduction of arousal with right vs. left hemisphere lesions are also unknown. Because lesions restricted to the right hemisphere could not directly interfere with the left hemisphere's corticopedal projections (i.e., the mesodiencephalic reticular system's influence on the left cortex), one would have to posit that the reduced arousal associated with right hemisphere lesions is related to the right hemisphere's privileged communications with the reticular activating system such that the bilateral arousal defect associated with right hemisphere lesions is related to a loss of the right hemisphere's corticofugal influence on the reticular formation. The mechanism for the increased arousal with left hemisphere lesions is probably related to some type of inhibitory control mediated by the left hemisphere. This control can theoretically be transcallosal or directly on the diencephalic and mesencephalic reticular systems.

There are several possible brain mechanisms that may account for the superiority of the right hemisphere in vigilance tasks. We have already discussed the right hemisphere's attentional superiority. In the discussion of the neural systems that mediate directed attention, I discussed the contribution of the frontal lobes. I mentioned that the frontal lobes appear to provide information to the attentional systems about the goals that are not motivated by immediate biological needs. In vigilance tasks, even in the absence of a stimulus, one has to continue to direct attention. Therefore, in contrast to directing attention to novel or biologically important stimuli, vigilance tasks may be heavily dependent upon the input of the frontal lobe into the attentional systems. Wilkens et al. (1987) found that it was primarily patients with right frontal lesions that were impaired on a monotonous signal detection task, and Cohen et al. (1988) used physiologic imaging to find that a patient's frontal cortex was activated by vigilance tasks.

Vigilance tasks are monotonous, and monotony is associated with reduced arousal. We have already discussed the role of the right hemisphere in mediating arousal. One of the reasons the right hemisphere may play a critical role in vigilance is because it is the hemisphere that also plays a dominant role in controlling arousal.

UP/DOWN AND CLOSE/FAR ATTENTIONAL ASYMMETRIES

Our prior discussion has primarily been directed at right/left asymmetries. Rapcsak, Cimino, and Heilman (1988) reported a patient with biparietal lesions who, when asked to bisect vertically oriented lines (in respect to both her body and gravity), bisected the lines above their true midpoint. When she was tested for vertical extinction, she was also unaware of the lower stimulus. Shelton, Bowers, and Heilman (1990) reported a patient with bilateral ventral temporo-occipital lesions who, in contrast to the patient of Rapcsak et al., had neglect of upper vertical space. When presented with radial lines, the patient of Shelton et al. erred by bisecting the line proximal to its actual midline or toward the patient's body (extrapersonal neglect). Mennemeier, Wertman, and Heilman (1992) tested the patient reported by Rapcsak et al. who had vertical neglect on a radial line bisection task, and, in contrast to the patient of Shelton et al., this patient erred by bisecting lines beyond their midpoint or away from her body (peripersonal neglect).

When normal controls were asked to bisect radial lines, they bisected lines slightly beyond their midpoint (Shelton et al., 1990). Based on this finding, Shelton et al. posited that normally visually directed attention is biased away from peripersonal space and toward extrapersonal space.

Normal subjects bisect vertical lines slightly above their midpoint (Rapcsak et al., 1988). Although one could also explain this bisection error by positing that, in normal subjects, visual attention is biased toward upper visual space, Geldmacher and Heilman (1992) sought a more parsimonious explanation. Ishiai, Furukawa, and Tsukagoshi (1989) demonstrated that normal subjects foveate the point on the line where they make their bisection mark. Therefore, when one attempts to bisect a vertical line the upper portion of this line is projecting to the lower portion of the retina (upper visual field) and the lower portion of the line is projecting to the upper retina or lower visual field. Studies of normal subjects have demonstrated that magnitude (e.g., length) estimates are related to the allocation of attention or to an attentional bias such that the portion of the line to which attention is directed appears longer than an equal length of line to which attention is not directed (Milner, Brechmann, and Pagliarini, 1992). Therefore, a systematic error on line bisection tasks suggest that one visual half-field may be attentively dominant over the other. In the case of vertical lines, it would suggest that the upper field is dominant over the lower. However, when one bisects a radial line below eye level, the proximal portion of the line projects to the upper retina or upper visual field. To learn if the radial attentional bias described by Shelton et al. (1990) was being induced by a bias toward extrapersonal vs. peripersonal space or was related to upper vs. lower visual-field bias, Geldmacher and Heilman (1992) had normal subjects bisect radial lines above and below eye level. In the below condition, Geldmacher and Heilman (1992) replicated Shelton's study. That is, normal subjects bisected lines distal to their true center. However, in the above condition the subjects erred by bisecting lines proximal to the true center. These results suggest that attention is biased toward the upper visual field or away from the lower visual field.

Geldmacher et al. (1991) also reported that, when normal subjects are performing a cancellation task, they have a propensity to make more errors in the section of the paper close to their body. Stimuli close to the body are more likely to fall into the lower visual field. Whereas both of these studies suggest that visual attention is biased toward the upper field, the neuronal mechanism underlying this bias remains unknown.

Heilman et al. (1993a) noted that whereas most of the visually mediated cognitive activities performed by the left hemisphere, such as reading, writing, and praxis, were performed close to the body or in peripersonal space, many of the visual cognitive activities performed by the right hemisphere, such as facial and emotional recognition and route finding, took place away from the body in extrapersonal space. To learn if there was a close anatomic relationship between the areas that mediate visual cognitive activities and those that direct attention such that they coinhabit the same hemisphere, Heilman et al. (1993a) studied normal subjects to learn if the left hemisphere has a propensity to direct attention toward the body and if the right hemisphere has a propensity to direct attention away from the body. To test this hypothesis, the subjects were asked to compare the size of radial lines placed in right or left hemispace. Because each half of the retina projects to the hemisphere on the same side when the subject gazes to the left, the portion of the line closest to the body projects primarily to the right hemisphere and the portion of the line farthest from the body projects primarily to the left hemisphere. When looking toward the right, the opposite occurs. If the left hemisphere directs attention to peripersonal space and the right to extrapersonal space, when subjects view lines in left hemispace, their attention would be directed to the center of the lines, and when subjects view lines in right hemispace, their attention would be directed to both ends of the line. When attention is directed to the center of the line they may be unaware of the full extent of the line and the line may appear shorter than when they attend to both ends of a line. Heilman et al. (1993a) found that when subjects looked leftward, lines appeared shorter than when they looked rightward. These results are consistent with the hypothesis that the right hemisphere directs attention to visual extrapersonal space and the left hemisphere directs attention to peripersonal space. The neuronal mechanisms underlying this dichotomy, however, remain to be determined.

REFERENCES

Albert, M. D. (1973). A simple test of visual neglect. *Neurology, 23,* 658–664.

Battersby, W. S., Bender, M. B., and Pollack, M. (1956). Unilateral spatial agnosia (inattention) in patients with cerebral lesions. *Brain, 79,* 68–93.

Bisiach, E., Geminiani, G., Berti, A., and Rusconi, M. L. (1990). Perceptual and premotor factors of unilatral neglect. *Neurology, 40,* 1278–1281.

Bowers, D., and Heilman, K. M. (1976). Material specific hemispheric arousal. *Neuropsychologia, 14,* 123–127.

Bowers, D., and Heilman, K. M. (1980). Pseudoneglect: Effects of hemispace on tactile line bisection task. *Neuropsychologia, 18,* 491–498.

Bradshaw, J. L., Nettleton, N. C., Nathan, G., and Wilson, L. E. (1985). Bisecting rods and lines: effects of horizontal and vertical posture on left sided underestimation by normal subjects. *Neuropsychologia, 23,* 421–426.

Brain, W. R. (1941). Visual disorientation with special reference to lesions of the right cerebral hemisphere. *Brain, 64,* 224–272.

Bushnell, M. C., Goldberg, M. E., and Robinson, D. L. (1981). Behavioral enhancement of visual responses in monkey cerebral cortex: I. Modulation of posterior parietal cortex related to selected visual attention. *Journal of Neurophysiology, 46,* 755–772.

Butter, C. M., Kirsch, N. L., and Reeves, G. (1990). The effect of lateralized dynamic stimuli on unilateral spatial neglect following right hemisphere lesions. *Restorative Neurology and Neuroscience, 2,* 39–46.

Chatterjee, A., Mennemeier, M., and Heilman, K. M. (1992). Search patterns in neglect. *Neuropsychologia, 30,* 657–672.

Cohen, R. M., Semple, W. E., Gross, M., Holocomb, H. J., Dowling, S. M., and Nordahl, T. E. (1988). Functional localization of sustained attention. *Neuropsychiatry, Neuropsychology and Behavioral Neurology, 1,* 3–20.

Coslett, H. B., Bowers, D., Fitzpatrick, E., Haws, B., and Heilman, K. M. (1990). Directional hypokinesia and hemispatial inattention in neglect. *Brain, 113,* 475–486.

Costa, L. D., Vaughan, H. G., Horowitz, M., and Ritter, W. (1969). Patterns of behavior deficit associated with visual spatial neglect. *Cortex, 5,* 242–263.

Critchley, M. (1966). *The parietal lobes.* New York, NY: Hafner Publishing Co.

Damasio, A. R. (1985). The frontal lobes. In K. M. Heilman and E. Valenstein (Eds.), *Clinical neuropsychology.* New York, NY: Oxford University Press.

Desimone, R. Wessinger, M., Thomas, L., and Schneider, W. (1990). Attentional control of visual perception. *Cold Spring Harbor Symposia on Quantitative Biology, 55,* 963–971.

Deutsch, G., Papanicolaou, A. C., Bourbon, W. T., and Eisenberg, H. M. (1987). Cerebral blood flow evidence of right frontal activation in attention demanding tasks. *International Journal of Neuroscience, 36,* 23–28.

Dimond, S. J. (1979). Performance by split-brain humans on lateralized vigilance tasks. *Cortex, 15,* 43–50.

Feinberg, T. E., Habor, L. D., Stacy, C. D. (1990). Ipsilateral extinction in the hemineglect syndrome. *Archives of Neurology, 47,* 803–804.

Fiorelli, M., Blin, J., Bakchine, S., LaPlane, D., and Baron, J. C. (1991). PET studies of cortical diaschisic in patients with motor hemi-neglect. *Journal of the Neurological Sciences, 104,* 135–142.

Gainotti, G., Messerli, P., and Tissot, R. (1972). Qualitative analysis of unilateral and spatial neglect in relation to laterality of cerebral lesions. *Journal of Neurology, Neurosurgery, and Psychiatry, 35,* 545–550.

Geldmacher, D., Doty, L., and Heilman, K. M. (1991). Attentional bias in normal elderly subjects on a letter cancellation task. *Neurology, 41,* 236.

Geldmacher, D. S., and Heilman, K. M. (1992). Differences in radial line bisection above and below eye level. *Journal of Clinical and Experimental Neuropsychology, 14,* 35.

Goldberg, M. E., and Robinson, D. C. (1977). Visual responses of neurons in monkey inferior parietal lobule. The physiological substrate of attention and neglect. *Neurology, 27,* 350.

Halligan, P. W., and Marshall, J. C. (1989). Laterality of motor response in visuospatial neglect. *Neuropsychologia, 27,* 1301–1308.

Heilman, K. M. (1979). Neglect and related disorders. In K. M. Heilman and E. Valenstein (Eds.), *Clinical neuropsychology* (pp 268–307). New York, NY: Oxford University Press.

Heilman, K. M., Bowers, D., and Watson, R. T. (1984). Pseudoneglect in patients with partial callosal disconnection. *Brain, 107,* 519–532.

Heilman, K. M., Chatterjee, A., and Doty, L. (1993a). Hemispheric asymmetries of spatial attention. *Journal of Clinical and Experimental Neuropsychology, 15,* 14.

Heilman, K. M., Pandya, D. N., and Geschwind, N. (1970). Trimodal inattention following parietal lobe abolations. *Transactions of the American Neurologic Association, 95,* 259–261.

Heilman, K. M., and Rothi, L. J. G. (1993). Apraxia. In K. M. Heilman and E. Valenstein (Eds.), *Clinical neuropsychology.* New York, NY: Oxford University Press.

Heilman, K. M., Schwartz, H. D., and Watson, R. T. (1978). Hypoarousal in patients with neglect syndrome and emotional indifference. *Neurology, 28,* 229–232.

Heilman, K. M., and Valenstein, E. (1972). Frontal lobe neglect in man. *Neurology, 22,* 660–664.

Heilman, K. M., and Valenstein, E. (1979). Mechanisms underlying hemispatial neglect. *Annals of Neurology, 5,* 166–170.

Heilman, K. M., Valenstein, E., and Watson, R. T. (1983). Localization of neglect. In A. Kertesz (Ed.), *Localization in neurology* (pp 471–492). New York, NY: Academic Press.

Heilman, K. M., Valenstein, E., and Watson, R. T. (1993b). Neglect and related disorders. In *Clinical Neuropsychology*. New York: Oxford University Press.

Heilman, K. M., and Van Den Abell, T. (1980). Right hemisphere dominance for attention: the mechanisms underlying hemispheric asymmetries of inattention (neglect). *Neurology, 30,* 327–330.

Heilman, K. M., and Watson, R. T. (1977). The neglect syndrome—a unilateral defect of the orienting response. In S. Hardned, R. W. Doty, L. Goldstein, J. Jaynes, and G. Kean Thamer (Eds.), *Lateralization in the nervous system.* New York, NY: Academic Press.

Heilman, K. M., and Watson, R. T. (1978). Changes in the symptoms of neglect induced by changes in task strategy. *Archives of Neurology, 35,* 47–49.

Heilman, K. M., and Watson, R. T. (1991). Intentional motor disorders. In H. S. Levin, H. M. Eisenberg and A. L. Benton (Eds.), *Frontal lobe function and dysfunction,* (pp 199–213). New York: Oxford University Press.

Ishiai, S., Furukawa, T., and Tsukagoshi, H. (1989). Visuospatial processes of line bisection and the mechanisms underlying unilateral spatial neglect. *Brain, 112,* 1485–1502.

Joanette, Y., Brouchon, M., Gauthier, L., and Samson, M. (1986). Pointing with left vs right hand in left visual field neglect. *Neuropsychologia, 24,* 391–396.

Kinsbourne, M. (1970). A model for the mechanism of unilateral neglect of space. *Transactions of the American Neurologic Association, 95,* 143.

Kinsbourne, M. (1974). Direction of gaze and distribution of cerebral thought processes. *Neuropsychologia, 12,* 270–281.

Kooistra, C. A., and Heilman, K. M. (1989). Hemispatial visual inattention masquerading as hemianopsia. *Neurology, 39,* 1125–1127.

Ladavas, E. (1987). Is the hemispatial deficit produced by right parietal damage associated with retinal or gravitational coordinates? *Brain, 110,* 167–180.

Ladavas, E., Petronio, A., and Umicta, C. (1990). The deployment of visual attention in the intact field of hemineglect patients. *Cortex, 26,* 307–312.

Lynch, J. C. (1980). The functional organization of posterior parietal association cortex. *Behavioral Brain Science, 3,* 485–534.

Mark, V. W., Kooistra, C. A., and Heilman, K. M. (1988). Hemispatial neglect affected by non-neglected stimuli. *Neurology, 38,* 1207–1211.

McCormick, D. A. (1989). Cholinergic and noradrenergic modulation of thalamocortical processing. *Trends in Neurology, 12,* 215–221.

Meador, K., Loring, D. W., Lee, G. P., Brooks, B. S., Thompson, W. O., and Heilman, K. M. (1988). Right cerebral specialization for tactile attention as evidenced by intracarotid sodium amytal. *Neurology, 38,* 1763–1766.

Mennemeier, M., Wertman, E., and Heilman, K. M. (1992). Neglect of near peripersonal space. *Brain, 115,* 37–50.

Mesulam, M., Van Hesen, G. W., Pandya, D. N., and Geschwind, N. (1977). Limbic and sensory connections of the inferior parietal lobule (area PG) in the rhesus monkey: a study with a new method for horseradish peroxidase histochemistry. *Brain Research, 136,* 393–414.

Milner, A. D., Brechmann, M., and Pagliarini, L. (1992). To halve and to halve not: an analysis of line bisection judgements in normal subjects. *Neuropsychologia, 30,* 515–526.

Moruzzi, G., and Magoun, H. W. (1949). Brainstem reticular formation and activation of the EEG. *Electroencephalography and Clinical Neurophysiology, 1,* 455–473.

Motter, B. C., and Mountcastle, V. B. (1981). The functional properties of the light sensitive neurons of the posterior parietal cortex studied in waking monkeys: foveal sparing and opponent vector organization. *Journal of Neuroscience, 1,* 3–26.

Nadeau, S. E., and Heilman, K. M. (1991). Gaze-dependent hemianopia without hemispatial neglect. *Neurology, 41,* 1244–1250.

Neville, H. J., and Lawson, D. (1987). Attention to central and peripheral visual space in a movement detection task: an event-related potential and behavioral study. I. Normal hearing adults. *Brain Research, 405*(2), 253–267.

Pandya, D. M., and Kuypers, H. G. J. M. (1969). Cortico-cortical connections in the rhesus monkey. *Brain Research, 13,* 13–36.

Pardo, J. V., Fox, P. T., and Raichle, M. E. (1991). Localization of a human system for sustained attention by positron emission tomography. *Nature, 349,* 61–64.

Posner, M. I., Walker, J., Friedrich, F. J., and Rafal, R. D. (1984). Effects of parietal lobe injury on covert orienting of visual attention. *Journal of Neuroscience, 4,* 163–187.

Rapcsak, S. Z., Cimino, C. R., and Heilman, K. M. (1988). Altitudinal neglect. *Neurology, 38,* 277–281.

Rapcsak, S. Z., Fleet, W. S., Verfaellie, M., and Heilman, K. M. (1989). Selective attention in hemispatial neglect. *Archives of Neurology, 46,* 178–182.

Rapcsak, S. Z., Watson, R. T., and Heilman, K. M. (1987). Hemispace-visual field interactions in visual extinction. *Journal of Neurology, Neurosurgery and Psychiatry, 50,* 1117–1124.

Reeves, A. G., and Hagamen, W. D. (1971). Behavioral and EEG asymmetry following unilateral lesions of the forebrain and midbrain of cats. *Electroencephalography and Clinical Neurophysiology, 39,* 83–86.

Riddoch, M. J., and Humphreys, G. (1983). The effect of cuing on unilateral neglect. *Neuropsychologia, 21,* 589–599.

Robinson, D. L., Goldberg, M. E., and Stanton, G. B. (1978). Parietal association cortex in the primate sensory mechanisms and behavioral modulations. *Journal of Neurophysiology, 41,* 910–932.

Rubens, A. B. (1985). Caloric stimulation and unilateral visual neglect. *Neurology, 35,* 1019–1024.

Sato, H., Hata, Y., Hagihara, K., and Tsumoto, T. (1987). Effects of cholinergic depletion on neuron activities in the cat visual cortex. *Journal of Neurophysiology, 58,* 781–794.

Scheibel, M. E., and Scheibel, A. B. (1966). The organization of the nucleus reticularis thalami: a Golgi study. *Brain Research, 1,* 43–62.

Schrandt, N. J., Tranel, D., and Domasio, H. (1989). The effects of total cerebral lesions on skin conductance response to signal stimuli. *Neurology, 39*(Suppl 1), 223.

Schwartz, A. S., Marchok, P. L., Kreinick, C. J., and Flynn, R. E. (1979). The asymmetric lateralization of tactile extinction in patients with unilateral cerebral dysfunction. *Brain, 102,* 669–684.

Shelton, P. A., Bowers, D., and Heilman, K. M. (1990). Peripersonal and vertical neglect. *Brain, 113*, 191–205.

Shute, C. C. D., and Lewis, P. R. (1967). The ascending cholinergic reticular system, neocortical olfactory and subcortical projections. *Brain, 90*, 497–520.

Steriade, M., and Glenn, L. (1982). Neocortical and caudate projections of intralaminer thalamic neurons and their synaptic excitation from the midbrain reticular core. *Journal of Neurophysiology, 48*, 352–370.

Stuss, D. T., and Benson, D. F. (1986). *The frontal lobes*. New York, NY: Raven Press.

Ungerleider, L. G., and Mishkin, M. (1982). Two cortical visual systems. In P. J. Ingle, J. W. Mansfield, and M. A. Goodale (Eds.), *Advances in the analysis of visual behavior*. Cambridge, MA: MIT Press.

Vallar, G., Bottini, G., Sterzi, R., Passerini, D., and Rusconi, M. L. (1991a). Hemianesthesia, sensory neglect and defective access to conscious experience. *Neurology, 41*, 650–652.

Vallar, G., Sandroni, P., Rusconi, M. L., and Barbieri, S. (1991b). Hemianopia, hemianesthesia, and spatial neglect: a study with evoked potentials. *Neurology, 41*, 1918–1922.

Vallar, G., Sterzi, R., Bottini, G., Cappa, S., and Rusconi, L. (1990). Temporary remission of left hemianesthesia after vestibular stimulation: a sensory neglect phenomenon. *Cortex, 26*, 123–131.

Watson, R. T., Heilman, K. M., Cauthen, J. C., and King, F. A. (1973). Neglect after cingulectomy. *Neurology, 23*, 1003–1007.

Watson, R. T., Heilman, K. M., Miller, B. D., and King, F. A. (1974). Neglect after mesencephalic reticular formation lesions. *Neurology, 24*, 294–298.

Weintraub, S., and Mesulam, M. M. (1987). Right cerebral dominance in spatial attention: further evidence based on ipsilateral neglect. *Archives of Neurology, 44*, 621–625.

Welch, K., and Stuteville, P. (1958). Experimental production of neglect in monkeys. *Brain, 81*, 341–347.

Whitehead, R. (1991). Right hemisphere processing superiority during sustained visual attention. *Journal of Cognitive Neuroscience, 3*, 329–334.

Wilkins, A. J., Shallice, T., and McCarthy, R. (1987). Frontal lesions and sustained attention. *Neuropsychologia, 25*, 359–366.

Yokoyama, K., Jennings, R., Ackles, P., Hood, P., and Boller, F. (1987). Lack of heart rate changes during an attention demanding task after right hemisphere lesions. *Neurology, 37*, 624–630.

10 Classical Conditioning and Implicit Learning: The Right Hemisphere Hypothesis

Kenneth Hugdahl

CLASSICAL CONDITIONING: IMPLICIT LEARNING

Classical conditioning is a basic form of learning wherein a weak sensory stimulus gains signaling qualities through repeated associations with a strong stimulus. The associative process thus transforms the weak stimulus into a conditioned stimulus (CS), eliciting a similar response as that elicited by the strong stimulus (unconditioned stimulus, UCS). The change in behavior that follows the presentation of the UCS is called the unconditioned response (UCR), and the response that accompanies the temporal pairing of the CS and UCS is called a conditioned response (CR). The choice of terminology reflects a behavioristic heritage (e.g., Spence, 1960); this, however, should not cloud the use of the conditioning paradigm for the study of cognitive functions like attention and short-term memory which mediate the building up of a learned association (cf. Öhman, 1983). Conditioning may also be a prototype for the study of brain functions involved in unconscious acquisition of knowledge (cf. Lazarus and McCleary, 1951). Classical conditioning allows for temporary behavioral and physiologic adaptations to an ever-changing environment. Classical conditioning also plays an important role in many psychopathologic disorders, including anxiety disorders (Seligman, 1971); modulation of immune system reactivity (Ader and Cohen, 1985); substance abuse (Stewart, de Wit, and Eikelboom, 1984; Hugdahl and Ternes, 1981); and placebo responses (Turkkan and Brady, 1985), just to mention a few. However, although research on classical conditioning in humans has a long history in psychology and psychiatry (Turkkan, 1989), we still know very little about the brain mechanisms involved. Data are presented in this chapter which show that the two hemispheres of the brain differ not only in perceptual analysis of sensory stimuli but that they also differentially regulate the formation of an association in memory. That the hemispheres differ in their capacity to form associations may have not only a basic research interest but may also be of critical importance for a neuropsychological understanding of learning disabilities.

The behavioristic tradition is probably to blame for the neglect by Western researchers on how conditional associations are stored and retrieved in the human brain. Instead, focus has traditionally been on the stimulus-response connection, with no role for the brain in this process. In contrast, it may be of interest to recall Pavlov's (1927) original view of conditional learning as a theoretical tool to explain the functioning of the cortical hemispheres. For Pavlov, studies of conditional learning provided insights into the functional properties of the nervous system, and particularly the cerebral hemispheres. For Pavlov, the establishment of a CR was a process described in terms of an association, or connection, between cortical centers on a neurophysiologic level (Windholz and Lamal, 1986; Windholz, 1992). This means that Pavlov looked at the CR as a result of a stimulus-stimulus (S-S) association, and not as a stimulus-response (S-R) association, which was later adapted as the model for associative learning among Western behaviorists (cf. Spence, 1960). Pavlov argued that when two cortical areas in the brain are excited, the excitation will irradiate until they merge as an excitation focus (Windholz, 1992). This would also hold for the case when, e.g., a word is associated with a light, and then the light is paired with a UCS, eliciting a CR. The CR will in this case also be elicited by the word. Pavlov called this phenomenon "association of associations." In other contexts it has variously been labeled "higher-order conditioning" or "second-order conditioning" (Rescorla, 1980).

Higher-order conditioning is based on the fact that a CS which is paired with a UCS a number of times can act as a UCS itself. The old CS is then presented after the new CS has been presented. A version of higher-order conditioning is *semantic generalization* and what Pavlov called the "second signal system." Semantic generalization studies have shown that a response can be conditioned to the meaning of a stimulus rather than to the stimulus itself (Razran, 1961). For example, if a response is conditioned to the number 4, a CR can be elicited also to stimuli such as $\sqrt{16}$, 2/8, etc. It is as if the brain is responding to the concept of "4-ness" rather than to the physical stimulus. Following these lines of argument, a recent view of classical conditioning stresses the correlational nature of the CS-UCS relationship as an important mediator of how an association is established and represented in the brain. Rescorla and Wagner (1972) and Rescorla (1980) have argued that in order for an association to occur, the CS must provide unique information about the presence of the UCS, i.e., the CS predicts the occurrence of the UCS. The importance with more modern views of conditioning is that concepts related to attention, expectancy, and memory are stressed, i.e., emphasizing an information-processing view (cf. Öhman, 1983; Davey, 1987). A process-oriented view of conditioning also provides a basis for relating conditioning to brain function. The view taken in this chapter is that classical conditioning under certain circumstances reflects the differential functioning of the cerebral hemispheres, and mainly activity within the right hemisphere.

Procedures and Terminology   There are a variety of different approaches and procedures to study human classical conditioning. Since two different approaches were used in the reported experiments, the discussion is constrained to these two procedures. The first approach involves a "within-subjects" design, in which each subject serves as his or her own control. Two different CS's are randomly mixed during the acquisition, or associative phase of the experiment. The two stimuli are usually within the same sensory modality, but differ with respect to content, shape, or pitch, etc. One of the two CS's, the CS+ is paired with the UCS, while the other, the CS−, is not. The response that follows the presentation of the CS+ should be greater than the response following CS− presentations in order for conditioning to have occurred. The other approach may be termed a "between-subjects" design. In this design, there is a single CS, and one group of subjects is presented with contingent CS-UCS pairings where the UCS follows in close temporal proximity to the presentation of the CS. The other group receives only CS presentations, or may have noncontingent presentations of the CS and UCS, i.e., the CS and UCS are not paired together. For conditioning to have been demonstrated, responses in the contingent CS-UCS group should be greater than responses in the CS-alone, or noncontingent, group (see Prokasy and Kumpfer, 1973; Boucsein, 1992, for further details).

The associative process should be distinguished from nonassociative processes, like arousal and perceptual priming, in order to demonstrate that conditioning has occurred. A critical methodologic procedure involves controlling for sensitization, or "pseudoconditioning" (Kimble, 1961) which means that the UCS may prime or sensitize a particular brain state, so that the subject responds to *any* weak stimulus that is presented, irrespective of whether it has been paired with the UCS or not. The effects of such perceptual saliency are controlled for in the between-subjects design by comparing responses a CS-alone group with the CS-UCS group.

Acquisition and Extinction

For both designs, there is typically an "acquisition," or learning phase, and an "extinction," or test phase. The UCS is only presented during the acquisition phase, while the CS is used as a probe during the extinction phase to elicit the CR on each trial for as long as possible. The extinction phase is therefore the actual test of the retrieval of the learned association. The extinction test is also used in the present experiments as a vehicle to reveal hemispheric differences in brain representation of the conditioned association by separately probing the left and right hemispheres (cf. Hugdahl et al., 1987). Often, there is an habituation, or adaptation, period before acquisition begins (Prokasy and Kumpfer, 1973). This is to allow for habituation of the orienting response (OR) (Sokolov, 1960) before conditioning starts (see Öhman, 1983 for a discussion of the role of the OR in electrodermal conditioning). In animal conditioning experiments, CR strength usually increases as a function of the number of CS-UCS presentations (Kimble, 1961). This is, however, not true for human autonomic conditioning, where there usually is an initial increase in responding, followed by a drop-off with further pairings. The decline in response magnitudes across trials has been explained through gradual build-up of conditioned inhibition (Kimmel, 1966), or as reduction of UCS arousal (Lykken, 1968).

LATERALITY AND AUTONOMIC FUNCTION

Laterality is a common term to denote that cognitive and affective functions are differentially represented in the two hemispheres of the brain. Although traditionally restricted to cortical function, laterality is used in a much broader sense in this chapter, implying not only subcortical functions (see Crosson, 1992) but also peripheral, autonomic, endocrine, and immune functions. Thus, in the present context, laterality goes beyond the more traditional meaning of specialization only for higher cognitive functions, like language and visuo-spatial processing (cf. Hellige, 1990). Recent advances in psychophysiologic research have revealed a number of important physiologic asymmetries, related to immune function (Barneoud et al., 1987), neuroendocrine responses (Wittling and Pfluger, 1990), and cardiovascular function (e.g., Weisz et al., 1992; Heller et al., 1990). For example, Wittling (1990) found that the cerebral hemispheres markedly differed in their capability to regulate blood pressure during emotionally laden situations. Both diastolic and systolic blood pressures were significantly increased for right hemisphere presentations of short film clips with emotional content (see also chapter 12). Furthermore, Hugdahl, Wahlgren, and Wass (1982) reported that habituation of the electrodermal orienting response was delayed when visual stimuli were unilaterally presented to the right as compared to the left hemisphere. The Hugdahl et al. (1982) study involved repeated presentations of visual shapes randomly in either the left or right visual half-field, i.e., with unilateral input to the right and left hemispheres of the brain. The reduction in response amplitude over trials (habituation) was more rapid on left as compared to right hemisphere presentations, indicating a delay in habituation when the shapes were presented to the right hemisphere. An important feature of the Hugdahl et al. (1982) study was that there were no significant differences in skin conductance amplitude between the right and left hand recordings (cf. Lacroix and Comper, 1979). Thus, the results indicated that while the electrodermal orienting (OR) system was differentially regulated from the two hemispheres of the brain, there was no indication of a lateralized effect in the electrodermal system in itself.

It may be speculated as to the nature of peripheral laterality, whether it reflects only subcortical influences or whether, e.g., peripheral autonomic functions also are influenced by the cortex. This is a difficult question to answer since central regulation of autonomic function is still unclear (see Cechetto and Saper, 1990). The view taken in this chapter is that activation of the autonomic nervous system may centrally be differentially controlled from the left and right hemispheres, (cf. Werntz et al., 1983). This was supported in the study by Heller et al. (1990) who showed that cardiovascular arousal was directly related to stimulation of the right hemisphere in a visual half-field paradigm. A right hemisphere effect was also reported by Hachinsky et al. (1992) in a conceptually important study in which rats had either the left or right middle cerebral artery experimentally occluded. Heart rate (HR), blood pressure, and plasma epinephrine and norepinephrine were monitored, among other variables. The results clearly showed greater sympathetic consequences after right hemisphere than after left hemisphere lesions. An untested prediction from the findings by Hachinsky et al. (1992) is that patients with right-sided cerebral stroke may be more susceptible to lethal consequences than patients with left-sided stroke. It could perhaps be argued that hospital records should be compared for patients with left- vs. right-sided ischemic stroke, looking for possible differences in severity of the insult, and differences in the progress of rehabilitation.

CLASSICAL CONDITIONING AS IMPLICIT LEARNING

Schacter (1987) and Graf and Schacter (1985) have coined the term *implicit memory* to refer to an experimental situation where information that was learned and encoded during a particular stage of an experiment is expressed at a later stage, without the subject having any explicit, or conscious, awareness of the learning situation. This means that a response to a current event can be influenced by a past event of which the subject is unaware (cf. Lockhart, 1989). A typical task for implicit memory is the priming stem completion task (Graf and Schacter, 1985). In a first phase of a stem completion experiment, the subject is shown a list of common words, such as "tower," "stable," etc. Each word is chosen so that it has about ten different possible completions. An equal number of similar words are also chosen but not presented during the first phase of the experiment. Following the first task, the subjects are shown a list of word stems such as "tow____," "cas____," "sta____," etc. They are asked to say the first word that comes to mind that would complete the stem and form a word. They are further told to respond as quickly as possible with whatever word that springs to mind. Half of the stems are taken from the words in the exposure list during the first phase of the experiment; the other half are not. The measure of priming is the difference between the number of stems completed to form words shown during the exposure phase and the number of stems completed to form words that were not shown during the exposure. From results like these it is inferred that exposure primes the subjects to complete the stems into those words because of implicit memory processes that the subject is unaware of.

The priming effect in implicit memory tasks represents a temporary connection or binding between past and present events and situations. Priming is therefore conceptually similar to the notion of a conditioned association between a salient and a neutral stimulus. The priming effect can be looked at as an example of second-order conditioning where the spontaneous response following the presentation of the word stem is the CR, and the word stem itself is the CS. An intriguing feature of implicit memory is that implicit stimulus connections are perhaps more common than explicit memories for which we can recall the background history. As put forward by Lockhart (1989): "Why ... should we be impressed by the fact that a response to a current stimulus can be influenced by a past event of which the subject is unaware. Isn't that how most organisms behave most of the time...?" (p. 6). One could add to this that such temporary unaware connections between events are necessary to keep order and stability in a changing environment. Isn't this how we cope with a constantly overwhelming information load? Behavior adaptations to changes in the environmental perceptual input are, to a great extent, "set" by past implicit memory processes, some of them in the framework of CRs. That a conditioning experience may be implicitly encoded was also acknowledged by Schacter (1987) who discussed several examples where subjects can learn contingencies between stimulus events without awareness of learning and, hence, without explicit memory for them. He also argued that subjects could acquire various types of classically conditioned responses without awareness of the conditioning contingencies. Thus, classical conditioning is under certain circumstances an example of implicit learning.

Studying implicit memory in a repetition priming paradigm with recordings of cerebral blood flow, Squire et al. (1992) found reduction of flow in the right posterior cortex. This might provide a clue to the neural basis of priming: after the presentation of a stimulus, less neural activity is required to process the same stimulus the second time it appears. An interesting question is whether similar changes in blood flow would occur in a classical conditioning experiment, considering that the CS would require less neural activity to be processed once the association has taken place. A blood flow study of human conditioning has, however, to my knowledge never been performed.

A typical implicit conditioning experiment was that of Lazarus and McCleary (1951) who conditioned subjects to visual presentations of nonsense syllables with shock to the hand as the UCS. When later tested with brief presentations of the conditioned syllables mixed with other syllables, subjects showed larger skin conductance responses (SCRs) to the CS syllables compared to the control stimuli, although they could not detect the presence of the stimuli. Unfortunately, subliminal implicit conditioning phenomena were left out from mainstream experimental psychology after the initial demonstration in the early 1950s. This was possibly a consequence of the criticism, voiced by, e.g., Eriksen (1960), about the nature of unaware learning. However, the available data from the early 1950s to date seem to indicate that CRs can sometimes be elicited by stimuli that the subject cannot recognize or remember ever having perceived (cf. Öhman, 1986).

Hemispheric Asymmetry and Implicit Learning

Although not unchallenged, several studies have shown a kind of implicit, unconscious learning, involving autonomic responses. In a now classic paper,

Tranel and Damasio (1985) tested two patients with prosopagnosia after occipitotemporal lesions involving the right hemisphere. Neither of the patients could overtly recognize pictures of familiar faces when mixed with presentations of unfamiliar faces. Nevertheless, they showed greater electrodermal responses to the familiar, compared to the unfamiliar, faces. In a conceptually similar study, Berti and Rizzolatti (1992) showed that five right hemisphere–lesioned neglect patients could make categorical judgments about objects presented in the neglected field if the stimuli had been primed before they were presented. The study involved presentation of words of different categories (animals and fruits) on a screen in front of the patient. One of the words within a category was a prime, the other a target to which the patient gave a verbal response. The prime was always presented in the right, unaffected visual field, the target always in the left, affected, field. Thus, patients with neglect after right-sided lesions (see Heilman et al., 1987 for a description of neglect) are able to implicitly process stimuli presented in the neglected visual field, even when they overtly deny ever having seen the stimuli. However, not all studies have found evidence of unaware, or implicit, learning in right hemisphere–lesioned patients. Sergent and Villemure (1989) studied a prosopagnostic woman (B.M.) after right hemispherectomy. B.M. showed no signs of implicit recognition of known faces in a learning task, and there was no indication that she could store facial information in memory. B.M. seems, though, to have had a different symptomatology than other prosopagnostic patients since she could easily evoke semantic information about familiar faces and retrieve their names when visually cued.

Studies of implicit processing in altered states of consciousness have also revealed a right hemisphere dominance. Spiegel et al. (1985) reported significantly reduced P3 amplitudes of the event-related potential (ERP) to visual stimuli in a situation where highly hypnotizable subjects were instructed that there was a hallucinated object blocking their view of the monitor where the stimuli were presented. The P3 effect was furthermore more marked over the right hemisphere. Similarly, Frumkin, Ripley, and Cox (1978) found greater right hemisphere involvement in a dichotic listening task when subjects were compared in normal and hypnotic consciousness. These findings were partially confirmed in a subsequent study by Levine, Kurtz, and Lauter (1984), although Crawford, Crawford, and Koperski (1983) failed to find evidence for right hemisphere involvement in hypnosis. Moreover, Putnam, Zahn, and Post (1990) showed that persons with multiple personality disorders produced consistent differences in electrodermal responses when they "changed" personality, which accompanied the separate cognitive and affective behaviors that these persons typically manifest when they alter personality states (see also Coons, Bowman, and Milstein, 1988).

Another area where autonomic responding to right hemisphere activation has been demonstrated is a classic study by Dimond and Farrington (1977) who used a specially designed lens to present film clips only to the left or right hemisphere. Negative emotional films had a greater impact on HR changes when presented to the right as compared to the left hemisphere.

Thus, implicit learning in classical conditioning may be mediated through right hemisphere processes. As discussed above, Squire et al. (1992) found unique changes in cerebral blood flow in the right compared to the left prefrontal and posterior cortices to a verbal stimulus that had been primed. A right hemisphere effect for implicit conditioning was also observed by Corteen and Wood (1972) who showed that electrodermal responses were greater to previously shocked names when they were presented dichotically to the left ear (right hemisphere) together with other nonshocked names, although the subjects were not aware of the presentation of the names.

The Corteen and Wood (1972) experiment consisted of two phases. In the first phase, subjects received an electric shock as the UCS contingent upon presentation of city names which served as CS's. The CS words were presented over headphones to the subjects. In the second phase, the conditioned words were presented to the left ear, mixed with other nonshocked names, while a prose passage was presented to the right ear in a dichotic shadowing task (cf. Broadbent, 1958). The subjects were instructed to attend only to the prose passage, ignoring the words presented to the other ear. The results showed that the previously shocked words yielded greater CRs than the nonshocked words. In order to make sure that the subjects had not noticed the unattended words, the authors interviewed their subjects after the experiment. Although the interviewing technique may be criticized as a measure of stimulus unawareness (see Dawson and Reardon, 1973; Holender, 1986), the results of the Corteen and Wood (1972) study indicated that an autonomic conditioned response may be elicited without the subject being aware of the CS-UCS contingency. The results were later confirmed by Dawson and Schell (1982), Martin et al. (1984), and by Wright, Andersson, and Stenman (1975).

In another attempt at replication, however, Wardlaw and Kroll (1976) failed to find evidence for unconscious conditioning. Interestingly, these authors counterbalanced the ear of presentation of the unattended conditioned and control words during the second phase of the experiment, with left ear presentations on half of the trials and right ear presentations on the other half. Corteen and Wood (1972), on the other hand, had only *left* ear presentations, which in a dichotic situation means primarily activating the right hemisphere. Thus, Wardlaw and Kroll (1976) might have seen evidence of discriminatory responding had they analyzed the left and right ear presentations separately. A similar observation was made by Dawson and Schell (1982) who also noticed that evidence for unconscious conditioning was present only when the ear of presentation of the CS was the left ear. The findings by Dawson and Schell thus support and reinforce the argument for a unique role for the right hemisphere in implicit associative learning.

As previously mentioned, a critical methodologic issue related to the use of dichotic stimulus presentations to unravel hemispheric differences in unconscious processing is the possibility that subjects may rapidly shift attention to the nonattended channel when the critical test stimuli are presented (see Dawson and Schell, 1982; Holender, 1986). Hugdahl and Andersson (1986) have shown that the standard dichotic procedure is sensitive to attentional influences, where a hemisphere-specific ear advantage may be shifted if attention is focused to the ipsilateral ear (see also Hugdahl, 1992). This was nicely controlled for in a recent study by Wexler et al. (1992) who used the dichotic fusing technique developed by Wexler and Halwes (1983) when presenting emotional and neutral words to either the left or right ear. The fused dichotic technique means that two different words, which differ only with respect to their initial consonant, are presented exactly at the same time, one in each ear. The temporal and spectral overlap between the two stimulus words usually results in a single "fused" percept. Hemispheric differences are observed by scoring frequency of correctly identified left vs. right ear words. In addition, Wexler et al. (1992) found that both electroencephalographic (EEG) and facial electromyelographic (EMG) responses were greater to unconsciously processed emotional words presented to the right hemisphere. That is, for trials in which the subject reported hearing the neutral word, there was greater physiologic activation when the emotional word was presented to the left ear. In a conceptually similar experiment, Wexler et al. (1986) showed that different personality characteristics (repressors, high-anxiety, low-anxiety subjects) interacted with the presentation of the fused emotional dichotic words. Highly anxious subjects and repressors showed initially a reduced right ear advantage to the words, probably indicating spontaneous overactivation of the right hemisphere.

RIGHT HEMISPHERE CONDITIONING: EXPERIMENTS

Drawing on the work of Marcel (1983), Öhman (e.g. 1986) has used brief presentations (<40 ms) of masked visual stimuli paired with shock in an electrodermal conditioning paradigm. The results have shown that near-subliminal presentations of angry faces that previously have been associated with shock yield greater electrodermal CRs than do control stimuli. Öhman has used a differential conditioning paradigm, with mixed presentations of the CS+ and CS− during the acquisition phase of his experiments. For half of the subjects, an angry face was the CS+, with a happy face as the CS−. The other half of the subjects had the order reversed. During the extinction phase, both the CS+ and the CS− were presented near subliminally while skin conductance responses were recorded.

Öhman (1986) has argued that CSs, and especially fear-relevant CSs, may become effective in engaging automatic, preattentive processing mechanisms, which may be particularly tuned into priming autonomic physiologic responses. Using Öhman's (1986) model of preattentive, automatic processing for fear conditioning, linking it to implicit learning in classical conditioning, we predicted that this type of learning should particularly implicate right hemisphere processing.

Although the final common pathways between the cerebral cortices and the autonomic nervous system are not known in detail (see Cechetto and Saper, 1990), electrodermal responses are under cortical as well as subcortical influences. Using magnetic resonance imaging (MRI), Raine, Reynolds, and Sheard (1991) found positive correlations between electrodermal responses and size of prefrontal areas. Moreover, skin conductance responses were diminished in monkeys after lateral frontal lesions, and absent after removal of the dorsolateral cortex (Bagshaw, Kimble, and Pribram, 1965). Finally, Cechetto and Saper argued that the medial prefrontal cortex, including the infralimbic parts, may act as an autonomic motor cortex (see also LeDoux, 1991). The electrodermal system is under two separate cortical influences: an ipsilateral system including the limbic structures and hypothalamus, and a contralateral system including the prefrontal cortex and the basal ganglia (Schliak and Schiffter, 1979; see also Boucsein, 1992). The argument here is that right hemisphere areas play a more active role than homologous left hemisphere areas in autonomic classical conditioning.

These predictions were put to a first empirical test in a pilot experiment (Öhman et al., 1988) in which subjects were conditioned to angry and happy faces with one of the faces (CS+) always followed by the shock UCS, and the other (CS−) never paired with shock. The extinction phase consisted of brief (30 ms) presentations of the happy and angry faces, immediately followed by a neutral masking face. Using the visual half-field technique (VHF), which allows for unilateral activation of each hemisphere separately (see McKeever, 1986), the previous CS+ and CS− were presented to the right hemisphere (left VHF) on half of the trials, and on the other half of trials they were presented to the left hemisphere (right VHF). A simplified outline of the basic design is seen in figures 10.1 and 10.2. Note that the faces used in the study were slides of real human faces taken from the Ekman, Friesen, and Ellsworth (1972) series of facial emotional expressions.

Skin conductance responses separated for the left and right hemisphere groups are seen in figure 10.3. The data in figure 10.3 are plotted as the average of the angry and happy face presentations. The results showed significant differentiation between the CS+ and the CS− only for right hemisphere presentations. In other words, the left hemisphere had obviously not "learned" that it was only the CS+ that previously was associated with shock, suppressing responses to the CS−. Consequently, the left hemisphere responded as much to the CS− as to the CS+ owing to their perceptual and attentional characteristics. There was also a clear tendency in the data for greater CS+-CS− discrimination in the group with the angry face as the CS+.

The results of this study were remarkable considering that the only difference between conditions was that on 50% of the trials the stimulus picture was moved to the right side of the screen, and on the other 50% of the trials it was moved to the left side. Since presentations were random with respect to the half-fields, the subjects could not know in advance which half-field the

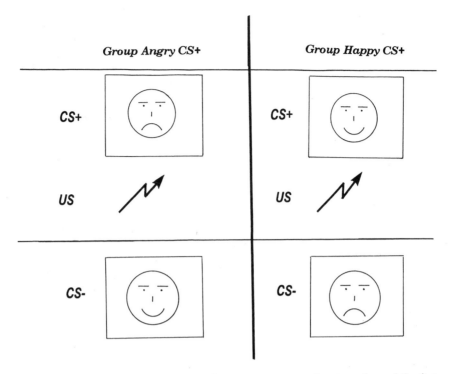

Figure 10.1 Outline of the design for the acquisition, or conditioning, phase of the first experiment. CS, conditioned stimulus; US, unconditioned stimulus (shock); CS+, CS paired with shock; CS−, CS not paired with shock.

stimulus would be presented in on a given trial. The results were also remarkable in the sense that the difference between the hemispheres was obtained *after learning had occurred*, i.e., during the extinction or, "probe," phase of the study. Presenting the CS+ probe for only 30 ms (and followed by the mask) still initiated retrieval of the encoded association from the right hemipsere.

Control Procedures

Although confirming our main predictions, the results of this pilot study should be interpreted cautiously. There are a number of methodologic issues that should be sorted out before a more coherent model of right hemisphere functioning in implicit learning and conditioning is presented (see Hugdahl and Johnsen, 1993). There are particularly two issues that should be addressed: the perceptual vs. associative basis for the right hemisphere effect, and a conditioning vs. sensitization or priming effect. The results of the pilot study could have been caused by a right hemisphere advantage for the *perception* of nonverbal, and particularly facial emotional expressions, considering the huge literature on right hemisphere dominance for visuospatial perception

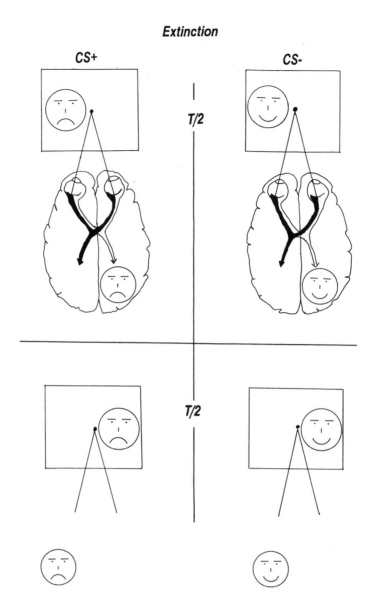

Figure 10.2 Outline of the design for the extinction, or test, phase of the first experiment. T/2, half of the trials.

(Hellige, 1990), and on perception of facial expressions (Suberi and McKeever, 1977). This could be tested by including two no-shock control groups in the experimental situation. If the right hemisphere no-shock group yields responses during the extinction phase that cannot be distinguished from the responses observed in the right hemisphere "conditioning" group, then the effect must have been a perceptual one. In a similar way, the right hemisphere may have been uniquely primed, or sensitized, by the shock UCS during the acquisition phase. If so, it could have shown greater reactivity to *any* stimulus configuration presented in the left half-field during the extinction test. This

Extinction Test

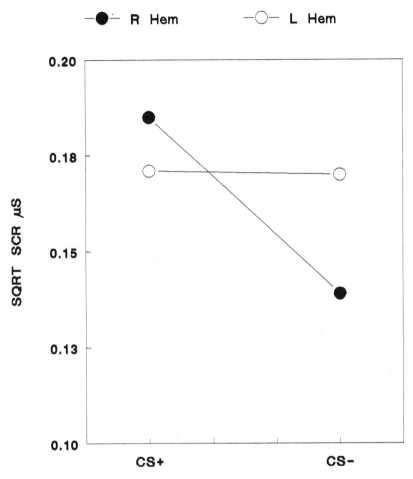

Figure 10.3 Square root–transformed skin conductance responses in microsiemens (SQRT SCR μS) to the CS+ and CS− for faces presented to the right and left hemispheres, respectively, in the first experiment. R Hem, right hemisphere; L Hem, left hemisphere. Data are averaged across angry/happy faces, and across left/right hand recordings. (Data from Öhman et al. (1988), reprinted with permisson from the publisher.)

could be tested by presenting a new stimulus during extinction that had never been paired with the UCS. If responses to the new stimulus were similar to responses to the conditioned stimulus, then the effect was a nonassociative sensitization effect.

Two other issues were also addressed in the present experiments: sex differences and other response systems. Sex differences were studied because they have been observed in other studies of brain laterality (McGlone, 1980). If there is a genuine hemispheric difference in implicit conditional learning, then males and females should differ in their responding. Other response systems included were stimulus-elicited HR responses, and event-related brain potentials (ERPs) recorded from the scalp. The new response measures were included as a test of the generality of the right hemisphere effect.

Common Methods

The subjects were female and male students at the University of Bergen, Norway, their ages varying between 19 and 35 years. All subjects were tested for right-handedness with a questionnaire containing 15 items related to manual preference, and one item related to pedal preference.

Bilateral phasic SCRs were recorded on a Beckman polygraph with two Beckman SCR couplers. The couplers each supplied a constant voltage of 0.5 V. To control for possible differences in voltage between the couplers, both couplers were randomly shifted between subjects for right- vs. left-hand recordings. Beckman 8-mm Ag and AgCl cup electrodes were filled with a 0.05 M NaCl Unibase concentration.

The stimuli were slides that were back-projected onto a 70- × 72-cm milkglass screen inside a sound-attenuating chamber. The slides were projected from two slide projectors, each fitted with a high-speed shutter in front of the lens. This was done in order to achieve maximum onset of slide presentation, and to control for short presentation times.

A plywood box was mounted inside the chamber, with the milk glass screen as the posterior wall with a small rubber mask opening for the eyes in the anterior wall. A 2-mm light-emitting diode (LED) was placed in the center of the milk-glass screen as a fixation point (when the LED was lighted during a trial).

The face stimuli were tachistoscopically projected either to the right or left side of the LED, i.e., either in the right or left VHF. Electric shocks, serving as UCS's, were randomly presented to the fourth and fifth fingers of the subject, and were generated from a DC shock generator. The shock generator was electrically shielded from all other equipment. Half of the subjects in each (condition) group had shock in their right hand, the other half in their left hand. The intensity of the electric shock was determined individually for each subject before the experiments started by delivering shocks of increasing intensity until the subject reported that the shock was "unpleasant but not painful." In the fifth experiment, white noise was used as the UCS instead of shock.

To control for involuntary eye movements during a trial, an electro-oculogram (EOG) was recorded from both eyes on a Beckman nystagmus coupler.

The pictures of facial emotional expressions were taken from the Ekman et al. (1972) standardized facial expressions set. The same models expressing either an angry (No. 105) or a happy (No. 101) expression were used. On unilateral trials, the slides were projected at about 2.5 degrees of visual angle either to the right or left of the central LED.

Generally, all experiments contained three phases: (1) a familiarization, or habituation, phase; (2) an association, or acquisition, phase when the CS was followed by the UCS; and (3) a test, or extinction, phase. To simplify presentation of the data across experiments, only the extinction data are presented, while data for the acquisition phase are described in the text.

Perceptual vs. Associative Laterality

Before any more definitive conclusions were reached concerning the right hemisphere effect in the study by Öhman et al. (1988), a control study was run to test whether the CS+-UCS *association* was encoded in the right hemisphere, or whether the angry face elicited larger responses because facial emotional expressions are more easily *perceived* by the right hemisphere. Thus, in the control study, we tried to disentangle associative from nonassociative factors (Johnsen and Hugdahl, 1993). We have previously argued that separating, e.g., perceptual from associative factors "is not an easy question to answer" (Johnsen and Hugdahl, 1991). Perceptual CS properties are often emphasized in modern theories of learning (e.g., Siddle and Remington, 1987), and superior conditioning for certain CS-UCS pairings may be due to a host of factors specifically related to the perceptual and motivational saliency of the CS. Thus, the CS may be biologically prepared to elicit a conditioned response, as in certain conditioned phobic reactions (Seligman, 1971; Hugdahl and Öhman, 1977), it may be more intense, or it may have been contextually primed to be associated with the UCS. Perceptual and attentional factors are thus closely interwoven with the connectiveness inherent in the CS-UCS association.

However, one way to separate nonassociative from associative processes in the present series of experiments would be to add a group of subjects that have everything equal to the conditioning groups, except that the shock UCS is omitted during the acquisition phase. These groups would be subjected to a "pseudoacquisition," or prolonged habituation phase, with no shocks presented in the interval when the conditioning groups received the UCS. If the no-shock angry CS group shows the same response magnitudes as the corresponding shock group, then the previously observed right hemisphere effect is nonassociative. However, if the groups differ in response amplitudes, then the effect is associative.

Another aspect that was added to the later experiments was that lateralized presentations of the CS's were moved from the extinction phase, as in the Öhman et al. (1988) study, to the acquisition, or conditioning, phase. The logic for the experimental setup was taken from the study by Hugdahl et al.(1987) where a compound CS (words and colors) was used, with one component of the compound being presented to the right VHF while the other

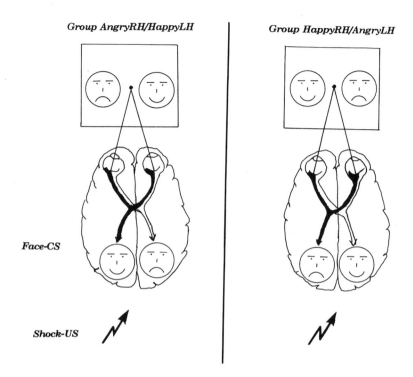

Figure 10.4 Outline of the design for the acquisition phase in the second experiment. RH, right hemisphere; LH, left hemisphere.

component was simultaneously presented to the other half-field. The compound was followed by an aversive white noise as the UCS during the acquisition phase of the experiment. Thus, one component of the compound CS was uniquely projected to the left hemisphere, and the other component was simultaneously projected to the right hemisphere. The question asked was which of the two CS components was associated with the UCS, the one in the left or the one in the right hemisphere. This was tested in the Hugdahl et al. (1987) study by taking the components apart during the extinction phase, presenting them separately and focally. The results showed that the color component that previously had been presented in the right hemisphere yielded greater responses than the word stimuli. The dichoptic paradigm developed by Hugdahl et al. (1987) was used in later experiments, with angry and happy faces presented simultaneously during the acquisition phase, one in each half-field, and both of them paired with shock during the acquisition phase. Half of the subjects had the angry face in the left half-field and the happy face in the right half-field (Group AngryRH/HappyLH). The other half of the subjects had the order of presentation reversed, the happy face in the

Group AngryRH/HappyLH | Group HappyRH/AngryLH

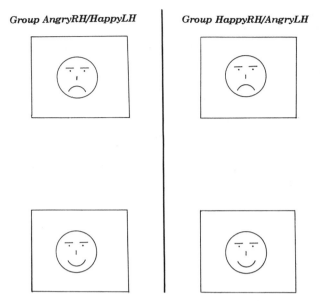

Figure 10.5 Outline of the design for the extinction phase of the second experiment. RH, right hemisphere presentation during acquisition; LH, left hemisphere presentation during acquisition.

left field, and the angry face in the right field (Group HappyRH/AngryLH). During the extinction phase, either an angry or a happy face was presented, with focal nonlateralized presentations. The experimental setup is seen in figures 10.4 and 10.5.

In our view, lateralized CS presentations during the acquisition phase are a more stringent test of the right hemisphere hypothesis. Since the only difference between the groups in the entire experiment was the right or left field position during the *acquisition* phase, any differences in responding to the faces during the *extinction* phase should be due to a specific associative capacity for the hemisphere that received this face during acquisition.

In addition to the right and left field conditioning groups, two yoked nonshock groups were added, being identical to the two conditioning groups except for the shocks during acquisition. Thus, the experiment consisted of four groups: two CS shock groups and two CS no-shock groups.

The compound CS was presented for 180 ms during the acquisition phase, and the single CS was presented for 30 ms during the extinction test phase. Thus, the presentation time during extinction was close to the subliminal presentation time, allowing for tests of lateralized unconscious classical conditioning. In comparison with the Öhman et al. (1988) study, the second experiment in the present series used *lateralized* and *above*-recognition threshold presentations during the acquisition phase, but *foveal* and *below*-recognition threshold presentations during the test phase. Phasic electrodermal responses were used as dependent measures. Responses were obtained from both hands, but since there were no theoretically interesting differences between the recordings from the two hands, data are presented as averages from the left and right hand recordings. There were 62 female subjects in the experiment. Nine trials of the compound CS were used in the acquisition phase, with ten trials of each face during the extinction phase. As in the Öhman et al. (1988) study, the faces were taken from the Ekman et al. (1972) series of facial pictures. Conditioning effects during the acquisition phase were evaluated as the average of the first two presentations each of the angry and happy face during the test phase. This is an unusual way of assessing conditioning effects, using the same data for the analysis of both acqustion and extinction. However, the very nature of the compound CS precludes conventional assessment procedures during the acquisition phase. Furthermore, the critical comparisons were between the shock vs. no-shock groups, and between the left vs. right half-field position of the face CS during acquisition. For both comparisons, using data from the first extinction trials to assess acquisition effects is an appropriate procedure. The results showed that significant conditioned associations had occurred for both the angry and happy faces. The results for the extinction phase are shown in figure 10.6. Figure 10.6 shows SCR magnitudes averaged across trials, separated for groups and conditions.

The data were evaluated in a three-way ANOVA (analysis of variance), with a posteriori follow-up tests. The most conspicuous finding was the absence of any effects for the no-shock conditions, seen in the significant main effect of shock vs. no shock. Moreover, as can be seen in figure 10.6, there were no differences between the two no-shock groups. However, there was a huge difference between the shock and no-shock groups, and especially for the group that had the angry face projected to the right hemisphere during acquisition. This was statistically corroborated in the significant two-way interaction of face Position (during acquisition) × Shock or No-shock. Finally, for both the angry and happy faces, right hemisphere projections during acquisition resulted in greater conditioned responses during extinction compared to the corresponding left hemisphere projections. The results thus supported an interpretation in terms of associative rather than perceptual processes since the no-shock right hemisphere groups did not respond with the same SCR magnitudes as the corresponding right hemisphere shock groups.

Right Hemisphere Sensitization

Although the findings in the second experiment supported an associative explanation, other confounding nonassociative factors cannot be completely ruled out. As previously discussed, the shock may have uniquely primed or

Extinction

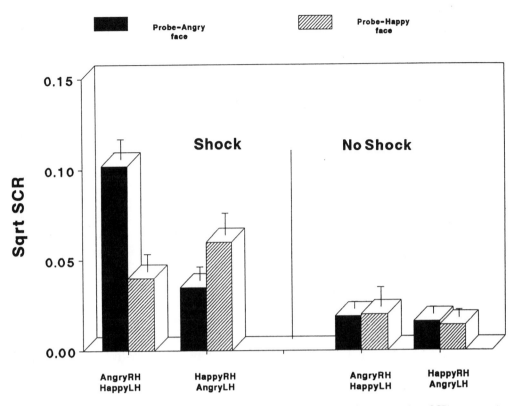

Figure 10.6 Square root–transformed skin conductance responses (Sqrt SCR) in microsiemens during the extinction phase of the second experiment. RH, right hemisphere presentation during acquisition; LH, left hemisphere presentation during acquisition. Data averaged across trials and hands. (Data from Johnsen and Hugdahl, 1993; reprinted with permission from the publisher.)

sensitized the right hemisphere, although half the subjects had shock in their right hand, and half in their left hand, and there were no significant differences between these conditions. A sensitization effect can be tested by including a new stimulus in the extinction phase that was not presented during the conditioning phase, and consequently never had been associated with the shock UCS. If responses to right hemisphere presentations of the new stimulus are equal to the responses to the face stimuli, then a priming confounding effect would exist. This was evaluated in a dichoptic paradigm similar to that used in the perceptual control experiment, with the exception that slides of a color bar were interspersed among the slides of the faces during the extinction phase. All stimuli were administered for 180 ms during acquisition and for 30 ms during extinction. The outcome of the ANOVA showed SCRs twice as large for the group with the angry face presented to the right hemisphere during acquisition. Interestingly, the color bar showed the smallest SCR amplitudes during the extinction phase of the experiment, particularly the group that had the angry face projected to the right hemisphere during acquisition. Thus, sensitization of the right hemisphere by shock during acquisition was not a major confounding factor for the right hemisphere effect in the first two experiments. This could be further elaborated in the sense that *if* UCS sensitization had primed the right hemisphere to respond to *any* kind of stimulus, then there should not have been a difference in response magnitudes when probing with the angry vs. the happy face CS in the second experiment.

Sex Differences

It has repeatedly been shown that the prevalence of phobic fears is higher in females than in males (e.g., Geer, 1965). Females also react with greater autonomic responses in fear conditioning (Fredrikson, Hugdahl, and Öhman, 1976). It could therefore be hypothesized that females would be more responsive in the present conditioning paradigms than males since shock was used as the UCS, eliciting conditioned fear responses. The same experimental design was used as in the previous experiment, with the addition of two male groups.

The results showed that only the females acquired the learned association during the acquisition phase. There was a clear difference between the female and male groups in right hemisphere responding during the extinction phase (figure 10.7).

Thus, probing the right hemisphere with the angry CS face yielded significantly larger responses in females as compared to males. The same occurred when probing with the happy CS face, although overall response magnitudes were smaller. This was statistically supported in the significant interaction of Sex × Face (right/left position during acquisition) × Emotion (happy/angry).

Other Measures Heart Rate Responses

Phasic HR responses are typically observed as a triphasic response complex during the CS-UCS interval in autonomic conditioning (e.g., Obrist, Webb, and Sutterer, 1969). There is usually an initial deceleration 1 to 3 seconds after CS onset, followed by an acceleration for about 3 to 4 seconds, with a second deceleration occurring at about the time when the UCS is presented (Bohlin and Kjellberg, 1979). The acceleration in response to the CS may be taken as an index of the conditioned response (Öhman, 1983).

Relating HR changes to sensory stimulation to laterality, several authors have suggested that HR changes are regulated from the right hemisphere (e.g., Walker and Sandman, 1979; Hugdahl et al., 1983). Yokoyama et al. (1987) showed that patients with right hemisphere lesions did not show the typical anticipatory HR response profile in a two-stimulus paradigm. Furthermore,

Sex Differences

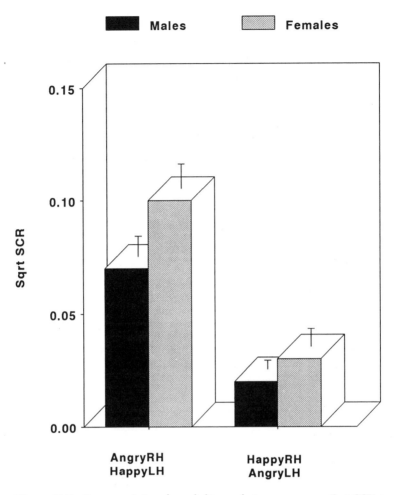

Figure 10.7 Square root–transformed skin conductance responses (Sqrt SCR) in microsiemens separated for males and females. Design is the same as in the second experiment. RH, right hemisphere presentation during acquisition; LH, left hemisphere presentation during acquisition. Data are averaged across trials and hands.

Rosen et al. (1982) reported that HR changes were smaller following right carotid injections of amobarbital sodium (Amytal Sodium) than those following left carotid injections. These observations fit the anatomy of the vagus nerve and the innervation of the sinoatrial (SA) node of the heart. It is the right branch of the vagus nerve that innervates the SA node, which is the primary pacemaker for the beating of the heart (Brodal, 1981). Analyzing existing empirical evidence, Porges and Maiti (1992) have recently developed a model of right hemisphere control of vagus outflow to the postganglionic nuclei in the SA and atrioventricular (AV) nodes.

Hugdahl: Laterality and Implicit Learning

Angry RH / Happy LH

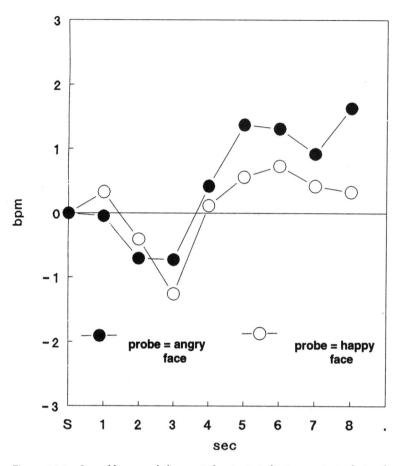

Figure 10.8 Second-by-second changes in heart rate in beats-per-minute during the extinction phase in the third experiment. Design is the same as for the second experiment. Data are averaged across trials. RH, right hemisphere presentation during acquisition; LH, left hemisphere presentation during acquisition.

Relating these findings to the present series of experiments, it could be predicted that acceleratory changes in HR after CS presentations should differ between the right and left hemisphere groups. Thus, a new study was run with the same paradigm as in the second and third experiments but in which HR was also recorded. Second-by-second changes in HR were scored as deviations in beats per minute (bpm) from the 3 seconds immediately preceding the presentation of the probe CS during the extinction phase.

The results are shown in figure 10.8, separated for the right and left hemisphere groups.

Happy RH / Angry LH

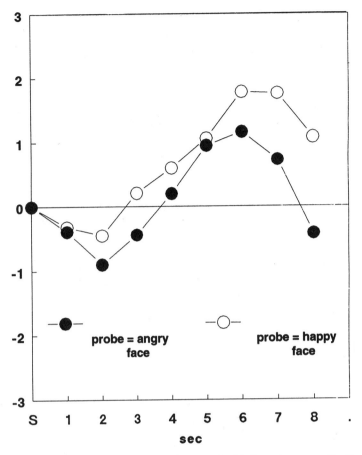

Once again, probing with the angry CS face during extinction resulted in significantly larger HR acceleration in the group that had the *angry* face projected to the right hemisphere during acquisition. Similarly, probing with the *happy* CS face resulted in significantly larger acceleration in the group with the happy face projected to the right hemisphere during acquisition. This can be seen in seconds 5 to 8 in figure 10.8.

Event-Related Potentials

The last experiment to be reported in this series involved recordings of ERPs from the scalp, time-locked to presentations of the CS's. This study differed from the other experiments in that auditory stimuli were used. The paradigm involved a dichotic listening (DL) situation to evaluate differential conditioning in the two hemispheres of the brain. The dichotic conditioning paradigm is described in detail in Hugdahl and Nordby (1991), and Hugdahl and Brobeck (1986). Therefore, only a summary is given here. The general outline of conditioning experiments using DL is that subjects are exposed to dichotic presentations of either consonant-vowel (CV) syllables or different tones, with one stimulus presented in the right ear and the other simultaneously presented in the left ear. Dichotic stimulus presentations provide an auditory "analog" to the VHF technique for visual stimulus presentations (see Springer, 1986, for a review). The rationale for inferring laterality differences from performance in the DL situation is that under conditions of competition between the ears, the contralateral projections from the cochlea in the ear to the primary auditory cortex in the temporal lobe will predominate (Rosenzweig, 1951; Connolly, 1985; Maximilian, 1982). The predominance of the contralateral cortical representation of each ear may possibly be a consequence of the ampler projection of second-order neurons to the inferior colliculus on the contralateral compared to the ipsilateral side (Brodal, 1981). The contralateral preponderance in DL results from the fact that a stronger projection from the right ear will suppress the weaker information coming from the left ear, and vice versa (Kimura, 1967). Thus, presenting a stimulus in the right ear will uniquely project initially only to the left hemisphere, and vice versa for left ear stimulus presentations.

The DL technique was used in the present conditioning experiment with an acquisition and extinction phase. During the acquisition phase, one group had two different CV syllables /ba/ and /pa/ randomly presented binaurally, one at a time. Another group had two tones differing in pitch, presented in the same manner as the syllables for the CV group. During the acquisition phase, one of the two stimuli was followed by an aversive white noise as the UCS; the other stimulus was never followed by noise. Thus, a differential within-subjects paradigm was used with the stimulus followed by the noise being turned into a conditioned stimulus (CS+), the other being turned into a sensitization control stimulus (CS−). After conditioning, the CS+ and CS− were presented together, dichotically. For half of the subjects in each group, the CS+ was presented in the left ear (right hemisphere projection); for the other half it was presented in the right ear (left hemisphere projection). The nature of the DL technique thus means that because the CS+ and the CS− are presented simultaneously and *together* at the level of the *ear*, they actually reach each hemisphere *separately* at the level of the *brain*. Thus, laterality effects in classical conditioning may be observed in another sensory modality than for the visual experiments. ERPs moreover allow the researcher to look at a central nervous system (CNS) measure of the associative process. An important feature of the dichotic conditioning paradigm, as well as of the dichoptic VHF paradigm, is that usually only *a single* manipulation separates the groups in the experiments: the reversal of the CS+ and CS− locations in the DL paradigm, and the reversal of half-field positions in the VHF paradigm.

Analysis of the ERP waveform with respect to time elapsed since the presentation of the stimulus may be classified along a continuum ranging from exogenous stimulus-elicited components to endogenous, more cognitive components (Donchin et al., 1986). A larger positive-going deflection of the ERP in the range of 300 to 500 ms after stimulus presentations, labeled P3, has been found to be sensitive to shifts of attention and to stimulus significance (Donchin, 1981), while the earlier components, e.g., the N1, are influenced by the physical characteristics of the stimulus (Näätänen, 1992). The process of conditioning implies that the same physical stimulus is transformed into a conditioned stimulus, gaining attentional and motivational saliency. It could therefore be predicted that the effects of laterality on the representation of the association in the brain should be revealed in the later, endogenous ERP components (cf. Hugdahl and Nordby, 1991).

ERPs were recorded from 19 leads on the scalp and were used as dependent measures. However, only data from the midline vertex recording (Cz) are presented here. There were 10 trials each of the CS+ and CS− during the acquisition phase, and 13 dichotic trials during extinction. The intertrial interval was varied between 5 and 9 seconds between stimulus presentations. The results from the extinction phase are shown in figure 10.9. Note that the data in figure 10.9 are averaged for both the CV syllables and tone groups.

As can be seen in figure 10.9, there were mainly two responses occurring in the scoring interval, an early N1 peak in the 100- to 150-ms window after stimulus presentations, and a P3 peaking in the 250- to 350-ms window. The increased response amplitudes in the P3 region 250 to 350 ms after CS presentation were larger for the two groups that had the CS+ presented to the left ear, i.e., to the right hemisphere. Thus, right hemisphere presentations of the CS+ elicited significantly greater ERPs in the P3 region than corresponding left hemisphere presentations. This means that probing the right hemisphere with the previously noise-reinforced CS yielded a greater P3 than probing the corresponding areas in the left hemisphere. Once again, it should be noted that the only difference between the groups in the entire experiment was the reversal of the headphones during extinction, with half of the subjects receiving the CS+ in the left ear, the other half receiving it in the right ear. All physical parameters were exactly the same between the groups, since the same stimuli were used for both laterality groups.

As argued by Wexler et al. (1986), the dichotic technique may trigger hemisphere-specific frontal attentional centers that facilitate processing of information in the left or right sensory half-field. It could be added that dichotic input in a conditioning paradigm may in addition trigger memory representations in temporofrontal brain areas. Within a conditioning paradigm, these representations may be specific to one hemisphere, depending on the nature of the conditioning task (Hugdahl et al., 1987). As previously described, Squire et al. (1992) showed that implicit repetition priming particularly activated the right hippocampal region in the brain. They found further

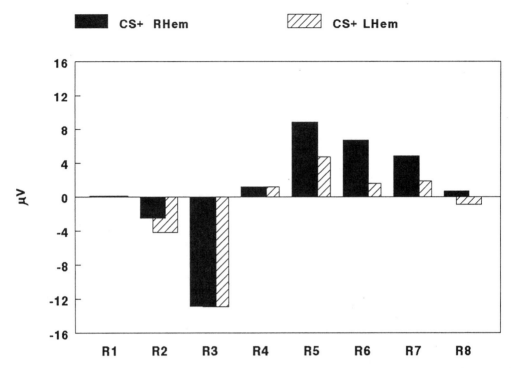

Figure 10.9 Event-related potential (ERP) peak amplitudes in microvolts as a function of scoring interval. R1, R2, ... = 50-ms interval window with R1 = 0–50 ms after stimulus presentation, R2 = 50–100 ms, etc. Maximum peak amplitude within a scoring range was used as raw data. RHem, right hemisphere; LHem, left hemisphere. (From Nordby and Hugdahl, unpublished data.)

changes in activity in the right prefrontal and posterior areas. Looking at the other EEG leads in the present study revealed that increased right hemisphere P3 amplitudes were also present at the temporal and frontal leads, which fit the observations made by Squire et al. (1992).

SUMMARY AND CONCLUSIONS

A series of experiments are reviewed wherein autonomic and CNS activity were used to index hemispheric differences in representation of conditioned responses to facial emotional expressions. Few studies of hemispheric specialization and lateralization have been directed to the question of laterality for simple associative conditioning, and whether the two hemispheres of the brain may be differentially involved in the establishment of conditioned associations. This probably reflects the decreased interest in learning theory over the past two decades, although the kind of implicit learning contingencies that are typical of a conditioned association probably are more common in everyday life than we usually are aware of. Thus, the decrease in interest among researchers in a certain area does not always match the importance of that same phenomenon in psychological functioning. A main argument in this chapter is that associative learning to emotionally relevant conditional stimuli are represented in the right hemisphere, particularly for negative, aversive stimuli. A major question that still remains open is what brain areas are specifically regulating human classical conditioning. As previously mentioned, LeDoux (1991) has shown that the medial and lateral parts of the amygdala seems to play an important role in the mediation of fear conditioning in rats. However, there are no data from humans showing that the same brain circuitry is involved in human conditioning. This could be tested by, for example, recordings of autonomic conditioned responses in humans with lesions to the amygdala. Tranel and Damasio (1989) showed normal SCRs to auditory stimuli in a patient with bilateral destruction of the amygdaloid complex. This does not, however, answer the question whether patients with amygdaloid lesions also would show a *conditioned* response to the pairing of, e.g., a tone with shock. If they show autonomic fear responses to mere presentations of negative stimuli, but fail to show evidence of a conditioned fear response, it could be possible to tease apart whether the amygdala system primarily is critical for conditioned responses or for nonassociative fear behavior in general. In addition to the involvement of limbic structures, there is evidence that human conditioning also involves both frontal and temporoparietal cortical areas.

The connection between higher cortical structures and electrodermal reactivity is far from known. Electrodermal activity is regulated from several different cortical areas involving both the frontal and temporal lobes. The link to the frontal lobes may be important in trying to track down a right hemisphere dominance for electrodermal responses to emotional stimuli. Cechetto and Saper (1990) have argued that the medial prefrontal cortex, including the infralimbic, may act as an autonomic motor cortex. This is an attractive hypothesis since limbic structures clearly are involved in the regulation of both electrodermal activity and emotional affect. It is further suggested that it is the right infralimbic cortex that regulates autonomic reactivity after a conditioned association has occurred, linking peripheral physiologic activity to cortical functioning. The brain mechanisms involved in cortical representation of a conditioned association may, however, be right hemisphere regions, particularly in the prefrontal and posterior areas (cf. Squire et al., 1992). The intricate play between cortical and peripheral mechanisms involved in human associative conditioning needs to be further delineated in future research, using modern brain imaging technology.

ACKNOWLEDGMENT

Research was supported financially by grants from the Norwegian Council for Research in the Social Sciences (NAVF-RFS).

REFERENCES

Ader, R., and Cohen, N. (1985). CNS-immune system interactions: Conditioning phenomena. *The Behavioral and Brain Sciences, 8,* 379–394.

Bagshaw, M. H., Kimble, D. P., and Pribram, K. H. (1965). The GSR of monkeys during orienting and habituation and after ablation of the amygdala, hippocampus, and inferotemporal cortex. *Neuropsychologia, 3,* 111–119.

Barneoud, P., Neveu, P. J., Vitiello, R., and LeMoal, M. (1987). Functional heterogeneity of the right and left neocortex in modulation of the immune system. *Physiology and Behavior, 41,* 525–530.

Berti, A., and Rizzolatti, G. (1992). Visual processing without awareness: Evidence from unilateral neglect. *Journal of Cognitive Neuroscience, 4,* 345–351.

Bohlin, G., and Kjellberg, A. (1979). Orienting activity in two-stimulus paradigms as reflected in heart rate. In H. D. Kimmel, E. H. van Olst, and J. F. Orlebeke (Eds.), *The orienting reflex.* Hillsdale, NJ: Lawrence Erlbaum Associates.

Boucsein, W. (1992). *Electrodermal activity.* New York, NY: Plenum Press.

Broadbent, D. (1958). *Perception and communication.* London: Pergamon Press.

Brodal, A. (1981). *Neurological anatomy in relation to clinical medicine,* (ed 3.). New York, NY: Oxford University Press.

Cechetto, D. F., and Saper, C. B. (1990). Role of the cerebral cortex in autonomic functioning. In A. D. Loewy and K. M. Spyer (Eds.), *Central regulation of autonomic functioning.* New York, NY: Oxford University Press.

Connolly, J. F. (1985). Stability of pathway-hemispheric differences in the auditory event-related potential (ERP) to monaural stimulation. *Psychophysiology, 22,* 87–96.

Coons, P. M., Bowman, E. L., and Milstein, V. (1988). Multiple personality disorder: A clinical investigation of 50 cases. *Journal of Nervous and Mental Disease, 176,* 519–527.

Corteen, R. S., and Wood, B. (1972). Automatic responses to shock-associated words in an unattended channel. *Journal of Experimental Psychology, 94,* 308–313.

Crawford, H. J., Crawford, K., and Koperski, B. J. (1983). Hypnosis and lateral cerebral function as assessed by dichotic listening. *Biological Psychiatry, 18,* 415–427.

Crosson, B. (1992). *Subcortical functions in language and memory.* New York, NY: Guilford Press.

Davey, G. L. C. (1987). *Cognitive processes and pavlovian conditioning.* Chichester, England: John Wiley & Sons.

Dawson, M. E., and Reardon, P. (1973). Construct validity of recall and recognition postconditioning measures of awareness. *Journal of Experimental Psychology, 98,* 308–315.

Dawson, M. E., and Schell, A. M. (1982). Electrodermal responses to attended and nonattended significant stimuli during dichotic listening. *Journal of Experimental Psychology: Human Perception and Performance, 8,* 315–324.

Dimond, S. J., and Farrington, L. (1977). Emotional response to films shown to the right or left hemisphere of the brain measured by heart rate. *Acta Psychologica, 41,* 255–260.

Donchin, E. (1981). Surprise.... Surprise! *Psychophysiology, 8,* 493–513.

Donchin, E., Karis, D., Bashore, T. R., Coles, M. G. H., and Gratton, G. (1986). Cognitive psychophysiology and human information processing. In M. Coles, E. Donchin, and S. W. Porges (Eds.), *Psychophysiology: Systems, processes, and applications.* Amsterdam: Elsevier.

Ekman, P., Friesen, W. V., and Ellsworth, P. (1972). *Emotion in the human face*. Elmsford, NY: Pergamon Press.

Eriksen, C. W. (1960). Discrimination and learning without awareness: A methodological survey and evaluation. *Psychological Review, 67*, 279–300.

Fredrikson, M., Hugdahl, K., and Öhman, A. (1976). Electrodermal conditioning to potentially phobic stimuli in male and female subjects. *Biological Psychology, 4*, 306–315.

Frumkin, L. R., Ripley, H. S., and Cox, G. B. (1978). Changes in cerebral hemispheric lateralization with hypnosis. *Biological Psychiatry, 13*, 741–750.

Geer, J. H. (1965). The development of a scale to measure fear. *Behaviour Research and Therapy, 3*, 45–53.

Graf, P., and Schacter, D. L. (1985). Implicit and explicit memory for new associations in normals and amnesic patients. *Journal of Experimental Psychology: Learning, Memory, and Cognition, 11*, 501–518.

Hachinsky, V. C., Oppenheimer, S. M., Wilson, J. X., Guiraudon, C., and Cechetto, D. F. (1992). Asymmetry of sympathetic consequences of experimental stroke. *Archives of Neurology, 49*, 697–702.

Heilman, K. M., Bowers, D., Valenstein, E., and Watson, R. T. (1987). Hemispace and hemispatial neglect. In M. Jeannerod (Ed.), *Neurophysiological and neuropsychological aspects of spatial neglect*. Amsterdam: North-Holland.

Heller, W., Lindsey, D. L., Metz, J., and Farnum, D. M. (1990). Individual differences in right-hemisphere activation are associated with arousal and autonomic response to lateralized stimuli. *Journal of Clinical and Experimental Neuropsychology, 13*, 95.

Hellige, J. B. (1990). Hemispheric asymmetry. *Annual Review of Psychology, 41*, 55–80.

Holender, D. (1986). Semantic activation without conscious identification in dichotic listening, parafoveal vision, and visual maksing: A survey and appraisal. *Behavioral and Brain Sciences, 9*, 1–66.

Hugdahl, K. (1992). Brain lateralization: Dichotic studies. In B. Smith and G. Adelman (Eds.), *Encyclopedia of neuroscience, supplementum 2*. Boston, MA: Birkhauser.

Hugdahl, K., and Andersson, L. (1986). The "forced-attention paradigm" in dichotic listening to CV-syllables: A comparison between adults and children. *Cortex, 22*, 417–432.

Hugdahl, K., and Brobeck, C. G. (1986). Hemispheric asymmetry and human electrodermal conditioning: The dichotic extinction paradigm. *Psychophysiology, 23*, 491–499.

Hugdahl, K., Franzon, M., Andersson, B., and Walldebo, G. (1983). Heart rate responses (HRR) to lateralized visual stimuli. *Pavlovian Journal of Biological Science, 18*, 186–198.

Hugdahl, K., and Johnsen, B. H. (1993). Brain asymmetry and autonomic conditioning: Skin conductance responses. In J. C. Roy, W. Boucsein, D. C. Fowles, and J. Gruzelier (Eds.), *Progress in electrodermal research* (pp 271–288). London: Plenum Press.

Hugdahl, K., Kvale, G., Nordby, H., and Overmier, J. B. (1987). Hemispheric asymmetry and human classical conditioning to verbal and nonverbal visual CSs. *Psychophysiology, 24*, 557–565.

Hugdahl, K., and Nordby, H. (1991). Hemisphere differences in conditional learning: An ERP study, *Cortex, 27*, 557–570.

Hugdahl, K., and Öhman, A. (1977). Effects of instruction on acquisition and extinction of electrodermal responses to fear-relevant stimuli. *Journal of Experimental Psychology: Human Learning and Memory, 3*, 608–618.

Hugdahl, K., and Ternes, J. (1981). An electrodermal measure of arousal in opiate addicts to drug-related stimuli. *Biological Psychology, 12,* 291–298.

Hugdahl, K., Wahlgren, C., and Wass, T. (1982). Habituation of the electrodermal orienting reaction is dependent on the cerebral hemisphere intially stimulated. *Biological Psychology, 15,* 49–62.

Johnsen, B. H., and Hugdahl, K. (1991). Hemispheric asymmetry in conditioning to facial emotional expressions. *Psychophysiolgy, 28,* 154–162.

Johnsen, B. H., and Hugdahl, K. (1993). Right hemisphere representation of autonomic conditioning to facial emotional expressions. *Psychophysiology, 30,* 274–278.

Kimble, G. A. (1961). *Hilgard and Marquis' conditioning and learning.* New York, NY: Appleton-Century-Crofts.

Kimmel, H. D. (1966). Inhibition of the unconditioned response in classical conditioning. *Psychological Review, 73,* 232–240.

Kimura, D. (1967). Functional asymmetry of the brain in dichotic listening. *Cortex, 3,* 163–168.

Lacroix, J. M., and Comper, P. (1979). Lateralization in the electrodermal system as a function of cognitive/hemispheric manipulation. *Psychophysiology, 16,* 116–129.

Lazarus, R. S., and McCleary, R. (1951). Autonomic discrimination without awareness: A study of subception. *Psychological Review, 58,* 113–122.

LeDoux, J. E. (1991). Emotion and the limbic system concept. *Concepts in Neuroscince, 2,* 169–199.

Levine, J. L., Kurtz, R. M., and Lauter, J. L. (1984). Hypnosis and its effects on left and right hemisphere activity. *Biological Psychiatry, 19,* 1461–1475.

Lockhart, R. S. (1989). The role of theory in understanding implicit memory. In S. Lewandowsky, J. C. Dunn, and K. Kirsner (Eds.), *Implicit memory: Theoretical issues.* Hillsdale, NJ: Lawrence Erlbaum Associates.

Lykken, D. T. (1968). Neuropsychology and psychophysiology in personality research. In E. F. Borgatta and W. W. Lambert (Eds.), *Handbook of personality theory and research: Part 2.* Chicago, IL: Rand McNally.

Marcel, A. (1983). Conscious and unconscious perception: An approach to the relations between phenomenological experience and perceptual processes. *Cognitive Psychology, 15,* 238–300.

Martin, D. G., Stambrook, M., Tataryn, D. J., and Biehl, H. (1984). Conditioning in the unattended left ear. *International Journal of Neuroscience, 23,* 95–102.

Maximilian, V. A. (1982). Cortical blood flow asymmetry during monaural verbal stimulation. *Brain and Language, 15,* 1–11.

McGlone, J. (1980). Sex differences in human brain asymmetry: A critical survey. *Behavioral and Brain Sciences, 3,* 127–138.

McKeever, W. F. (1986). Tachistoscopic methods in neuropsychology. In J. F. Hannay (Ed.), *Experimental techniques in human neuropsychology.* New York, NY: Oxford University Press.

Näätänen, R. (1992). *Attention and brain function.* Hillsdale, NJ: Lawrence Erlbaum Associates.

Obrist, P. A., Webb, R. A., and Sutterer, J. R. (1969). Heart rate and somatic changes during aversive conditioning and a simple reaction time task. *Psychophysiology, 5,* 696–723.

Öhman, A. (1983). The orienting response during pavlovian conditioning. In D. Siddle (Ed.), *Orienting and habituation—Perspectives in humna research*. Chichester, England: John Wiley & Sons.

Öhman, A. (1986). Face the beast and fear the face: Animal and social fears as prototypes for evolutionary analyses of emotion. *Psychophysiology, 23,* 123–146.

Öhman, A., Esteves, F., Parra, C., Soares, J., and Hugdahl, K. (1988). Brain lateralization and preattentive elicitation of conditioned skin conductance responses. *Psychophysiology, 25,* 473.

Pavlov, I. P. (1927). *Conditioned reflexes.* G. V. Anrep (Trans.). New York, NY: Dover Publications.

Porges, S. W., and Maiti, A. K. (1992). The smart and vegetative vagi: Implications for specialization and laterality of function. Paper presented at the 32nd Annual Meeting of the Society for Psychophysiological Research, San Diego, CA, October 15–20.

Prokasy, W. F., and Kumpfer, K. L. (1973). Classical conditioning. In W. F. Prokasy and D. C. Raskin (Eds.), *Electrodermal activity in psychological research.* New York, NY: Academic Press

Putnam, F. W., Zahn, T. P., and Post, R. M. (1990). Differential autonomic nervous system activity in multiple personality disorder. *Psychiatry Research, 31,* 251–260.

Raine, A., Reynolds, G. P., and Sheard, C. (1991). Neuroanatomical correlates of skin conductance orienting in humans: A magnetic resonance imaging study. *Psychophysiology, 28,* 548–558.

Razran, G. (1961). The observable unconscious and the inferable conscious in current Soviet psychophysiology. *Psychological Review, 68,* 81–147.

Rescorla, R. A. (1980). *Pavlovian second-order conditioning.* New York, NY: Academic Press.

Rescorla, R. A., and Wagner, A. R. (1972). A theory of pavlovian conditioning: Variations in the effectiveness of reinforcement and nonreinforcement. In A. Black and W. F. Prokasy (Eds.), *Classical conditioning II: Current theory and research.* New York, NY: Appleton-Century-Crofts.

Rosen, A. D., Gur, R. C., Sussman, N. M., Gur, R. E., and Hurtig, H. (1982). Hemispheric asymmetry in the control of heart rate. *Neuroscience Abstracts, 8,* 917.

Rosenzweig, M. R. (1951). Representations of the two ears at the auditory cortex. *American Journal of Physiology 167,* 147–214.

Schacter, D. L. (1987). Implicit memory: History and current status. *Journal of Experimental Psychology: Learning, Memory, and Cognition, 13,* 501–518.

Schliack, H., and Schiffter, R. (1979). Neurophysiologie und Pathophysiologie der Schweissensekretion. In E. Schwartz, H. W. Spier, and G. Stüttgen (Eds.), *Handbuch der Haut- und Geschlechtskrankheiten: Vol 1/4A. Normale und pathologische Physiologie der Haut.* Berlin: Springer-Verlag.

Seligman, M. E. P. (1971). Phobias and preparedness. *Behavior Therapy, 2,* 307–321.

Sergent, J., and Villemure, J.-G. (1989). Prospagnosia in a right hemispherectomized patient. *Brain, 112,* 975–995.

Siddle, D. A. T., and Remington, B. (1987). Latent inhibition and human pavlovian conditioning: Research and relevance. In G. L. C. Davey (Ed.), *Cognitive processes and pavlovian conditioning in humans.* Chichester, England: John Wiley & Sons.

Sokolov, E. N. (1960). Neuronal models in the orienting reflex. In M. A. Brazier (Ed.), *The central nervous system and behavior.* New York, NY: Macy Foundation.

Spence, K. W. (1960). *Behavior theory and conditioning.* New Haven, CT: Prentice-Hall.

Spiegel, D., Cutcomb, S., Ren, C., and Pribram, K. (1985). Hypnotic hallucination alters evoked potentials. *Journal of Abnormal Psychology, 94,* 249–255.

Springer, S. P. (1986). Dichotic listening. In J. Hannay (Ed.), *Experimental techniques in human neuropsychology.* New York, NY: Oxford University Press.

Squire, L. R., Ojemann, J. G., Miezin, F. M., Petersen, S. E., Videen, T. O., and Raichle, M. E. (1992). Activation of the hippocampus in normal humans: A functional anatomical study of memory. *Poceedings of the National Academy of Sciences of the United States of America, 89,* 1837–1841.

Stewart, J., de Wit, H., and Eikelboom, R. (1984). The role of unconditioned and conditioned drug effects in the self-administration of opiates and stimulants. *Psychological Review, 91,* 251–268.

Suberi, M., and McKeever, W. F. (1977). Differential right hemisphere memory storage of emotional and non-emotional faces. *Neuropsychologia, 15,* 757–768.

Tranel, D., and Damasio, A. R. (1985). Knowledge without awareness: An autonomic index of facial recognition by prosopagnosics. *Science, 228,* 1453–1454.

Turkkan, J. S. (1989). Classical conditioning: The new hegenomy. *Behavioral and Brain Sciences, 12,* 121–179.

Turkkan, J. S., and Brady, J. (1985). Meditational theory of the placebo effect: Discussion. In L. White, B. Tursky, and G. E. Schwartz (Eds.), *Placebo: Theory, research and mechanisms.* New York, NY: Guilford Press.

Walker, B. B., and Sandman, C. A. (1979). Human visual evoked responses are related to heart rate. *Journal of Comparative and Physiological Psychology, 93,* 717–729.

Wardlaw, K. A., and Kroll, N. E. (1976). Autonomic responses to shock-associated words in nonattended message: A failure to replicate. *Journal of Experimental Psychology: Human Perception and Performance, 2,* 357–360.

Weisz, J., Szilagyi, N., Lang, E., and Adam, G. (1992). The influence of monocular viewing on heart period variability. *International Journal of Psychophysiology, 12,* 11–18.

Werntz, D. A., Bickford, R. G., Bloom, F. E., and Shannahof-Khalsa, D. S. (1983). Alternating cerebral hemispheric activity and the lateralization of autonomic nervous function. *Human Neurobiology, 2,* 39–43.

Wexler, B. E., and Halwes, T. G. (1983). Increasing the power of dichotic methods; the fused rhymed words test. *Neuropsychologia, 21,* 59–66.

Wexler, B. E., Schwartz, G. E., Warrenburg, S., Servis, M., and Tarlatzis, I. (1986). Effects of emotion on perceptual asymmetry: Interactions with personality. *Neuropsychologia, 24,* 699–710.

Wexler, B. E., Warrenburg, S., Schwartz, G. E., and Janer, L. D. (1992). EEG and EMG responses to emotion-evoking stimuli processed without conscious awareness. *Neuropsychologia, 30,* 1065–1079.

Windholz, G. (1992). Pavlov's conceptualization of learning. *American Journal of Psychology, 105,* 459–469.

Windholz, G., and Lamal, P. A. (1986). Pavlov and the concept of association. *Pavlovian Journal of Biological Science, 21,* 12–14.

Wittling, W., and Pfluger, M. (1990). Neuroendocrine hemisphere asymmetries: Salivary cortisol secretion during lateralized viewing of emotion-related and neutral films. *Brain and Cognition, 14,* 243–265.

Wittling, W. (1990). Psychophysiological correlates of human brain asymmetry: Blood pressure changes during lateralized presentation of an emotionally laden film. *Neuropsychologia, 28,* 457–470.

Wright, J. M. von, Andersson, K., and Stenman, U. (1975). Generalizationb of conditioned GSRs in dichotic listening. In P. M. Rabbit and S. Dornic (Eds.), *Attention and performance,* Vol. 5. London: Academic Press.

Yokoyama, K., Jennings, R., Ackles, P., Hood, P., and Boller, F. (1987). Lack of heart rate changes during an attention-demanding task after right hemisphere lesions. *Neurology, 36,* 624–630.

V Central-Autonomic Integration

11 Hemispheric Asymmetry, Autonomic Asymmetry, and the Problem of Sudden Cardiac Death

Richard D. Lane and J. Richard Jennings

Bart Giamatti was a Renaissance scholar and former president of Yale University who became commissioner of baseball. He brought to the position the wit and wisdom of an accomplished academic, the experience of a seasoned administrator who was no stranger to controversy, and a boyhood passion for the Boston Red Sox. The position of commissioner was created to uphold the integrity of the national pastime, and indeed, Bart Giamatti faced a crisis that required his full energies: Pete Rose, perhaps the greatest hitter in the history of baseball, was accused of gambling on baseball games. After months of investigation, Bart Giamatti announced that Pete Rose was permanently banned from baseball and would not be eligible for induction into the Hall of Fame. Several days after this announcement, Bart Giamatti died suddenly of a heart attack.

Cases in which emotional stress seems to play a role in sudden cardiac death (SCD) are not unusual. Engel (1971) reviewed over 500 examples of emotion-induced sudden death from history and recent newspaper accounts, following Cannon's (1942) classic study of voodoo death, in which tribesmen were observed to die within hours of being cursed by a medicine man. The possibility that emotional stress can kill people suddenly through cardiovascular mechanisms appears to be plausible. But are we really sure that psychological influences can kill people suddenly? If so, what are the psychological triggers of such events? What are the biological mechanisms involved? What can be done to prevent this from happening?

The importance of psychological factors in SCD has been established in animal experiments that have demonstrated that emotional stress can significantly lower the threshold for ventricular fibrillation, the most common terminal event in SCD (Lown, Verrier, and Rabinowitz, 1977; Lown, 1979; Lown et al., 1980). Studies in mammals as varied as pigs, dogs, and mice have demonstrated that stress may induce ventricular fibrillation and myocardial ischemia (MI). Furthermore, selective central (CNS) (Skinner and Reed, 1981) and peripheral nervous system interventions (Schwartz, 1984; Schwartz and Priori, 1990) successfully alter such fibrillation and ischemia. Thus, it is reasonable to conclude that brain mechanisms mediating emotion can be a contributing factor in inducing sudden death.

The significance of this conclusion becomes evident from an epidemiologic perspective. SCD is the leading cause of death in the industrialized world. It is estimated that about 300,000 people die from SCD each year in the United States alone (Myerburg, Kessler, and Castellanos, 1993), and that emotion plays a significant role in about 20% of cases (Cottington et al. 1980; Meyers and Dewar, 1975; Reich et al., 1981; Rissanen, Romo, and Siltanen, 1978)—a rate of sudden death in the United States related to emotion that is comparable to the death rate due to acquired immunodeficiency syndrome (AIDS) (about 35,000 annually) (Centers for Disease Control and Prevention, 1993) and suicide (about 30,000 annually) (*Accident Facts*, 1992) combined.

The precise definition of SCD varies between studies. Typically, definitions require that all cases of death occur within 24 hours or less of symptom onset and often require that death occurs out of hospital or in the absence of any previously recognized or documented symptoms of heart disease. SCDs are typically found to account for approximately one fourth of new coronary events (Kuller, Cooper, and Perper, 1972) and half of all cardiac deaths. Ventricular fibrillation is by far the most common terminal event in SCD, but SCDs due to bradyarrhythmias also occur (Myerburg et al., 1990).

It was previously thought that SCD was an inevitable result of progressive heart disease. However, while most SCD victims have organic heart disease, only about one third of SCD victims show evidence of an acute coronary occlusion (myocardial infarction) (Dimarco and Haines, 1990). It is now recognized that SCD is an electrical accident (Lown et al., 1980). If victims can be resuscitated, appropriate clinical management is largely successful in preventing recurrent lethal arrhythmias. A better understanding of how the brain regulates cardiovascular function can therefore have a major impact on public health.

For cardiologists, the challenge that remains in this area of research is to identify the mechanisms influencing vulnerability to ventricular fibrillation so that preventive interventions can be made (Dimarco and Haines, 1990). Sudden death is a phenomenon with a multifactorial etiology that can be divided into substrates and triggers (Keefe, Schwartz, and Somberg, 1987). Substrates refer to the underlying myocardial disease and include presence of coronary artery disease (CAD), previous MI, and low ejection fraction. Triggers include ventricular arrhythmias, hypercoagulable states, electrolyte disturbances, elevated circulating catecholamines, and autonomic nervous system (ANS) activity (Keefe et al., 1987). A role for both sympathetic and parasympathetic mechanisms and their interaction is well documented (Verrier, 1990).

An intriguing observation within this area of research has been that stimulation of the left sympathetic nerves to the heart lowers ventricular fibrillation threshold more than does stimulating the right side (Lown et al., 1977; Verrier, Thompson, and Lown, 1974). Given the finding that cerebral hemispheric asymmetries exist in the mediation of emotion (Silberman and Weingartner, 1986), Lane and Schwartz (1987) hypothesized that the minority of people who are more lateralized to the left hemisphere (LH) during emotion channel this activation ipsilaterally to induce a lateralized imbalance in sympathetic input to the heart, increasing the likelihood of ventricular fibrillation and sudden death. This "brain-heart laterality (BHL) hypothesis" was stimulated in part by Galin's (1974) suggestion that activity in each cerebral hemisphere might be expressed in a distinctive pattern of autonomic activity, given the existence of autonomic asymmetries.

New research on the cardiovascular effects of lateralized brain activity (e.g., Zamrini et al., 1990) has recently been conducted that potentially has important implications for research on the functional neuroanatomy and psychophysiology of emotion. This work in turn has called attention to past and present psychophysiologic research examining the differential influence of the two cerebral hemispheres on autonomic function (Zoccolotti, Scabini, and Violani, 1981; Zoccolotti et al., 1986). The latter suggests that the right hemisphere (RH) has a preferential influence in regulating autonomic function. Thus, there are two converging areas of research involving asymmetry in the autonomic nervous system: that pertaining to sudden death and that pertaining to autonomic correlates of lateralized hemispheric activity. The BHL hypothesis therefore has relevance not only to sudden death but to the research on hemispheric laterality in general.

The cornerstone of this chapter is therefore the BHL hypothesis. The role of psychological factors in SCD, an overview of CNS control of autonomic function, and the existence of asymmetries in autonomic control of the heart are reviewed, followed by presentation of the BHL hypothesis. Next, a critique of the methods available for testing the BHL hypothesis are presented, followed by a review of relevant findings. The review includes both studies in which hemispheric activity has been unilaterally altered and noninvasive hemispheric laterality studies that have incorporated cardiovascular measures with implications for autonomic asymmetry. The chapter concludes with an agenda for future research in this area.

THE ROLE OF PSYCHOLOGICAL FACTORS IN SUDDEN CARDIAC DEATH

Psychosocial and neurophysiologic influences on SCD that are lateralized should be understood within the more general context of evidence for psychosocial influences on SCD which has not explicitly considered laterality. Kamarck and Jennings (1991) recently reviewed evidence illustrating how psychosocial factors could influence SCD. The case for such influences are briefly reviewed here in order to place the BHL hypothesis in context.

Figure 11.1 reprints the diagram from Kamarck and Jennings (1991) which provides a useful, organizing view of SCD. Psychological influences contribute to the pathophysiology of SCD at multiple points. Atherosclerosis is seen as the core disease—one that develops over a long period of time and is thus portrayed as a background factor. In the presence of atherosclerotic disease, other acute factors may prime the system, predisposing it toward lethal

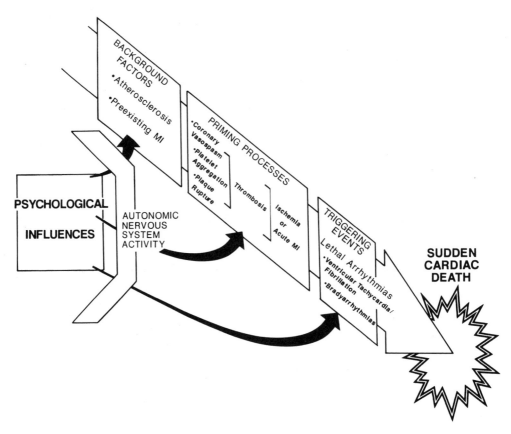

Figure 11.1 Pathways of psychological influences in sudden cardiac death. MI, myocardial infarction. (From Karmarck and Jennings, 1991.)

events; e.g., narrowing of the coronary arteries (vasoconstriction), particularly in the presence of blood clotting (thrombosis), will induce a reduced oxygen supply to the heart (ischemia). The final trigger to the vulnerable substrate is electrical instability resulting in cardiac arrhythmia and sudden death.

Long-term influences, captured by life stress and dispositional personality measures such as the type A coronary-prone behavior pattern, seem likely to contribute to atherosclerosis directly or by influencing positive health maintenance behaviors (Krantz and Manuck, 1984; Jennings, 1982). Priming and triggering processes are suitable for laboratory as well as correlational studies. The results of these studies and the concepts behind them will now be summarized.

Long-term psychological stress, as defined by life stress inventories and life condition, such as low socioeconomic class, has been consistently related to increased prevalence of SCD (Kamarck and Jennings, 1991). This supports the common belief of a link between stress and SCD. A close examination of the studies in this area raises some concerns, however. The absolute number of studies is relatively surprising; relatively few studies have specifically addressed this issue. Among available studies some are retrospective and some do not differentially examine sudden and nonsudden cardiac death. Given the weaknesses of the studies, it is often hard to ensure that the relationships are specific to SCD as opposed to reflecting an overall relationship with heart disease incidence.

Assessment of how long-term stress translates into cardiac end points would be aided by studies showing that daily, stressful events induce pathologic processes in the heart, such as myocardial ischemia (sometimes experienced as angina or chest pain) and cardiac arrhythmia—particularly ventricular fibrillation.

Examining myocardial ischemia first, the literature on the psychological induction of cardiac ischemia is rapidly expanding as ambulatory measurement permits the assessment of electrocardiographic (ECG) indices of ischemia in real-life situations. At present, however, published reports of personality type, emotional ratings, and acute emotional events are somewhat sparse because of the recency of clinical techniques to detect ambulatory myocardial ischemia. Available studies show some correlation of stressful events and myocardial ischemia but many cardiac events occur in the absence of any stressful event (Kamarck and Jennings, 1991).

A larger literature has examined myocardial ischemia in response to laboratory stressors. This literature is almost unanimous in showing that a significant portion of patients with heart disease (but not controls) show ischemia during the performance of challenging tasks (Rozanski et al., 1988; Legault et al., 1993). A particularly interesting development in this literature is the demonstration that acute stressors can induce vasoconstriction of the coronary arteries. Such vasoconstriction would restrict blood flow to the heart and thus induce myocardial ischemia. This has been shown by Yeung et al. (1991) among humans with CAD, and in animal models. Verrier and Dickerson (1991) demonstrated that dogs acutely angered by food withdrawal showed a marked vasoconstriction of the coronary arteries after transient reactions to anger shown in heart rate (HR) and blood pressure (BP). Elimination of noradrenergic input via stellectomy was shown to eliminate the vasoconstriction. These studies suggest that myocardial ischemia can be directly induced psychologically; studies using other techniques have shown that psychological factors can increase the work demanded of the heart by increasing HR and BP, thereby indirectly inducing ischemia. Similar studies have produced conflicting evidence about whether stressors can be related to platelet aggregation.

Turning to cardiac arrhythmia, studies in both animals and humans verify that psychological stress seems to be related to an increase in both spontaneously occurring ventricular arrhythmia as well as a decrease in the threshold for triggering ventricular arrhythmia. The human studies examined behavioral dispositions, such as type A, ratings of stress and distress, and also specific acute emotional events. The expected relationships were generally observed, i.e., type A, greater stress, and emotionally traumatic events were associated with a greater incidence of arrhythmia. Animal studies in dogs and pigs have been relatively successful in inducing arrhythmia. For example, using a pig model, Skinner, Lie, and Entman (1975) combined the stress of a novel environment with an artificial induction of reduced coronary blood flow (via a snare device). Ventricular fibrillation was induced in pigs in the novel environment but not in pigs that had been adapted to the environment prior to the same induction of ischemia. Attempts to induce arrhythmia in humans in response to specific stressors have been less successful. Arrhythmias typically occur only in those with organic heart disease (Natelson, 1985), and it is difficult to isolate the initiating event. Similarly, controlling arrhythmia via operant learning has proved difficult (Weiss et al., 1985), suggesting that, as with cardiac ischemia, much more needs to be learned about how psychological stress and arrhythmia are related.

An interesting recent development has been the realization that cardiac deaths, infarctions, and incidents of myocardial ischemia are more likely in the early morning hours. A special issue of the *American Journal of Cardiology* (Muller and Tofler, 1990) reviewed not only these circadian patterns but also included a number of articles on triggers for ischemia, arrhythmia, and MI. We do not know as yet whether behavioral factors or rhythmic biological factors account for the rather striking morning prevalence of cardiac symptomatology. A number of papers in the issue relate the circadian patterning to sympathetic nervous system activity, however.

This overview of the literature suggests that psychological factors, stress in particular, can induce significant changes in cardiac function that can contribute significantly to the pathogenesis of coronary heart disease. Given such a relationship, exactly what physiologic changes are induced by these psychological factors? Can psychophysiologic mechanisms be identified which relate particular psychological processes to particular physiologic and pathophysiologic processes? Work on these questions is in its infancy. Current concepts of the mechanisms underlying SCD should be considered useful working hypotheses that capture important segments of current available data.

A primary notion is that much of the psychological influence on the acute expression of cardiovascular disease is mediated by the activation of the sympathetic nervous system and its subsequent influence on adrenal medullary hormones (e.g., Manuck and Krantz, 1986). Sympathetic activation induces change both directly through the synaptic release of norepinephrine (NE, an α and β_1-adrenergic substance) and through action on the adrenal medulla primarily releasing epinephrine (similar to NE, with greater β_2-adrenergic activity). These two actions will synergistically increase, among other things, HR, BP, and peripheral vascular resistance. In vulnerable persons, cardiac ischemia has been associated with increases in both α- and β-adrenergic activation (e.g., Heusch, 1990; Egstrup, 1991; Olsson and Ryden, 1991). However, rises in catecholamine levels alone do not account sufficiently for mechanisms of stress-induced arrhythmia. For example, Taggert, Carruthers, and Somerville (1973) observed that with the stress of public speaking to a medical audience, NE levels rose in 21 of 23 normal physicians, but frequent ventricular premature beats occurred in only 6, and were multifocal (more pathologic) in only 2.

In contrast, activation of the vagus nerve generally induces, among other actions, cholinergically mediated slowing of the HR and decreases in cardiac contractility, the latter occurring primarily through indirect effects by counteracting sympathetic influences. In animal models vagal activation seems protective in the face of induced ischemia and arrhythmia (e.g., Cerati and Schwartz, 1991; DeFerrari et al., 1991). Again, these general principles must be tempered with the understanding that interactions between sympathetic and vagal influences can be more arrhythmogenic than sympathetic influences alone (Verrier, 1990).

Another perspective on mechanisms of SCD is that offered by authors such as Winfree (1983) who emphasize the importance of timing or phase in cardiac control. From this perspective the heart is viewed as a cyclically controlled organ, which is reset to different periods by external events, e.g., neural stimulation. The mechanism of heart beat generation appears to permit resetting more readily at some points in the cycle than others. Winfree (1983, 1987) reviewed data suggesting that resetting at certain points in the cycle can lead to instability and even the termination of the heart beat in simple cardiac preparations. It is well known clinically that a premature wave of ventricular depolarization occurring during repolarization, the so-called R-on-T phenomenon, can induce malignant ventricular arrhythmias. However, these observations are also consistent with currently popular discussions of chaotic dynamics of control. These and their application to heart beat timing and sudden death are reviewed in Glass and MacKay (1988).

Finally, emotional factors are increasingly being recognized as predictors of sudden death. Hostility, anger, and impatience have emerged from studies of cardiovascular risk due to the type A coronary-prone behavior pattern. In their widely known work Friedman and Rosenman (1974) identified a complex of behavior and attitudes that was prospectively associated with heart disease. Since the initial studies, both conceptual and empirical motives have emerged for specifying more precisely what was coronary-prone within the complex of type A behavior. A variety of clinical and experimental studies in humans now indicate the possible important role of anger, hostility, and impatience in predicting sudden death (Williams et al., 1980). These studies are supplemented by work in animals showing specifically that anger induction can induce myocardial ischemia (such as that discussed above; Verrier and Dickerson, 1991). Another set of findings indicates that depression or depressed affect are significant predictors of subsequent cardiac events, including SCD, in post-MI patients (Ahern et al., 1990; Almada et al., 1991; Carney et al., 1988; Frasure-Smith, 1991; Frasure-Smith et al., 1993). Together, these findings highlight the plausibility of hypothesizing that the way in which the brain mediates emotion may influence susceptibility to SCD.

In sum, psychological stress has been shown to influence myocardial ischemia, cardiac arrhythmia, and perhaps platelet aggregation. The critical variables within the complex of events termed *psychological stress* have not been clearly identified, but current interest is focused on anger, hostility, and depression. Pathophysiologic effects on the heart and coronary vessels seem at present to be primarily related to sympatheticoadrenal influences held in check by vagal restraint. Both conceptual and empirical work is called for by the very promising work done to date. The current development of the BHL hypothesis is one effort in this direction.

CENTRAL NERVOUS SYSTEM REGULATION OF CARDIOVASCULAR FUNCTION

The literature just reviewed indicates that psychological factors appear to play a role in SCD and that they exert their effects primarily through the ANS. It is therefore pertinent to consider what is known about how the brain regulates the ANS. The following is offered for its heuristic value, as any summary this brief on an area so complex and incompletely understood is inevitably subject to additional caveats and alternative interpretations.

Autonomic activity is believed to be controlled by multiple integrative sites within the CNS that are hierarchically arranged (Natelson, 1985; Talman, 1985; Smith and DeVito, 1984; Cechetto and Saper, 1990; Oppenheimer, Cechetto, and Hachinski, 1990). The exact functional pathways involved are not clearly understood. However, a roadmap of anatomic connections between structures provides our best evidence of the structures involved. The roadmap will point out monosynaptic, polysynaptic, and integrative components. Monosynaptic connections between two structures suggest an important functional relationship. Polysynaptic connections may be important as well but are harder to study and therefore less well understood. Exactly what role each integrative structure within the CNS plays is not known at this time. Autonomic pathways have both afferent and efferent components. Traditional concepts have centered on the efferent component, but our increasing knowledge of afferent components has led to concepts of dynamic control of cardiovascular function based on feedback and oscillatory control.

The broad outlines of CNS control of sympathetic outflow are as follows (Smith and DeVito, 1984; Natelson, 1985). The preganglionic sympathetic neurons arise in the intermediolateral (IML) cell columns of the spinal cord. These neurons synapse with postganglionic neurons in sympathetic ganglia such as the stellate ganglia. Monosynaptic connections exist between various nuclei in the medulla, pons, and diencephalon and the IML cell columns. These nuclei include the ventrolateral reticular formation (including the NE-containing A5 neurons in the ventral pons, and the NE-containing A1 neurons in the caudal ventrolateral medulla); the NE-containing neurons of the locus caeruleus in the medulla; the epinephrine-containing C1 neurons of the rostral ventral medulla; the serotonin-containing neurons in the raphe nucleus extending from the caudal medulla to the mesencephalon; the parabrachial complex; central gray area; zona incerta; and paraventricular nucleus of the hypothalamus. All of these structures have direct connections to IML cell columns and to one another. Smith and DeVito (1984) argue that the "head ganglion" of the sympathetic nervous system is the perifornical region of the lateral hypothalamus because of its direct connections to each of these nuclei and to the IML cell columns.

Preganglionic parasympathetic neurons that influence the heart arise in the medulla and synapse with postganglionic neurons adjacent to the heart. Parasympathetic fibers emanate from the nucleus tractus solitarius, dorsal vagal nucleus, and nucleus ambiguus and course to the periphery through the ninth (glossopharyngeal) and tenth (vagus) cranial nerves. These medullary nuclei also send fibers to the IML cell columns and other brainstem nuclei regulating sympathetic function.

Less well understood is the role of the cerebral cortex in regulating autonomic function (Cechetto and Saper, 1990). However, the existence of direct projections to subcortical structures regulating autonomic function, as well as neurophysiologic studies showing autonomic changes with stimulation or inactivation of these structures, supports their important role in autonomic regulation. These areas include the medial prefrontal cortex, the cingulate gyrus, the insula, the temporal pole, and possibly primary sensory and motor cortex (Cechetto and Saper, 1990; Mesulam, 1985). The first three areas in particular have direct connections to amygdala, hypothalamus, brainstem, and spinal cord areas involved in autonomic control. Their important role in autonomic regulation does not necessarily reflect a primary autonomic function. These higher centers coordinate autonomic outflow with higher mental functions, emotional reactions, and homeostatic needs of the internal environment.

The foregoing discussion indicates that structures at multiple levels of the neuraxis form highly interconnected bidirectional circuits. It is noteworthy that with the exception of certain midline nuclei in the brainstem such as the raphe nucleus and locus ceruleus, the principal structures regulating autonomic function, including the IML cell columns, the parasympathetic nuclei in the medulla, the hypothalamic nuclei regulating sympathetic function, the amygdala, the insula and the medial prefrontal cortex all are bilateral structures. The possibility therefore exists that relative activation lateralized to one side may get transmitted to end organs such as the heart in a lateralized manner. A key factor may be the algebraic sum of activating and inhibiting influences impinging on the midbrain and brainstem centers controlling autonomic function on each side.

Clearly, much remains to be learned about how the CNS regulates autonomic function. Some of the important questions to be answered in the present context include: (1) Do anterior and posterior cortical structures reciprocally inhibit one another when activated? (2) Does each hemisphere reciprocally inhibit structures in the homotopic area of the other hemisphere when activated? (3) When activated, do cortical structures themselves activate or inhibit subcortical structures? (4) What neuronal events determine whether the sympathetic system is activated or inhibited? (5) What neuronal events determine whether the parasympathetic system is activated or inhibited? Answers to these questions will make it possible to determine how psychological functions such as emotion lead to coordinated autonomic activity.

ASYMMETRY IN THE AUTONOMIC INNERVATION OF THE HEART

Conclusions about the anatomic distribution of the right and left sympathetic limbs to the heart are based primarily on physiologic findings rather than methods that trace the topography of the nerve fibers themselves. Current evidence suggests that the right postganglionic sympathetics, which emanate from sympathetic ganglia, including the stellate ganglia, innervate the atria and the anterior surfaces of the right and left ventricles, while the left sympathetics have a more posterolateral distribution and predominate in supplying the atrioventricular (AV) node and left ventricle (Randall and Ardell, 1990; Levy, Ng, and Zieske, 1966).

Less work has been completed on the parasympathetic innervation of heart (Levy and Martin, 1984). In general, the right and left vagi appear to roughly follow the distribution of the right and left sympathetics. However, the vagi predominate over the sympathetics in the atria, thus exerting a greater influence over sinus node–generated HR, for example, than do the sympathetics, while the vagi have minor effects on the ventricles and exert their influence on the ventricles predominantly through counteracting sympathetic effects (Rardon and Bailey, 1983). Furthermore, vagal influences in the atria may be more symmetric than sympathetic influences in the atria (Randall and Ardell, 1990). However, sectioning of right-sided vagal fibers induces greater acceleration of HR than does sectioning of left-sided vagal fibers (Hamlin and Smith, 1968).

Levy and colleagues (1966) observed in dogs that stimulation of the right and left stellate ganglia, the origin of most of the postganglionic sympathetic fibers emanating to the heart, had very different effects. These investigators observed that right stellate stimulation had primarily chronotropic effects, inducing a major increase in HR, while left stellate stimulation had primarily inotropic (contractility) effects, inducing a major increase in systolic BP. As is typical in studies comparing the two sides of the sympathetic nervous system, stimulation of the contralateral side resulted in minor effects in the same direction, e.g., a slight increase in HR with left stellate stimulation.

Yanowitz, Preston, and Abildskov (1966) observed that right stellate stimulation increased HR, lowered T-wave amplitude, and did not change the QT interval, while left stellate stimulation did not change HR, increased T-wave amplitude, and increased the QT interval. Changes in T-wave amplitude and prolongation of the QT interval are clinically relevant as they reflect repolarization phenomena that are associated with life-threatening arrhythmias and SCD (Schwartz et al., 1990; Zipes, 1991).

Other studies in dogs (Verrier et al., 1974; Lown et al., 1977) have shown that stimulation of either stellate ganglion significantly reduces ventricular fibrillation threshold, but the magnitude of reduction on the left is nearly twice that of the right (Natelson, 1985). Furthermore, ablation of the right stellate ganglion significantly lowers ventricular fibrillation threshold (Schwartz, 1984), while left stellate ganglion ablation has a protective effect (Schwartz et al., 1991). However, bilateral is more effective than left stellate stimulation in lowering ventricular fibrillation threshold.

Asymmetric sympathetic activation is believed to lower ventricular fibrillation threshold by increasing the dispersion of refractory periods in the ventricle (Schwartz, 1984). When neurogenic sympathetic input to the ventricle is imbalanced, those areas of the ventricle that receive sympathetic stimulation repolarize more quickly than adjacent areas that were not so stimulated. Adjacent areas that are still depolarized can prematurely depolarize the adjacent ventricular areas that have repolarized, a phenomenon known as *reentry*. This mechanism can induce a circus of aberrant conduction which can disrupt the normal depolarization-repolarization cycle and deteriorate into ventricular fibrillation. Interestingly, Han and Moe (1964) demonstrated in dogs that the infusion of exogenous catecholamines decreased the dispersion of refractory periods and the propensity for reentrant arrhythmias created by unilateral stimulation of the stellate ganglia.

To our knowledge, the right and left sympathetic pathways to the heart have not been traced in humans. Rogers and colleagues (1978) observed in pain patients undergoing stellate ganglion block that right stellate block resulted in bradycardia, while left stellate block resulted in no significant change in HR, consistent with the findings in dogs.

The animal findings pertaining to ventricular repolarization and ventricular fibrillation threshold have achieved clinical relevance in the congenital long QT syndrome, in which a deficit in right-sided sympathetics yielding an imbalance favoring the left has been found (Schwartz et al., 1990). Left stellate ganglion ablation has been used to treat patients with the long QT syndrome who have recurring life-threatening arrhythmias that are refractory to pharmacologic intervention (Schwartz et al., 1991). Schwartz and colleagues (1985) have also observed in a follow-up study of anterior MI patients that survival rates of patients randomly assigned to left stellate ganglion ablation or β-blocker treatment were equivalent and superior to those of patients given placebo. The reasons for this greater effect of left-sided sympathetics is not completely understood, but may be because of a quantitatively greater adrenergic influence on the ventricles compared to the right (Zipes, 1991).

In summary, these studies indicate that physiologically important autonomic asymmetries exist. However, most of this work has been done in animals, and virtually nothing is known about the degree to which interindividual differences are present in the extent of autonomic asymmetries in humans.

THE BRAIN-HEART LATERALITY (BHL) HYPOTHESIS

While behavioral scientists are generally aware that the cerebral hemispheres are asymmetric in their mediation of certain mental functions, the existence of autonomic asymmetries is less generally known. Similarly, cardiologists and cardiovascular researchers are generally familiar with autonomic asymmetries, but tend to know less about cerebral laterality. The BHL hypothesis is truly interdisciplinary in the sense that it draws on two bodies of knowledge developed in separate domains, the significance of which in each case is extended by the other.

Behavioral scientists know that mental events triggered by environmental cues can have deleterious effects on physical health. A vexing problem is how to identify the mechanistic links between mental events and physiologic changes. One valid approach is to characterize the psychological phenomenon first and then correlate that with peripheral mediators of a pathophysiologic process, setting aside for the time being the problem of identifying the brain mechanisms linking the psychological and the physiologic. This is the approach that has been taken with type A and CAD. An alternative approach is to specify the relationship between a pattern of brain activity and its physiologic effects. If the relationship can be demonstrated, the psychological correlates of the brain activity pattern in question can be identified at a later time. The BHL hypothesis is an example of the latter approach.

The basic BHL hypothesis can be stated as follows: emotional arousal triggers ventricular fibrillation and sudden death in a vulnerable individual (with organic heart disease) through asymmetric activation of the cerebral hemispheres, which is transmitted through the autonomic nervous system to induce a net lateralized imbalance in sympathetic input to the heart. Sympathetic activation lateralized to the left is more arrhythmogenic than sympathetic activation lateralized to the right, but an imbalance in either direction can significantly lower ventricular fibrillation threshold. Figure 11.2 is a schematic representation of the BHL hypothesis.

Given that only a minority of SCD events occur in the context of emotional arousal, individual differences in lateralization for emotion are pertinent. If one assumes that the RH is typically more active than the LH during emotional arousal (Davidson et al., 1990), and that individual differences in this characteristic are present (Tomarken et al., 1992; Wheeler, Davidson, and Tomarken, 1993), then the minority of persons who are more LH-activated during emotion are at greater risk for sudden death if asymmetric hemispheric arousal is transmitted ipsilaterally. Evidence of ipsilateral transmission is presented below.

There are many combinations of changes in the brain that can result in lateralized sympathetic input to the heart. Focusing for the moment on a sympathetic imbalance to the left, assuming ipsilateral transmission, and that activation or deactivation in a hemisphere induces similar changes in sympathetic or parasympathetic activity, a left-sided sympathetic imbalance can be

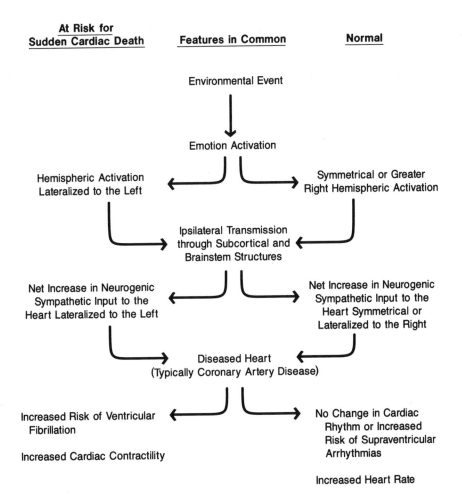

Environmental Event

Emotion Activation

Hemispheric Activation
Lateralized to the Left

Symmetrical or Greater
Right Hemispheric Activation

Ipsilateral Transmission
through Subcortical and
Brainstem Structures

Net Increase in Neurogenic
Sympathetic Input to the
Heart Lateralized to the Left

Net Increase in Neurogenic
Sympathetic Input to the
Heart Symmetrical or
Lateralized to the Right

Diseased Heart
(Typically Coronary Artery Disease)

Increased Risk of Ventricular
Fibrillation

No Change in Cardiac
Rhythm or Increased
Risk of Supraventricular
Arrhythmias

Increased Cardiac Contractility

Increased Heart Rate

Figure 11.2 Schematic repesentation of hypothesized hemispheric influence on cardiac rhythm during emotion.

induced by: (1) LH activation stimulating left-sided sympathetic activity; (2) LH deactivation decreasing left-sided parasympathetic activity; (3) RH deactivation decreasing right-sided sympathetic activity; and (4) RH activation increasing right-sided parasympathetic activity.

These mechanisms make it readily apparent that we must be more precise about exactly which structures in each hemisphere are activated or deactivated. It is entirely possible, for example, that deactivation of inhibitory structures can have a net ipsilateral activation effect. Furthermore, given that both callosal fibers (Cook, 1984; Trevarthen, 1984) and frontal-hypothalamic fibers (Brutkowski, 1964) are primarily inhibitory, it is also possible that activation of one hemisphere may lead to contralateral autonomic activation. The possibilities are numerous and cannot be further limited until additional research is completed.

While the BHL hypothesis was formulated in an attempt to explain how emotion could induce SCD, it is possible that any mental state or personality disposition that induces lateralized hemispheric activation could conceivably alter ventricular fibrillation threshold. Thus, the incidence of SCD induced by lateralized mechanisms could conceivably be higher than the 20% incidence of SCD associated with emotion. What role, if any, individual differences in the distribution of the right and left sympathetic and parasympathetic pathways play remains to be determined.

Available evidence for the BHL hypothesis will be detailed below after considering the methodologic problems associated with the necessary research. To date, support for the BHL hypothesis is provided by human studies showing that the RH appears to play a greater role in the regulation of HR (under right autonomic control) than the LH, and animal studies showing that left hypothalamic stimulation induces changes in repolarization and contractility similar to left sympathetic stimulation. Intriguing but inconclusive observations also include left hypothalamic stimulation lowering ventricular fibrillation threshold in dogs (Verrier, Calvert, and Lown, 1975) and experimental ischemia in the distribution of the left middle cerebral artery in cats inducing life-threatening arrhythmias (Weidler, Das, and Sodeman, 1976).

CRITIQUE OF METHODS AVAILABLE TO TEST THE BHL HYPOTHESIS

A variety of methods can be used to explore the relevant issues. Indeed, since each approach has its advantages and disadvantages, no one method can be used to answer all of the questions.

It might seem at first glance that animal studies could easily be designed to definitively determine whether asymmetric hemispheric activation induces lateralized autonomic activity. However, if our interest is in mental activities in humans that are associated with hemispheric arousal asymmetries, the difficulty of simulating such events with electrical stimulation of the brain in animals should be evident. Clearly, differences between animals along the phylogenetic scale are pertinent, particularly in the frontal cortex. Based on our limited knowledge of brain structures involved in cardiovascular regulation, deciding which areas of the brain to electrically stimulate is not obvious.

Other potential pitfalls that have plagued earlier animal studies of brain influences on autonomic function include the need to: (1) specify the site of stimulation based on recognized architectonic boundaries; (2) verify that cell bodies originating at the site in question are being stimulated rather than fibers of passage; (3) minimize voltage so as to avoid current spread to adjacent structures; and (4) differentiate primary autonomic effects from those secondary to somatic and motor reflexes. In addition, differences in species, anesthetic technique, and experimental protocols may limit the generalizability of findings (Cechetto and Saper, 1990).

Furthermore, no one animal species is ideal for study from the standpoint of both the CNS and ANS. More is known about the autonomic innervation of the heart in the dog than in other animals (Randall and Ardell, 1990), and the dog is commonly used in experimental studies of ventricular fibrillation. The brain of the pig is more like that of man than the dog, but the pig's heart is more electrically unstable and prone to ventricular fibrillation (and resistant to defibrillation) with minor perturbations than the dog's.

Be that as it may, there remain many advantages to animal studies. One can select specific CNS structures to activate, inactivate, or ablate. It is possible to verify on postmortem examination exactly where the stimulating electrodes were placed. Techniques such as horseradish peroxidase labeling can also be used to trace neuronal pathways. In the living animal it is also possible to control variables not permissible in man, such as keeping HR and BP constant during the testing of ventricular fibrillation threshold. Furthermore, sudden death research in man must necessarily be observational, while repeated induction of ventricular fibrillation followed by defibrillation is ethically permissible in animals.

A variety of patient models are available for laterality research which have yielded important insights. These can be divided into conditions that either suppress or activate brain structures. The main problem here is that patients typically have abnormal brains, either because of known brain lesions or psychiatric conditions such as depression that are probably associated with lateralized abnormalities. Each clinical setting has its own advantages and disadvantages. Table 11.1 summarizes the strengths and weakeness of the various patient groups for examining the BHL hypothesis.

Patients with strokes are numerous and have a high incidence of cardiovascular abnormalities induced by the stroke (Oppenheimer and Hachinski, 1992). The location of the stroke can be well characterized with magnetic resonance imaging (MRI) and clinical examination, but previous brain lesions, preexisting cardiovascular abnormalities, and medications such as β blockers which affect both heart and brain function are commonly used.

Patients with epilepsy that are at risk for sudden death (Leestma et al., 1984) may undergo continuous electroencephalographic (EEG) and cardiac monitoring to verify that seizures are present, and to characterize their type and location. Electrodes implanted in the brain or electrode grids placed on the brain surface, when used, are far more accurate than EEGs obtained with scalp electrodes. The major difficulty is that abnormal brain tissue is present, which may be underactive or overactive at different times. The etiology and age of onset of seizures are critical features which have an enormous impact on possible reorganization of brain function. In many cases one or more anticonvulsants are being used, which may have cardiac as well as neural effects. Seizures themselves usually start in one hemisphere; they may remain localized to one hemisphere or become generalized. Generalized seizures, which are more common, have both direct neurogenic and indirect endocrine effects.

Table 11.1 Strengths and weaknesses of various clinical groups for examining the brain-heart laterality hypothesis

Patient group	Strength	Weakness
Stroke	Increased incidence of arrhythmias Lesion location can be well-defined	Premorbid baseline data typically missing Medications affecting brain and heart often given Multiple lesions common
Epilepsy	EEG, ECG routinely monitored simultaneously Increased risk of sudden cardiac death	Abnormal brain tissue present Brain reorganization with early age-of-onset seizures Most seizures generalized
Wada test	Can observe effects of inactivating one hemisphere only Each side is sequentially inactivated	Abnormal brain tissue present Brain reorganization with early age-of-onset seizures
Intraoperative brain stimulation	Can activate discrete points in brain	Only one side typically accessible Surface, not deep structures, typically accessible Brain usually abnormal
Electroconvulsive therapy	Asymmetric activation induced by unilateral electrode placement Right and left unilateral stimulation can be used in same course of treatment Regional, not point, activation Structural brain disease typically absent	Pretreatment hemisphere arousal; asymmetries may be present in depressed patients Brain structures activated are relatively nonspecific
Stellate ganglion blockade	Temporary unilateral inactivation of major sympathetic nerves to heart	Blockade typically on one side only Patients with reflex sympathetic dystrophy have abnormal sympathetic function on side of block No premorbid baseline
Heart transplant	Autonomic nerves to heart removed	Regrowth of autonomic innervation can occur
Postmyocardial infarction	Abundant supply of patients Increased risk of sudden cardiac death	Medications affecting brain and heart often used Large patient sample needed
Lost QT syndrome	Sympathetic imbalance present Increased risk of sudden cardiac death	Condition is rare

Patients that need neurosurgery for intractable epilepsy often first undergo the Wada test. Sodium amobarbital is injected into a carotid artery to produce temporary inactivation of one hemisphere at a time. The major limitations to the test are those associated with epilepsy. The neuropsychological testing conducted following injection is essentially the same for each side, but the activity induced may differ depending on the functional capability (inherent capacity and decrements due to disease) of the nonsuppressed tissue.

Direct intraoperative stimulation of the brain for the purpose of observing cardiovascular effects has recently been reported (Oppenheimer et al., 1992), indicating that problems associated with obtaining informed consent are not insurmountable. In fact, neurosurgeons commonly electrically stimulate the motor strip intraoperatively, and stimulating other areas is not fundamentally different. This clearly has the advantage of studying lateralized effects induced by stimulation rather than inactivation. The major limitations are that the operative exposure to the brain usually only permits stimulation on one side, eliminating the possibility of within-subject comparisons of right- and left-sided stimulation. Furthermore, access to structures deep in the brain are relatively uncommon compared to those on the brain surface.

Another model involving stimulation is unilateral electroconvulsive therapy (ECT) in the treatment of depression. Although right unilateral ECT is used more commonly than left unilateral ECT because of memory and language effects associated with the latter, these effects are transient. The two methods are equally efficacious and can be used consecutively within the same course of treatment in a given patient (Abrams, 1988). There are several advantages of ECT for testing the BHL hypothesis. ECT provides regional rather than point activation in persons that typically do not have coarse brain disease. ECT is given under general anesthesia, and the vagolytic medications given for the purpose of preventing cardiac standstill and preventing the drying of secretions render the cardiovascular effects of ECT readily interpretable as sympathetic effects (Swartz et al., 1994). Furthermore, the time course of cardiovascular effects makes it possible to disentangle neurogenic from adrenal sympathetic effects. On the other hand, possible hemispheric arousal asymmetries associated with depression (Henriques and Davidson, 1991) again impose constraints on the interpretation of results.

Other clinical populations can be useful in further exploring the effects of the autonomic innervation of the heart. Patients with reflex sympathetic dystrophy are sometimes treated with stellate ganglion blockade (Rogers et al., 1978). Typically one side only is blocked in a given patient. The effects on sympathetic function of abnormalities within the system are unknown. Patients who undergo heart transplant have denervated hearts, which makes it possible to identify purely adrenal effects (Sloan, Shapiro, and Gorman, 1990). Heart transplant patients therefore constitute a useful comparison group for exploring the cardiovascular effects of hemispheric arousal asymmetries. It has also been observed that regrowth of autonomic innervation has occurred, so caution is needed.

Psychophysiologic techniques have the great advantage of being applicable to subjects with normal brains and hearts. Lateralized stimulus input, as with the visual half-field technique or dichotic listening, have many advantages for exploring subtleties of higher cognitive and emotional functioning. However, the major problems in the present context are that the structures in the brain that are activated are not known precisely, interhemispheric transfer does occur, and the transient nature of the effects and the mild stimulus intensity induce only minor perturbations in cardiovascular activity. While statistically significant and scientifically important findings may be obtained, more profound effects that are demonstrable in the individual patient may be needed if one is interested in using what is known in day-to-day clinical decision making in the clinical cardiologic setting.

Another behavioral technique which may be promising in this context is the Levy Chimeric Faces Test. To the extent that the more activated hemisphere is dominant in the judgment of which chimeric face in each pair looks happier (Levy et al., 1983), it is a very simple, inexpensive, and useful method. Support for the validity of the Levy Chimeric Faces Test as a measure of hemispheric arousal asymmetry comes from the work of O'Boyle, Alexander, and Benbow (1991), who observed EEG activation consistent with this interpretation in a study of mathematically gifted children.

Among brain-mapping techniques, EEG is useful for measuring asymmetries in hemispheric activation, but the source of the signals detected on the scalp surface remains unknown and the technique when used alone cannot distinguish deep from superficial activity. Skinner, Beckman, and Gray (1987) have shown that a correlation exists between the magnitude of the contingent negative variation (CNV) and the frequency of extrasystoles on Holter monitor. Although no attempt was made to examine laterality effects in this work, such an approach is possible. Nevertheless, event-related potential (ERP) studies are comparable to EEG studies in precision of localization.

More precise localization of brain activity in normal persons is increasingly attainable with the evolution of new brain imaging techniques. Positron emission tomography (PET) is among the most promising, with maximal spatial resolution of about 5 mm and a temporal resolution of about 1 minute using radiotracers such as $H_2^{15}O$ (Fox and Mintun, 1989). Coregistration with MRI is possible, although the technical difficulties with this have not yet been fully overcome. Advantages include the precise localization of cerebral blood flow, a good index of local metabolic activity, visualization of cortical and subcortical structures, and the possibility of performing within-subject studies. The major disadvantages are the expense, currently about $2000 per PET session, the relative scarcity of PET centers (about 50 in the United States), and the limitations imposed by utilizing stimulation methods that must be sustained for at least 1 minute. Single photon emission computed tomography (SPECT) is far cheaper and more readily available, its temporal resolution is comparable using the radiotracer HM-PAO, but the spatial resolution currently is about 2 cm (Innis, 1992).

New techniques under development include functional brain imaging with ecoplanar MRI (Stehling, Turner, and Mansfield, 1991) and magnetoencephalography. These techniques have enormous potential for naturalistic study of mental states as their temporal resolution is on the order of milliseconds. The former is especially promising in that it can visualize superficial as well as deep brain structures.

With regard to cardiovascular techniques, noninvasive measures of chronotropy (sinus HR) and inotropy (e.g., systolic BP, preejection period, ejection fraction) are readily available. Regarding measures relevant to sudden death in man, we are restricted to clinical observational studies such as cardiac electrophysiologic studies, in which an attempt is made to induce life-threatening arrhythmias in a controlled setting for the purpose of finding an effective treatment in patients who have had an episode of "sudden death" from which they have been successfully resuscitated (Dimarco and Haines, 1990).

It is also possible to follow patients who are at high risk for sudden death, such as those who have sustained an MI. Depending on the specific clinical situation, the estimated cardiac mortality in these patients can be as low as 5% annually, requiring a large patient population to detect statistically significant effects.

Yet another model is to study patients with the idiopathic long QT syndrome in whom a sympathetic imbalance is present. The clinical manifestations of this syndrome are variable, but the role of CNS factors in this variability has not been studied.

EVIDENCE OF LATERALIZED HEMISPHERIC CONTROL OF CARDIOVASCULAR FUNCTION

Until recently, systematic studies examining the cardiovascular consequences of lateralized brain function have not been undertaken. This work is still in its infancy, and important studies, such as a systematic comparison of the arrhythmogenic effects of stimulating homologous structures on the right and left sides of the brain, have not been undertaken. However, because sinus HR is influenced more by right than left autonomic activity, studies of lateralized brain function that include HR as a dependent variable shed light on this issue.

Henry and Calaresu (1974) observed in vagotomized cats that stimulation of 56% of sites in the right medulla induced changes in HR, while only 3% of left-sided stimulations did so, consistent with the right-sided predominance in sympathetic input to the sinoatrial (SA) node. Rogers, Abildskov, and Preston (1973) found that stimulation of either the right or left hypothalamus in cats with intact vagi produced T-wave changes characteristic of stellate ganglion stimulation on the same side. Furthermore, ECG effects of unilateral hypothalamic stimulation could be abolished by removal of the ipsilateral stellate ganglion. Fang and Wang (1962) observed in vagotomized dogs that right hypothalamic stimulation produced primarily cardioacceleration while left hypothalamic stimulation primarily augmented myocardial contractility, entirely consistent with the findings of Levy and colleagues (1966) in their studies of the effects of unilateral stellate stimulation. Unilateral activation of the brain appears to be transmitted to the heart ipsilaterally in animals.

Animal studies of ventricular fibrillation provide partial support for the BHL hypothesis, but definitive studies remain to be done. Verrier et al. (1975) observed in dogs that electrical stimulation of the left posterior hypothalamus lowered ventricular fibrillation threshold by 40%, a decrease which was abolished by β-blockade but not by cervical vagotomy or bilateral adrenalectomy. Comparison stimulation of the right posterior hypothalamus was not undertaken

(R. Verrier, personal communication, February 1993). Weidler et al. (1976) demonstrated that ligation of the left middle cerebral artery induced "major arrhythmias" over the next 3 days in 7 of 12 cats but in 0 of 6 sham-operated cats ($P < .025$). Comparison intervention on the right side was not undertaken. Skinner and Reed (1981) demonstrated in pigs that bilateral inactivation of the pathways from the frontal lobes to the hypothalamus and brainstem prevented the induction of ventricular fibrillation when the animals were exposed to the stress of a novel environment during experimental coronary artery ligation. This same experiment with unilateral inactivation has not been undertaken (J. E. Skinner, personal communication, May 1992).

Hachinski and colleagues (1992) observed in rats that right middle cerebral artery occlusion produced a greater increase in plasma NE than left middle cerebral artery occlusion without concomitant differences in HR or BP. This may reflect a differential influence of the two hemispheres on adrenal catecholamines. If so, this would add to our understanding of the mechanisms mediating the differential influence of the cerebral hemispheres on the heart. Given that Han and Moe (1964) have shown that exogenous infusion of catecholamines decreases the dispersion of refractory periods, additional complexity is added to the problem of understanding whether the two hemispheres have a differential influence in cardiovascular regulation.

Findings across species must be viewed with caution. While the findings cited above are internally consistent, T-waves changed in the opposite direction in the cat and the dog, and comparable studies have not been performed in the rat. It is not known with certainty whether humans are more similar to cats, dogs, or rats, or manifest their own unique pattern.

The results of human studies are consistent with animal studies, but have typically utilized models of asymmetry involving inactivation rather than activation. Yokoyama and colleagues (1987) compared the HR changes during a video game task in patients with RH strokes, LH strokes, and normal controls. They observed that the vagally mediated deceleration in HR following a warning tone was absent in RH patients and exaggerated in LH patients compared with controls. Zamrini and colleagues (1990) reported in 25 patients undergoing the Wada test that differential HR changes were observed as a function of side of injection: HR decreased with right-sided injection and increased with left-sided injection. If one assumes (by virtue of the distribution of the anterior and middle cerebral arteries in man) that the effects of amobarbital injection are sympathetically mediated, and that HR is under predominantly right autonomic control, this study suggests that RH inactivation suppresses and that LH inactivation disinhibits right-sided autonomic function. Clearly, results from studies of this sort will be difficult to interpret unless sympathetic and parasympathetic functions are measured or otherwise controlled in the same patients.

Lane and colleagues (1989) have also completed a study similar to that of Zamrini, examining HR changes in 13 patients with temporal lobe epilepsy undergoing the Wada test. Like Zamrini et al., these investigators found that HR increased following LH injection. They also found that this HR increase was significant in patients with LH epileptic foci but not in those with RH epileptic foci. Since epileptic lesions are hypometabolic interictally (Engle, Kuhl, and Phelps, 1982), amobarbital and epileptic focus may have similar effects in suppressing ipsilateral sympathetic tone.

In a study involving a within-subjects comparison of HR changes during right-unilateral (R-U) and left-unilateral (L-U) ECT for the treatment of depression, Swartz and colleagues (in press) demonstrated that the HR increase was greater with R-U than with L-U ECT. Since this effect occurred during the seizure, and since patients were pretreated with vagolytic agents, these findings appear to confirm a model of ipsilateral transmission of lateralized hemispheric activation through the sympathetic chain to the heart. Consistent with these results, Oppenheimer and colleagues (1992) performed 39 right insular cortex stimulations in three patients and 31 left insular cortex stimulations in two other patients during the course of epilepsy surgery. Decreases in HR and BP were more frequently observed during left insular cortex stimulation and increases in HR and BP were more frequently observed during right insular cortex stimulation.

In 1979, Jannetta and Gendell reported a possible etiologic connection between essential hypertension and intraoperatively observed neurovascular compression of the ventrolateral medulla at the level of the root entry zone of the ninth and tenth cranial nerves on the left. Recently, Naraghi and colleagues (1992) performed an autopsy study which revealed that all 24 patients with a history of essential hypertension manifested this left-sided neurovascular compression at the level of the brainstem, while none of 10 patients with renal hypertension and none of 21 normotensive control patients showed such a pattern. These findings are consistent with suppression of vagal activity on the left leading to increased sympathetic activity on that side.

Observational studies of lateralized lesions in man with dependent variables relevant to sudden death have been very limited. Yamour and colleagues (1980) observed prolonged QT intervals or neurogenic T waves, or both, in five of six patients with nontraumatic left frontal lobe hemorrhage, repolarization changes similar to those observed with left sympathetic stimulation. In the only study to date in man examining the differential influence of the two hemispheres on ventricular arrhythmogenesis, Lane et al. (1992) conducted a retrospective examination of Holter monitor results in 38 patients with RH or LH strokes (n = 19 in each group) obtained within 2 weeks of admission to a stroke unit. They found that all four cases of supraventricular tachycardia occurred in patients with RH strokes ($P = .05$), consistent with a model of ipsilateral vagal inhibition with stroke. There was a nonsignificant trend for an association between LH stroke and multifocal premature ventricular contractions (PVCs) or nonsustained ventricular tachycardia. However, differences between RH and LH groups in medications and previous lateralized strokes prevented definitive conclusions.

Barron and colleagues (1994) tested the hypothesis of ipsilateral vagal inhibition with stroke by comparing spectral analyses of heart rate variability in patients with RH or LH strokes to those of normal controls. All stroke patients manifested decreases in the purely parasympathetic component of heart rate variability due to respiration relative to controls, but the decreases in RH stroke patients were significantly greater than those in LH stroke patients, supporting the conclusions of Lane et al. (1992).

It should be noted that while few studies have been designed specifically to examine the differential influence of the two hemispheres on the heart, investigators may have examined data collected for other purposes to answer this question and not observed lateralized effects. For example, in a personal communication related to a paper (Blumhardt, Smith, and Owen, 1986) on ECG accompaniments of temporal lobe epileptic seizures, it was reported that mean HR change in right unilateral seizures was 12 beats per minute higher than in left unilateral seizures (n = 21 in each group), but the differences were not significant owing to the magnitude of variance in relation to mean HR change. It is not known how many such unreported findings there are.

PSYCHOPHYSIOLOGIC MEASURES IN HEMISPHERIC LATERALITY STUDIES

It is fascinating to compare and contrast related studies in the field of psychophysiology, because they are derived from a theoretical and empirical foundation that is different in several important ways from those conducted within medical specialties such as cardiology, neurology, and psychiatry. First, much of this work has been aimed at elucidating the differences in cognition and emotion between the two hemispheres, with autonomic variables being used to confirm whether hypothesized differences exist between the cerebral hemispheres, rather than focusing on CNS-ANS interactions per se. Indeed, it was from this tradition that Galin (1974) made his suggestion that was the origin of the BHL hypothesis. Secondly, while most work cited has been based on a model of descending influences of the brain on the heart, the James-Lange model of sensory processes determining the nature of emotional experience has led to a focus on the afferent influences from the heart and other viscera on brain function. It is remarkable that areas of convergence exist between studies from the medical tradition and those from the psychophysiologic tradition. Cross-fertilization of ideas and methods will no doubt lead to extension and enrichment of each body of work.

When autonomic variables such as HR and electrodermal activity (EDA) are used as indices of hemispheric activation, there is the implicit assumption that each hemisphere is functioning as a unit to drive autonomic activity. While this is clearly simplistic, our understanding of how the brain coordinates and directs autonomic activity, as discussed above, is quite incomplete. Therefore, psychophysiologic research findings may indeed be useful in extending knowledge on the lateralization of CNS-ANS interactions.

Dimond and colleagues (1976, 1977) helped to put the dominant role of the RH in emotional judgments on a solid empirical footing by showing film clips with different emotional valence to each hemisphere with special contact lenses. The major finding was that films were rated as more unpleasant when viewed by the RH. While HRs differed significantly across the film conditions, mean HRs with LH viewing were higher than those with RH viewing for two films rated as pleasant, with HR higher with RH viewing for the film rated most unpleasant. Indices of left-sided autonomic function were not examined.

Walker and Sandman (1979, 1982) examined averaged evoked potentials (AEPs) in the occipital area during spontaneously occurring fast, slow, and midrange HRs, and during the systolic and diastolic phases of the cardiac cycle. In a complex set of findings, the main conclusion was that evoked potentials in the RH varied significantly as a function of HR while those in the LH did not. P1 and P2 amplitudes were larger during slow HRs than during fast HRs, consistent with a restriction in sensory intake with higher HRs. Furthermore, components of the ERP occurring 200 to 300 ms after stimulation were enhanced in the RH during diastole and in the LH during systole. Since these findings could not rule out the possibility that cardiovascular activity was under brain control rather than the reverse, these findings stimulated new psychophysiologic investigations of functional hemispheric asymmetries.

Using the visual half-field technique with stimuli exposed exclusively to the RH in half the subjects and the LH in the other half, Hugdahl and colleagues (1983) observed that there was an anticipatory acceleration in HR in the RH group and an anticipatory deceleration of HR in the LH group 3 to 5 seconds before slide onset. The HR differences observed were a function of the hemisphere to which the stimuli were presented, not the verbal or visuospatial nature of the visual stimuli.

Studies of EDA response to emotional and nonemotional stimuli in patients with unilateral brain lesions indicate that emotional responses and EDA were decreased in patients with lesions in the RH but not in normal controls or those with LH lesions (Zoccolotti et al., 1981, 1986). These findings, as well as those showing an association between RH activity and HR, have contributed to the prevailing model among many psychophysiologists of the predominant role of the RH in the control of autonomic function. However, these studies illustrate that if autonomic variables such as EDA are used to establish that one hemisphere is preferentially specialized to mediate a particular function, they cannot also be used to determine what autonomic functions are controlled by each hemisphere independent of the quality of the stimulus, particularly if variables reflective of left-sided autonomic activity (such as measures of cardiac contractility) are not also included.

In 1984 Hugdahl reviewed 51 studies up to 1982 involving bilateral EDA recordings during studies of functional hemispheric asymmetry. Bilateral differences in EDA were small and subject to distortion owing to variations in the experimental conditions. Although some findings were contradictory, and some studies showed no left-right differences in EDA, the data were more consistent with a model of contralateral inhibition than one of contralateral excitation. The distinction between contralateral inhibition and ipsilateral activation was not explicitly discussed, based in part on evidence of inhibitory cortical control of EDA in animal experiments.

In an investigation involving continuous presentation of an emotionally positive 3-minute film to one visual half-field at a time, Wittling (1990) found that postfilm systolic and diastolic BP changes relative to prefilm baseline were greater with RH presentation than with LH presentation. Interestingly, hemispheric asymmetry for BP changes were present in women but not in men.

Heart rate changes during attention are relevant because the RH appears to predominate in the mediation of attention. Attentive observation of the environment, particularly in anticipation of an important event, is known to slow HR via a vagal mechanism (Lacey and Lacey, 1974). The hemispheric mediation of this phenomenon was examined in the Yokoyama et al. (1987) report discussed above. HR deceleration prior to the stimulus for a speeded reaction was virtually eliminated in patients with RH lesions, but clearly present in those with LH lesions. These results suggest that the organization of behavior, perhaps primarily affective-emotional behavior, in the RH extends to the organization of the autonomic changes supporting those behaviors.

Werntz and colleagues (1983, 1987), Shannahoff-Khalsa (1991), and Backon and colleagues (1990a,b) have conducted EEG studies suggesting that there is an ultradian rhythm of alternating dominance or lateralization of cerebral activation that is tightly coupled to a nasal cycle of alternating shifts in airflow to the right and left nostrils. If the technique of selective hemispheric stimulation with unilateral forced nostril breathing could be further validated, it would be a useful tool in the exploration of the BHL hypothesis. This work could also conceivably relate to findings of circadian patterns in the incidence of sudden death.

Recent findings by Tomarken and colleagues (Tomarken et al., 1992; Wheeler, Davidson, and Tomarken, 1993) suggest that stable individual differences exist in the degree of asymmetry of frontal activation as measured by EEG that can be used to predict the intensity of emotional responses to films. Less well founded but potentially relevant is the "hemisphericity" research suggesting that stable individual differences exist in cognitive style (Yeap, 1989). O'Boyle and colleagues (1991) have observed that mathematically gifted children appear to have stable patterns of hemispheric arousal asymmetry that are more lateralized to the right hemisphere than in children with average mathematical ability. If confirmed, specific predictions could be made about the patterns of autonomic activity to be observed based on these stable individual differences in hemispheric arousal asymmetry.

The literature on hemispheric asymmetry and emotion concerns issues such as whether some or all emotion functions are lateralized to the RH, which structures are involved in mediating each function, whether the emotions are differentially lateralized to the hemispheres based on an underlying principle such as positive vs. negative or approach vs. withdrawal, and whether cortical or subcortical structures are responsible for the association between valence and hemisphere (Borod, 1992). Until these issues are resolved it is not possible to determine whether current findings regarding the cardiovascular correlates of different primary emotions are consistent with a model of ipsilateral transmission of hemispheric activation or not. However, resolution of these issues will make it possible to identify those emotional states that may put vulnerable persons, such as those with CAD, at even higher risk for sudden death.

FUTURE RESEARCH AGENDA

This review has made it clear that there are many gaps in our knowledge. Perhaps the best way to begin to define research priorities in this area is to identify the key questions that remain unanswered. These include:

1. Does activation of the left cerebral cortex have effects on the heart that are reliably distinguishable from those due to activation of the right cerebral cortex?

a. If so, does transmission of lateralized hemispheric activation occur ipsilaterally?

b. What is the role of interhemispheric transfer?

c. Precisely which cortical structures can induce lateralized autonomic activation?

d. What are the roles of vagal and sympathetic effects in this phenomenon?

e. What are the relative contributions of neurogenic and endocrine effects?

2. If present, is this phenomenon relevant to the problem of SCD?

3. What is the profile of psychological states or traits that influence sudden death risk, and to what extent is there a common substrate involving hemispheric laterality?

All of these questions can be addressed in empirical research. The first priority is to establish in animals that lateralized brain mechanisms can lower ventricular fibrillation threshold. For example, Skinner and Reed's (1981) work in pigs involved bilateral inactivation of the pathways connecting the frontal lobes to the hypothalamus and brainstem. The BHL hypothesis would predict that inactivation on the left will have a protective effect while inactivation on the right will not. Another example is the work of Verrier and colleagues (1975), who demonstrated that stimulation of the left posterior hypothalamus lowered ventricular fibrillation threshold. The efficiency of left compared to right posterior hypothalamic stimulation in lowering ventricular fibrillation threshold needs to be determined.

The next logical step would be to conduct epidemiologic surveys in patients at risk for sudden death, such as those who have recently sustained an MI, to determine whether aspects of hemispheric lateralization can predict survival. Indices of hemispheric asymmetry such as handedness could be useful for this purpose, given the evidence that left-handers do not live as long as right-handers (Coren and Halpern, 1991), and evidence that the rate of left-handedness (23.1%) among 26 resuscitated victims of sudden death was significantly greater than the expected rate (5%) based on norms in the general population, while the rate among 26 control patients (7.7%) did not differ from that of the general population (Lane et al., 1994). Another related approach would be to determine whether psychological variables that have been linked with sudden death, including depression and hostility, are so linked because of mechanisms involving cerebral laterality.

If it could be established that a link exists between lateralized brain mechanisms and sudden death, the mechanisms mediating this link would need to be elucidated. A program of research would be needed to examine autonomic and CNS asymmetries and the links between them.

Much more needs to be learned about the anatomy of the autonomic nerves innervating the heart in man. Are the distribution patterns of the right and left sympathetics similar to those seen in the dog? How variable are these patterns? Do vagal fibers follow a course parallel to the sympathetics? If patterns of autonomic innervation of the heart are relatively invariant, the importance of variability in hemispheric arousal asymmetry will be heightened.

In contrast to laterality research designed to elucidate the functional capabilities of each hemisphere, methods for preferentially activating one hemisphere or the other, particularly in frontal areas, are needed. Frontal activation asymmetries could be measured with EEG, SPECT, or PET. Dependent variables would include HR and indices of contractility such as preejection period or systolic BP. Methods for disentangling sympathetic from parasympathetic effects could be used, such as spectral analysis of HR variability.

The next phase of research would involve identifying states and traits associated with asymmetric patterns of hemispheric activation. Once behavioral markers were established for these patterns, methods of intervention could be developed to alter the underlying activation asymmetries.

Assuming it were possible to identify persons at risk for SCD based on their pattern of hemispheric lateralization during emotion or other mental states, of what clinical benefit would this be? Such a measure would be of use to cardiologists in assisting with management decisions of patients with CAD, such as whether to study a patient electrophysiologically for inducibility (and reversibility) of arrhythmias (see above), or providing a new indication for existing treatment modalities, such as left stellate ganglion ablation or implantation of an antitachycardia device such as the automatic implantable cardioverter defibrillator. Furthermore, because SCD may be the first manifestation of CAD, such a capability would likely lead primary care providers to advise their patients with the laterality pattern in question to make every effort possible to reduce or eliminate risk factors for CAD, such as smoking, obesity, elevated cholesterol, and hypertension. Given recent evidence that an 8-week aerobic exercise training program decreases EEG alpha laterality and increases vagal tone (Kubitz and Landers, 1993), the importance of implementing an aerobic exercise program would be further reinforced.

AFTERWORD

One of the implications of this work is that it may shed light on why emotion may be lateralized to the RH. If our hypothesis is correct, activation of the LH during emotion could induce sudden death, perhaps at an early age. (Schwartz and colleagues [1982] have found evidence of sympathetic imbalance to the left in sudden infant death syndrome.) Natural selection would have conferred greater survival value on persons whose brains mediated emotion on the right.

How then may we explain how laterality has come to play a role in sudden death? The answer may lie in the survival value conferred independently by both autonomic asymmetry and hemispheric asymmetry. The ability to increase myocardial contractility (left-sided sympathetics) while maintaining a steady HR (right-sided autonomics) could have survival value by maximizing cardiac output in emergency situations: if HR increases too much, the ventricles will not have adequate filling time. It may also be assumed that asymmetry of the brain in itself conferred upon man enhanced cognitive abilities (Levy, 1969), ultimately enabling man to survive longer. With prolonged survival, new disease processes became prevalent, but were no longer subjected to natural selection because they did not affect the ability to procreate.

In this light, it is interesting to note that sudden death occurs in man typically in middle age (Lown, 1979), considerably older than the life span of humans until the modern era. Sudden death also typically occurs in persons with diseased hearts such as CAD. Thus, the forces of natural selection acted to enhance survival by promoting autonomic and cerebral laterality, only to create mechanisms *through their interaction* that could contribute to man's demise in the context of disease processes that natural selection could not anticipate.

REFERENCES

Abrams, R. (1988). *Electroconvulsive therapy*. New York, NY: Oxford University Press.

Accident facts (1992). Chicago: National Safety Council.

Ahern, D. K., Gorkin, L., Anderson, J. L., Tierney, C., Hallstlrom, A., Ewart, C., Capone, R. J., Schron, E., Kornfield, D., Herd, J. A., Richardson, D. W., and Follick, M. J. (1990). Biobehavioral variables and mortality or cardiac arrest in the cardiac arrhythmia pilot study (CAPS). *American Journal of Cardiology, 66*, 59–62.

Almada, S. J., Zonderman, A. B., Shekelle, R. B., Dyer, A. R., Daviglus, M. L., and Costa P. T., Jr. (1991). Neuroticism and cynicism and risk of death in middle-aged men: the Western Electric Study. *Psychosomatic Medicine, 53*, 165–175.

Backon, J. (1990b). Forced unilateral nostril breathing: a technique that affects brain hemisphericity and autonomic activity. *Brain and Cognition, 12,* 155–157.

Backon, J., Matamoros, N., Ramirez, M., Sanchez, R. M., Ferrer, J., Brown, A., and Ticho, U. (1990a). A functional vagotomy induced by unilateral forced right nostril breathing decreases intraocular pressure in open and closed angle glaucoma. *British Journal of Ophthalmology, 74,* 607–609.

Barron, S. A., Rogovski, Z., and Hemli, J. (1994). Autonomic consequences of cerebral hemisphere infarction. *Stroke, 25,* 113–116.

Blumhardt, L. D., Smith, P. E. M., and Owen, L. (1986). Electrocardiographic accompaniments of temporal lobe epileptic seizures. *Lancet, 1,* 1051–1056.

Borod, J.C. (1992). Interhemispheric and intrahemispheric control of emotion: a focus on unilateral brain damage. *Journal of Consulting and Clinical Psychology, 60,* 339–348.

Brutkowski, A. (1964). Prefrontal cortex and drive inhibition. In J. Warren and K. Akert (Eds.), *The frontal granular cortex and behavior.* New York, NY: McGraw-Hill Book Co.

Cannon, W. B. (1942). "Voodoo" death. *American Anthropologist, 44,* 182–190.

Carney, R. M., Rich, M. W., Freedland, K. E., Saini, J., TeVelde, A., Simeone, C., and Clark, K. (1988). Major depressive disorder predicts cardiac events in patients with coronary artery disease. *Psychosomatic Medicine, 50,* 627–633.

Cechetto, D., and Saper, C. (1990). Role of the cerebral cortex in autonomic function. In A. Loewy and K. Spyer (Eds.), *Central regulation of autonomic functions* (pp 208–223). New York, NY: Oxford University Press.

Centers for Disease Control and Prevention (1993). HIV/AIDS Surveillance Report, 5(3), p 12.

Cerati, D., and Schwartz, P. J. (1991). Single cardiac vagal fiber activity, acute myocardial ischemia, and risk for sudden death. *Circulation, 69,* 1389–1401.

Cook, N. (1984). Homotopic callosal inhibition. *Brain and Language, 23,* 116–125.

Coren, S., and Halpern, D. F. (1991). Left-handedness: a marker for decreased survival fitness. *Psychological Bulletin, 109,* 90–106.

Cottington, E. M., Matthews, K. A., Talbott, E., and Kuller, L. H. (1980). Environmental events preceding sudden death in women. *Psychosomatic Medicine, 42,* 567–574.

Davidson, R. J., Ekman, P., Saron, C., Senulis, J., and Friesen, W. V. (1990). Approach/withdrawal and cerebral asymmetry: Emotional expression and brain physiology, I. *Journal of Personality and Social Psychology, 58,* 330–341.

DeFerrari, G. M., Vanoli, E., Stramba-Badiale, M., Hull, S. S. Jr., Foreman, R. D., and Schwartz, P. J. (1991). Vagal reflexes and survival during acute myocardial ischemia in conscious dogs with healed myocardial infarction. *American Journal of Physiology, 261,* H63–H69.

Dimarco, J. P., and Haines, D. E. (1990). Sudden cardiac death. *Current Problems in Cardiology,* 183–232.

Dimond, S. J., and Farrington, L. (1977). Emotional response to films shown to the right or left hemisphere of the brain measured by heart rate. *Acta Psychologica, 41,* 255–260.

Dimond, S. J., Farrington, L., and Johnson, P. (1976). Differing emotional response from right and left hemispheres. *Nature, 261,* 690–692.

Engel, G. L. (1971). Sudden and rapid death during psychological stress. *Annals of Internal Medicine, 74,* 771–782.

Engle, J., Kuhl, D. E., and Phelps, M. E. (1982). Patterns of human local cerebral glucose metabolism during epileptic seizures. *Science, 218,* 64–66.

Egstrup, K. (1991). Silent ischemia and beta-blockade. *Circulation, 84,* VI-84–VI-92.

Fang, H. S., and Wang, S. C. (1962). Cardioaccelerator and cardioaugmentor points in hypothalamus of the dog. *American Journal of Physiology, 203,* 147–150.

Fox, P. T., and Mintun, M. A. (1989). Noninvasive fucntional brain mapping by change-distribution analysis of averaged PET images of $H_2^{15}O$ tissue activity. *Journal of Nuclear Medicine, 30,* 141–149.

Frasure-Smith, N. (1991). In-hospital symptoms of psychological stress as predictors of long-term outcome after acute myocardial infarction in men. *American Journal of Cardiology, 67,* 121–126.

Frasure-Smith, N., Lespérance, F., and Talajic, M. (1993). Depression following myocardial infarction—impact on 6-month survival. *Journal of the American Medical Association, 270,* 1819–1825.

Friedman, M., and Rosenman, R. H. (1974). *Type A behavior and your heart.* New York, NY: Alfred A. Knopf.

Galin, D. (1974). Implications for psychiatry of left and right cerebral specialization. *Archives of General Psychiatry, 31,* 572–583.

Glass, L., and MacKay, M. C. (1988). *From clocks to chaos: The rhythms of life.* Princeton, NJ: Princeton University Press.

Hachinski, V. C., Oppenheimer, S. M., Wilson, J. X., Guiraudon, C., and Cechetto, D. F. (1992). Asymmetry of sympathetic consequences of experimental stroke. *Archives of Neurology, 49,* 697–702.

Hamlin, R. L., and Smith, C. R. (1968). Effects of vagal stimulation on S-A and A-V nodes. *American Journal of Physiology, 215,* 560–568.

Han, J., and Moe, G. K. (1964). Nonuniform recovery of excitability in ventricular muscle. *Circulation Research, 14,* 44–60.

Henriques, J. B., and Davidson, R. J. (1991). Left frontal hypoactivation in depression. *Journal of Abnormal Psychology, 100,* 535–545.

Henry, J. L., and Calaresu, F. R. (1974). Excitatory and inhibitory inputs from medullary nuclei projecting to spinal cardioacceleratory neurons in the cat. In O. Creutzfeldt and D. R. Curtis (Eds.), *Experimental brain research.* New York, NY: Springer-Verlag.

Heusch, G. (1990). Alpha-adrenergic mechanisms in myocardial ischemia. *Circulation, 81,* 1–13.

Hugdahl, K. (1984). Hemispheric asymmetry and bilateral electrodermal recordings: a review of the evidence. *Psychophysiology, 21,* 371–393.

Hugdahl, K., Franzon, M., Andersson, B., and Walldebo, G. (1983). Heart-rate responses (HRR) to lateralized visual stimuli. *Pavlovian Journal of Biological Science, 18,* 186–198.

Innis, R. B. (1992). Neuroreceptor imaging with SPECT. *Journal of Clinical Psychiatry, 53[11, suppl],* 29–34.

Jannetta, P. J., and Gendell, H. M. (1979). Clinical observations on etiology of essential hypertension. *Surgical Forum, 30,* 431–432.

Jennings, J. R. (1982). Attention and coronary heart disease. In D. S. Krantz, A. Baum, and J. E. Singer (Eds.), *Handbook of psychology and health III: Cardiovascular disorders and behavior* (pp 85–124). Hillsdale, NJ: Lawrence Erlbaum Associates.

Kamarck, T., and Jennings, J. R. (1991). Biobehavioral factors in sudden cardiac death. *Psychological Bulletin, 109*, 42–75.

Keefe, D. L., Schwartz, J., and Somberg, J. C. (1987). The substrate and the trigger: the role of myocardial vulnerability in sudden cardiac death. *American Heart Journal, 113*, 218–225.

Krantz, D. S., and Manuck, S. B. (1984). Acute psychophysiological reactivity and risk of cardiovascular disease: A review and methodological critique. *Psychological Bulletin, 96*, 435–464.

Kubitz, K. A., Landers, D. M. (1993). The effects of aerobic training on cardiovascular responses to mental stress: an examination of underlying mechanisms. *Journal of Sport and Exercise Psychology, 15*, 326–337.

Kuller, L. H., Cooper, M., and Perper, J. (1972). Epidemiology of sudden death. *Archives of Internal Medicine, 129*, 714–719.

Lacey, B. C., and Lacey, J. I. (1974). Studies of heart rate and other bodily processes in sensorimotor behavior. In P. A. Obrist, A. Black, J. Brener, and I. DiCara (Eds.), *Cardiovascular psychophysiology: current issues in response mechanisms, biofeedback and methodology*. Chicago: Aldine-Atherton.

Lane, R. D., Caruso, A. C., Brown, V. L., Axelrod, B., Schwartz, G. E., Sechrest, L., and Marcus, F. I. (1994). Effects of non-right-handedness on risk for sudden death associated with coronary artery disease. *American Journal of Cardiology* (in press).

Lane, R., Novelly, R., Cornell, C., Zeitlin, S., and Schwartz, G. (1989, May). *Asymmetrical hemispheric control of heart rate*. Paper presented at the Annual Meeting of the Society for Psychophysiological Research, San Francisco, CA, October 1988, and the Annual Meeting of the American Psychiatric Association, San Francisco, CA.

Lane, R., and Schwartz, G. (1987). Induction of lateralized sympathetic input to the heart by the CNS during emotional arousal: A possible neurophysiologic trigger of sudden cardiac death. *Psychosomatic Medicine, 49*, 274–284.

Lane, R. D., Wallace, J. D., Petrosky, P. P., Schwartz, G. E., and Gradman, A. H. (1992). Supraventricular tachycardia in patients with right hemisphere strokes. *Stroke, 23*, 362–366.

Leestma, J. E., Kalelkar, M. B., Teas, S. S., Jay, G. W., and Hughes, J. R. (1984). Sudden unexplained death associated with seizures: analysis of 66 cases. *Epilepsia, 25*, 84–88.

Legault, S. E., Breissblatt, W. M., Jennings, R. J., Manuck, S. B., and Follansbee, W. P. (1993). Myocardial ischemia during mental stress testing: is the mechanism different from exercise-induced ischemia? *Homeostasis in Health and Disease, 39*, 252–265.

Levy, J. (1969). Possible basis for the evolution of lateral specialization of the human brain. *Nature, 224*, 614–615.

Levy, J., Heller, W., Banich, M. T., and Burton, L. A. (1983). Are variations among right-handed individuals in perceptual asymmetries caused by characteristic arousal differences between hemispheres? *Journal of Experimental Psychology: Human Perception and Performance, 9*, 329–359.

Levy, M. N., and Martin, P. (1984). Parasympathetic control of the heart. In W. C. Randall W. C. (Ed.), *Nervous control of cardiovascular function*. New York, NY: Oxford University Press.

Levy, M. N., Ng, M. D., and Zieske, H. (1966). Functional distribution of the peripheral cardiac sympathetic pathways. *Circulation Research, 14*, 650–661.

Lown, B. (1979). Sudden cardiac death: the major challenge confronting contemporary cardiology. *American Journal of Cardiology, 43*, 313–328.

Lown, B., DeSilva, R. A., Reich, P., and Murawski, B. J. (1980). Psychophysiologic factors in sudden cardiac death. *American Journal of Psychiatry, 137,* 1325–1335.

Lown, B., Verrier, R., and Rabinowitz, S. (1977). Neural and psychologic mechanisms and the problem of sudden cardiac death. *American Journal of Cardiology, 39,* 890–902.

Manuck, S. B., and Krantz, D. S. (1986). Psychophysiologic reactivity in coronary heart disease and essential hypertension. In V. A. Matthews, S. M. Weiss, T. Detre, T. M. Dembroski, B. Falkner, S. B. Manuck, and R. B. Williams, Jr. (Eds.), *Handbook of stress, reactivity and cardiovascular disease* (pp 11–34). New York, NY: John Wiley & Sons.

Mesulam, M.-M. (1985). *Principles of behavioral neurology.* Philadelphia, PA: F. A. Davis Co.

Meyers, A., and Dewar, H. (1975). Circumstances attending 100 sudden deaths from coronary artery disease and coroner's necropsies. *British Heart Journal, 37,* 1133–1143.

Muller, J. E., and Tofler, G. H. (1990). A symposium: Triggering and circadian variation of onset of acute cardiovascular disease. *American Journal of Cardiology, 66,* 1G–70G.

Myerburg, R. J., Kessler, K. M., and Castellanos, A. (1993). Sudden cardiac death: epidemiology, transient risk and intervention assessment. *Annals of Internal Medicine, 119,* 1187–1197.

Myerburg, R. J., Kessler, K. M., Interian, A., Fernandez, P., Kumura, S., Kozlovskis, P. L., Furukawa, T., Basset, A. L., and Castellanos, A. (1990). Clinical and experimental pathophysiology of sudden cardiac death. In D. P. Zipes and J. Jalife (Eds.), *Cardiac electrophysiology.* Philadelphia, PA: W. B. Saunders Co.

Naraghi, R., Gaab, M. R., Walter, G. F., and Kleinberg, B. (1992). Arterial hypertension and neurovascular compression at the ventrolateral medulla: A comparative microanatomical and pathological study. *Journal of Neurosurgery, 77,* 103–112.

Natelson, B. H. (1985). Neurocardiology—an interdisciplinary area for the 80s. *Archives of Neurology, 42,* 178–184.

O'Boyle, M. W., Alexander, J. E., and Benbow, C. P. (1991). Enhanced right hemisphere activation in the mathematically precocious: a preliminary EEG investigation. *Brain and Cognition, 17,* 138–153.

Olsson, G., and Ryden, L. (1991). Prevention of sudden death using beta-blockers. *Circulation, 84,* VI-33–VI-37.

Oppenheimer, S. M., Cechetto, D. F., and Hachinski, V. C. (1990). Cerebrogenic cardiac arrhythmias. *Archives of Neurology, 47,* 513–519.

Oppenheimer, S. M., Gelb, A., Girvin, J. P., and Hachinski, V. C. (1992). Cardiovascular effects of human insular cortex stimulation. *Neurology, 42,* 1727–1732.

Oppenheimer, S. M., and Hachinski, V. C. (1992). The cardiac consequences of stroke. *Neurological Clinics, 10,* 167–176.

Randall, W. C., and Ardell, J. L. (1990). Nervous control of the heart: anatomy and pathophysiology. In D. P. Zipes and J. Jalife (Eds.), *Cardiac electrophysiology.* Philadelphia, PA: W. B. Saunders Co.

Rardon, D., and Bailey, J. (1983). Parasympathetic effects on electrophysiologic properties of cardiac ventricular tissue. *Journal of the American College of Cardiology, 2,* 1200–1209.

Reich, P., Desilva, R., Lown, B., and Murawski, B. J. (1981). Acute psychological disturbances preceding life-threatening ventricular arrhythmias. *Journal of the American Medical Association, 246,* 233–235.

Rissanen, V., Romo, M., and Siltanen, P. (1978). Premonitory symptoms and stress factors preceding sudden death from ischaemic heart disease. *Acta Medica Scandinavica, 204,* 389–396.

Rogers, M., Abildskov, J., and Preston, J. (1973). Neurogenic ECG changes in critically ill patients: an experimental model. *Critical Care Medicine, 1,* 192–196.

Rogers, M. C., Battit, G., McPeek, B., and Todd, D. (1978). Lateralization of sympathetic control of the human sinus node: ECG changes of stellate ganglion block. *Anesthesiology, 48,* 139–141.

Rozanski, A., Bairey, C. N., Krantz, D. S., Friedman, J., Resser, K. J., Morell, M., Hilton-Chalfen, S., Hestrin, L., Bietendorf, J., and Berman, D. S. (1988). Mental stress and the induction of silent myocardial ischemia in patients with coronary artery disease. *New England Journal of Medicine, 318,* 1005–1012.

Schwartz, P. (1984). Sympathetic imbalance and cardiac arrhythmias. In W. Randall (Ed.), *Nervous control of cardiovascular function.* New York, NY: Oxford University Press.

Schwartz, P. J., Locati, E. H., Moss, A. J., Crampton, R. S., Trazzi, R., and Ruberti, U. (1991). Left cardiac sympathetic denervation in the therapy of congenital long QT syndrome—a worldwide report. *Circulation, 84,* 503–511.

Schwartz, P. J., Locati, E., Priori, S. G., and Zaza, A. (1990). The long Q-T syndrome. In D. P. Zipes and J. Jalife (Eds.), *Cardiac electrophysiology.* Philadelphia, PA: W. B. Saunders Co.

Schwartz, P. J., Montemerlo, M., Facchini, J., Salice, P., Rosti, D., Poggio, G., and Giorgetti, R. (1982). The QT interval throughout the first six months of life: a prospective study. *Circulation, 66,* 496–501.

Schwartz, P. J., Motolese, M., Pollavini, G., Malliani, Bartorelli, C., and Zanchetti, A. (1985). Surgical and pharmacological antiadrenergic interventions in the prevention of sudden death after a first myocardial infarction. *Circulation, 72,* III-358.

Schwartz, P. J., and Priori, S. G. (1990). Sympathetic nervous system and cardiac arrhythmias. In D. P. Zipes and J. Jalife (Eds.), *Cardiac electrophysiology.* Philadelphia, PA: W. B. Saunders Co.

Shannahoff-Khalsa, D. (1991). Lateralized rhythms of the central and autonomic nervous systems. *International Journal of Psychophysiology, 11,* 225–251.

Silberman, E. K., and Weingartner, H. (1986). Hemispheric lateralization of functions related to emotion. *Brain and Cognition, 5,* 322–353.

Skinner, J. E., Beckman, K. J., and Gray, C. M. (1987). Detection of the cardiac patient at risk using the event-related slow potential. In R. Johnson, J. W. Rohrbaugh, and R. Parasuraman (Eds.), *Current trends in event-related potentials research* (pp 543–548). Amsterdam: Elsevier.

Skinner, J. E., Lie, J. T., and Entman, M. L. (1975). Modification of ventricular fibrillation latency following coronary artery occlusion in the conscious pig. The effects of psychological stress and beta-adrenergic blockade. *Circulation, 51,* 656–667.

Skinner, J. E., and Reed, J. C. (1981). Blockade of frontocortical-brain stem pathway prevents ventricular fibrillation of ischemic heart. *American Journal of Physiology, 249,* H156–H163.

Sloan, R. P., Shapiro, P. A., and Gorman, J. M. (1990). Psychophysiological reactivity in cardiac transplant patients. *Psychophysiology, 27,* 187–194.

Smith, O. A., and DeVito, J. L. (1984). Central neural integration for the control of autonomic reponses associated with emotion. *Annual Review of Neuroscience, 7,* 43–65.

Stehling, M. K., Turner, R., and Mansfield, P. (1991). Echo-planar imaging: magnetic resonance imaging in a fraction of a second. *Science, 254,* 43–50.

Swartz, C. M., Abrams, R., Lane, R. D., DuBois, M. A., and Srinivasaraghavan, J. (1994). Heart rate differences between right and left hand unilateral electroconvulsive therapy. *Journal of Neurology, Neurosurgery and Psychiatry, 57,* 97–99.

Taggart, P., Carruthers, M., and Somerville, W. (1973). Electrocardiogram, plasma catecholamines and lipids, and their modifications by oxprenolol when speaking before an audience. *Lancet, 2,* 341–346.

Talman, W. T. (1985). Cardiovascular regulation and lesions of the central nervous system. *Annals of Neurology, 18,* 1–12.

Tomarken, A. J.,Davidson, R. J., Wheeler, R. E., and Doss, R. C. (1992). Individual differences in anterior brain asymmetry and fundamental dimensions of emotion. *Journal of Personality and Social Psychology, 62,* 676–687.

Trevarthen, C. (1984). Functional relations of disconnected hemispheres with the brain stem and with each other: monkey and man. In M. Kinsbourne and W. Smith (Eds.), *Hemispheric disconnection and cerebral function.* Springfield, IL: Charles C Thomas.

Verrier, R., Thompson, P., and Lown, B. (1974). Ventricular vulnerability during sympathetic stimulation: role of heart rate and blood pressure. *Cardiovascular Research, 8,* 602–610.

Verrier, R. L. (1990). Behavioral stress, myocardial ischemia, and arrhythmias. In D. P. Zipes and J. Jalife (Eds.), *Cardiac electrophysiology.* Philadelphia, PA: W. B. Saunders Co.

Verrier, R. L., Calvert, A., and Lown, B. (1975). Effect of posterior hypothalamic stimulation on ventricular fibrillation threshold. *American Journal of Physiology, 228,* 923–927.

Verrier, R. L., and Dickerson, L. W. (1991). Autonomic nervous system and coronary blood flow changes related to emotional activation and sleep. *Circulation, 83* (Suppl 2), II-81–II-89.

Walker, B. B., and Sandman, C. A. (1979). Human visual evoked responses are related to heart rate. *Journal of Comparative Physiology and Psychology, 93,* 717–729.

Walker, B. B., and Sandman, C. A. (1982). Visual evoked potentials change as heart rate and carotid pressure change. *Psychophysiology, 19,* 520.

Weidler, D. J., Das, S. K., and Sodeman, T. M. (1976). Cardiac arrhythmias secondary to acute cerebral ischemia: prevention by autonomic blockade. *Circulation, 53,* II-102.

Weiss, T., Cheatle, M. D., Rubin, S. I., Reichek, N., and Brady, J. P. (1985). Effects of repeated ambulatory ECG monitoring and relaxation practice on premature ventricular contractions. *Psychosomatic Medicine, 47,* 446–450.

Werntz, D. A., Bickford, R., Bloom, F., and Shannahoff-Khalsa, D. (1983). Alternating cerebral hemispheric activity and the lateralization of autonomic nervous function. *Human Neurobiology, 2,* 39–43.

Werntz, D., Bickford, R., and Shannahoff-Khalsa, D. (1987). Selective hemispheric stimulation by unilateral forced nostril breathing. *Neurobiology, 6,* 165–171.

Wheeler, R. E., Davidson, R. J., and Tomarken, A. J. (1993). Frontal brain asymmetry and emotional reactivity: a biological substrate of affective style. *Psychophysiology, 30,* 82–89.

Williams, R. B. J., Haney, T. L., Lee, K. L., Kong, Y., Blumenthal, J. A., and Whalen, R. E. (1980). Type A behavior, hostility, and coronary atherosclerosis. *Psychosomatic Medicine, 42,* 539–549.

Winfree, A. T. (1983). Sudden cardiac death: A problem in topology. *Scientific American, 248,* 144–161.

Winfree, A. T. (1987). *When time breaks down.* Princeton, NJ: Princeton University Press.

Wittling, W. (1990). Psychophysiological correlates of human brain asymmetry: blood pressure changes during lateralized presentation of an emotionally laden film. *Neuropsychologia, 28,* 457–470.

Yamour, B. J., Sridharan, M. R., Rice, J. R., and Flower, N. C. (1980). Electrocardiographic changes in cerebrovascular hemorrhage. *American Heart Journal, 99,* 294–300.

Yanowitz, F., Preston, J. B., and Abildskov, J. A. (1966). Functional distribution of right and left stellate innervation to the ventricles: production of neurogenic electrocardiographic changes by unilateral alteration of sympathetic tone. *Circulation Research, 28,* 416–428.

Yeap, L. L. (1989). Hemisphericity and student achievement. *International Journal of Neuroscience, 48,* 225–232.

Yeung, A. C., Vekshtein, V. I., Krantz, D. S., Vita, J. A., Ryan T. J., Jr., Ganz, P., and Selwyn, A. P. (1991). The effect of atherosclerosis on the vasomotor response of coronary arteries to mental stress. *New England Journal of Medicine, 325,* 1551–1556.

Yokoyama, K., Jennings, J. R., Ackles, P., Hood, P., and Boiler, F. (1987). Lack of heart rate changes during an attention-demanding task after right hemisphere lesions. *Neurology, 37,* 624–630.

Zamrini, E. Y., Meador, K. J., Loring, D. W., Nichols, F. T., Lee, G. P., Figueroa, R. E., and Thompson, W. O. (1990). Unilateral cerebral inactivation produces differential left/right heart rate responses. *Neurology, 40,* 1408–1411.

Zipes, D. P. (1991). The long QT interval syndrome: a Rosetta Stone for sympathetic related ventricular tachyarrhythmias. *Circulation, 84,* 1414–1419.

Zoccolotti, P., Caltagirone, C., Benedetti, N., and Gainotti, G. (1986). Perturbation des réponses végétatives aux stimuli émotionnels au cours des lésions hémisphériques unilaterales. *L'Encéphale, 12,* 263–268.

Zoccolotti, P., Scabini, D., and Violani, C. (1981). Electrodermal responses in patients with unilateral brain damage. *Journal of Clinical Neuropsychology, 4,* 143.

12 Brain Asymmetry in the Control of Autonomic-Physiologic Activity

Werner Wittling

Since Roger Sperry's pioneering work on the functioning of the surgically disconnected hemispheres in split-brain patients, the functional asymmetry of the cerebral hemispheres has been one of the most extensively studied aspects of the brain. It is now a well-established fact that the hemispheres clearly differ in their basic mode of cognitive processing (Trevarthen, 1990). In more recent times, Gainotti (1972, 1983) and other authors have advocated the view that emotion-related processes, too, are lateralized within the brain. Although the laterality model underlying brain control of emotional processes is somewhat disputed (Gainotti, 1989; Silberman and Weingartner, 1986), the fundamental assumption of asymmetric regulation of affect has received support from a vast number of experimental and clinical studies. In contrast, the considerable methodologic demands and the unjustified assumption that physiologic processes subjected largely to subcortical control cannot be regulated in an asymmetric manner have, in the past, prevented an extensive study of brain asymmetry in the control of autonomic-physiologic functions. In the first comprehensive review of this field of research, an attempt is undertaken in this chapter to characterize the state of research with respect to some of the most fundamental physiologic systems and to provide empirical and theoretical evidence supporting the view that brain asymmetry is a universal phenomenon characterizing functioning of the whole neural system.

ASYMMETRY IN NEUROTRANSMITTER ACTIVITY

Neurotransmitters are chemical substances that are used by any particular nerve cell to transmit electrical nerve impulses and to communicate with other cells. They play a critical role in the transmission of nerve impulses both in peripheral parts of the body, especially in the sympathetic and parasympathetic nervous system, and in the brain itself. Among the central neurotransmitters, the brain monoamines norepinephrine, serotonin, and dopamine are of critical importance for the regulation of a wide spectrum of human and animal behavior, including cognitive and emotional responses, but also arousal and autonomic-physiologic processes.

Noradrenergic Activity

Noradrenergic neurons have their cell bodies mainly in the pontine locus ceruleus. The major efferent pathway projects to widespread regions in the mesencephalon, thalamus, and limbic system including the amygdaloid body, hippocampus, entorhinal cortex, and septum. The majority of neocortical innervation derives from fibers that enter the cortex at the frontal pole, the great bulk originating in the ipsilateral locus ceruleus. There is a homogeneous and moderately to highly dense innervation of the whole cortical matter with an especially dense distribution of noradrenergic fibers in the cingulate gyrus and prefrontal orbital cortex (Fallon and Loughlin, 1987).

The noradrenergic system seems to be of central importance for the cerebral regulation of arousal, attention-related functions, and adaptive responses of the organism to stress and environmental stimulation. This has been demonstrated by studies showing that discharge rates of central noradrenergic cells in the locus ceruleus are significantly elevated in situations that imply a physiologic challenge to the organism (Morilak, Fornal, and Jacobs, 1987), evoke orienting behavior, or require selective attention to novel or relevant environmental information (Clark, Geffen, and Geffen, 1987). Aside from its arousing effects, norepinephrine seems to be involved in the modulation of affective behavior. Brain norepinephrine is decreased in some types of depression, and antidepressant drugs, which increase the amount of norepinephrine acting on the postsynaptic receptors, have ameliorative influences on the depressive symptomatology (Schildkraut, 1965; Garver and Zemlan, 1986). The role of central norepinephrine in immunoregulation is somewhat unclear. Although its main effects seem to be immunosuppressive, at least some aspects of immune function may be enhanced by central noradrenergic activity (Dunn, 1989; Besedovsky, del Rey, and Sorkin, 1985).

Studies assessing *asymmetries* in noradrenergic brain innervation are of two different types. In one approach, norepinephrine distribution is measured biochemically by means of high-pressure liquid chromatography in bilaterally symmetric brain dissections of either human postmortem brains or brain tissues of normal untreated animals. The other approach, using the same biochemical measurement technique, studies the effects of symmetrically placed left- or right-sided lesions on the norepinephrine content in brain dissections of the animal's ipsilateral or contralateral hemisphere.

Oke et al. (1978) were the first to study norepinephrine concentration in the thalamus of five human brains obtained after routine autopsy. With the exception of the pulvinar region, which had a higher norepinephrine concentration on the left brain side, the whole thalamus showed a clearly higher norepinephrine concentration on the right side. Similar findings were reported by Oke, Lewis, and Adams (1980) for the rat thalamus, with higher left-sided values in some anterior regions and a right-sided norepinephrine lateralization extending over the middle and posterior thalamic regions. Likewise, Barnéoud, Le Moal, and Neveu (1990) found higher norepinephrine values in the right anterior hypothalamus of the mouse brain, whereas Kabani, Reader, and Dykes (1990) could not extend these results to the rat cortex.

The asymmetric distribution of brain norepinephrine, reported in most of the above-mentioned studies, is confirmed by studies assessing the effects of unilateral brain lesions on noradrenergic activity. To determine whether there are asymmetries in the biochemical consequences of right as opposed to left hemisphere infarction, Robinson (1979) compared the effects of right vs. left middle cerebral artery ligation in rats. Radioenzyme assays measuring brain norepinephrine revealed that right hemisphere infarction led to a significant reduction of norepinephrine in the lesioned cortex as well as in the unlesioned posterior cortex and locus ceruleus of the ipsilateral hemisphere, amounting to up to 30% in comparison with sham-operated animals. Norepinephrine concentration was also clearly reduced in the frontotemporal and posterior cortex of the contralateral hemisphere. In contrast, left hemisphere infarction exerted no significant effects on norepinephrine concentration, neither in the ipsilateral nor in the contralateral cortex or locus ceruleus.

These findings have been consistently confirmed by other studies of the same research group using either middle cerebral artery ligation or small cortical suction lesions to induce cerebral damage (Dewberry et al., 1986; Moran et al., 1986; Pearlson and Robinson, 1981), as well as by recently performed studies of other research groups (Barnéoud, Le Moal, and Neveu, 1991; Hachinski et al., 1992). On the whole, the above-mentioned results, derived from two different experimental approaches, present a quite consistent picture suggesting that the noradrenergic innervation—the biochemical substrate of arousal (Tucker and Williams, 1984)—shows a clear right hemisphere asymmetry.

Serotonergic Activity

Serotonin or 5-hydroxytryptamine (5-HT) innervation in the brain is derived mainly from neurons located in the dorsal, and to a lesser extent, in the median raphe nuclei of the mesencephalon. The projections of the 5-HT cells of the raphe nuclei are predominantly ipsilateral, running through the median forebrain bundle (Fallon and Loughlin, 1987). The serotonergic innervation is widespread, supplying nearly all regions of the hypothalamus, thalamus, amygdala, and hippocampus, as well as the mesencephalon and cerebellum. The cortical innervation is especially dense and uniform, with highly dense innervation in the frontal and visual cortex and lower innervation in the primary motor cortex (Fallon and Loughlin, 1987).

It is generally believed that serotonin is an inhibitory neurotransmitter depressing the discharge rate of cerebral neurons, reducing arousal, and inhibiting the activity of the noradrenergic system (Birbaumer and Schmidt, 1991). As for its role in modulating immunity, most data indicate that serotonin exerts a net immunosuppressive effect (Hall and Goldstein, 1985). There is also a considerable body of research examining the potential role of serotonin in the regulation of affective states, behavior, and psychopathologic disorders (Spoont, 1992). Although there are contradictory findings, the prevailing hypothesis suggests that serotonergic dysfunction may contribute to depressive disorders and suicidal behavior (Arora and Meltzer, 1989a,b; Asberg et al., 1987; Meltzer and Lowy, 1987). Especially in postmortem studies, lower concentrations of 5-HT and 5-HIAA (5-hydroxyindoleacetic acid), the major metabolite of 5-HT, have been reported in midbrain raphe nuclei of suicide victims, as opposed to normal control subjects.

The existence of an *asymmetric distribution* of serotonergic innervation and activity has been studied in human postmortem brain tissue samples as well as in the living brains of normal and brain-damaged subjects.

Mayberg et al. (1988) measured cortical S2 serotonin receptor binding by means of positron emission tomography (PET) in normal control subjects and patients with either right or left hemisphere strokes. Whereas no right-left asymmetry was found in receptor binding in any of the cortical regions in control subjects and left hemisphere stroke patients, right hemisphere stroke patients showed a significantly higher S2 serotonin receptor binding in the noninjured temporal and parietal regions of the damaged right hemisphere, as opposed to the symmetric regions of the nondamaged left hemisphere. The authors postulated that the observed upregulation of cortical S2 receptors in the damaged right hemisphere is due to a much greater extent of serotonin depletion by right hemisphere stroke. Therefore, the results point to a greater right hemisphere involvement in serotonergic brain activity.

At present, the most extensive findings on serotonergic asymmetry come from research done in postmortem specimens from brains of suicide victims and humans who died from natural causes. Although there are contradictory findings, and asymmetry in serotonergic activity has not been found in all studies (Arora and Meltzer, 1991), there is a clear tendency toward a right hemisphere serotonin lateralization in normal nondepressive humans and toward a reversed lateralization in suicide victims. In the first study of this type, Arató and colleagues (1987) measured 5-HT and 5-HIAA content as well as the number of ^{3}H-imipramine binding sites (B max) in the frontal cortex and hippocampus of suicide victims and normal controls. ^{3}H-Imipramine binding sites are present on serotonergic neurons in the brain and are believed to be allosteric regulators of the 5-HT uptake sites (Marcusson, Backstrom, and Ross, 1986). Whereas 5-HT and 5-HIAA contents did not differ between the hemispheres, the number of imipramine binding sites was significantly higher in the right as opposed to the left frontal cortex of normal controls. According to the authors, this finding indicates an increased net serotonergic transmission and hence a higher serotonergic activity in the right hemisphere of normal subjects. In contrast, suicide victims showed a significantly higher B max for imipramine binding in the left as compared with the right hemisphere.

Subsequent studies by Tekes et al. (1988), Demeter et al. (1989), and Arató et al. (1991a) in adult human subjects consistently supported the above-mentioned finding, indicating a right hemisphere asymmetry of serotonergic activity in normal humans and a reversed neurotransmitter pattern in suicide victims. As reported by Arató et al. (1991b), higher B max values of imipramine binding have been found in 87% of the biochemically analyzed brains of 62 normal human subjects studied to date. Since right hemisphere serotonin lateralization has already been demonstrated in neonates (Frecska et al., 1990) it seems to be an inborn feature of human brain organization. Unfortunately, there are no handedness data to date.

Altogether, there are strong indications that serotonin, too, shows a right hemisphere lateralization. Therefore, it may be assumed that both neurotransmitter substances being mostly involved in the upregulation (norepinephrine) and downregulation (serotonin) of arousal, and having reciprocally inhibitory relations (Flor-Henry, 1986), are asymmetrically distributed, favoring the right side of the brain. Moreover, it cannot be excluded that alterations of this normal innervation pattern are correlated with affective and behavioral abnormalities.

Dopaminergic Activity

Dopaminergic brain innervation arises from neurons located in the ventral mesencephalon, forming two subsystems. In the cortex there is dense dopamine innervation in prefrontal, premotor, and motor areas and a relatively sparse innervation in posterior regions. Generally, there is a preferential innervation of motor vs. sensory cortices and association areas vs. primary sensory areas (Fallon and Loughlin, 1987). Therefore, it is assumed that dopamine is involved in higher integrative cortical functions and in the regulation of cortical output activity, especially in motor control. The above conclusions, based on anatomic studies, are corroborated by findings from lesion and pharmacologic studies (Clark, Geffen, and Geffen, 1987), indicating that the integrity of the dopaminergic pathways is critical for the selection and carrying out of appropriate motor responses and for the coordination of motor output with sensory input.

Since dopamine seems to be closely involved in the control of motor activity, *asymmetric dopamine innervation* should favor the hemisphere primarily responsible for motor control. Therefore, in humans, showing an overwhelming majority of right-handedness in population, a higher dopamine concentration should be expected in the contralateral left hemisphere. This is exactly what has been found in empirical studies.

Glick, Ross, and Hough (1982) reanalyzed data on neurotransmitter concentrations in the left and right sides of various brain regions collected by Rossor, Garrett, and Iversen (1980) in postmortem studies of 14 normal human subjects. Results demonstrate that dopamine content is significantly higher in the left globus pallidus than in the right globus pallidus. Although handedness data were lacking, it should be assumed that most subjects were right-handed. Likewise, PET imaging of dopamine receptors in the living brain revealed higher concentrations of dopamine terminals in the left than in the right basal ganglia in a human case study (Wagner et al., 1983).

Results obtained in human studies are corroborated by animal studies. Asymmetries have been found in the striatum and cortex of rat and mice brains with respect to dopamine content (Glick et al., 1980; Zimmerberg, Glick, and Jerussi, 1974), dopamine metabolism (Yamamoto and Freed, 1984), dopamine-stimulated adenylate cyclase activity (Glick et al., 1983), and striatal dopamine receptors (Schneider, Murphy, and Coons, 1982). These asymmetries in dopaminergic innervation are related to various kinds of motor-behavioral asymmetries (Castellano et al., 1989). The great majority of studies suggest that dopamine concentration is significantly higher in the neostriatum contralateral to the animal's side or hand preference, asymmetry amounting to 10% to 15% in experimentally naive animals (Zimmerberg et al., 1974). However, it must be mentioned that there are contradictory results, too, either finding no consistent relationship between behavioral and biochemical asymmetries in male animals or revealing two subpopulations of rats differing in their relationship between dopamine asymmetry and behavioral responses (Glick et al., 1987; Shapiro, Camarota, and Glick, 1987).

The main conclusion that can be drawn from the above data is that lateralization of brain neurotransmitters seems to take place in close correspondence with lateralization in other physiologic and psychological functions. Neurotransmitters such as norepinephrine and serotonin, being closely involved in the upregulation or downregulation of autonomic and psychological arousal, show a relatively higher concentration in the right side of the human and animal brain, emphasizing the right hemisphere's well-known role in cerebral control of arousal. In contrast, neurotransmitters such as dopamine, being more intimately involved in the control of motor behavior and higher integrative functions, obviously favor the left side of the human brain, whose leading role in the control of these functions is undisputed.

ASYMMETRY IN NEUROENDOCRINE ACTIVITY

Aside from the neural system, the hormonal system is the second main control system of the body, regulating a wide spectrum of miscellaneous biological processes in the organism. In contrast to the neural system, transmitting information along fixed pathways by the aid of chemical neurotransmitters, the hormonal system makes use of blood circulation to send information to the target organs where it is decoded by hormone-specific receptors. There is extensive reciprocal influence between both systems. Cerebral control of hormonal activity is mainly provided by the hypothalamus, being itself under the influence of the midbrain, the limbic system, the amygdala, and the frontal cortex (Feldman, 1989; Schmidt and Thews, 1989).

Animal research on lateralization of neuroendocrine control has largely been associated with the laboratory of Gerendai, and detailed reviews of these research approaches have been presented by Gerendai (1984, 1987). Asymmetry in endocrine brain mechanisms has for the first time been demonstrated in a study by Gerendai et al. (1978). These authors observed that in intact female rats concentration of hypothalamic *luteinizing hormone–releasing hormone (LHRH)* was significantly higher in the right mediobasal hypothalamus than in the left. As stated by the authors, the asymmetry proved to be unexpectedly stable with no reversal in direction or absence of difference in any animal.

Results supporting these observations and presenting further evidence for a hypothalamic laterality in the regulation of LHRH release and in the control of gonadal function in rodents have subsequently been reported by several research groups. Bakalkin and colleagues (1984) found a significantly higher content of LHRH in the right as opposed to the left side of the hypothalamus in rats. Fukuda and co-workers (1984) showed that the ovarian compensatory hypertrophy in female rats was effectively suppressed by unilateral lesions of the right side of the hypothalamus. Finally, in a more recent study by Inase and Machida (1992) LHRH-immunoreactive cells were found to be more numerous in the right side of the brain than in the left side in male mice. In addition, they found that right-sided but not left-sided hemiorchidectomy caused a decrease in the amount of LHRH in the mouse brain.

Further studies by Gerendai and collaborators revealed that *prolactin secretion*, too, seems to be predominantly controlled by the right brain in male rats (Gerendai et al., 1985b). However, no evidence of asymmetric control of *thyrotropin releasing hormone (TRH) secretion* has been found by Gerendai et al. (1985a).

A further finding reported by Gerendai (1984) deserves mention, although it is not exclusively related to the topic of neuroendocrine control. Animals with experimental unilateral lesions of the medial preoptic area, lower brainstem, or medial basal hypothalamus had two to three times higher mortality rates if the lesions were performed in the right brain than if identical lesions were performed in the left brain. Although these brain regions are known to play a critical role in the regulation of neuroendocrine functions, they exert control on many other vital functions, too. Therefore, it cannot be decided whether this effect is caused by damage to neuroendocrine or to other physiologic mechanisms. Nevertheless, the results seem to support the conclusion that the right brain is more critically involved in vital functions than the left.

Asymmetry in cerebral regulation of cortisol secretion in humans has recently been studied for the first time by Wittling and Pflüger (1990). One hundred twenty-three normal right-handed subjects were shown either an emotionally aversive or a neutral film in their left or right visual hemifield. Both films were black-and-white video films, lasted 3 minutes, and were presented without sound. In the aversive film the electroconvulsive treatment of a patient was shown, whereas the neutral film showed a group of alpinists walking along a snowed-up but undangerous mountain pass. The technique of lateralized film presentation developed in our laboratory is based on the principle that an electronic mask that is yoked to the subject's eye movements recorded by an infrared oculometer moves horizontally on the video monitor and masks off the vertical meridian and either the left or right visual hemifield irrespective of the eye movement. Therefore, the film can only be perceived in one preselected visual hemifield. Moreover, in previous studies by our team it has been regularly found that cerebral asymmetry in the control of various physiologic functions such as cortisol (Roschmann, Wittling, and Pflüger, 1992; Wittling, 1990b), blood pressure (Wittling, 1990a), or heart rate (Wittling and Schweiger, 1992a) is markedly enhanced if lateralized visual input is combined with lateralized motor responding to the film's content. The observed asymmetry is highest if the hemisphere which laterally perceives the film is caused to engage more actively in processing the film's content by simultaneously carrying out a film-related response by the corresponding contralateral hand. Therefore, in the present study only completely lateralized experimental conditions were compared, with both visual perception and motor responding being bound to the same hemisphere. To accomplish lateralized motor responding, subjects were instructed to judge the film's content continuously with respect to the emotional arousal they felt at any moment by turning a small revolving disk in a semicircular direction with the forefinger of the hand being controlled by the film-perceiving hemisphere. Film-related changes of cortisol secretion relative to a prefilm baseline were determined by salivary cortisol radioimmunoassay.

Results indicate that with respect to the whole group cortisol secretion is distinctly affected by the film's emotion-related attributes. The aversive film, judged as emotionally arousing, led to significantly higher cortisol increases than the neutral control film, which had been judged to elicit only weak feelings of subjective arousal. Right hemisphere presentation of the emotionally aversive film went along with significantly higher increases of cortisol secretion than left hemisphere presentation of the same film. These differences occured within a time period of 5 to 40 minutes after film presentation, reaching their peak values 15 to 30 minutes after the end of the film. No such differences could be detected with respect to the neutral film, indicating that hemispheric differences in response to the emotional film are not caused by differing responses to visual stimulation, in general. Comparing the effects of the two films separately for each hemisphere revealed that only the right hemisphere is able to respond neuroendocrinologically in a different manner to emotional and nonemotional stimuli, showing clearly higher cortisol responses to the emotional film. In contrast, with the left hemisphere film presentation no differences could be observed in cortisol response to both films. Therefore, it can be concluded that cortical regulation of cortisol secretion in emotion-related situations is under the primary control of the right hemisphere, whereas the left hemisphere seems to play only a subordinate role.

As was only briefly mentioned in the original paper (Wittling and Pflüger, 1990, p. 260) we additionally tried to decide on the question whether the observed asymmetry is the direct result of an asymmetric efficiency of the cerebral mechanisms involved in cortisol regulation or only the indirect consequence of higher subjective-emotional arousal often associated with right hemisphere stimulation. Therefore, subjects' emotional responses to the presented films were evaluated by means of 10-point rating scales assessing the degree of general emotional arousal brought forth by the films, the emotional valence of the films, and the degree of ten specific emotions felt during film presentation (Wittling and Pflüger, 1990, p. 245). Each film was rated immediately after the end of the film by those subjects who had seen the respective film under lateralized viewing conditions. The end points of the rating scales were verbally defined as "extremely low" (0) vs. "extremely high" (10). Data were analyzed by means of 2- × 2- × 2-factor ANOVAs (analyses of variance) with the independent variables Film (aversive, neutral), Hemisphere (left, right), and Gender (male, female). In table 12.1, mean values of subjective-emotional responses are depicted together with the respective F values for the main effects of Hemisphere and the interaction effects of Hemisphere × Film, being particularly relevant in this connection.

As can be seen from table 12.1, ANOVAs do not shield any significant differences between left hemisphere and right hemisphere film presentation (main effect of the variable Hemisphere). Moreover, contrary to the cortisol data, there is no evidence pointing to a stronger right hemisphere superiority in response to the emotionally aversive film as opposed to the neutral film (Hemisphere × Film interaction). Therefore, the above-presented data provide some indirect evidence favoring the hypothesis that the observed asymmetry in neuroendocrine regulation is likely to be a *self-reliant process* not depending on subjective-emotional asymmetry.

More direct evidence in favor of this hypothesis has recently been found in a yet unpublished study by me. Forty subjects were presented in their left visual hemifield an emotionally aversive film showing traffic accidents and their victims and a second film matched with respect to contents and emotion-related qualities was presented in their right visual hemifield. Intraindividual difference scores were calculated for the strength of cortisol responses measured under both conditions of lateralized film presentation. Likewise, intraindividual difference scores were calculated for the strength of subjective-emotional arousal assessed on-line and continuously during both conditions of lateralized film presentation by means of our manual-motor rating technique (e.g., Wittling and Roschmann, 1993). Preliminary results reveal that intraindividual asymmetry scores for cortisol responses and subjective-emotional arousal were not correlated ($r = -.052$) and that more than 40% of subjects showing right hemisphere superiority with respect to cortisol regulation failed to show right hemisphere superiority with respect to subjective-emotional arousal. This result indicates that brain asymmetry in cortisol regulation can hardly be attributed to hemispheric differences in subjective-emotional arousal.

Having shown that cerebral regulation of cortisol secretion is normally characterized by a functional asymmetry favoring right hemisphere control,

Table 12.1 Retrospective ratings of subjective-emotional responses to the emotionally aversive film and the neutral control film

Emotional quality	Neutral film		Aversive film		$F\,(1,\,115)$	
	Left hemisphere	Right hemisphere	Left hemisphere	Right hemisphere	Main effect Hemisphere	Hemisphere × film interaction
General emotional arrousal	1.4	2.5	6.1	6.3	2.53	0.58
Positive valence	5.8	5.9	2.1	2.1	0.00	0.02
Compassion	0.9	1.6	6.1	6.9	2.69	0.15
Disgust	0.4	0.7	5.9	6.7	1.83	0.64
Anger	0.6	1.1	4.7	5.7	2.13	0.39
Anxiety	0.9	1.5	3.6	3.9	1.58	0.25
Sadness	0.9	1.5	4.9	3.7	0.43	3.45
Aesthetic sensation	5.5	4.7	2.1	1.9	0.73	0.12
Relaxation	4.7	3.7	0.7	0.4	3.37	0.48
Tenderness	0.6	1.3	0.7	0.6	0.67	1.44
Joy	2.3	3.4	0.4	0.2	1.15	2.59
Well-being	3.7	3.5	0.2	0.3	0.08	0.47

we recently started a series of studies examining the association between *alterations of brain asymmetry in cortisol regulation* and physical well-being and health. The impetus to these studies was given by the unique role cortisol plays in the regulation of human behavior and in the pathogenesis of disease, recognized by most biopsychological disease models of the present (Reinert and Wittling, 1980). We know that chronically elevated cortisol levels are associated with the development of various diseases such as atherosclerosis (Troxler et al., 1977) and neoplastic disease (Sklar and Anisman, 1981). On the other hand, an adequate level of cortisol seems to be a necessary prerequisite to guaranteeing an undisturbed functioning of the organism, increasing resistance to stress (Munck, Guyre, and Holbrook, 1984), enhancing immunoreactivity (Cupps and Fauci, 1982; Dunn, 1989), and preventing disease (Munck et al., 1984). Therefore, cortisol secretion is enhanced in a wide variety of stress-related situations of a physical or psychosocial nature ranging from emotional threats and challenges to work stress, noxious stimuli, antigen challenge, and illness. The physiologic function of these stress-induced increases in corticosteroid levels is mainly to protect the organism against its own normal defense reactions that are activated by stress and, if not damped or switched off, would damage the organism in a variety of ways (Munck et al., 1984). By exerting suppressive effects on virtually every phase and component of the immune and the inflammatory response, as well as by its impact on metabolic, renal, endocrine, and neural functions (Meyer, 1985), cortisol prevents defense reactions from overshooting and threatening homeostasis. Therefore, both a chronically elevated and an abnormally low cortisol level should be associated with disturbed physiologic functioning and health problems.

Preliminary evidence has been obtained suggesting that in left-handers both normal right hemisphere lateralization of cortisol regulation seems to be altered (Wittling and Schweiger, 1992b) and cortisol response to psychosocial stress in natural situations is clearly reduced as compared to right-handers (Wittling and Schweiger, 1992a). Since left-handers are suspected of having more serious health problems (Coren and Halpern, 1991; Schweiger, Wittling, and Roschmann, 1992) and a higher number of immune disorders (Geschwind and Behan, 1982, 1984), it seems not illogical to assume that alterations of brain asymmetry in the control of cortisol secretion possibly go along with less efficient and less adaptive neural mechanisms of cortisol regulation, and consequently with a greater amount of health problems. To study this hypothesis in a more general way, asymmetry in cerebral control of cortisol secretion was assessed in normal right-handed subjects reporting a "high degree of physical complaints" as compared with subjects reporting only a "low degree of physical complaints" (Wittling and Schweiger, 1993a). They were selected according to their values in the scale "physical complaints" of the Freiburger Personality Inventory (Fahrenberg, Hampel, and Selg, 1984). The scale is based on self-report and allows the calculation of a total score representing the degree of subjective complaints in several functional systems of the body (vasomotor, gastrointestinal, cardiovascular, neuromuscular,

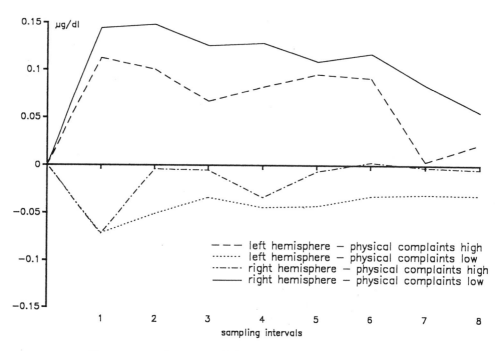

Figure 12.1 Salivary cortisol changes in the groups with high vs. low physical complaints following left hemisphere vs. right hemisphere film presentation.

pain-related, and sleep disorders). Prior studies have shown that the scale clearly discriminates between healthy persons and patients treated in psychosomatic hospitals. To obtain additional information about their physical health status, all subjects were administered a disease questionnaire assessing both incidence and recurrence of specific diseases in 12 different disease categories during the last year as well as the degree of subjective impairment and the number of visits to the physician during this time span. The groups with a high as opposed to a low degree of physical complaints were significantly different with respect to all measures of this disease questionnaire.

To assess hemispheric asymmetry in cortisol regulation, subjects (n = 56) were presented the emotionally aversive film, used in the above reported study, either in their left or right visual hemifield. The technical procedure also corresponded to that used in the previous study. In order to control for the well-known effect that cortisol concentration continuously decreases during an experimental session, cortisol values were represented as difference scores to the corresponding values of a control group (n = 68) viewing a neutral control film, but being identical with the experimental subjects in all control variables assessed. Film-related cortisol changes were determined at eight sampling intervals during a period of 80 minutes after the end of the film presentation.

As may be seen from figure 12.1, there is a clear relationship between physical complaints and asymmetry in cerebral regulation of cortisol. The overall test of interaction between the variables Film-Perceiving Hemisphere and Degree of Physical Complaints reveals highly significant differences, as do the single tests of interaction for six out of eight sampling intervals. Subjects with a low degree of physical complaints are characterized by the expected pattern of brain asymmetry already found in the above-reported study (Wittling and Pflüger, 1990). As a group, they respond with clearly higher cortisol increases if the emotionally aversive film is presented laterally to the visual areas of the right cerebral hemisphere than if the same film is presented laterally to the left hemisphere's visual areas. In contrast, subjects with a high degree of physical complaints show an altered pattern of cerebral cortisol regulation. In this group of subjects, normal right hemisphere dominance in brain control of cortisol secretion is lost and clear expression of brain asymmetry is lacking. Moreover, there is a statistically insignificant tendency for brain asymmetry to be reversed in direction, with the left brain side showing relatively stronger cortisol responses.

In this study, too, the potential relationship between cortisol-related brain asymmetry and asymmetry in subjective-emotional arousal was examined, using the same retrospective ratings of subjective-emotional responses as in the aforementioned study by Wittling and Pflüger (1990; see table 12.1). Analysis of subjects' emotional responses to lateralized film presentation by means of 2- × 2- × 2-factor ANOVAs with the independent variables Hemisphere (left, right), Physical Complaints (high, low), and Gender (male, female) revealed that the differences in brain asymmetry of cortisol regulation found between subjects with a high vs. a low degree of physical complaints are self-reliant mechanisms and are, obviously, neither the results of differences in emotional reactivity nor in emotion-related brain asymmetry between both groups of subjects. Whereas subjects with a high vs. a low degree of physical complaints differ significantly in their patterns of cortisol-related brain asymmetry, they show no differences in their amount of emotional responsiveness to the presented film and, particularly, in their emotion-related brain asymmetry.

It should be remembered that the indices of cerebral asymmetry used in the above-described study are based on a comparison between different groups of subjects, one group of subjects being examined under left hemisphere lateralization conditions, the other group being examined under right hemisphere lateralization conditions. Moreover, subjects were selected according to the criterion Physical Complaints. The disadvantage of this proceeding is to be seen in the fact that it does not permit a direct examination of the effects of various asymmetry patterns, and in particular that it does not allow a statement about the risk of developing physical problems that is associated with altered brain asymmetry. In a recently completed study we dealt with this problem, trying to predict physical complaints from the individual's specific pattern of brain asymmetry in cortisol regulation. Intraindividual brain asymmetry scores were determined by calculating differences in cortisol responses to cognitively activating tasks (block design tasks), which subjects had to perform both under completely lateralized right hemisphere and under completely lateralized left hemisphere stimulus-response conditions. Depending on whether right hemisphere or left hemisphere task completion led to relatively stronger cortisol responses, subjects were classified as either right hemisphere–dominant or left hemisphere–dominant in cortisol regulation. Results indicate that strongly lateralized subjects clearly differ in the degree of self-reported physical complaints (Wittling and Schweiger, 1992b, 1993b). In accord with the above-presented findings, strongly lateralized left hemisphere–dominant subjects reported a significantly greater number of physical complaints than strongly lateralized right hemisphere–dominant subjects. In addition, the subject's specific pattern of neuroendocrine brain asymmetry could be used with relatively good success to separate individuals with high vs. low degrees of physical complaints. Therefore, the possibility cannot be excluded that alterations in cerebral control of cortisol secretion indeed influence physical well-being in a clinically relevant manner.

ASYMMETRY IN NEUROIMMUNOLOGIC ACTIVITY

The immune system has traditionally been assumed to be a self-monitoring system performing host defense to a great extent in an autoregulated way. Now that the intricate interactions of the cellular immune mechanisms with a plentitude of other physiologic processes have become obvious, the autonomy confered to immune processes is thought to be quite restricted. During the last decade, compelling evidence for a close *bidirectional communication* between the immune and the nervous systems has accumulated, indicating that the brain plays a decisive role in the modulation of immune functions (Calabrese, Kling, and Gold, 1987; Daruna and Morgan, 1990; Dunn, 1989). There are two different *mechanisms* enabling the brain to exert its control over the immunologic apparatus. Firstly, it may influence immunoresponsiveness directly via neural pathways of the sympathetic and parasympathetic nervous system innervating lymphoid tissues such as the thymus, spleen, bone marrow, or lymph nodes. In this case, neurotransmitters may locally regulate immune responses. Secondly, brain modulation of the immune response may be mediated indirectly by neuroendocrine pathways under hypothalamic and cortical control and exposed to regulatory feedback from the immune system. Especially, the corticosteroids of the hypothalamic-pituitary-adrenal axis seem to play a critical role in immunomodulation, having mainly immunosuppressive effects on several facets of the human and animal cellular immune response (Tsokos and Balow, 1986).

Since there is widespread evidence that lateralization is a main characteristic of anatomic and functional brain organization, and that several mechanisms involved in brain immunomodulation, such as emotional arousal, sympathetic innervation, neurotransmitter concentration, and neuroendocrine activity, are clearly lateralized, it seems most likely that the brain modulates immune response in an *asymmetric* manner.

The vast majority of studies examining brain asymmetry in neuroimmuno-modulation has been done with animals (mice or rats), using a lesion approach. In most of these studies, the influence of the neocortical hemispheres on immune functioning was investigated, whereas lateralized immunomodulation in subcortical structures has been investigated in only a few recently performed studies. As a rule, animals were randomly assigned to one of four surgical procedures: (1) partial right neocortical ablation, (2) partial left neocortical ablation, (3) sham operation, or (4) no surgery. In the majority of studies, unilateral lesions extended to about a third of the right or left hemisphere, involving the dorsal and lateral aspects of the frontal, parietal, and occipital cortex, without penetrating the corpus callosum (Renoux and Bizière, 1986). Immunologic testing was usually done 8 to 10 weeks after surgery to minimize the consequences of surgical stress on neuroendocrine and immunologic functions.

In one of the first studies, Bardos and colleagues (1981) found that natural killer (NK) cell activity of mouse spleen cells, thought to be indicative of spontaneous resistance against tumor cells, was significantly impaired following left cortical lesions, whereas right cortical lesions exerted no observable influence on NK cell activity, as compared with sham-operated or normal control animals. Similar findings were obtained by Renoux et al. (1983a) with respect to the capacity of the serum from left vs. right decorticated mice to release factors inducing the acquisition of cytotopic T-cell markers. The most extensive study on lateralized neocortical immunomodulation, confirming and extending prior results, has been done by Renoux et al. (1983b), who examined a broad spectrum of immune-related functions in mice (see also Bizière et al., 1985, and Renoux and Bizière, 1986): (1) Unilateral neocortical ablation of the dorsal and lateral aspects of the frontal, parietal, and occipital regions affected the development of lymphoid organs resulting in markedly reduced spleen and thymus weights in left-lesioned mice and in a significantly enhanced thymus weight in right-lesioned mice, compared to sham-operated animals. (2) The number of splenic T (Thy-1$^+$) cells was reduced in left-lesioned mice to about 50% of that of sham-operated mice, whereas it was unchanged in right-lesioned mice. In contrast, splenic B (sIg$^+$) cells were unaffected by either left or right decortication. (3) Functional immunocompetence of antibody-secreting spleen cells was determined by enumeration of plaque-forming spleen cells (PFCs) of the IgG and IgM class developed in response to immunization with sheep red blood cells (SRBCs). The number of IgG-PFCs, a T cell–dependent response, was significantly depressed following left cortical ablation and significantly elevated following right cortical ablation when compared with sham-operated animals. The number of IgM-PFCs, a B cell–dependent response, was not affected by either left or right hemisphere ablation. (4) In order to measure the capacity of T cells and B cells to respond to antigens, lymphocyte proliferation in response to mitogenic stimulation by phytohemagglutinin (PHA), concanavalin A (ConA), and pokeweed mitogen (PWM) was evaluated. Left cortical ablation significantly depressed the ability of splenic lymphocytes to be stimulated by the T cell–specific mitogens PHA and ConA, whereas right cortical ablation markedly enhanced lymphoproliferative responses to these mitogens. Neither right nor left hemisphere lesions affected responses to PWM, a B cell–specific mitogen.

The above findings were confirmed by other research groups using mice or rats as experimental animals (Barnéoud et al., 1988a,b). They indicate strongly that at least T cell–mediated immunity is modulated by the asymmetrically balanced activity of both hemispheres, probably playing opposite roles in neuroimmunomodulation. Whereas left hemisphere activity usually seems to enhance responsiveness of several T cell–dependent immune parameters, right hemisphere activity seems to be predominantly immunosuppressive. B cell–dependent processes do not seem to be critically influenced by cortical mechanisms, although there are some conflicting results (LaHoste et al., 1989; Neveu, 1988).

However, caution must be taken against generalizing the above results prematurely, as has been pointed out by Neveu (1992a,b). Firstly, all results are derived from animal studies and it remains to be determined whether they also hold for human immunity. Secondly, little is known about the cellular target of cortical immunomodulation, as well as about the pathophysiologic and clinical effects of experimental modulation of various immunologic parameters by lateralized neocortical lesions. Thirdly, the respective role of each hemisphere in neocortical immunomodulation is still controversial. Whereas most findings seem to support the assumption that both hemispheres are directly active on the immune system but in an opposite way, some authors have postulated that the right hemisphere only plays an indirect role in neuroimmunomodulation by controlling and inhibiting the left hemisphere's inductive signals, which in turn modulate immunoreactivity in a direct way (Renoux and Bizière, 1986; Renoux et al., 1987). Fourthly, findings have been presented suggesting that immune responses are not only influenced by the laterality of brain lesions but also by the intrahemispheric localization of neocortical ablation. Whereas in the above-mentioned studies lesions were rather extensive involving lateral frontal areas thought to be particularly critical for the cerebral regulation of vital functions, two further studies restraining lesions to parieto-occipital regions obtained diverging results with lymphoproliferation being more depressed following right cortical lesions than following left cortical lesions (LaHoste et al., 1989; Neveu, 1988). This indicates that cortical immunomodulation is much more complex than was thought and that each hemisphere probably contains both activating and suppressing areas which may communicate not only via commissural pathways (right-left axis) but also via associational corticocortical interconnections (anteroposterior axis). Fifthly, results obtained with the lesion approach may be affected by some built-in methodologic problems such as neuronal reorganization and other secondary functional changes taking place in the postoperative period and masking the hemisphere's normal role in immunomodulation (Barnéoud et al.,

1988a), as well as alterations in immunoregulatory feedback circuits modifying the immune-related activity of unlesioned brain regions (Neveu, 1992a,b).

To our knowledge, only one study to date has examined the relationship between brain asymmetry and immune function in *humans*. Kang and colleagues (1991) assessed immune responses in a group of 20 normal right-handed females, selected from an original sample of 90 right-handed females on the basis of extreme and stable patterns of hemispheric activation in the frontal scalp region. Hemispheric activation was measured electroencephalo-graphically (EEG) and defined by regional alpha power density, a measure that is inversely related to emotional or cognitive brain activation (R. J. Davidson, 1988). Asymmetry in hemispheric activation was computed as the difference between right hemisphere and left hemisphere frontal alpha power. Subjects scoring in the top or bottom 25th percentile of the distribution were selected and assigned to the left hemisphere or right hemisphere activation group. Measuring immunoresponsiveness, the groups did not differ in lymphocyte proliferation in response to the mitogens ConA, PHA, and PWM, or in the percentages of T-cell subsets, as would have been expected from animal results. However, both groups differed markedly in their NK cell activity, subjects with extreme left frontal activation showing significantly higher levels of NK cell activity than subjects with extreme right frontal activation. This finding, being in accord with the above-presented animal results, suggests that conclusions drawn from animal studies may hold for human immune responses too.

Finally, at least a brief comment on the relationship between *altered brain asymmetry* and *immune functioning* should be added. The studies reported above have shown that changes of hemispheric balance in neuroimmunomodulation, either by neocortical ablation of one hemisphere (as in animal research) or by a relatively higher activation of the other hemisphere (as in the study of Kang et al., 1991), have been found to result in altered immunoresponsiveness. Therefore, it should be expected that left-handedness, known to be associated with altered brain asymmetry, at least with respect to motor and language functions, may possibly be related to immunoresponsiveness in a significant way. Although we are at present not in a position to decide whether left-handers differ from right-handers in their specific pattern of immune-related brain asymmetry (e.g., Neveu et al., 1991), there is some evidence suggesting that right-handers and left-handers probably differ in *immunoresponsiveness*. Most of the relevant studies have been done with mice selected for right- or left-handedness by means of a paw preference test (Betancur et al., 1991; Fride et al., 1990; Neveu et al., 1988, 1991) or with New Zealand black mice known to spontaneously develop autoimmune disease such as lupuslike glomerulonephritis and hemolytic anemia (Neveu et al., 1989). Only very few studies have been done with humans (Burke et al., 1988; Chengappa et al., 1992). The results are highly complex and indicate that the assumed relationship between handedness and immunoresponsiveness is not only strain-dependent in animals but is, additionally, influenced by variables such as sex, strength of hand preference, and the specific immunologic parameters studied.

Inspired by some provocative articles by Geschwind and collaborators (Geschwind and Behan, 1982, 1984), considerable efforts have been made to study the association between left-handedness and *vulnerability to immune disorders in humans*. But results have been conflicting until now (Bryden, McManus, and Steenhuis, 1991; McManus, Naylor, and Brooker, 1990; Searleman and Fugagli, 1987; Smith, 1987) owing both to methodologic problems inherent in most studies and in lacking the validity of Geschwind's highly complex and speculative system of assumptions (Geschwind and Galaburda, 1985, 1987; McManus and Bryden, 1991; Wofsy, 1984). In our opinion, the main problem of this research approach may be seen in the fact that it is a somewhat isolated and premature attempt to relate handedness to clinically relevant aspects of immunity without (a) making due allowance for the above-presented body of basic animal research on immune-related brain asymmetry, (b) having knowledge about the relationship between variations of handedness and immune-related brain asymmetry, and (c) having adequate information about the possible consequences that alterations of the normal patterns of immune-related brain asymmetry will exert on various parameters of the individual's immunoreactivity. A better understanding of the relationships between handedness and immune disorders can only be expected if this research approach discontinues its present strategy and attempts to integrate itself into the body of basic research on neuroimmunomodulation asymmetry.

ASYMMETRY IN NEUROCARDIOLOGIC ACTIVITY

The brain controls cardiovascular processes primarily by modulating the outflow of sympathetic and parasympathetic pathways innervating the heart and blood vessels. *Sympathetic outflow* originates in neurons located in the dorsolateral and ventrolateral parts of the bulb and the medulla oblongata, known as vasomotor centers. Most sympathetic fibers innervating the heart funnel through the stellate ganglion (Levy and Martin, 1979). *Parasympathetic outflow* to the heart originates in preganglionic neurons of the dorsal motor nucleus of the vagus and the nucleus ambiguus, both being located in the medulla oblongata. Postganglionic sympathetic and parasympathetic fibers innervate the pacemaker cells of the sinoatrial (SA) node, the atrial myocardium, and the atrioventricular (AV) node. The ventricular myocardium is predominantly innervated by sympathetic fibers (Johnson, Lambie, and Spalding, 1984).

Sympathetic and parasympathetic regulation of cardiovascular processes is modulated by various descending pathways originating primarily in the hypothalamus and in the amygdala and projecting both to the bulbomedullary nuclei concerned with cardiovascular control and more directly to the preganglionic sympathetic neurons located in the intermediolateral cell column of the spinal cord (Price and Amaral, 1981; Spyer, 1989). There is now unequivocal evidence that not only subcortical structures but also the *cerebral cortex* are critically involved in the process of neurocardiomodulation. Firstly, studies using electrical stimulation in animals have revealed some major cortical regions where alterations in a wide spectrum of cardiovascular functions can be elicited reliably (Delgado, 1960; Hall, Livingstone, and Bloor, 1977; Hoff, Kell, and Carroll, 1963). Secondly, descending fibers have been identified that originate in the "visceral areas" of the cerebral cortex and project to brainstem areas concerned with cardiovascular regulation (Korner, 1979; Shipley, 1982; Wall and Davis, 1951). Thirdly, in animals, brain injury induced by cranial trauma, epidural and subdural compression, or experimental ischemic and hemorrhagic stroke has amply been documented to lead both to myocardial damage and to cardiac arrhythmias (Norris and Hachinski, 1987). Fourthly, in humans, electrocardiographic (ECG) abnormalities and cardiac arrhythmias have regularly been observed in patients with various kinds of brain damage (Norris and Hachinski, 1987; Talman, 1985).

Neural control of cardiovascular functions is a lateralized phenomenon which manifests itself at both the peripheral and central levels of the regulatory processes.

Peripheral Autonomic Control of Cardiac Activity

There is widespread evidence that both sympathetic and parasympathetic innervation of the heart are lateralized, influencing cardiac activity in an asymmetric manner. Neural control of *heart rate* is achieved mainly by sympathetic and parasympathetic innervation of the SA node. Sympathetic outflow results in accelerated heart rate, whereas parasympathetic outflow leads to heart rate deceleration. It has been shown that the distribution of sympathetic fibers to pacemaker tissues of the SA node consistently varies between the right and left sympathetic pathways (Randall, 1977). Most fibers innervating the SA node are carried by the right stellate cardiac nerves, whereas there is only a sparse supply from the left stellate cardiac nerves (Mizeres, 1958). A similar distribution is found with respect to parasympathetic innervation, supply to the SA node being mainly through the right vagus (Levy and Martin, 1979). In accord with lateralized SA innervation, autonomic control of the heart rate also works in an asymmetric manner. Cardiac acceleration resulting from stimulation of the right stellate ganglion in dogs is several times higher than acceleration produced by stimulation applied to the left sympathetic pathway (Kamosinska, Nowicki, and Szulczyk, 1989; Levy, Ng, and Zieske, 1966; Randall, 1977). Likewise, following right stellate ganglion block in humans, heart rate decreases considerably, whereas left stellate ganglion block fails to produce significant heart rate slowing (Rogers et al., 1978). Similar effects have been consistently found in dogs or cats after unilateral stellate ganglion block or unilateral stellate ganglionectomy (Schwartz, Stone, and Brown, 1976). Parasympathetic control of heart rate, too, is clearly more efficient when mediated by right vagal pathways. Therefore, heart rate deceleration is considerably more marked upon stimulation of the right vagus than upon left vagal stimulation (Hageman, Randall, and Armour, 1975; Irisawa, Caldwell, and Wilson, 1971). Similarly, transection of the right vagus nerve results in significantly greater heart rate acceleration than transection of the left vagus (Hamlin and Smith, 1968).

As has been shown repeatedly, *AV conduction time* is reduced by sympathetic and increased by parasympathetic innervation of the AV node. In contrast to the control of heart rate, the neural control of AV conduction seems to be mediated more efficiently by sympathetic and parasympathetic pathways running on the left side (Levy and Martin, 1979). Stimulation of the left stellate ganglion results in shorter AV conduction time than comparable stimulation of the right stellate ganglion (Goldberg and Randall, 1973; Irisawa et al., 1971). Left vagal stimulation causes prolongation of AV conduction time more consistently than right vagal stimulation and seems to induce first- and second-degree heart block (Hageman et al., 1975; Hamlin and Smith, 1968).

Myocardial contractility seems to be more efficiently controlled by sympathetic outflow resulting from the left sympathetic pathway. Left ventricular systolic pressure, a measure of contractile force, has been shown to rise much more following left as opposed to right stellate ganglion stimulation (Furnival, Linden, and Snow, 1973; Levy et al., 1966). Similarly, shortening of ventricular refractory periods is more marked following left than following right stellate ganglion stimulation (Haws and Burgess, 1978).

In recent years additional evidence has accumulated indicating that the right and left sympathetic pathways are asymmetrically involved in the genesis of cardiac *arrhythmias* and *ECG abnormalities* (Malliani, Schwartz, and Zanchetti, 1980; Schwartz, 1976). Electrical stimulation of the left cardiac sympathetic nerves often results in ventricular and supraventricular arrhythmias as well as in ectopic heart beats (Armour, Hageman, and Randall, 1972; Hageman et al., 1973). These abnormalities are only rarely observed following comparable stimulation of the right cardiac sympathetic nerves or following bilateral stimulation. Furthermore, left but not right stellate ganglion stimulation has been found to lead to prolonged QT intervals, an abnormality that is associated with ventricular arrhythmias and sudden cardiac death (Yanowitz, Preston, and Abildskov, 1966). Moreover, stimulation of the left stellate ganglion seems to be associated with vulnerability to ventricular fibrillation since it leads to a more marked decrease in ventricular fibrillation threshold than comparable right stellate ganglion stimulation (Lown, Verrier, and Rabinowitz, 1977).

Especially interesting are studies examining the effects of unilateral stellate ganglion blockade or unilateral stellectomy on the pathogenesis of arrhythmias. Schwartz, Stone, and Brown (1976) compared the effects of left vs. right stellate ganglion block in dogs in which small coronary arteries had been occluded to increase the risk of cardiac arrhythmias. It was found that blockade of the right stellate ganglion during coronary arterial occlusion increased the occurrence of cardiac arrhythmias such as ventricular tachycardia, ventricular fibrillation, and ectopic beats, as compared to control animals which had merely received coronary artery occlusion. In contrast, left stellate ganglion block had a protective effect on cardiac activity, consistently reducing or abolishing occlusion-induced arrhythmias. Asymmetric effects of left vs. right stellate ganglion block in line with the above-mentioned results have been observed with respect to other ECG abnormalities. Among other things, it has been found that the ventricular fibrillation threshold is decreased by ablating or cooling the right stellate ganglion and increased by ablating or cooling the left stellate ganglion (Schwartz, 1976; Schwartz, Snebold, and Brown, 1975). Also, rhythmic alterations in the polarity of the T waves have been repeatedly observed following right stellate block (Schwartz, Stone, and Brown, 1976) or other manipulations inducing left sympathetic dominance (Schwartz and Malliani, 1975). Finally, human as well as animal studies have demonstrated that unilateral stellate ganglion block asymmetrically affects the QT interval, in that right stellate ganglion block leads to QT prolongation, whereas left stellate ganglion block either has no effect or reduces the QT interval (Cinca et al., 1985; Moss and McDonald, 1971; Schwartz et al., 1976; Yanowitz et al., 1966). Physiologic mechanisms which may provide a working hypothesis to explain both the protective effects of left stellectomy and the paradoxical arrhythmogenic effects of right stellectomy have been proposed by Schwartz (1984). In view of the above-mentioned results, left sympathectomy has been used therapeutically to prevent lethal arrhythmias and sudden death in patients with a long QT syndrome (Malliani et al., 1980; Schwartz, 1984; Schwartz, Periti, and Malliani, 1975).

On the whole, findings on peripheral autonomic control of cardiac activity suggest that chronotropic cardiac activity, as manifested by heart rate changes, is predominantly and more efficiently controlled by sympathetic and parasympathetic pathways running on the right side. Ionotropic and dromotropic cardiac activity, such as AV conduction and ventricular contractility, instead seem to be more closely associated with autonomic outflow passing on the left side. Imbalance in cardiac sympathetic innervation with left-sided dominance, resulting from stimulation of the left stellate ganglion and blocking or ablation of the right stellate ganglion, seems to be a pathogenetic mechanism leading to various cardiac arrhythmias (Lane and Schwartz, 1987; Schwartz, 1984).

Cardiac Effects of Lateralized Cerebral Damage, Inactivation, and Stimulation

In view of the fact that pathways concerned with sympathetic and parasympathetic control of cardiac activity descend primarily on the ipsilateral side both within the brain and the spinal cord (Johnson et al., 1984), it should be expected that asymmetries characterizing peripheral autonomic control of cardiac activity may be observed at the level of subcortical and cortical brain structures involved in cardiovascular control. This has been confirmed by several studies using both animal and human subjects.

Animal studies with cats and dogs using either unilateral electrical stimulation (Chai and Wang, 1962; Fang and Wang, 1962) or unilateral injection of γ-aminobutyric acid (GABA) into sympathoexcitatory neuronal structures (Shapoval, Sagach, and Pobegailo, 1991) have shown that at the levels of the dorsal medulla (Chai and Wang, 1962), the ventrolateral medulla (Shapavol et al., 1991), and the hypothalamus (Fang and Wang, 1962), the left brain is more effectively involved in neural control of myocardial contractility, whereas the right brain is clearly more effective in the regulation of heart rate. At the level of the cerebral cortex, effects of experimental stroke induced by left or right middle cerebral artery occlusion and involving the insula and portions of the perirhinal, frontolateral, motor, and sensory cortex (Hachinski et al., 1992) have been found to affect mean arterial pressure and the QT interval of the ECG more strongly if the right brain as opposed to the left brain was involved.

With few exceptions (e.g., Yamour et al., 1980) most studies examining the cardiac effects of *unilateral brain damage in human subjects* have been concerned with alterations of heart rate. The most extensive and influential studies have been done by Italian research workers (Caltagirone et al., 1989; Zoccolotti et al., 1986). Caltagirone et al. (1989) measured heart rate changes in 40 right-handed patients with unilateral right or left brain damage and in 20 normal controls while subjects were viewing short 20-second sequences of either an emotionally negative or a neutral film. Generally, compared to baseline values, heart rate decelerated during film presentation in all groups, an effect that may have been expected from Lacey's intake-rejection hypothesis (Green, 1980; Lacey and Lacey, 1978). But, remarkably, left brain–damaged patients and control subjects displayed a significantly higher decelerative response to the emotionally negative film than to the neutral film. Right brain–damaged patients, on the contrary, did not differ in their cardiac responses to the films and had a clearly smaller decelerative response to the emotional film than both other groups. Therefore, parasympathetic control of heart rate is thought to be impaired in right brain–damaged patients.

Results obtained from brain-damaged patients suggesting right hemisphere superiority in heart rate control are supported by studies examining cardiac effects of *unilateral hemispheric inactivation* by intracarotid amobarbital injection. Rosen et al. (1982), studying heart rate responses in five patients, found heart rate increases to be higher in all patients following left hemisphere inactivation than following right hemisphere inactivation. Lane et al. (1989) assessed heart rate in 13 patients with temporal lobe epilepsy undergoing unilateral intracarotid amobarbital injection. These authors found that heart rate increased merely during left hemisphere inactivation, favoring patients with left hemisphere as opposed to right hemisphere damage (Lane and Schwartz, 1990). In a recently published study, Zamrini et al. (1990) reported results on 25 patients undergoing unilateral cerebral inactivation as preoperative evaluation for epilepsy surgery. Heart rate was measured during the 1 minute immediately preceding amobarbital injection and during a 3-minute period immediately following completion of the injection. There was a significant difference in heart rate changes following left vs. right intracarotid injection. Mean heart rate increased up to four beats per minute (bpm) during left hemisphere inactivation and decreased up to 2.4 bpm during right hemisphere inactivation. Interestingly, no significant relation could be observed between overt emotional responses and right-left differences in heart rate changes, indicating that there may be a dissociation in brain control for behavioral-emotional and autonomic processes.

Cardiovascular Consequences of Lateralized Stimulus Presentation

To date, only a few studies have examined the cardiovascular consequences of lateralized stimulus presentation in normal subjects. Two different approaches have been used. Hugdahl et al. (1983) exposed subjects either to a fear-related or a neutral slide, presented repeatedly to the left or right visual half-field by means of short-time tachistoscopic exposure. Subjects were told that the·slide would always appear in the same visual hemifield. To control for foveal fixation, eye movements were recorded by means of electro-oculography. Slide onset was signaled by a light-emitting diode (LED) which served as a fixation point and which always went on 5 seconds prior to slide presentation. Heart rate changes were assessed during 10 seconds after LED onset and were computed as second-by-second deviations from a baseline phase immediately prior to LED onset. Whereas heart rate deceleration, being a function of slide onset, was observed with both left and right visual hemifield stimulation, anticipatory heart rate acceleration prior to slide onset was observed only if the stimuli were expected to appear in the left hemifield, that is, in the right hemisphere. According to the authors, the findings imply that the right cerebral hemisphere is more efficiently primed by motivational and emotional aspects of stimulation. On the other hand, it must be noted that both emotional and neutral slides provoked right hemisphere—dependent acceleration. Therefore, it is also possible that right hemisphere priming as such provokes stronger heart rate changes, irrespective of the emotional or neutral nature of stimulation. The latter assumption receives some support from another experiment by Hugdahl and Franzon (1987) in which heart rate changes were recorded in discrete-trial Stroop paradigms presented either to the right or left visual hemifield. Significant heart rate deceleration, being associated with slide onset, was only observed if the stimuli were presented to the left visual hemifield (right hemisphere). Since Stroop-like tasks are likely to involve cognitive stress rather than affective responses, the results are in line with the assumption, already suggested by the aforementioned amobarbital study (Zamrini et al., 1990), that the right hemisphere's dominance in heart rate control may be independent of emotional processes and emotion-related asymmetries.

Dimond and Farrington (1977) used a contact lens technique which allowed lateralized presentation of a whole film sequence. Twenty-one subjects were presented three films with emotionally negative, positive, or neutral contents either in their left or right visual hemifield, while heart rate was recorded. Whereas no significant differences were found with respect to the neutral film, heart rate was significantly higher during right as opposed to left hemisphere presentation of the emotionally negative film and during left as opposed to right hemisphere presentation of the emotionally positive film. Though these results were interpreted by the authors as indication of a differential emotion-related specialization of the hemispheres, there are some problems complicating interpretation. Heart rate differences are only minimal (1–2 bpm) between hemisphere groups, and baseline values are not referred to. Moreover, in view of the findings mentioned by Caltagirone et al. (1989), suggesting heart rate deceleration during film viewing, there is no straightforward conclusion that can be drawn from the results. Finally, unavoidable lens slippage, optical diffraction around the edge of the slit, and the very small display area of about 1 mm make the contact lens technique somewhat suspect.

In a yet unpublished study by our research group (for preliminary results, see Wittling and Schweiger, 1992a), we tried to deal with some of the problems encountered by Dimond and Farrington (1977). Using the above-described technique of lateralized film presentation, 60 normal right-handed subjects were shown the emotionally aversive film (electroconvulsive therapy) either in their left or right visual hemifield. Heart rate (R-R interval) was recorded continuously, both immediately prior to film onset, with no significant differences being observed, and during the whole period of film presentation. Moreover, subjects' self-reported emotional arousal during film viewing was assessed continuously by means of the above-described manual-motor rating technique. Half the subjects performed the rating with the hand being directly controlled by the film-perceiving hemisphere (left visual field/left hand or right visual field/right hand), whereas the other half of the subjects performed the rating with the hand not being directly controlled by the film-perceiving hemisphere (left visual field/right hand or right visual field/left hand). Both heart rate values and rating values were subsequently averaged over 2-second intervals. In this way, two time-related response curves with an equal number of synchronous time points were obtained for each subject.

It was hypothesized that with respect to changes in heart rate and subjective arousal a distinction must be drawn between the time-related trends of a response curve and phasic fluctuations of the response data superimposed on the trends. The trends of a response curve are thought to characterize slow shifts in tonic basal arousal due to a variety of nonspecific factors of the experimental situation such as the necessity to attend and respond to visual stimuli in sensory intake tasks, to be observed by the experimenter, or to be confronted with emotionally laden material in general. In contrast, phasic fluctuations are short-term deviations from the trend lines, which typically have a rather rapid onset and an equally rapid return to baseline. They are superimposed on the trends and can be distinguished against the ongoing tonic level of activity by clearly identifiable patterns of change. It is thought that these phasic responses are evoked by specific changes in contents of stimulation and may be regarded as specific emotional responses to specific film scenes.

Evaluating time-related *slow shifts* of tonic basal arousal by means of three-factor ANOVAs with the independent variables Film-Perceiving Hemisphere and Rating-Performing Hand and with repeated measures on the within-subjects variable Time (86 time intervals) revealed opposing shifts with respect to heart rate and subjective arousal. Self-reported arousal significantly increased over the whole film period with higher arousal values accompanying right hemisphere film viewing but just failing to reach statistical significance. Heart rate changed only insignificantly, showing a slight drop after the beginning of the film and a recovery to the initial values during the second half of the film. No significant effects of film lateralization could be observed with respect to heart rate changes.

To examine whether lateralized film presentation influenced *phasic* heart rate responses, thought to be evoked by the emotion-related content of specific film scenes, correlations were calculated between phasic heart rate changes and phasic changes in self-reported arousal. To arrive at a measure of phasic changes, best-fitting (fourth-degree) orthogonal polynomial curves (Lienert, 1978) were adapted to each group's mean response curves of heart rate and self-reported arousal. For each time point of both response curves the differences between the empirically obtained raw scores and the respective mathematically calculated values of the orthogonal polynomial curve were determined. These (detrented) difference scores were used to calculate correlations and lag correlations between heart rate and self-reported arousal.

Generally, results reveal a tendency toward a higher correspondence between heart rate changes and changes in subjective arousal if the film is presented to the right than to the left hemisphere. These hemispheric differences are accentuated if only those subgroups are compared in which both lateralized film presentation and lateralized motor rating performance are bound to the same hemisphere (figure 12.2). The respective Pearson coefficients of correlation (without time lag) are $r = .47$ ($P < .0001$) with right hemisphere and $r = .09$ (NS) with left hemisphere film viewing, the difference being highly significant. Moreover, there is evidence that the hemispheres differ also with respect to time-related factors of covariation. Calculating lag correlations reveals that with right hemisphere film presentation, correspondence between heart rate and self-reported arousal is highest if there is no time lag between both response curves. With left hemisphere film viewing, however, the response latency of the rating is always longer than that of the heart rate changes. Lag correlation with respect to figure 12.2 is highest ($r = .27$, $P < .05$) if the response curve of heart rate changes is temporally displaced backward up to 6 seconds. This effect probably suggests that with left hemisphere film presentation, self-report of emotional states occurs in a

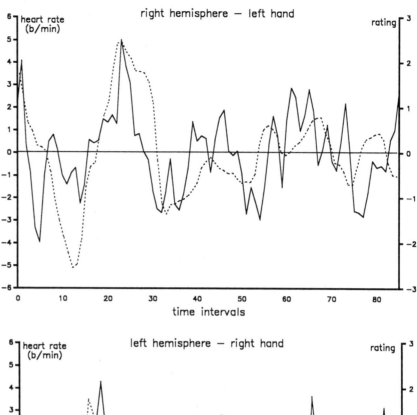

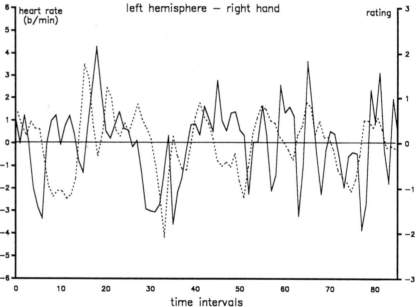

Figure 12.2 Response curves of phasic heart rate changes (solid lines) and phasic changes in self-reported arousal (dotted lines) during lateralized film presentation after elimination of trend components. Lateralized film presentation and lateralized rating performance are either bound to the right hemisphere (*upper*) or to the left hemisphere (*lower*).

Central-Autonomic Integration

more controlled and less spontaneous fashion causing changes in self-reported arousal to lag behind heart rate changes, whereas with right hemisphere film viewing no differences in response latency can be observed between both response parameters. However, it should be remembered that the above results are merely based on the correlational analysis of the groups' mean response curves. Therefore, no conclusions can be drawn about possible hemispheric differences in the strength of correspondence between heart rate changes and subjective-emotional changes at the level of single subjects.

To our knowledge, only one study to date (Wittling, 1990a) has examined brain asymmetry in the modulation of *blood pressure*. Using the above-mentioned video technique for lateralized film presentation, 50 adult subjects were shown a 3-minute sexually arousing scene from the film *Don't Look Now*, judged as emotionally positive by retrospective ratings on ten emotional qualities. Half the subjects watched the film in the left visual hemifield; the other half of the subjects watched the same film in the right visual hemifield. To examine, furthermore, whether blood pressure regulation would not only be influenced by lateralized presentation of visual input but, additionally, by lateralized motor responding to the film's content, half the subjects of each visual laterality group performed the rating with the hand being directly controlled by the film-perceiving hemisphere. The other half of the subjects performed the rating with the hand being controlled by the other hemisphere receiving film information only after callosal relay.

It was found that only right hemisphere film presentation resulted in statistically significant increases in systolic and diastolic blood pressure, whereas left hemisphere film presentation caused only minimal and insignificant changes. These differences were further increased if lateralized film presentation and lateralized motor responding to the film's content were combined within the same hemisphere, thereby enhancing unilateral processing. Mean systolic and diastolic changes were 12.42 mm Hg and 6.25 mm Hg with right hemisphere film presentation and 0.43 mm Hg and −0.21 mm Hg with left hemisphere film presentation. This asymmetry is reflected also by the distribution of individual subjects' change scores. Considerable increases in systolic (> 10 mm Hg) and diastolic blood pressure (> 5 mm Hg) were found in only 14% and 21% of the subjects viewing the film in the left hemisphere, but in 67% and 58% of the subjects viewing the film in the right hemisphere. Systolic and diastolic pressure remained unchanged or even decreased in 43% and 64% of the subjects viewing the film in the left hemisphere, but in only 17% and 8% of the subjects viewing the film in the right hemisphere. However, it seems worth mentioning that there was a significant two-factor interaction between the variables Film-Perceiving Hemisphere and Gender, revealing that brain asymmetry in regulating blood pressure favoring the right hemisphere is significantly more pronounced in females than in males.

Again, neither the main effect, indicating stronger blood pressure responses during right hemisphere film viewing, in general, nor the interaction effect, revealing a more pronounced asymmetry in females, can be explained by differences in subjective-emotional responses to the presented film as assessed by the aforementioned retrospective rating scales (see table 12.1). On the one hand, despite large differences observed in blood pressure responses, ratings of subjective-emotional arousal were only slightly and insignificantly higher with right hemisphere as opposed to left hemisphere film presentation. On the other hand, although brain asymmetry favoring right hemisphere regulation of blood pressure was significantly more pronounced in females than in males, no comparable differences could be detected with respect to subjective-emotional responses. Females especially, while being characterized by a very strong right hemisphere superiority in the regulation of blood pressure, did not show any indication of hemispheric differences in subjectively felt emotional arousal.

Cerebral Feedback of Cardiovascular Processes

Both anatomic and physiologic evidence has been found indicating that brain activity is modulated by cardiovascular processes via afferent feedback circuits predominantly mediated by the baroreceptors and relayed through the nucleus tractus solitarius of the medulla. These feedback circuits seem to be lateralized, favoring right hemisphere feedback. The two main research strategies used to examine asymmetry in cardiovascular feedback are EEG recording of cardiovascular-related brain activity and behavioral assessment of autonomic discrimination and interoceptive feedback.

Walker and Sandman (1979) were the first to study the relationship between spontaneous changes in heart rate and human visual evoked potentials. Subjects with variable heart rates (interbeat intervals) were presented flashes of light during fast, midrange, and slow heart beats, while evoked responses were recorded over the left and right occipital lobes. Spontaneous changes in heart rate were found to be related to visual evoked potentials, but cortical reflection of heart rate changes proved to be different for the two hemispheres. Potentials recorded during high vs. slow heart rate could be differentiated from one another by waveform if recording was done over the right hemisphere. In contrast, potentials were not related to heart rate if recorded from the left hemisphere. In a subsequent study, Walker and Sandman (1982) examined whether there are differences in the waveforms of visual evoked potentials recorded during periods of systolic vs. diastolic carotid pressure, assuming that baroreceptor activity is differentially influenced by changes in blood pressure. Once again, it was found that merely sensory evoked activity recorded from the right hemisphere differed significantly between systolic and diastolic pressure phases.

There are two possible explanations that may account for these results. On the one hand, it is possible that neuronal activity of brain cells controlling cardiovascular activity may operate on electrocortical activity, altering EEG responses evoked by sensory input. Although highly speculative, the assumption is supported by findings showing that in the cat's amygdala, neurons discharge phasically with cardiac and respiratory cycles and that tonic discharge rates correlate with spontaneous changes in blood pressure and rate of respiration (Frysinger, Zhang, and Harper, 1988). Moreover, Frysinger and Harper (1989, 1990) recently demonstrated that single-unit activity in human amygdala and hippocampus shows discharge patterns that have a timing relationship with the cardiac cycle and are correlated with spontaneous changes in heart rate or respiratory periods. On the other hand, a hypothesis favored by most authors (Elbert et al., 1991; Walker and Sandman, 1982) posits that cardiovascular changes exert a widespread influence on cortical and subcortical brain structures via afferent feedback circuits. Especially changes in baroreceptor activity relayed through the nucleus tractus solitarius are thought to modulate brain activity (Walker and Sandman, 1982).

The feedback hypothesis has received support from studies showing that subjective heartbeat perception is accompanied by a specific electrocortical potential appearing most clearly over the frontal lobes. This potential, known as "heartbeat evoked potential," is typically characterized by a prominent negative component 200 to 400 ms following the ECG R wave and is influenced by good vs. poor heartbeat perception as well as by the motivation to discriminate heartbeat activity (Weitkunat and Schandry, 1990). It has been shown that the amplitude of the heartbeat evoked potential recorded from the right frontal area is positively correlated with the accuracy of subjective heartbeat discrimination (Weitkunat, Cestaro, and Katkin, 1989). Moreover, the influence of motivation on the amplitude of the heartbeat evoked potential is strongest in the right frontal area (Weitkunat and Schandry, 1990). Therefore, we may assume that afferent feedback from cardiovascular structures to the brain is more effectively processed in the right cerebral hemisphere.

Asymmetry in cerebrocardiovascular feedback favoring the right hemisphere has also been found in behavioral studies assessing accuracy of heartbeat discrimination. Davidson and colleagues (1981), exploring differences in time relationship between left- vs. right-hand finger-tapping and heartbeat, found that left-hand tapping was significantly closer to the immediately preceding R spike than right-hand tapping. Although this finding is consistent with the notion of a right hemisphere superiority in the processing of afferent cardiac feedback, the methodologic approach based on heartbeat-contingent motor responses has recently been criticized by Flynn and Clemens (1988).

Modified approaches to assess heartbeat perception have been used by several other authors. Montgomery and Jones (1984) assessed cardiac awareness by means of the Whitehead heartbeat discrimination procedure, requiring the subject to decide whether light flashes occurring either 128 ms or 384 ms after each R spike represented an immediate (true) or delayed (false) heartbeat feedback. Dividing subjects into good or poor heartbeat perceivers, the authors found that good heartbeat perceivers made significantly more left lateral eye movements in response to 20 questions than poor perceivers. Since conjugate lateral eye movements to the left are thought to indicate right hemisphere activation (Ehrlichman and Weinberger, 1978; Katkin and Reed, 1988), this would indicate that heartbeat perception is more accurate during right than during left hemisphere activation. Similar results were obtained by Hantas, Katkin, and Reed (1984), Katkin and Reed (1988), and Weisz et al. (1990) determining the influence of asymmetric hemispheric activation as assessed by conjugate lateral eye movements on heartbeat perception. In all studies "left movers" performed better on heartbeat perception than "right movers." Leaving the somewhat questionable validity of conjugate lateral eye movements out of account, these results, too, are in line with the notion of a right hemisphere superiority in the processing of afferent cardiac feedback.

ASYMMETRY IN PAIN SENSITIVITY

Noxious peripheral stimulation is processed in neurons of the medial and lateral thalamus, receiving noxious information both by direct projection from the spinal cord (spinothalamic pathways) or by pathways relayed through the reticular formation of the brainstem (spinoreticular pathways). From the thalamus, information about noxious stimulation is sent to the cortex, where it reaches conscious awareness. Pain modulation is achieved by an ascending pathway from the midbrain periaqueductal gray to the medial thalamus and by a descending pathway from the pericruciate cortex to the thalamus, both being able to inhibit nociceptive neural activity and to reduce pain perception (Andersen, 1986). Afferent pain stimulation is predominately transmitted via crossed contralateral pathways (Stein, Price, and Gazzaniga, 1989; Talbot et al., 1991). In human cortex, processing of painful stimuli is restricted to the anterior cingulate cortex, an area involved in the regulation of emotion-related arousal, as well as to the secondary and primary somatosensory cortices (Talbot et al., 1991).

There is evidence from experimental and clinical studies that pain sensitivity is lateralized in humans, with the right hemisphere showing relatively higher pain sensitivity than the left hemisphere. In *experimental studies* pain sensitivity is determined by assessing either pain threshold, pain tolerance, or pain endurance to a variety of pain-inducing procedures such as local pressure or local heating, electrical current, submaximal effort tourniquet test, or cold pressure test applied to the left or right side of the body. Göbel and Westphal (1987) have listed 15 experimental studies examining pain threshold or pain tolerance. The vast majority of studies reveal a relatively lower pain threshold or pain tolerance if noxious stimuli are applied to the left side of the body in right-handers, indicating a higher pain sensitivity in the right hemisphere. In left-handers, pain sensitivity is reversed in most cases (Göbel and Westphal, 1987). Using lateralized presentation of visual and auditory stimuli to assess hemispheric activation, Otto, Dougher, and Yeo (1989), moreover, observed that prior exposure to pain resulted in increased right hemisphere activation, suggesting that pain perception is more closely associated with the right than with the left hemisphere.

With respect to *clinical studies*, results are somewhat more ambiguous. Cubelli, Caselli, and Neri (1984) studied pain endurance in left brain–damaged and right brain–damaged patients. In accord with experimental results, pain endurance was found to be significantly higher in right brain–damaged patients as compared to both a normal control group and left brain–damaged patients. Neri, Vecchi, and Caselli (1985), additionally, demonstrated that right brain damage affected pain sensitivity both in the contralateral paralyzed arm and in the ipsilateral healthy arm, whereas in left brain–damaged patients only the contralateral paralyzed arm was affected. Given that the right hemisphere is more closely involved in pain perception and that pain pathways are crossed, it should be assumed that in pain patients pain is preferentially lateralized at the left side of the body. This hypothesis has been supported by Merskey and Watson (1979), who reviewed a series of ten studies on patients with psychogenic pain, rheumatic pain, and hysterical conversion reactions. Pain, when lateralized in these patients, occurred consistently more often at the left side of the body. Subsequent studies in patients with pain due to illness, trauma, carcinoma, and surgery could not replicate these results and found no evidence for preferential left lateralization of pain (Hall and Clarke, 1982; Hall, Hayward, and Chapman, 1981).

CONCLUSIONS

Theoretical Considerations

The main conclusion that can be drawn from the above-presented survey is that brain asymmetry is a *universal phenomenon* characterizing not only cerebral control of cognitive functions or subjectively experienced emotional states but cerebral regulation of autonomic-physiologic processes as well. In view of the remarkable consistency and strength of asymmetric control revealed by the great bulk of the studies, the assumption seems justified that the manifestation of brain laterality in the control of bodily processes is at least as pronounced as that of cognitive and emotional functions.

Lateralization of neural control has been observed at all levels of the nervous system ranging from peripheral pathways to lower brainstem, midbrain, hypothalamus, thalamus, basal ganglia, amygdala, and the prefrontal and orbitofrontal regions of the cortex.

Physiologic functions found to be asymmetrically controlled include a broad spectrum of chemical and physical events ranging from neurotransmitter activity to neuroendocrine activity, immunomodulatory activity, and cardiovascular activity. Additionally, cerebral asymmetry has been found to extend to other functional systems not explicitly discussed in this review, such as electrodermal activity (Caltagirone et al., 1989; Davidson et al., 1992; Heilman, Schwartz, and Watson, 1978; Hugdahl, 1984; Morrow et al., 1981; Schrandt, Tranel, and Damasio, 1989; Schuri and von Cramon, 1982;

Zoccolotti, Scabini, and Violani, 1982), skin temperature (Harrison, 1990), and vasomotor activity (Varni, Doerr, and Franklin, 1971).

Whereas dopaminergic activity is predominately left-lateralized as is neural control of AV conduction and myocardial contractility, all the other functions are predominantly right-lateralized, including noradrenergic and serotonergic neurotransmitter activity, most neuroendocrine activity, chronotropic cardiac activity, arterial blood pressure, cardiac feedback and discrimination, skin conductance response, and pain sensitivity. This indicates that there is a differential specialization of the two brain sides with respect to the control of different functional systems or single functions within a functional system, one brain side being more critically involved in the regulation of some particular functions, the other side being of higher importance for the control of other functions.

Attempting to characterize the *basic role of each brain side* in the regulation of physiologic functions, we may tentatively assume that the left brain is not only involved in the control of motor behavior and higher integrative functions, as revealed by its higher dopaminergic innervation, but is also of critical importance for the regulation of the organism's defense responses against invading agents, as is illustrated by its effects on immunomodulation. Its role in the control of other physiologic functions, e.g., cardiac activity, is difficult to characterize at present. The right brain seems to be primarily involved in the control of vital functions supporting survival and enabling the organism to cope actively with stress and external challenges. This has especially been suggested by Gerendai's findings, showing higher mortality rates following damage to the right brain, as well as by human and animal studies revealing a stronger involvement of the right brain in noradrenergic and serotonergic neurotransmitter activity, in the regulation of the stress hormone cortisol, in the control of blood pressure and chronotropic cardiac activity, and in sensitivity to pain-related and noxious stimuli. Although most studies have examined the activating and arousing effects of right brain activity, causing some authors to assume right hemisphere superiority in the regulation of sympathetic activity (Hachinski et al., 1992), there is evidence that right-lateralized control extends to both upregulation and downregulation of autonomic-physiologic arousal. Support for this assumption is especially provided by studies demonstrating higher serotonergic activity in the right brain as well as stronger effects on parasympathetic heart rate slowing and a higher heart rate variability during situations of changing emotional content.

Having established that the two brain sides are differentially specialized with respect to the control of different physiologic functions does not imply that a single function is exclusively controlled by one hemisphere or the other. Examining the *interaction between both brain sides* during the control of a single physiologic function reveals two different regulatory mechanisms. Whereas with respect to most functions both brain sides seem to differ only in strength or efficiency of their regulatory activity, other functions, particularly immunomodulatory processes, are obviously controlled in a reciprocally inhibitory way by both brain sides, one exerting enhancing effects, the other exerting inhibitory effects on physiologic functioning. It must be emphasized, however, that reciprocal functional inhibition is not restrained to interhemispheric communication but may also be assumed to occur between activating and suppressing areas within the same hemisphere (e.g., Neveu, 1988, 1992a,b).

A last issue deserving consideration is whether the observed asymmetries in different physiologic functions are *self-reliant mechanisms* or are dependent on asymmetries existing in other functional systems. We are not aware of any studies that have explored the correspondence between asymmetries in different functional systems in any detail. Therefore, no empirically substantiated answer can be given, although on theoretical grounds, correspondence between different systems should be expected. An asymmetric distribution of neurotransmitters in both sides of the brain should be expected to be related to asymmetries found in other aspects of behavior, such as emotional, neuroendocrine, cardiovascular, or immunologic processes.

At least with respect to the correspondence between subjective-emotional and physiologic asymmetries, some indirect empirical evidence has accumulated indicating that asymmetries reported for the control of autonomic-physiologic functions are likely to be independent of asymmetries characterizing subjective-emotional processing. Firstly, autonomic asymmetries have been found in situations in which activation has been provoked by cognitive effort not associated with emotional responses, such as block-design tasks (Wittling and Schweiger, 1993b) or Stroop-like tasks (Hugdahl and Franzon, 1987). Secondly, autonomic asymmetries have repeatedly been reported in neutral measurement conditions uninfluenced by emotional or cognitive arousal, such as biochemical determination of neurotransmitter concentration in postmortem brains, assessment of lesion-dependent immunoresponsiveness in normal laboratory situations, measurement of event-related potentials evoked by cardiovascular activity, or peripheral stimulation or blocking of sympathetic and parasympathetic cardiac pathways. Thirdly, studies reporting on the relationship between lateralized cerebral control of autonomic functions and subjective-emotional responses shown in the same experimental situations were unable to find any significant correlations between brain asymmetries of both response systems (Kang et al., 1991; Wittling, 1990a; Wittling and Pflüger, 1990; Wittling and Schweiger, 1993a; Zamrini et al., 1990). Taken together, contrary to the prevailing view, we may assume that brain asymmetries in the control of autonomic-physiologic functions are likely to be independent of emotion-related brain asymmetry.

Methodologic Considerations

Methodologic approaches applied to the study of lateralized control of physiologic functions embrace a wide *spectrum of multifarious techniques* stipulated by the enormous variety of physiologic processes to be investigated, such as (a) biochemical determinations of neurotransmitter contents of the brain either by means of high-pressure liquid chromatography in bilateral dissections of postmortem brains of normal subjects or experimentally lesioned animals, or by PET imaging of neurotransmitter receptor binding in the living human brain; (b) bioelectrical recording of event-related potentials assessing either cardiovascular-related brain activity or electrocortical effects of neurotransmitter-related medication; (c) lateralized electrical stimulation of neural structures involved in the control of physiologic functions, such as peripheral autonomic pathways or regions in the lower brainstem or hypothalamus; (d) lateralized sensory stimulation using either short-term or prolonged visual exposition or noxious and pain-related stimuli; (e) lateralized elimination or inhibition of neural structures either by unilateral brain lesions, unilateral ablation or blocking of peripheral autonomic pathways, or by unilateral hemispheric inactivation using intracarotid amobarbital injection; and (f) measurement of physiologic effects of naturally occurring lateralized brain activation, established by means of either EEG power analysis or conjugate lateral eye movements.

Given the wide spectrum of diverse methodologic approaches, ranging from biochemical determinations to neuropsychological procedures, a detailed evaluation of the assumptions, advantages, and methodologic problems associated with each individual approach is beyond the scope of this chapter. On the other hand, some fundamental assumptions are common to all procedures irrespective of diversities in technical details. The most central question applying to the procedures listed above is: *What are the basic assumptions* justifying the hope that a lateralized manipulation of neural tissue, whether by electrical stimulation, functional inactivation, lesioning, or sensory stimulation, will lead to asymmetric effects on the measured physiologic functions, given the exceptional profusion of reciprocal connections characterizing neural communication in the brain?

An inevitable prerequisite allowing lateralized manipulation of neural tissue to result in asymmetric physiologic changes is, of course, the existence of lateral differences in the efficiency of cerebral control of physiologic functions. To enable assessment of these existing asymmetries in brain control of physiologic functions by unilateral manipulations, some further assumptions are necessary. Besides the fact that unilateral manipulation should, indeed, be primarily restricted to only one side of the brain, neural activity influenced by unilateral manipulation is assumed to remain lateralized during the completion of the multistage control process implying several hierarchically ordered brain structures. To warrant this, it seems necessary to assume that descending pathways engaged in the respective control process project ipsilaterally, at least at brain level. In addition, horizontal spread of neural activity transmitted by commissural fibers should be minimal as far as functionally relevant activity is concerned. Relying on *lateralized visual stimulation* as an example, a short evaluation of these basic assumptions will be given.

There is compelling evidence from anatomic, electrophysiologic, and behavioral studies that the left hemiretina of each eye projects to the striate cortex of the left hemisphere, whereas the right hemiretina projects to the striate cortex of the right hemisphere. Therefore, with due control for eye movements, *visual input to the cortex* resulting from hemifield stimulation is split, with probably only a narrow strip at the vertical meridian projecting to both hemispheres (Bunt, Minckler, and Johanson, 1977; Fendrich and Gazzaniga, 1989; Stone, 1966; Stone, Leicester, and Sherman, 1973; Wittling, 1976).

Visual areas in the occipital and inferotemporal cortex are arranged in hierarchic sequences. Higher-order areas receive topographically organized connections from the striate cortex, emphasizing serial processing of information from lower to higher visual areas (Kaas, 1986; Pandya and Yeterian, 1986; Weller and Kaas, 1981). Analysis of form-related visual information is largely completed in the rostral inferotemporal cortex, where single cells have been found which respond selectively to specific faces or facial expressions (Kendrick and Baldwin, 1987). Most areas implicated in sequential processing have only sparse interhemispheric connections. Only the inferotemporal higher-order areas have callosal connections sufficiently widespread and dense to allow visual information to be efficiently transferred to the other hemisphere (Cusick and Kaas, 1986; Kaas, 1986). This suggests that callosal relay favors the transfer of visual information that has already been processed in the main visual areas of the directly stimulated hemisphere.

Although anatomic conditions in the inferotemporal cortex allow processed visual information to transfer to the other hemisphere, it is by no means self-evident that *callosally relayed information* is of functional relevance for cerebral control of physiologic processes under these experimental conditions. Interhemispheric transmission is a very time-consuming process, as is revealed by simple response time tasks (Bashore, 1981; Saron and Davidson, 1989; Wittling, 1973). This marked disadvantage is potentiated if not only a single stimulus but a complex sequence of continuously changing stimuli is to be conveyed. We could recently show (Wittling, 1992) that the time needed to complete a visuomotor tracking task was increased by 27% if the stimulus pattern, laterally presented to the left visual hemifield, had to be callosally transmitted to enable manual-motor responding by the right hand, compared to an experimental condition in which the visual stimulus pattern was laterally presented to the right visual hemifield. In addition, the percentage of errors increased by 42% if the information had to be continuously transmitted along the corpus callosum.

Further doubt as to the functional relevance of callosally conveyed information is raised by other experimental results. Doty, Negrao, and Yamaga (1973) provide consistent evidence from their own experimental results (Doty, 1969; Doty and Negrao, 1973; Negrao and Doty, 1969) and work done by others (Gazzaniga, 1963; Kaas, Axelrod, and Diamond, 1967), that memory traces in monkeys are commonly laid down unilaterally in a single trained or dominant hemisphere and do not pass spontaneously into the other hemisphere. Finally, it should be remembered that the commonly used procedure to estimate interhemispheric transmission time—calculating reaction time differences between responses initiated by the hemisphere being directly stimulated as compared to the hemisphere receiving stimulus input only after transcallosal relay (Bashore, 1981)—demonstrates that at least under time pressure stimulus processing and response execution is induced immediately by the directly stimulated hemisphere, not delaying response until information is conveyed to the other hemisphere.

The functional relevance of callosally transmitted information is further reduced by experimental approaches combining lateralized sensory input with lateralized motor responding by the contralateral hand, thus additionally enhancing stimulus-related activity in the directly stimulated hemisphere. This has been proved in the three aforementioned studies of our team, showing that cerebral asymmetry in the control of various physiologic functions is markedly enhanced under these conditions. Further support is derived from a study by Ely, Graves, and Potter (1989). Using a new dichotic listening technique based on a psychophysical threshold procedure, the authors found that emotional words elicited a right ear advantage when responses were performed verbally (thus favoring left hemisphere output), but a left ear advantage when responses were performed manually with left hand key presses (favoring right hemisphere output). Similar effects were reported by Bradshaw and Gates (1978) with respect to visual hemifield stimulation and in a more indirect manner by Halligan and Marshall (1989), Joanette et al. (1986), and Robertson (1991), demonstrating that the use of the contralateral arm in performing stimulus-related tasks may reduce the degree of visual neglect shown by hemi-inattentive patients.

On the whole, the above data seem to play down the functional relevance of callosally conveyed information in experimental approaches using lateralized sensory stimulation. Taking these results into consideration, it seems not improbable that neural activity evoked by unilateral visual stimulation remains largely lateralized after having been processed in the main visual areas of the directly stimulated hemisphere. There are two main pathways relating neural discharge from the inferotemporal cortex to ipsilateral cortical and subcortical areas intimately involved in the regulation of autonomic-physiologic processes. *Afferents from the inferotemporal cortex*, conveying visual information, project directly to the prefrontal cortex and the orbitofrontal regions (Pandya and Yeterian, 1986; Fuster, 1986), which have been shown to be of central importance for the cerebral regulation of nearly all physiologic functions discussed in this chapter. From there, descending pathways run to the amygdala, the hypothalamus, and other subcortical and lower brainstem areas involved in autonomic regulation. A second major pathway linking the visual areas in the inferotemporal areas with brain centers involved in autonomic physiologic control is to the amygdala (Horel, 1988). Interestingly, in the amygdala too, interhemispheric transmission of neural discharge is severely reduced. On the one hand, anatomic findings indicate that commissural connections in the amygdala and in the hippocampus are sparse or totally absent (Pandya and Rosene, 1985; Pandya and Seltzer, 1986). On the other hand, electrophysiologic findings in humans and monkeys suggest that electrical activity in one amygdaloid body is not transmitted to the other. Thus, local afterdischarge resulting from seizure activity or electrical stimulation, although spreading to ipsilateral brain structures, does not cross to the contralateral amygdala (Poblete, Ruben, and Walker, 1959; Wada, Mizoguchi, and Komai, 1981). Also, stimulation of one amygdaloid body does not elicit a defense reaction in animals if the ipsilateral ventral amygdalofugal pathway is interrupted, indicating that even under these conditions a functionally relevant transmission of impulses to the contralateral amygdala is lacking (Doty, 1989; Hilton and Zbrozyna, 1963).

A last mechanism supporting lateralized brain control of autonomic functions in experimental approaches using laterally presented sensory stimulation is given by the fact that *descending fibers engaged in autonomic control take predominantly an ipsilateral route.* There is overwhelming evidence from numerous anatomic and electrophysiologic studies that neural connections between brain structures involved in the multistage control process are either restricted to the ipsilateral side or are clearly more dense and more efficient at the ipsilateral side. This refers to virtually all autonomic functions controlled by the brain and to connections at virtually all brain levels, including amygdalofugal and amygdalopetal connections with cortical areas (Iwai and Yukie, 1987), amygdaloid connections with hypothalamus, thalamus, midbrain, pons, and medulla (Cechetto, Ciriello, and Calaresu, 1983; Price and Amaral, 1981; Sakarana, Shibasaki, and Lederis, 1986), and direct hypothalamoautonomic pathways connecting hypothalamic areas with preganglionic nuclei of the sympathetic and parasympathetic systems (Saper et al., 1976).

All in all, the anatomic and physiologic findings listed above lend support to the assumption that asymmetries in cerebral control of autonomic-physiologic functions reported here are scarcely due to methodologic artifacts, but are well founded on basic anatomic and physiologic features of the brain.

Perspectives

Compared to laterality research in the cognitive, emotional, and behavioral domains, the study of lateralized cerebral control of autonomic-physiologic functions is at its very beginning. Therefore, the number of unanswered questions in this field of research excels the number of solved problems by far.

There are a vast number of functional systems that have only received marginal attention or have even been spared so far, such as vasomotor responses, gastrointestinal responses, urogenital responses, temperature, pain, and endocrinologic and metabolic processes (e.g., Shannahoff-Khalsa, 1991). Other functional systems, such as immunologic and neurotransmitter activity, have mainly been explored in animals and await generalization of results to human subjects.

Little is known about the consistency of the measured asymmetries, about possible causes of reversed asymmetries, and, above all, about the distribution and variability of asymmetries at the level of the individual. Moreover, there is only preliminary information about the effects that variations in lateralized cerebral control of physiologic functions exert upon basic mechanisms of physiologic functioning such as strength, duration, course, adequacy, and lability of the respective responses.

Apart from these unanswered questions, which will probably become the targets of research within the next few years, we are strongly convinced that within the next decade research on lateralized cerebral control of autonomic-physiologic functions will open a *new way to the understanding of physical disease*, integrating two complementary fields of central importance for health research: neuropsychological brain research, on the one hand, and behavioral medicine, or psychosomatics, on the other (Reinert and Wittling, 1980; Wittling, 1980, 1990b, 1991, 1993; Wittling and Schweiger, in 1993a,b).

Irrespective of results on asymmetric control, this review has repeatedly presented empirical evidence that a wide spectrum of physiologic functions such as neurotransmitter activity, neuroendocrine activity, immuneorespon-siveness, cardiovascular activity, and pain sensitivity are modulated by the cortex. In this way, physiologic functions are subjected to direct influences exerted by a multitude of psychosocial, stress-related, and emotion-related events impinging on the brain along neurosensory pathways. This means that the brain is a central moderator variable mediating psychosocial effects to peripheral physiologic systems. As has been shown repeatedly in this survey, the consequences of this mediatory process are not only determined by the specific nature of sensory information impinging on the brain but also by functional characteristics of the brain and of the whole neural system in general. Abnormalities in brain functioning by morphologic brain damage, cerebral inactivation, or altered neurotransmitter concentrations have been shown to result in a variety of immunologic, cardiovascular, and related physiologic disorders.

Remarkably, modern biopsychological disease models have not yet made adequate allowance for this modulatory role of functional brain characteristics for the pathogenesis of psychosomatic disorders. Behavioral medicine, although emphasizing the role of neuroendocrine and neuroimmunologic mechanisms as mediating processes in explaining psychosocial influences on physical disease, does not attribute an independent and significant moderating impact to functional characteristics of the brain itself.

One of the main reasons for the neglect of the brain's modulating impact on pathogenesis may be seen in the fact that the neurosciences have hardly succeeded in defining attributes of brain functioning that meet the following requirements: (1) They should be defined in a concrete operational manner and subjected to rigid measurement procedures. (2) They should be expected to vary reliably between different individuals. (3) Variations should be related to the individual's physiologic functioning or physical health in a valid and predictable way.

We think it possible that brain asymmetry in the control of autonomic-physiologic functions is a variable that may succeed in fulfilling these requirements within the next decade. We have demonstrated that lateralized control of peripheral physiologic functions is a universal phenomenon in humans. There is preliminary evidence also that asymmetry varies among individuals both in strength and direction and that it is possible to quantify intraindividual asymmetry in brain control reliably by means of diverse experimental procedures (Wittling and Schweiger, 1993a,b) or EEG measures (Kang et al., 1991; Roschmann and Wittling, 1992). Moreover, there are some indications that variations or reversals of brain asymmetry may be related to vulnerability to various physical disorders: (1) Reversed or altered asymmetry in cerebral control of cortisol secretion has been found to be associated with a high degree of physical complaints (Wittling and Schweiger, 1993a,b). (2) Subjects with a high level of physical complaints are also characterized by weaker or absent asymmetries of event-related potentials evoked by emotion-related stimuli (Wittling, Roschmann, and Schweiger, 1993). (3) Extreme right frontal activation has been found to be associated with significantly lower NK cell activity than extreme left frontal activation (Kang et al., 1991). (4) Reversed asymmetry in serotonergic activity seems to be related to affective and behavioral abnormalities, reduced impulse control, and suicidal behavior (Arató et al., 1991a,b). (5) Alexithymia, a common feature of psychosomatic patients, is suspected of being associated with either an imbalance between right vs. left hemisphere activation or with a deficit in interhemispheric interaction (Dewaraja and Sasaki, 1990; Hoppe and Bogen, 1977; TenHouten et al., 1988; Zeitlin et al., 1989). (6) Cardiac arrhythmias, ECG abnormalities, and sudden death seem to be related to alterations of lateralized sympathetic control of cardiac activity (Lane and Schwartz, 1987, 1990; Malliani, Schwartz, and Zanchetti, 1980; Moss and Schwartz, 1979; Schwartz, 1976, 1984; Schwartz and Malliani, 1975; Vincent, 1986). Perhaps similar relationships may be detected with respect to alterations of parasympathetic control (Berntson, Cacioppo, and Quigley, 1993; Pfeifer and Peterson, 1987). (7) Left-handedness, probably going along with abnormal asymmetries in neural control of peripheral physiologic functions (Wittling and Schweiger, 1992b), seems to be associated with altered physiologic functioning such as reduced cortisol secretion during stress-related situations (Wittling and Schweiger, 1992a), as well as with immunologic (Geschwind and Behan, 1982, 1984; McManus and Bryden, 1991) and other physical disorders (Kramer, Albrecht, and Miller, 1985; London and Albrecht, 1991; Schweiger, Wittling, and Roschmann, 1992; Senie et al., 1980) and with reduced longevity (Coren and Halpern, 1991; Halpern and Coren, 1990).

Although the above instances of recent research work can at best provide restricted and preliminary evidence for a possible correspondence between variations of brain asymmetry and vulnerability to physical disorders, they give rise to the hope that future work will open a new perspective in medical and biopsychological thinking providing for a better understanding of physical disease in the light of recent brain research.

REFERENCES

Andersen, E. (1986). Periaqueductal gray and cerebral cortex modulate responses of medial thalamic neurons to noxious stimulation. *Brain Research, 375,* 30−36.

Arató, M., Frecska, E., Tekes, K., and MacCrimmon, D. J. (1991a). Serotonergic interhemispheric asymmetry: Gender difference in the orbital cortex. *Acta Psychiatrica Scandinavica, 84,* 110−111.

Arató, M., Tekes, K., Palkovits, M., Demeter, E., and Falus, A. (1987). Serotonergic split-brain and suicide. *Psychiatry Research, 21,* 355−356.

Arató, M., Tekes, K., Tóthfalusi, L., Magyar, K., Palkovits, M., Frecska, E., Falus, A., and MacCrimmon, D. J. (1991b). Reversed hemispheric asymmetry of imipramine binding in suicide victims. *Biological Psychiatry, 29,* 699−702.

Armour, J. A., Hageman, G. R., and Randall, W. C. (1972). Arrhythmias induced by local cardiac nerve stimulation. *American Journal of Physiology, 223,* 1068.

Arora, R. C., and Meltzer, H. Y. (1989a). Serotonergic measures in the brains of suicide victims: 5-HT$_2$ binding sites in the frontal cortex of suicide victims and control subjects. *American Journal of Psychiatry, 146,* 730−736.

Arora, R. C., and Meltzer, H. Y. (1989b). ^{3}H-Imipramine binding in the frontal cortex of suicides. *Psychiatry Research, 30,* 125−135.

Arora, R. C., and Meltzer, H. Y. (1991). Laterality and ^{3}H-imipramine binding: Studies in the frontal cortex of normal controls and suicide victims. *Biological Psychiatry, 29,* 1016−1022.

Asberg, M., Schalling, D., Traskman-Bendz, L., and Wagner, A. (1987). Psychobiology of suicide, impulsivity and related phenomena. In H. Y. Meltzer (Ed.), *Psychopharmacology: The third generation of progress* (pp 655−668). New York, NY: Raven Press.

Bakalkin, G. Y., Tsibezov, V. V., Sjutkin, E. A., Veselova, S. P., Novikov, I. D., and Krivosheev, O. G. (1984). Lateralization of LH-RH in rat hypothalamus. *Brain Research, 296,* 361−364.

Bardos, P., Degenne, D., Lebranchu, Y., Biziere, K., and Renoux, G. (1981). Neocortical lateralization of NK activity in mice. *Scandinavian Journal of Immunology, 13,* 609−611.

Barnéoud, P., Le Moal, M., and Neveu, P. J. (1990). Asymmetric distribution of brain monoamines in left- and right-handed mice. *Brain Research, 520,* 317−321.

Barnéoud, P., Le Moal, M., and Neveu, P. J. (1991). Asymmetrical effects of cortical ablation on brain monoamines in mice. *International Journal of Neuroscience, 56,* 283−294.

Barnéoud, P., Neveu, P. J., Vitiello, S., and Le Moal, M. (1988a). Early effects of right or left cerebral cortex ablation on mitogen-induced spleen lymphocyte DNA synthesis. *Neuroscience Letters, 90,* 302−307.

Barnéoud, P., Neveu, P. J., Vitiello, S., Mormède, P., and Le Moal, M. (1988b). Brain neocortex immunomodulation in rats. *Brain Research, 474,* 394−398.

Bashore, T. R. (1981). Vocal and manual reaction time estimates of interhemispheric transmission time. *Psychological Bulletin, 89,* 352−368.

Berntson, G. G., Cacioppo, J. T., and Quigley, K. S. (1993). Respiratory sinus arrhythmia: Autonomic origins, physiological mechanisms, and psychophysiological implications. *Psychophysiology, 30*, 183−196.

Besedovsky, H. O., del Rey, A. E., and Sorkin, E. (1985). Immune-neuroendocrine interactions. *Journal of Immunology, 135*, 750−754.

Betancur, C., Neveu, P. J., Vitiello, S., and LeMoal, M. (1991). Natural killer cell activity is associated with brain asymmetry in male mice. *Brain, Behavior, and Immunity, 5*, 162−169.

Birbaumer, N., and Schmidt, R. F. (1991). *Biologische Psychologie.* Berlin: Springer-Verlag.

Biziére, K., Guillaumin, J. M., Degenne, D., Bardos, P., Renoux, M., and Renoux, G. (1985). Lateralized neocortical modulation of the T-cell lineage. In R. Guillemin, M. Cohn, and T. Melnechuk (Eds.), *Neural modulation of immunity* (pp 81−91). New York, NY: Raven Press.

Bradshaw, J. L., and Gates, E. A. (1978). Visual field differences in verbal tasks: Effects of task familiarity and sex of subject. *Brain and Language, 5*, 166−187.

Bryden, M. P., McManus, J. C., and Steenhuis, R. E. (1991). Handedness is not related to self-reported disease incidence. *Cortex, 27*, 605−611.

Bunt, A. H., Minckler, D. S., and Johanson, G. W. (1977). Demonstration of bilateral projection to the central retina of the monkey with horseradish peroxidase neuronography. *Journal of Comparative Neurology, 171*, 619−630.

Burke, H. L., Yeo, R. A., Vranes, L., Garry, P. J., and Goodwin, J. S. (1988). Handedness, developmental disorders, an in vivo and in vitro measurements of immune responses. *Developmental Neuropsychology, 4*, 103−115.

Calabrese, J. R., Kling, M. A., and Gold, P. W. (1987). Alterations in immunocompetence during stress, bereavement, and depression: Focus on neuroendocrine regulation. *American Journal of Psychiatry, 144*, 1123−1187.

Caltagirone, C., Zoccolotti, P., Originale, G., Daniele, A., and Mammucari, A. (1989). Autonomic reactivity and facial expression of emotion in brain-damaged patients. In G. Gainotti and C. Caltagirone (Eds.), *Emotions and the dual brain* (pp 204−221). Berlin: Springer-Verlag.

Castellano, M. A., Diaz-Palarea, M. D., Barroso, J., and Rodriguez, M. (1989). Behavioral lateralization in rats and dopaminergic system: Individual and population laterality. *Behavioral Neuroscience, 103*, 46−53.

Cechetto, D. F., Ciriello, J., and Calaresu, F. R. (1983). Afferent connections to cardiovascular sites in the amygdala: A horseradish peroxidase study in the cat. *Journal of the Autonomic Nervous System, 8*, 97−110.

Chai, C. Y., and Wang, S. C. (1962). Localization of central cardiovascular control mechanism in lower brain stem of the cat. *American Journal of Physiology, 202*, 25−30.

Chengappa, K. N., Ganguli, R., Yang, Z. W., Schurin, G., Cochran, J., Brar, J. S., and Rabin, B. (1992). Non-right sidedness: An association with lower IL-2 production. *Life Sciences, 51*, 1843−1849.

Cinca, J., Evangelista, A., Montoyo, J., Barutell, C., Figueras, J., Valle, V., Rius, J., and Soler-Soler, J. (1985). Electrophysiologic effects of unilateral right and left stellate ganglion block on the human heart. *American Heart Journal, 109*, 46−54.

Clark, C. R., Geffen, G. M., and Geffen, L. B. (1987). Catecholamines and attention I: Animal and clinical studies. *Neuroscience and Biobehavioral Reviews, 11*, 341−352.

Coren, S., and Halpern, D. F. (1991). Left-handedness: A marker for decreased survival fitness. *Psychological Bulletin, 109*, 90−106.

Cubelli, R., Caselli, M., and Neri, M. (1984). Pain endurance in unilateral cerebral lesions. *Cortex, 20,* 369–375.

Cupps, T. R., and Fauci, A. S. (1982). Corticosteroid-mediated immunoregulation in man. *Immunological Reviews, 65,* 133–155.

Cusick, C. G., and Kaas, J. H. (1986). Interhemispheric connections of cortical sensory and motor representations im primates. In F. Leporé, M. Ptito, and H. H. Jasper (Eds.), *Two hemispheres—one brain. Functions of the corpus callosum* (pp 83–102). New York, NY: Alan R. Liss.

Daruna, J. H., and Morgan, J. E. (1990). Psychosocial effects on immune function: Neuroendocrine pathways. *Psychosomatics, 31,* 4–12.

Davidson, R. A., Fedio, P., Smith, B. D., Aureille, E., and Martin, A. (1992). Lateralized mediation of arousal and habituation: Differential bilateral electrodermal activity in unilateral temporal lobectomy patients. *Neuropsychologia, 30,* 1053–1063.

Davidson, R. J. (1988). EEG measures of cerebral asymmetry: Conceptual and methodological issues. *International Journal of Neuroscience, 39,* 71–89.

Davidson, R. J., Horowitz, M. E., Schwartz, G. E., and Goodman, D. M. (1981). Lateral differences in the latency between finger tapping and the heart beat. *Psychophysiology, 18,* 36–41.

Delgado, J. M. R. (1960). Circulatory effects of cortical stimulation. *Physiological Reviews, 40* (Suppl 4), 146–171.

Demeter, E., Tekes, K., Majorossy, K., Palkovits, M., Soos, M., Magyar, K., and Somogyi, E. (1989). The asymmetry of ^{3}H-imipramine binding may predict psychiatric illness. *Life Sciences, 44,* 1403–1410.

Dewaraja, R., and Sasaki, Y. (1990). A left to right hemisphere callosal transfer deficit of nonlinguistic information in alexithymia. *Psychotherapy and Psychosomatics, 54,* 201–207.

Dewberry, R. G., Lipsey, J. R., Saad, K., Moran, T. H., and Robinson, R. G. (1986). Lateralized response to cortical injury in the rat: Interhemispheric interaction. *Behavioral Neuroscience, 100,* 556–562.

Dimond, S. J., and Farrington, L. (1977). Emotional response to films shown to the right or left hemisphere of the brain measured by heart rate. *Acta Psychologica, 41,* 255–260.

Doty, R. W. (1969). Electrical stimulation of the brain in behavioral context. *Annual Review of Psychology, 20,* 289–320.

Doty, R. W. (1989). Some anatomical substrates of emotion, and their bihemispheric coordination. In G. Gainotti and C. Caltagirone (Eds.), *Experimental brain research series 18* (pp 56–82). Berlin: Springer-Verlag.

Doty, R. W., and Negrao, N. (1973). Forebrain commissures and vision. In R. Jung (Ed.), *Handbook of sensory physiology, VII/3B* (pp 543–582). Berlin: Springer-Verlag.

Doty, R. W., Negrao, N., and Yamaga, K. (1973). The unilateral engram. *Acta Neurobiologae Experimentalis, 33,* 711–728.

Dunn, A. J. (1989). Psychoimmunology for the psychoneuroendocrinologist: A review of animal studies of nervous system-immune system interactions. *Psychoneuroendocrinology, 14,* 251–274.

Ehrlichman, H., and Weinberger, A. (1978). Lateral eye movements and hemispheric asymmetry: A critical review. *Psychological Bulletin, 85,* 1080–1101.

Elbert, T., Tafil-Klawe, M., Rau, H., and Lutzenberger, W. (1991). Cerebral and cardiac responses to unilateral stimulation of carotid sinus baroreceptors. *Journal of Psychophysiology, 5,* 327–335.

Ely, P. W., Graves, R. E., and Potter, S. M. (1989). Dichotic listening indices of right hemisphere semantic processing. *Neuropsychologia, 27,* 1007–1015.

Fahrenberg, J., Hampel, R., and Selg, H. (1984). *Das Freiburger Persönlichkeitsinventar (FPI-R).* Göttingen: Hogrefe.

Fallon, J. H., and Loughlin, S. E. (1987). Monoamine innervation of cerebral cortex and a theory of the role of monoamines in cerebral cortex and basal ganglia. In A. Peters and E. G. Jones (Eds.), *Cerebral cortex,* Vol 6 (pp 41–127). New York, NY: Plenum Press.

Fang, H. S., and Wang, S. C. (1962). Cardioaccelerator and cardioaugmentor points in hypothalamus of the dog. *American Journal of Physiology, 203,* 147–150.

Feldman, S. (1989). Afferent neural pathways and hypothalamic neurotransmitters regulating adrenocortical secretion. In H. Weiner, I. Florin, R. Murison, and D. Hellhammer (Eds.), *Frontiers of stress research* (pp 201–207). Lewiston, NY: Hans Huber Publishers.

Fendrich, R., and Gazzaniga, M. S. (1989). Evidence of foveal splitting in a commissurotomy patient. *Neuropsychologia, 27,* 273–281.

Flor-Henry, P. (1986). Observations, reflections and speculations on the cerebral determinants of mood and on the bilaterally asymmetrical distributions of the major neurotransmitter systems. *Acta Neurologica Scandinavica, 74* (Suppl 109), 75–89.

Flynn, D. M., and Clemens, W. J. (1988). On the validity of heartbeat tracking tasks. *Psychophysiology, 25,* 92–96.

Frecska, E., Arató, M., Tekes, K., and Powchik, P. (1990). Lateralization of ^{3}H-IMI binding in human frontal cortex. *Biological Psychiatry, 27* (9A), 72.

Fride, E., Collins, R. L., Skolnick, P., and Arora, P. K. (1990). Immune function in lines of mice selected for high or low degrees of behavioral asymmetry. *Brain, Behavior, and Immunity, 4,* 129–138.

Frysinger, R. C., and Harper, R. M. (1989). Cardiac and respiratory correlations with unit discharge in human amygdala and hippocampus. *Electroencephalography and Clinical Neurophysiology, 72,* 463–470.

Frysinger, R. C., and Harper, R. M. (1990). Cardiac and respiratory correlations with unit discharge in epileptic human temporal lobe. *Epilepsia, 31,* 162–171.

Frysinger, R. C., Zhang, J., and Harper, R. M. (1988). Cardiovascular and respiratory relationships with neuronal discharge in the central nucleus of the amygdala during sleep-waking states. *Sleep, 11,* 317–332.

Fukuda, M., Yamanouchi, K., Nakano, Y., Furuya, H., and Arai, Y. (1984). Hypothalamic laterality in regulating gonadotropic function: Unilateral hypothalamic lesion and ovarian compensatory hypertrophy. *Neuroscience Letters, 51,* 365–370.

Furnival, C. M., Linden, R. J., and Snow, H. M. (1973). Chronotropic and inotropic effects on the dog heart of stimulating the efferent cardiac sympathetic nerves. *Journal of Physiology, 230,* 137–153.

Fuster, J. M. (1986). The prefrontal cortex and temporal integration. In A. Peters and E. G. Jones (Eds.), *Cerebral cortex,* Vol 4 (pp 151–177). New York, NY: Plenum Press.

Gainotti, G. (1972). Emotional behavior and hemispheric side of lesion. *Cortex, 8,* 41–55.

Gainotti, G. (1983). Laterality of affect. The emotional behavior of right and left brain-damaged patients. In M. S. Myslobodsky (Ed.), *Hemisyndromes: Psychobiology, neurology, psychiatry* (pp 175–192). New York, NY: Academic Press.

Gainotti, G. (1989). The meaning of emotional disturbances resulting from unilateral brain injury. In G. Gainotti and C. Caltagirone (Eds.), *Emotions and the dual brain* (pp 147–167). Berlin: Springer-Verlag.

Garver, D. L., and Zemlan, F. P. (1986). Receptor studies in diagnosis and treatment of depression. In A. J. Rush and K. Z. Altshuler (Eds.), *Depression. Basic mechanisms, diagnosis, and treatment* (pp 143–170). New York, NY: Guilford Press.

Gazzaniga, M. S. (1963). Effects of commissurotomy on a preoperatively learned visual discrimination. *Experimental Neurology, 8,* 14–19.

Gerendai, I. (1984). Lateralization of neuroendocrine control. In N. Geschwind and A. M. Galaburda (Eds.), *Cerebral dominance. The biological foundations* (pp 167–178). Cambridge, MA: Harvard University Press.

Gerendai, I. (1987). Laterality in the neuroendocrine system. In D. Ottoson (Ed.), *Duality and unity of the brain: Unified functioning and specialisation of the hemispheres* (pp 17–28). New York, NY: Plenum Press.

Gerendai, I., Nemeskéri, A., Faivre-Bauman, A., Grouselle, D., and Tixier-Vidal, A. (1985a). Effects of unilateral or bilateral thyroidectomy on TRH content of hypothalamus halves. *Journal of Endocrinological Investigation, 8,* 321–323.

Gerendai, I., Prato, A., Clementi, G., and Scapagnini, U. (1985b). Effect of unilateral or bilateral mastectomy on prolactin secretion in male rats. *Neuroendocrinological Letters, 7,* 31–36.

Gerendai, I., Rotsztejn, W., Marchetti, B., Kordon, C., and Scapagnini, U. (1978). Unilateral ovariectomy induced luteinizing hormone–releasing hormone content changes in the two halves of the mediobasal hypothalamus. *Neuroscience Letters, 9,* 333–336.

Geschwind, N., and Behan, P. O. (1982). Left-handedness: Association with immune disease, migraine and developmental learning disorder. *Proceedings of the National Academy of Sciences of the United States of America, 79,* 5097–5100.

Geschwind, N., and Behan, P. O. (1984). Laterality, hormones and immunity. In N. Geschwind and A. M. Galaburda (Eds.), *Cerebral dominance* (pp 211–224). Cambridge, MA: Harvard University Press.

Geschwind, N., and Galaburda, A. M. (1985). Cerebral lateralization: Biological mechanisms, associations and pathology: II. A hypothesis and a program for research. *Archives of Neurology, 42,* 521–552.

Geschwind, N., and Galaburda, A. M. (1987). *Cerebral lateralization.* Cambridge, MA: MIT Press.

Glick, S. D., Carlson, J. N., Drew, K. L., and Shapiro, R. M. (1987). Functional and neurochemical asymmetry in the corpus striatum. In D. Ottoson (Ed.), *Duality and unity of the brain: Unified functioning and specialisation of the hemispheres* (pp 3–16). New York, NY: Plenum Press.

Glick, S. D., Meibach, R. C., Cox, R. D., and Maayani, S. (1980). Phencyclidine-induced rotation and hippocampal modulation of nigrostriatal asymmetry. *Brain Research, 196,* 99–107.

Glick, S. D., Meibach, R. C., Cox, R. D., and Maayani, S. (1983). Multiple and interrelated functional asymmetries in rat brain. *Life Sciences, 32,* 2215–2221.

Glick, S. D., Ross, D. A., and Hough, L. B. (1982). Lateral asymmetry of neurotransmitters in human brain. *Brain Research, 234,* 53–63.

Göbel, H., and Westphal, W. (1987). Die laterale Asymmetrie der menschlichen Schmerzempfindlichkeit. *Der Schmerz, 1,* 114–121.

Goldberg, J. M., and Randall, W. C. (1973). Dromotropic effects of stellate stimulation on the AV node and internodal pathways. *Proceedings of the Society for Experimental Biology and Medicine, 143,* 623–628.

Green, J. (1980). A review of the Lacey's physiological hypothesis of heart rate change. *Biological Psychology, 11,* 63–80.

Hachinski, V. C., Oppenheimer, S. M., Wilson, J. X., Guiraudon, C., and Cechetto, D. F. (1992). Asymmetry of sympathetic consequences of experimental stroke. *Archives of Neurology, 49,* 697–702.

Hageman, G. R., Goldberg, J. M., Armour, J. A., and Randall, W. C. (1973). Cardiac dysrhythmias induced by autonomic nerve stimulation. *American Journal of Cardiology, 32,* 823.

Hageman, G. R., Randall, W. C., and Armour, J. A. (1975). Direct and reflex cardiac bradydysrhythmias from small vagal nerve stimulations. *American Heart Journal, 89,* 338–348.

Hall, N. R., and Goldstein, A. L. (1985). Neurotransmitters and host defense. In R. Guillemin, M. Cohn, and T. Melnechuk (Eds.), *Neural modulation of immunity* (pp 143–154). New York, NY: Raven Press.

Hall, R. E., Livingstone, R. B., and Bloor, C. M. (1977). Orbital cortical influences on cardiovascular dynamics and myocardial structure in conscious monkeys. *Journal of Neurosurgery, 46,* 638–647.

Hall, W., and Clarke, I. M. C. (1982). Pain and laterality in a British pain clinic sample. *Pain, 14,* 63–66.

Hall, W. D., Hayward, L. D., and Chapman, C. R. (1981). On "the lateralization of pain." *Pain, 10,* 337–351.

Halligan, P. W., and Marshall, J. C. (1989). Laterality of motor response in visuo-spatial neglect: A case study. *Neuropsychologia, 27,* 1301–1307.

Halpern, D. F., and Coren, S. (1990). Laterality and longevity: Is left-handedness associated with a younger age at death? In S. Coren (Ed.), *Left-handedness. Behavioral implications and anomalies* (pp 509–545). Amsterdam: Elsevier North Holland.

Hamlin, R. L., and Smith, C. R. (1968). Effects of vagal stimulation on S-A and A-V nodes. *American Journal of Physiology, 215,* 560–568.

Hantas, M. N., Katkin, E. S., and Reed, S. D. (1984). Cerebral lateralization and heartbeat discrimination. *Psychophysiology, 21,* 274–278.

Harrison, D. W. (1990). The vascular orienting response and the law of initial values. *Biological Psychology, 31,* 149–155.

Haws, C. W., and Burgess, M. J. (1978). Effects of bilateral and unilateral stellate stimulation on canine ventricular refractory periods at sites of overlapping innervation. *Circulation Research, 42,* 195–198.

Heilman, K. M., Schwartz, H. D., and Watson, R. T. (1978). Hypoarousal in patients with the neglect syndrome and emotional indifference. *Neurology, 28,* 229–232.

Hilton, S. M., and Zbrozyna, A. W. (1963). Amygdaloid region for defence reactions and its efferent pathway to the brain stem. *Journal of Physiology, 165,* 160–173.

Hoff, E. C., Kell, J. F., and Carroll, M. N. (1963). Effects of cortical stimulation and lesions on cardiovascular function. *Physiological Reviews, 43,* 68–114.

Hoppe, K. D., and Bogen, J. E. (1977). Alexithymia in twelve commissurotomized patients. *Psychotherapy and Psychosomatics, 28,* 148–155.

Horel, J. A. (1988). Limbic neocortical interrelations. *Comparative Primate Biology, 4,* 81–97.

Hugdahl, K. (1984). Hemispheric asymmetry and bilateral electrodermal recordings: A review of the evidence. *Psychophysiology, 21,* 371–393.

Hugdahl, K., and Franzon, M. (1987). Heart-rate indices of hemispheric asymmetry in a discrete-trials stroop-paradigm. *Perceptual and Motor Skills, 64,* 1203–1211.

Hugdahl, K., Franzon, M., Andersson, B., and Walldebo, G. (1983). Heart-rate responses (HRR) to lateralized visual stimuli. *Pavlovian Journal of Biological Science, 18,* 186–198.

Inase, Y., and Machida, T. (1992). Differential effects of right-sided and left-sided orchidectomy on lateral asymmetry of LHRH cells in the mouse brain. *Brain Research, 580,* 338–340.

Irisawa, H., Caldwell, W. M., and Wilson, M. F. (1971). Neural regulation of atrioventricular conduction. *Japanese Journal of Physiology, 21,* 15–25.

Iwai, E., and Yukie, M. (1987). Amygdalofugal and amygdalopetal connections with modality-specific visual cortical areas in macques (*Macaca fuscata, M. mulatta,* and *M. fascicularis*). *The Journal of Comparative Neurology, 261,* 362–387.

Joanette, Y., Brouchon, M., Gauthier, L., and Samson, M. (1986). Pointing with left versus right hand in left visual field neglect. *Neuropsychologia, 24,* 391–396.

Johnson, R. H., Lambie, D. G., and Spalding, J. M. K. (1984). *Neurocardiology.* London: W. B. Saunders Co.

Kaas, J. H. (1986). The structural basis for information processing in the primate visual system. In J. D. Pettigrew, K. J. Sanderson, and W. R. Levick (Eds.), *Visual neuroscience* (pp 315–340). Cambridge, England: Cambridge University Press.

Kaas, J. H., Axelrod, S., and Diamond, I. T. (1967). An ablation study of the auditory cortex in the cat using binaural tonal patterns. *Journal of Neurophysiology, 30,* 710–724.

Kabani, N. J., Reader, T. A., and Dykes, R. W. (1990). Monoamines and their metabolites in somatosensory, visual, and cingulate cortices of adult rat: Differences in content and lack of sidedness. *Neurochemical Research, 15,* 1031–1036.

Kamosinska, B., Nowicki, D., and Szulczyk, P. (1989). Control of the heart rate by sympathetic nerves in cats. *Journal of the Autonomic Nervous System, 26,* 241–249.

Kang, D. H., Davidson, R. J., Coe, C. L., Wheeler, R. E., Tomarken, A. J., and Ershler, W. B. (1991). Frontal brain asymmetry and immune function. *Behavioral Neuroscience, 105,* 860–869.

Katkin, E. S., and Reed, S. D. (1988). Cardiovascular asymmetries and cardiac perception. *International Journal of Neuroscience, 39,* 45–52.

Kendrick, K. M., and Baldwin, B. A. (1987). Cells in temporal cortex of conscious sheep can respond preferentially to the sight of faces. *Science, 236,* 448–450.

Korner, P. I. (1979). Central nervous control of autonomic cardiovascular function. In R. M. Berne and N. N. Sperelakis (Eds.), *Handbook of physiology.* Sect 2: *The cardiovascular system,* Vol 1 (pp 691–739). Bethesda, MD: American Physiological Society.

Kramer, S. M. A., Albrecht, S., and Miller, R. A. (1985). Handedness and the laterality of breast cancer in women. *Nursing Research, 34,* 333–337.

Lacey, B. C., and Lacey, J. I. (1978). Two-way communication between the heart and the brain. Significance of time within the cardiac cycle. *American Psychologist, 33,* 99–113.

LaHoste, G. J., Neveu, P. J., Mormède, P., and Le Moal, M. (1989). Hemispheric asymmetry in the effects of cerebral cortical ablations on mitogen-induced lymphoproliferation and plasma prolactin levels in female rats. *Brain Research, 483,* 123–129.

Lane, R. D., Novelly, R., Cornell, C., Zeitlin, S., and Schwartz, G. E. (1989). Asymmetrical hemispheric control of heart rate (abstract). *Psychophysiology, 25,* 464.

Lane, R. D., and Schwartz, G. E. (1987). Induction of lateralized sympathetic input to the heart by the CNS during emotional arousal: A possible neurophysiologic trigger of sudden cardiac death. *Psychosomatic Medicine, 49,* 274–284.

Lane, R. D., and Schwartz, G. E. (1990). The neuropsychophysiology of emotion. *Functional Neurology, 5,* 263–266.

Levy, M. N., and Martin, P. J. (1979). Neural control of the heart. In R. M. Berne and N. N. Sperelakis (Eds.), *Handbook of physiology*, Sect 2: *The cardiovascular system*, Vol 1 (pp 581–620). Bethesda, MD: American Physiological Society.

Levy, M. N., Ng, M. L., and Zieske, H. (1966). Functional distribution of the peripheral cardiac sympathetic pathways. *Circulation Research, 19,* 650–661.

Lienert, G. A. (1978). *Verteilungsfreie Methoden in der Biostatistik*, Vol 2. Meisenheim: Hain.

London, W. P., and Albrecht, S. A. (1991). Breast cancer and cerebral laterality. *Perceptual and Motor Skills, 72,* 112–114.

Lown, B., Verrier, R., and Rabinowitz, S. (1977). Neural and psychological mechanisms and the problem of sudden cardiac death. *American Journal of Cardiology, 39,* 890–902.

Marcusson, J. O., Backstrom, J. T., and Ross, S. B. (1986). Single-site model of the neuronal 5-hydroxytryptamine uptake and imipramine-binding site. *Molecular Pharmacology, 30,* 121–128.

Malliani, A., Schwartz, P. J., and Zanchetti, A. (1980). Neural mechanisms in life-threatening arrhythmias. *American Heart Journal, 100,* 705–715.

Mayberg, H. S., Robinson, R. G., Wong, D. F., Parikh, R., Bolduc, P., Starkstein, S. E., Price, T., Dannals, R. F., Links, J. M., Wilson, A. A., Ravert, H. T., and Wagner, H. N. (1988). PET imaging of cortical S2 serotonin receptors after stroke: Lateralized changes and relationship to depression. *American Journal of Psychiatry, 145,* 937–943.

McManus, J. C., and Bryden, M. P. (1991). Geschwind's theory of cerebral lateralization: Developing a formal, causal model. *Psychological Bulletin, 110,* 237–253.

McManus, J. C., Naylor, J., and Booker, B. L. (1990). Left-handedness and myasthenia gravis. *Neuropsychologia, 28,* 947–955.

Meltzer, H. Y., and Lowy, M. T. (1987). The serotonin hypothesis of depression. In H. Y. Meltzer (Ed.), *Psychopharmacology: The third generation of progress* (pp 513–526). New York, NY: Raven Press.

Merskey, H., and Watson, G. D. (1979). The lateralization of pain. *Pain, 7,* 271–280.

Meyer, J. S. (1985). Biochemical effects of corticosteroids on neural tissues. *Physiological Reviews, 65,* 946–1020.

Mizeres, N. J. (1958). The origin and course of the cardioaccelerator fibers in the dog. *Anatomical Record, 132,* 261–279.

Montgomery, W. A., and Jones, G. E. (1984). Laterality, emotionality, and heartbeat perception. *Psychophysiology, 21,* 459–465.

Moran, T. H., Zern, K. A., Pearlson, G. D., Kubos, K. L., and Robinson, R. G. (1986). Cold water stress abolishes hyperactivity produced by cortical suction lesions without altering noradrenergic depletion. *Behavioral Neuroscience, 100,* 422–426.

Morilak, D. A., Fornal, C. A., and Jacobs, B. L. (1987). Effects of physiological manipulations on locus coeruleus neuronal activity in freely moving cats. II. Cardiovascular challenge. *Brain Research, 422,* 24–31.

Morrow, L., Vrtunski, P. B., Kim, Y., and Boller, F. (1981). Arousal responses to emotional stimuli and laterality of lesion. *Neuropsychologia, 19,* 65–71.

Moss, A. J., and McDonald, J. (1971). Unilateral cervicothoracic sympathetic ganglionectomy for the treatment of long Q-T interval syndrome. *New England Journal of Medicine, 285,* 903.

Moss, A. J., and Schwartz, P. J. (1979). Sudden death and the idiopathic long Q-T syndrome. *American Journal of Medicine, 66,* 6–7.

Munck, A., Guyre, P. M., and Holbrook, N. J. (1984). Physiological functions of glucocorticoids in stress and their relation to pharmacological actions. *Endocrine Reviews, 5,* 25–44.

Negrao, N., and Doty, R. W. (1969). Laterality of engram in macaques trained to respond to local electrical excitation of area striata. *Federation Proceedings, 28,* 647.

Neri, M., Vecchi, G. P., and Caselli, M. (1985). Pain measurements in right-left cerebral lesions. *Neuropsychologia, 23,* 123–126.

Neveu, P. J. (1988). Cerebral neocortex modulation of immune functions. *Life Sciences, 42,* 1917–1923.

Neveu, P. J. (1992a). Asymmetrical brain modulation of the immune response. *Brain Research Reviews, 17,* 101–107.

Neveu, P. J. (1992b). Asymmetrical brain modulation of immune reactivity in mice: A model for studying interindividual differences and physiological population heterogeneity? *Life Sciences, 50,* 1–6.

Neveu, P. J., Barnéoud, P., Vitiello, S., Betancur, C., and Le Moal, M. (1988). Brain modulation of the immune system: Association between lymphocyte responsiveness and paw preference in mice. *Brain Research, 457,* 392–394.

Neveu, P. J., Betancur, C., Barnéoud, P., Preud'homme, J. L., Aucouturier, P., LeMoal, M., and Vitiello, S. (1989). Functional brain asymmetry and murine systemic lupus crythematosus. *Brain Research, 498,* 159–162.

Neveu, P. J., Betancur, C., Barnéoud, P., Vitiello, S., and Le Moal, M. (1991). Functional brain asymmetry and lymphocyte proliferation in female mice: Effects of right and left cortical ablation. *Brain Research, 550,* 125–128.

Norris, J. W., and Hachinski, V. C. (1987). Cardiac dysfunction following stroke. In A. J. Furlan (Ed.), *The heart and stroke* (pp 171–183). Berlin: Springer-Verlag.

Oke, A., Keller, R., Mefford, J., and Adams, R. N. (1978). Lateralization of norepinephrine in human thalamus. *Science, 200,* 1411–1413.

Oke, A., Lewis, R., and Adams, R. N. (1980). Hemispheric asymmetry of norepinephrine distribution in rat thalamus. *Brain Research, 188,* 269–272.

Otto, M. W., Dougher, M. J., and Yeo, R. A. (1989). Depression, pain, and hemispheric activation. *Journal of Nervous and Mental Disease, 177,* 210–218.

Pandya, D. N., and Rosene, D. L. (1985). Some observations on trajectories and topography of commissural fibers. In A. G. Reeves (Ed.), *Epilepsy and the corpus callosum* (pp 21–39). New York, NY: Plenum Press.

Pandya, D. N., and Seltzer, B. (1986). The topography of commissural fibers. In F. Leporé, M. Ptito, and H. H. Jasper (Eds.), *Two hemispheres—one brain. Functions of the corpus callosum* (pp 47–73). New York, NY: Alan R. Liss.

Pandya, D. N., and Yeterian, E. H. (1986). Architecture and connections of cortical association areas. In A. Peters and E. G. Jones (Eds.), *Cerebral cortex*, Vol 4 (pp 3–61). New York, NY: Plenum Press.

Pearlson, G. D., and Robinson, R. G. (1981). Suction lesions of the frontal cortex in the rat induce asymmetrical behavioral and catecholaminergic responses. *Brain Research, 218,* 233–242.

Pfeifer, M. A., and Peterson, H. (1987). Cardiovascular autonomic neuropathy. In P. J. Dyck, P. K. Thomas, A. Asbury, A. J. Winegard, and D. Porte (Eds.), *Diabetic neuropathy* (pp 122–133). Philadelphia, PA: W. B. Saunders Co.

Poblete, R., Ruben, R. J., and Walker, A. E. (1959). Propagation of after-discharge between temporal lobes. *Journal of Neurophysiology, 22,* 538–553.

Price, J. L., and Amaral, D. G. (1981). An autoradiographic study of the projections of the central nucleus of the monkey amygdala. *Journal of Neuroscience, 1,* 1242–1259.

Randall, W. C. (1977). Sympathetic control of the heart. In W. C. Randall (Ed.), *Neural regulation of the heart* (pp 43–94). New York, NY: Oxford University Press.

Reinert, G., and Wittling, W. (1980). Klinische Psychologie: Konzepte und Tendenzen. In W. Wittling (Ed.), *Handbuch der klinischen Psychologie*, Vol 1 (pp 14–80). Hamburg: Hoffmann & Campe.

Renoux, G., and Bizière, K. (1986). Brain neocortex lateralized control of immune recognition. *Integrative Psychiatry, 4,* 32–40.

Renoux, G., Bizière, K., Renoux, M., Bardos, P., and Degenne, D. (1987). Consequences of bilateral brain neocortical ablation on imuthiol-induced immunostimulation in mice. In B. D. Jancovic, B. M. Markovic, and N. H. Spector (Eds.), *Neuroimmune interactions: Proceedings of the Second international Workshop on Neuroimmunomodulation* (pp 346–353). New York, NY: The New York Academy of Sciences.

Renoux, G., Bizière, K., Renoux, M., and Guillaumin, J. M. (1983a). The production of T-cell-inducing factors in mice is controlled by the brain neocortex. *Scandinavian Journal of Immunology, 17,* 45–50.

Renoux, G., Bizière, K., Renoux, M., Guillaumin, J. M., and Degenne, D. (1983b). A balanced brain asymmetry modulates T cell-mediated events. *Journal of Neuroimmunology, 5,* 227–238.

Robertson, I. (1991). Use of left vs. right hand in responding to lateralized stimuli in unilateral neglect. *Neuropsychologia, 29,* 1129–1135.

Robinson, R. G. (1979). Differential behavioral and biochemical effects of right and left hemispheric cerebral infarction in the rat. *Science, 205,* 707–710.

Rogers, M. C., Battit, G., McPeek, B., and Todd, D. (1978). Lateralization of sympathetic control of the human sinus node: ECG changes of stellate ganglion block. *Anesthesiology, 48,* 139–141.

Roschmann, R., and Wittling, W. (1992). Topographic brain mapping of emotion-related hemisphere asymmetries. *International Journal of Neuroscience, 63,* 5–16.

Roschmann, R., Wittling, W., and Pflüger, M. (1992). Visumotorische Langzeitlateralisierung als Methode zur Untersuchung funktionaler Hemisphärenasymmetrien (abstract). In L. Montada (Ed.), *Bericht über den 38. Kongress der deutschen Gesellschaft für Psychologie in Trier 1992*, Vol 1 (p 831). Göttingen: Hogrefe.

Rosen, A. D., Gur, R. C., Sussman, N., Gur, R. E., and Hurtig, H. (1982). Hemispheric asymmetry in the control of heart rate. *Abstracts of Social Neuroscience, 8,* 917.

Rossor, M., Garrett, N., and Iversen, L. (1980). No evidence for lateral asymmetry of neurotransmitters in post-mortem human brain. *Journal of Neurochemistry, 35,* 743–745.

Sakanaka, M., Shibasaki, T., and Lederis, K. (1986). Distribution and efferent projections of corticotropin-releasing factor-like immunoreactivity in the rat amygdaloid complex. *Brain Research, 382,* 213–238.

Saper, C. B., Loewy, A. D., Swanson, L. W., and Cowan, W. M. (1976). Direct hypothalamo-autonomic connections. *Brain Research, 117,* 305–312.

Saron, C. D., and Davidson, R. J. (1989). Visual evoked potential measures of interhemispheric transfer time in humans. *Behavioral Neuroscience, 103,* 1115–1138.

Schildkraut, J. (1965). The catecholamine hypothesis on affective disorders: A review of supporting evidence. *American Journal of Psychiatry, 122,* 509–522.

Schmidt, R. F., and Thews, G. (Eds.) (1989). *Human physiology.* Berlin: Springer-Verlag.

Schneider, L. H., Murphy, R. B., and Coons, E. E. (1982). Lateralization of striatal dopamine (D2) receptors in normal rats. *Neuroscience Letters, 33,* 281–284.

Schrandt, N. J., Tranel, D., and Damasio, H. (1989). The effect of focal cerebral lesions on skin conductance responses to "signal" stimuli. *Neurology, 39* (Suppl 1), 223.

Schuri, U., and von Cramon, D. (1982). Electrodermal response patterns in neurological patients with disturbed vigilance. *Behavioural Brain Research, 4,* 95–102.

Schwartz, P. J. (1976). Cardiac sympathetic innervation and the sudden infant death syndrome. *The American Journal of Medicine, 60,* 167–172.

Schwartz, P. J. (1984). Sympathetic imbalence and cardiac arrhythmias. In W. C. Randall (Ed.), *Nervous control of cardiovascular function* (pp 225–252). New York, NY: Oxford University Press.

Schwartz, P. J., and Malliani, A. (1975). Electrical alternation of the T-wave: Clinical and experimental evidence of its relationship with the sympathetic nervous system and with the long Q-T syndrome. *American Heart Journal, 89,* 45–50.

Schwartz, P. J., Periti, M., and Malliani, A. (1975). The long Q-T syndrome. *American Heart Journal, 89,* 378–390.

Schwartz, P. J., Snebold, N. G., and Brown, A. M. (1975). Effects of unilateral cardiac sympathetic denervation on the ventricular fibrillation threshold (abstract). *American Journal of Cardiology, 35,* 169.

Schwartz, P. J., Stone, H. L., and Brown, A. M. (1976). Effects of unilateral stellate ganglion blockade on the arrhythmias associated with coronary occlusion. *American Heart Journal, 92,* 589–599.

Schweiger, E., Wittling, W., and Roschmann, R. (1992). *Left-handedness and psychosomatic disorder.* Paper presented at the Second International Congress of Behavioral Medicine, Hamburg, Germany, July 15–18, 1992.

Searleman, A., and Fugagli, A. K. (1987). Suspected autoimmune disorders and left-handedness: Evidence from individuals with diabetes, Crohn's disease and ulcerative colitis. *Neuropsychologia, 25,* 367–374.

Senie, R. T., Rosen, P. P., Schottenfeld, D., and Lesser, M. L. (1980). Epidemiological factors related to laterality in breast carcinoma. *Clinical Bulletin, 10,* 30–33.

Shannahoff-Khalsa, D. (1991). Lateralized rhythms of the central and autonomic nervous system. *International Journal of Psychophysiology, 11,* 225–251.

Shapiro, R. M., Camarota, N. A., and Glick, S. D. (1987). Nocturnal rotational behavior in rats: Further neurochemical support for a two-population model. *Brain Research Bulletin, 19,* 421–427.

Shapoval, L. N., Sagach, V. F., and Pobegailo, L. S. (1991). Chemosensitive ventrolateral medulla in the cat: The fine structure and GABA-induced cardiovascular effects. *Journal of the Autonomic Nervous System, 36*, 159–172.

Shipley, M. T. (1982). Insular cortex projection to the nucleus of the solitary tract and brainstem visceromotor regions in the mouse. *Brain Research Bulletin, 8*, 139–148.

Silberman, E. K., and Weingartner, H. 1986. Hemispheric lateralization of functions related to emotion. *Brain and Cognition, 5*, 322–353.

Sklar, L. S., and Anisman, H. (1981). Stress and cancer. *Psychological Bulletin, 89*, 369–406.

Smith, J. (1987). Left-handedness: Its association with allergic disease. *Neuropsychologia, 25*, 665–674.

Spoont, M. R. (1992). Modulatory role of serotonin in neural information processing: Implications for human psychopathology. *Psychological Bulletin, 112*, 330–350.

Spyer, K. M. (1989). Neural mechanisms involved in cardiovascular control during affective behaviour. *Trends in Neurosciences, 12*, 506–513.

Stein, B. E., Price, D. D., and Gazzaniga, M. S. (1989). Pain perception in a man with total corpus callosum transection. *Pain, 38*, 51–56.

Stone, J. (1966). The naso-temporal division of the cat's retina. *Journal of Comparative Neurology, 136*, 585–600.

Stone, J., Leicester, J., and Sherman, S. M. (1973). The naso-temporal division of the monkey retina. *Journal of Comparative Neurology, 150*, 333–348.

Talbot, J. D., Marrett, M. S., Evans, A. C., Meyer, E., Bushnell, M. C., and Duncan, G. H. (1991). Multiple representations of pain in human cerebral cortex. *Science, 251*, 1355–1358.

Talman, W. T. (1985). Cardiovascular regulation and lesions of the central nervous system. *Annals of Neurology, 18*, 1–12.

Tekes, K., Tóthfalusi, L., Arató, M., Palkovits, M., Demeter, E., and Magyar, K. (1988). Is there a correlation between serotonin metabolism and ^{3}H-imipramine binding in the human brain? Hemispheric lateralization of imipramine binding sites. *Pharmacological Research Communications, 20* (Suppl 1), 41–42.

TenHouten, W. D., Walter, D. O., Hoppe, K. D., and Bogen, J. E. (1988). Alexithymia and the split brain: VI. Electroencephalographic correlates of alexithymia. *Psychiatric Clinics of North America, 11*, 317–329.

Trevarthen, C. (Ed.). (1990). *Brain circuits and functions of the mind. Essays in honor of Roger W. Sperry*. Cambridge, England: Cambridge University Press.

Troxler, R. G., Sprague, E. A., Albanese, R. A., and Thompson, A. J. (1977). The association of elevated plasma cortisol and early atherosclerosis as demonstrated by coronary angiography. *Atherosclerosis, 26*, 151–162.

Tsokos, G. C., and Balow, J. E. (1986). Regulation of human cellular immune responses by glucocorticosteroids. In N. P. Plotnikoff, R. E. Faith, A. J. Murgo, and R. A. Good (Eds.), *Enkephalins and endorphins. Stress and the immune system* (pp 159–171). New York, NY: Plenum Press.

Tucker, D. M., and Williams, P. A. (1984). Asymmetric neural control systems in human self-regulation. *Psychological Review, 91*, 185–215.

Varni, J. G., Doerr, H. O., and Franklin, J. R. (1971). Bilateral differences in skin resistance and vasomotor activity. *Psychophysiology, 8*, 390–400.

Vincent, G. M. (1986). The heart rate of Romano-Ward syndrome patients. *American Heart Journal, 112,* 61–64.

Wada, J. A., Mizoguchi, T., and Komai, S. (1981). Cortical motor activation in amygdaloid kindling: Observations in nonepileptic rhesus monkeys with anterior two thirds callosal bisection. In J. A. Wada (Ed.), *Kindling 2* (pp 235–248). New York, NY: Raven Press.

Wagner, H. N., Burns, D. H., Dannals, R. F., Wong, D. F., Langstrom, B., Duelfer, T., Frost, J. J., Ravert, H. T., Links, J. M., Rosenbloom, S. B., Lucas, S. E., Kramer, A. V., and Kuhlar, M. J. (1983). Imaging dopamine receptors in the human brain by positron tomography. *Science, 221,* 1264–1266.

Walker, B. B., and Sandman, C. A. (1979). Human visual evoked responses are related to heart rate. *Journal of Comparative and Physiological Psychology, 93,* 717–729.

Walker, B. B., and Sandman, C. A. (1982). Visual evoked potentials change as heart rate and carotid pressure change. *Psychophysiology, 19,* 520–527.

Wall, P. D., and Davis, G. D. (1951). Three cerebral cortical systems affecting autonomic function. *Journal of Neurophysiology, 14,* 507–517.

Weisz, J., Balazs, L., Lang, E., and Adam, G. (1990). The effect of lateral visual fixation and the direction of eye movements on heartbeat discrimination. *Psychophysiology, 27,* 523–527.

Weitkunat, R., Cestaro, V., and Katkin, E. S. (1989). Evidence for a lateralized heartbeat evoked potential (abstract). *Psychophysiology, 26,* 65.

Weitkunat, R., and Schandry, R. (1990). Motivation and heartbeat evoked potentials. *Journal of Psychophysiology, 4,* 33–40.

Weller, R. E., and Kaas. J. H. (1981). Cortical and subcortical connections of visual cortex in primates. In C. N. Woolsey (Ed.), *Cortical sensory organization, Vol 2: Multiple visual areas* (pp 121–155). Clifton, NJ: Humana Press.

Wittling, W. (1973). *Funktionle Hemisphären-Spezialisierung: Theorien, Methoden und Ergebnisse neuropsychologischer Forschung.* Dissertation, University of Mannheim, Germany.

Wittling, W. (1976). *Einführung in die Psychologie der Wahrnehmung.* Hamburg: Hoffmann & Campe.

Wittling, W. (1980). Klinische Psychologie im Rahmen medizinischer Probleme und Institutionen. In W. Wittling (Ed.), *Handbuch der klinischen Psychologie, Vol 6* (pp 341–407). Hamburg: Hoffmann & Campe.

Wittling, W. (1990a). Psychophysiological correlates of human brain asymmetry: Blood pressure changes during lateralized presentation of an emotionally laden film. *Neuropsychologia, 28,* 457–470.

Wittling, W. (1990b). Sind biopsychologische Störungsmodelle hirnlos? Plädoyer für eine Integration von Neuropsychologie und Gesundheitspsychologie (abstract). In D. Frey (Ed.), *Bericht über den 37. Kongress der deutschen Gesellschaft für Psychologie in Kiel 1990, Vol 1* (pp 695–696). Göttingen: Hogrefe.

Wittling, W. (1991). Emotionale Hemisphärenasymmetrien: Neue Forschungsansätze und ihre Bedeutung für die psycho-somatische Reaktivität. In D. Frey (Ed.), *Bericht über den 37. Kongress der deutschen Gesellschaft für Psychologie in Kiel 1990, Vol 2* (pp 656–659). Göttingen: Hogrefe.

Wittling, W. (1992). Hemisphäreninteraktion, Leistung und Belastung: Was "nützt" die Hirnforschung der Arbeitswissenschaft? In H. Bubb and W. v. Eiff (Eds.), *Innovative Arbeitssystemgestaltung—Mensch, Organisation, Information und Technik in der Wertschöpfungskette* (pp 21–35). Cologne: Wirtschaftsverlag Bachem.

Wittling, W. (1993). Asymmetrien der zerebralen Kontrolle autonomer Körperprozesse und psychosomatische Störungsanfälligkeit. In L. Montada (Ed.), *Bericht über den 38. Kongress der deutschen Gesellschaft für Psychologie in Trier 1992*, Vol 2. Göttingen: Hogrefe.

Wittling, W., and Pflüger, M. (1990). Neuroendocrine hemisphere asymmetries: Salivary cortisol secretion during lateralized viewing of emotion-related and neutral films. *Brain and Cognition, 14,* 243–265.

Wittling, W., and Roschmann, R. (1993). Emotion-related hemisphere asymmetry: Subjective emotional responses to laterally presented films. *Cortex, 29,* 431–448.

Wittling, W., Roschmann, R., and Schweiger, E. (1993). Topographic brain mapping of emotion-related hemisphere activity and susceptibility to psychosomatic disorders. In K. Maurer (Ed.), *Imaging of the brain in psychiatry and related fields* (pp 271–276). Berlin: Springer-Verlag.

Wittling, W., and Schweiger, E. (1992a). *Brain asymmetry in the regulation of autonomic arousal in emotion-related situations.* Presented at the International Neuropsychological Symposium, Schluchsee, Germany, June 22–26, 1992.

Wittling, W., and Schweiger, E. (1992b). *Neuroendocrine brain asymmetry and physical health.* Presented at the First International Symposium on Psychobiology, Giessen, Germany, November 19–21, 1992.

Wittling, W., and Schweiger, E. (1993a). Neuroendocrine brain asymmetry and physical complaints. *Neuropsychologia, 31,* 591–608.

Wittling, W., and Schweiger, E. (1993b). Alterations of neuroendocrine brain asymmetry: A neural risk factor affecting physical health. *Neuropsychobiology, 28,* 25–29.

Wofsy, D. (1984). Hormones, handedness and autoimmunity. *Immunology Today, 5,* 169–170.

Yamamoto, B. K., and Freed, C. R. (1984). Asymmetric dopamine and serotonin metabolism in nigrostriatal and limbic structures of the trained circling rat. *Brain Research, 297,* 115–119.

Yamour, B. J., Sridharan, M. R., Rice, J. F., and Flowers, N. C. (1980). Electrocardiographic changes in cerebrovascular hemorrhage. *American Heart Journal, 99,* 294–300.

Yanowitz, F., Preston, J. B., and Abildskov, J. A. (1966). Functional distribution of right and left stellate innervation to the ventricles. *Circulation Research, 18,* 416–428.

Zamrini, E. Y., Meador, K. J., Loring, D. W., Nichols, F. T., Lee, G. P., Figueroa, R. E., and Thompson, W. O. (1990). Unilateral cerebral inactivation produces differential left/right heart rate responses. *Neurology, 40,* 1408–1411.

Zeitlin, S. B., Lane, R. D., O'Leary, D. S., and Schrift, M. J. (1989). Interhemispheric transfer deficit and alexithymia. *American Journal of Psychiatry, 146,* 1434–1439.

Zimmerberg, B., Glick, S. D., and Jerussi, T. P. (1974). Neurochemical correlate of a spatial preference in rats. *Science, 185,* 623–625.

Zoccolotti, P., Caltagirone, C., Benedetti, N., and Gainotti, G. (1986). Perturbation des réponses végétatives aux stimuli émotionnels au cours des lésions hémisphériques unilatérales. *L'Encéphale, 12,* 263–268.

Zoccolotti, P., Scabini, D., and Violani, C. (1982). Electrodermal responses in patients with unilateral brain damage. *Journal of Clinical Neuropsychology, 4,* 143–150.

VI Emotional Lateralization

13 Cerebral Asymmetry, Emotion, and Affective Style

Richard J. Davidson

Emotion is a class of behavior that has invited the consideration of its underlying biological substrates since the time it was first studied. Probably more than any other class of behavior, emotion often involves frank biological changes that are frequently perceptible to the person in whom the emotion arises as well as to an observer (e.g., facial blood flow changes, as in "white with fear"). For much of its relatively short history in scientific psychology, the focus of research on the biological substrates of emotion was mostly on the autonomic changes that accompany emotion in humans or the subcortical limbic system circuits that mediate specific emotional behaviors in animals. Both of these research endeavors have yielded important insights about the nature of emotion. However, it is clear that in more complex animals, and especially in humans, the cerebral cortex plays an important role in aspects of emotional behavior and experience (Kolb and Taylor, 1990). In particular, anterior cortical regions, which have extensive anatomic reciprocity with both subcortical centers and with posterior cortical circuits, are critically implicated in emotional behavior. These anterior cortical zones are the brain regions which have shown more dramatic growth in relative size over the course of phylogeny compared with other brain regions (see Luria, 1973; Jerison, 1973, for reviews).

The focus of this chapter is on asymmetries in anterior cortical function that have been implicated in different forms of emotional behavior. Among the earliest suggestions regarding the importance of hemispheric asymmetries for emotional behavior were observations on patients with unilateral cortical lesions (e.g., Jackson, 1878). The majority of these reports indicated that damage to the left hemisphere was more likely to lead to what has been termed a *catastrophic-depressive reaction* compared with comparable damage to the right hemisphere (e.g., Goldstein, 1939). More recent studies have confirmed this basic observation (e.g., Gainotti, 1972; Sackeim et al., 1982). Of particular importance for the research to be reviewed in this chapter are studies by Robinson and his colleagues (1984). They have reported that it is damage specifically to the left frontal lobe which results in depressive symptomatology. They found that among left brain–damaged patients, the closer the lesion was to the frontal pole, the more severe the depressive symptomatology. Patients that developed mania subsequent to brain injury were much more likely to have sustained damage to the right hemisphere, sparing the left. These and other observations have provided the basis for our studies of anterior activation asymmetries associated with emotion and affective style. In the next part of this chapter, I sketch the major elements of the theoretical model that motivates the research to be presented. The methods that are common to our studies and the unique methodologic requirements of this research are then described. Research on anterior asymmetries associated with the phasic arousal of emotion are presented, followed by a summary of our findings on the relations between individual differences in baseline asymmetry and affective reactivity. The chapter ends with a discussion of some unanswered questions which are posed by this work.

THE ROLE OF THE CEREBRAL HEMISPHERES IN EMOTIONAL PROCESSING: A THEORETICAL ACCOUNT

That a fundamental asymmetry in the control of functions related to emotion is present is not surprising in light of speculations concerning the evolutionary advantages of cerebral asymmetry (e.g., Levy, 1972). In searching for the basis of the asymmetry underlying emotion, it is instructive to recall that investigators in comparative psychology, (Schneirla, 1959), behavioral neuroscience (Stellar and Stellar, 1985), and child development (Kagan et al., 1988) all agree that approach and withdrawal are fundamental motivational dimensions which may be found at any level of phylogeny where behavior itself is present. In several previous articles (e.g., Davidson, 1984, 1987, 1988; Davidson et al., 1990b; Davidson and Tomarken, 1989), my colleagues and I have suggested that the anterior regions of the left and right hemispheres are specialized for approach and withdrawal processes, respectively. The bases upon which this suggestion are made are as follows: First, the left frontal region has been described as an important center for intention, self-regulation, and planning (Luria, 1973). The functions which have been ascribed to this area are those which historically have been assigned to the *will*, a hypothetical structure of central import to approach-related behavior. Second, over the course of ontogeny, the infant and toddler will approach and reach out to objects of interest using its right hand much more often than its left (e.g., Young et al., 1983). It would be of interest to examine whether episodes of right-handed reaching and grasping are in fact associated with expressive signs of positive affect (e.g., smiling). Right-handed reaching and positive affect are taken to be the collective manifestation of a brain circuit mediating approach behavior, with the left frontal region serving as a "convergence zone" for this circuit (see Damasio, 1989, for a description of convergence zones, and Davidson, 1992a,b, for their application to the frontal emotion circuit). Third, as I have noted above, damage to the left frontal region results in behavior and experience which might best be characterized as a deficit in approach. Patients with damage to this brain region are apathetic, experience loss of interest and pleasure in objects and people, and have difficulty initiating voluntary action (i.e., psychomotor retardation). Thus, hypoactivation in this region should be associated with a lowered threshold for the experience of sadness and depression. The claim that the right anterior region is specialized for withdrawal is based upon a less extensive, but growing corpus of evidence. The most compelling evidence are the data on normal humans involving electrophysiologic measures of regional hemispheric activation. These findings, which are reviewed in detail in later sections, indicate that during the experimental arousal of withdrawal-related emotional states (e.g., fear and disgust), the right frontal and anterior temporal regions are selectively activated. In addition, subjects with baseline tonic activation in these regions show a propensity to respond with accentuated withdrawal-related negative affect to appropriate emotion elicitors. Such persons also report greater dispositional negative affect.

Recently, Morris and colleagues (1991) studied a patient with a right temporal lobectomy using psychophysiologic measures of affective reactivity in response to standardized laboratory elicitors of positive and negative emotion. The resection was performed to remove an arteriovenous malformation in the right temporal lobe and included the anterior portion of the temporal lobe and the whole right amygdala. The stimuli presented to the patient were slides which differed in valence, but which were matched on overall saliency. They recorded the skin conductance response to these slide stimuli. They found that the skin conductance response to the positive stimuli was equivalent in magnitude to that observed in normals. However, skin conductance responses to the negative slides were markedly attenuated. Using measures of regional cerebral blood flow derived from positron emission tomography (PET), Reiman and colleagues (1984) reported accentuated activation during a resting baseline in a right hemisphere subcortical site which projects to the amygdala in panic-prone patients. Taken together, these observations suggest a specialization for certain anterior cortical and subcortical right hemisphere regions in the mediation of withdrawal-related negative affect. Precisely what the differential role of the anterior temporal and frontal regions is in the mediation of the negative affective responding is not clear from the available evidence.

Some of the evidence referred to above is derived from the study of patients with unilateral lesions. Other findings come from the assessment of regional brain activation in neurologically intact subjects. In light of the assumption that lesions result in selective deficits in activation in the lesioned area (e.g., Burke et al., 1982), the findings described above support the following hypotheses regarding the anterior hemispheric substrates of emotion and emotion-related processes. Activation in the left anterior region is associated with approach-related emotions; deficient activation in this region is associated with emotion-related phenomena that might best be described as reflecting approach-related deficits such as sadness and depression; and activation in the right anterior region is associated with withdrawal-related emotions such as fear and disgust and withdrawal-related psychopathologic states such as anxiety. Two additional conceptual issues deserve emphasis. The first concerns the subcomponents of emotion which I address in this chapter and in the research that is described. The focus here is on the experience and expression of emotion. The hemispheric substrates of perceiving emotional information are likely to be different from those involved in actual emotional experience. Similarly, the underlying neural controls for the communication of information *about* emotion are likely to be different from those implicated in the experience and expression of *actual* emotion. In this regard it is instructive to note that some investigators have argued for a more general role for the right hemisphere in all emotion (e.g., Borod et al., 1986; Etcoff, 1986). However, it is imperative to emphasize that data upon which this claim is based are largely studies of the perception of emotional information (e.g., facial expressions) where the weight of the evidence does indeed suggest that the right *posterior* region is specialized for the perception of emotional information irrespective of valence. This fact underscores the importance of differentiating among different components of emotional functioning, most importantly between the perception of emotion and the experience or expression of emotion. In addition to my own writing on this issue (e.g., Davidson, 1984, 1988), a number of other commentators who have reviewed this literature have reached similar conclusions (e.g., Leventhal and Tomarken, 1986; Silberman and Weingartner, 1986).

The second issue concerns the importance of specifying the hypothesized logical status of the relation between asymmetric anterior activation and emotion-related processes. Failure to consider this problem has been a source of considerable confusion in previous reviews of this topic (see Davidson, 1993, for an extensive discussion of this issue). Although a large number of reports indicate that damage to the left hemisphere, particularly in the anterior regions, results in depressive symptomatology far more frequently than damage to corresponding regions of the right hemisphere, some investigators have underscored the fact that a number of reports have appeared which have shown no clear difference in the incidence or severity of depressive symptomatology in left brain–vs. right brain–damaged patients (e.g., House et al., 1990; see review by Gainotti, 1989). In addition to the obvious fact that many of the studies cited by Gainotti (1989) combined patients with both anterior and posterior damage, there is another crucial point in the interpretation of such data which has not been explicit in most of the reviews on this subject. We have proposed that anterior activation asymmetry functions as a diathesis which predisposes an individual to respond with predominantly positive or negative affect, *given an appropriate emotion elicitor*. In the absence of a specific elicitor, differences in affective symptomatology among persons with different patterns of anterior activation asymmetry or asymmetry of anterior brain lesions would not be expected. Consistent with this prediction is our observation that while baseline anterior asymmetry predicts reactivity to an affective challenge, it is unrelated to measures of the individual's current, unprovoked emotional state (e.g., Davidson and Fox, 1989; Tomarken, Davidson, and

Henriques, 1990; Wheeler, Davidson, and Tomarken, 1993).[1] Thus, in a patient with left anterior damage, depressive symptomatology would be expected only if that patient were exposed to the requisite environmental stresses. Left anterior damage is not in itself *sufficient* for the production of depressive symptomatology. We would therefore *not* expect *all* patients with left frontal damage to show depressive symptomatology. Only those exposed to an appropriate set of environmental stresses would be expected to show the hypothesized final state.[2]

CEREBRAL PSYCHOPHYSIOLOGIC METHODS IN THE STUDY OF HEMISPHERIC ASYMMETRY RELATED TO EMOTION AND AFFECTIVE STYLE

Several important considerations apply to the choice of methods for studying regional brain activity that underlies emotion. Many of the core phenomena of emotion are brief and therefore require measures that have a very fast time resolution. Moreover, periods of peak emotional intensity are unpredictable. They can occur at different points in time for different subjects in response to the same emotional stimulus. For example, some facial expressions of emotion are present for as little as 1 to 2 seconds. An ideal method would be one which could resolve activity as brief as the behavioral manifestations of emotion. It is also important to be able to record physiologic activity over much longer time intervals. This is needed when subjects are presented with affect elicitors that last several minutes, requiring physiology to be integrated over the entire period of the eliciting stimulus. In addition, as I describe in detail below, one of the most exciting new areas in psychophysiologic research on emotion is the study of the biological bases of individual differences in emotional reactivity. Such studies often require baseline physiology to be integrated over several minutes in order to obtain a reliable estimate of an individual's characteristic pattern. Thus, with respect to time resolution, the ideal measure would range from subsecond intervals to several minutes.

Another important consideration is related to the first. Data must be stored in a form which will permit post hoc extraction of epochs of varying durations. The capacity for post hoc data extraction is required so that physiology coincident with objective measures of emotional state (e.g., facial expressions of emotion) can be examined. In some of the research to be described below, brain activity coincident with the display of spontaneous facial expressions of emotion is extracted for analysis. Other measures of emotional state might also be utilized in a similar fashion, including vocal indices and on-line self-report. This requirement presupposes the accurate synchronization of the behavioral and physiologic data streams. Modern computer and video technology allow for this possibility.

Another essential requirement of any measure of regional brain activity used in the study of emotion is that it be relatively noninvasive. There are three major reasons for this. First, the more intrusive a method, the greater will be the interference with the elicitation of actual emotion. For example, certain types of PET scan protocols are highly intrusive and it is difficult to override the anxiety which is an inherent side effect of the procedure. It would likely be very difficult to elicit strong positive affect in many subjects undergoing a PET scan. The second important reason for limiting measures of regional brain activation to those that are relatively noninvasive is the need to study individuals over time as they undergo several different emotional states. It is crucial that psychophysiologic studies of emotion compare between at least two different emotions and a baseline period (see Davidson et al., 1990b, for a complete discussion of methodologic desiderata in psychophysiologic studies of emotion). Such comparisons enable the investigator to determine if the physiologic pattern observed during the emotion period differs from baseline, and if the pattern is simply characteristic of emotion per se (in which case the pattern associated with each of the two different emotions will not differ) or is emotion-specific. The third reason for preferring relatively noninvasive procedures is the possibility of using them with infants and young children. These age groups are particularly important in research on the biological bases of emotion, and the methods used must be appropriate for this population. In light of the considerations noted above, we have been using scalp-recorded brain electrical activity to make inferences about regional brain activation during the experimental arousal of acute emotions and emotion-related patterns of brain activity during resting baselines. The electroencephalogram (EEG) meets all of the requirements noted above. It is noninvasive, has a fast time resolution, and can be effectively synchronized with a behavioral data stream which permits extraction of data based upon post hoc specification of periods of intense behavioral signs of emotion. We have used recordings of brain electrical activity to make inferences about regional brain activation both during baseline periods as well as in response to a variety of emotion elicitors in adults, toddlers, and infants. We can examine brain activity during very brief epochs of emotion (1 second), provided that periods of the same emotion type occur sufficiently frequently within an individual. To obtain stable estimates of spectral power from which measures of activation are derived, one needs a minimum of approximately 10 to 15 seconds of activity. The individual epochs themselves can be as brief as 1 second, but when aggregated together, their sum must exceed approximately 10 seconds in length (Davidson, 1988; Tomarken et al., 1992). Movement and muscle activity frequently accompany the generation of emotion. We have developed procedures to partial out statistically the contributions of the muscle activity from the EEG (see Davidson, 1988, for a description of the method, and Henriques and Davidson, 1990, for the application of the method in an actual experiment). Finally, we use an electrode cap for EEG recording (Blom and Anneveldt, 1982). Such a cap permits accurate and rapid placement of electrodes and is particularly useful in studies with infants and children, with whom rapid application of electrodes is essential.

The principal measure extracted from the EEG in the studies I present in this chapter is power in the alpha band, which in adults represents activity between 8 and 13 Hz.[3] A wealth of evidence indicates that power in this frequency band is inversely related to activation in adults (e.g., Shagass, 1972). In the studies I describe on infants, we have used power in a lower frequency band as our dependent measure since this represents the functional equivalent of adult alpha activity (see, e.g., Davidson and Fox, 1989; Davidson and Tomarken, 1989). Our measures of band power are computed from the output of a fast Fourier transform (FFT) which decomposes the brain activity into its underlying frequency components.

Below I briefly review the findings from several recent studies performed in our laboratory where we examined brain activity during the experience or expression of experimentally aroused positive and negative emotion.

ANTERIOR ASYMMETRIES DURING THE EXPERIMENTAL AROUSAL OF APPROACH- AND WITHDRAWAL-RELATED EMOTION

We recently completed a collaborative study with Ekman and Friesen and others (Davidson et al., 1990b) in which adult subjects were exposed to short film clips designed to induce approach-related positive emotion and withdrawal-related negative emotion. Happiness and amusement were the positive, approach-related emotions and disgust was the negative, withdrawal-related emotion. Subjects were presented with two positive and two negative film clips in a darkened room while we videotaped their facial behavior unobtrusively. We also recorded brain electrical activity from the left and right frontal, central, anterior temporal, and parietal regions. An important consideration in research on emotion is that when two or more emotions are compared for their effects on either physiologic or behavioral-dependent variables, the intensities of the elicited emotion must be comparable. If the emotions differ in intensity, then any differences found between them could be attributed to intensity per se, rather than the qualitative nature of the emotion aroused. Accordingly, our positive and negative films were carefully matched on the intensities of the primary emotion elicited by each (amusement for the positive films and disgust for the negative films) as determined by self-report.

The video record of each subject was coded with Ekman and Friesen's (1978) *Facial Action Coding System (FACS)*. FACS distinguishes 44 action units, the minimal units anatomically separable and visually distinctive. Any facial movement can be described in terms of the particular action unit, or units, that produced it. The scorer identifies the action units, such as the one which lowers the brow or pulls the lip corners up, rather than making inferences about underlying emotional states such as anger or happiness. FACS scoring of the facial data from this experiment revealed that the two types of expression which occurred with the most frequency were happy expressions in

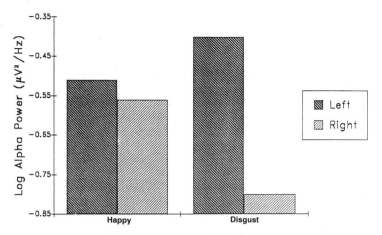

Figure 13.1   Mean log-transformed alpha power (in μV²/Hz) for the left and right midfrontal regions (F3 and F4) during happy and disgust facial expression conditions. (More negative numbers indicate less alpha power. The negative numbers are a function of the log transformation. Lower numbers (i.e., more negative) are associated with increased activation). (From Davidson et al., 1990b.)

response to the positive film clips and disgust expressions in response to the negative film clips. For each subject, the onset and offset of each happy and disgust expression was identified with FACS. These times were then entered into the computer so that EEGs coincident with these expressions could be extracted.

Following removal of eye movement, muscle, and gross movement artifact, the EEG during periods of happy and disgust facial expressions was Fourier-transformed and power in different frequency bands was calculated. Based upon the theory and evidence reviewed above, we hypothesized that the disgust periods would be associated with greater right-sided anterior activation compared with the happy periods, and that the happy periods would be associated with greater left-sided activation compared with the disgust periods. Figure 13.1 presents the alpha power data for the frontal leads. As can be seen from the figure, disgust is associated with less alpha power (i.e., *more* activation) in the right frontal lead compared with happiness, while happiness is associated with less alpha power in the left frontal lead compared with disgust. The Hemisphere × Valence interaction was highly significant ($P <$ .0005). This pattern of greater right-sided activation during disgust compared with happiness was also found in the anterior temporal electrodes. Importantly, there were no significant Hemisphere × Valence interactions in the central or parietal regions, underscoring the specificity of the valence-related asymmetry to anterior brain regions.

We examined frontal asymmetry on an individual subject basis to determine how consistent the difference was between happy and disgust epochs.

For each subject, we calculated an asymmetry index which expressed the asymmetry of frontal alpha power in a single metric. The index was log right minus log left alpha power. Higher numbers on this index denote greater relative left-sided activation. We computed this index separately for the happy and disgust periods. We found that 100% of the subjects showed a lower score on this index during the disgust compared with the happy periods. The direction of this difference indicates greater right-sided frontal activation during the disgust than during the happy conditions. We also found that there were large differences among individuals in their average asymmetry score (across emotion conditions). The difference between happy and disgust conditions appears to be superimposed upon subjects' basal levels of asymmetry. In the next part of this chapter, we show how such individual differences in asymmetry are related to characteristic differences in mood and affective reactivity, in short, to affective style.

In order to examine whether the procedures we used to verify the presence of an emotion (i.e., facial expression) actually made an important difference in uncovering patterns of asymmetry, we performed the type of analysis which is more typical in research on the psychophysiology of emotion. We simply compared all artifact-free EEG epochs extracted from the positive film clips with the comparable epochs extracted from the negative film clips. The epochs used for this analysis were selected irrespective of the subject's facial behavior. While the means were in the expected direction for the frontal leads, with the negative film clips producing more right-sided activation compared with the positive clips, we found no significant differences between these conditions on any of the measures of asymmetry. The lack of significant effects when the analyses were performed independent of facial behavior suggests that our method of using facial expressivity to flag epochs of peak emotional state was effective. In this study, significant between-condition differences in asymmetry were obtained only when facial expression was used to verify the presence of emotional states.

In a companion study with Ekman (Ekman, Davidson, and Friesen, 1990), we compared brain electrical activity during two very similar-appearing expressions. Each of these expressions was a smile, but only one was predicted to be associated with genuine happiness, while the other was thought to be more of a social smile. More than 100 years ago, the French anatomist Duchenne (1862) speculated that smiles that included contraction of the eye muscles in addition to the cheek muscles were the mark of frank joy, in contrast to smiles that included only the cheek muscles. Darwin's (1872) observations were consistent with Duchenne's and more recently, Ekman and Friesen (1982) have confirmed that smiles comprised of both zygomatic and orbicularis oculi activity were more highly correlated with self-reports of happiness than smiles that included only zygomatic activity. In our joint study with Ekman (Ekman et al., 1990), we compared epochs during which each of these two smile types was present in response to an amusing film clip that elicited both types of smile. Replicating Ekman's previous finding, we found that the longer subjects' displayed smiles with both muscles contracted, the greater was their intensity of self-reported positive affect. When we compared frontal brain activity during each smile type, we found that the smiles with both muscles active (which we termed "Duchenne smiles") were associated with significantly greater left-sided activation in the frontal and anterior temporal regions. A similar pattern was found in a study of these two types of smile that 10-month old infants exhibited in response to mother approach and stranger approach (Fox and Davidson, 1988). Other studies in our laboratory (e.g., Davidson and Fox, 1982) and in other laboratories (e.g., Ahern and Schwartz, 1985; Tucker et al., 1981) have found EEG differences between positive and negative emotional states without using facial expressive measures as an index of peak emotional intensity. Thus, the extraction of data during the presence of discrete facial expressions of emotion does not appear to be *necessary* for the emergence of hemispheric asymmetries relevant to emotion.

We recently completed a study where robust differences in frontal brain asymmetry emerged during approach- and withdrawal-related emotion in the absence of extraction of epochs based upon facial behavior (Sobotka, Davidson, and Senulis, 1992). In this experiment, we manipulated reward and punishment contingencies in the context of a video game—like task. The task consisted of a series of 400 trials, presented over the course of two experimental sessions, in blocks of 20 trials each. Half of the trials were potential reward trials and half were potential punishment trials. Each trial began with the presentation of a fixation point, followed between 2 and 4 seconds later by an arrow. The arrow was either in the up or down position. An up arrow denoted that the trial was a potential reward trial and a down arrow indicated that the trial was a potential punishment trial. Four seconds following the presentation of the arrow stimulus, a square was presented in the center of the screen. This was the imperative stimulus to which the subject was required to respond as quickly as possible. The outcome of each trial was based upon the subjects' reaction time to the imperative stimulus. There were two possible outcomes on each trial. For reward trials, subjects could either win money or have no change in their earnings. For punishment trials, subjects could either lose money or have no change in their earnings. The amount of money which was won or lost on each trial was always 25 cents. Subjects were told that they would receive $5 at the beginning of each session which represented their starting sum of money in the game they were about to play. Subjects were instructed that they could win additional money as well as lose money from the $5 starting amount. They were also told that the amount of money they ended up with following the completion of the game would be theirs to keep.

For subjects to win money in the reward trials and stay even (i.e., not lose money in the punishment trials), they were required to have a reaction time that was faster than the median reaction time from the previous block of trials. The computer which acquired the reaction time data thus updated the criterion reaction time on each trial block. We recorded brain electrical activity

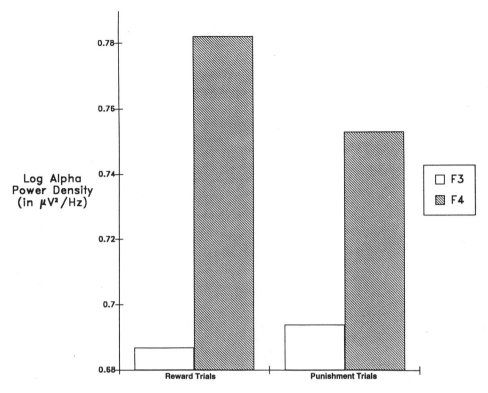

Figure 13.2 Mean log-transformed alpha power for the left and right midfrontal regions (F3 and F4) during reward and punishment conditions. (From Sobotka, Davidson, and Senulis, 1992.)

from most of the standard 10/20 locations during the performance of the task. Of major interest to us was the frontal brain activity during the preparatory interval between the arrow and imperative stimuli. The EEG during this period was Fourier-transformed and power in the alpha band was extracted as described in the experiment above. As predicted, we found a significant Valence × Hemisphere interaction, with greater right frontal activation (i.e., less alpha power) during the punishment compared with the reward trials. This interaction was significant in both the midfrontal (F3/4) and lateral frontal (F7/8) sites. These findings are displayed in figures 13.2 and 13.3. As can be seen from these figures, in both frontal regions the punishment condition is associated with less alpha power (i.e., more activation) in the right frontal lead compared with the reward condition. These data indicate that when reward and punishment contingencies are directly manipulated, frontal brain asymmetry changes in the direction of prediction, with greater right-sided activation present during the punishment condition compared with the reward condition. We also examined the contingent negative variation (CNV) during the 4-second preparatory interval. The CNV is a waveform which arises between a warning and imperative stimulus in a reaction time paradigm and

Davidson: Cerebral Asymmetry, Emotion, and Affective Style

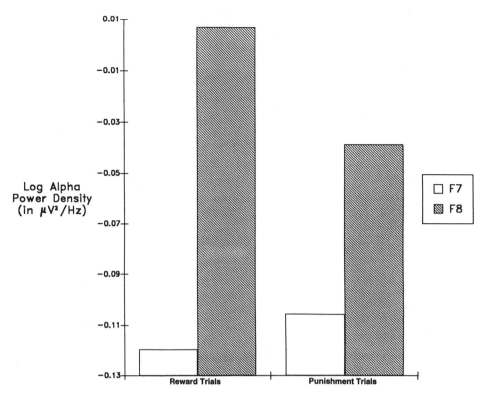

Figure 13.3 Mean log-transformed alpha power for the left and right lateral frontal regions (F7 and F8) during reward and punishment conditions. (From Sobotka, Davidson, and Senulis, 1992.)

represents a slow negative potential that peaks at the point of responding. No reliable asymmetries were observed in the CNV in this paradigm.

INDIVIDUAL DIFFERENCES IN ANTERIOR ASYMMETRY: A NEURAL SUBSTRATE FOR AFFECTIVE STYLE

In the first study described in the previous section, I noted that although 100% of the subjects showed a difference in the predicted direction between happy and disgust periods, these emotion-related differences were superimposed upon large individual differences in the overall magnitude and direction of asymmetry. In other research, we have found that a subject's overall (across-task) EEG asymmetry during task performance is highly correlated with his or her asymmetry during a resting baseline (e.g., Davidson, Taylor, and Saron, 1979) and that anterior asymmetries during resting baselines are stable over time (Tomarken et al., 1992), with test-retest correlations ranging between .66 and .73 for different measures of anterior activation asymmetry. Such measures also show excellent internal consistency reliability, with coefficient alphas (based upon eight separate 1-minute trials) in the .85 range. Over the past several years, we have performed several studies in both adults and infants which have examined the relation between individual differences in anterior activation asymmetry and dispositional mood, affective reactivity, and psychopathologic states. I present highlights of several components of this research effort below.

We began our studies of individual differences in anterior asymmetry by comparing subjects that differed in dispositional depressive mood. We (Schaffer, Davidson, and Saron, 1983) selected subjects on the basis of their scores on the Beck Depression Inventory and compared a group of high and stable scorers with a group of low and stable scorers on resting frontal asymmetry. We found that the depressed subjects had less left frontal activation compared with the nondepressed subjects. We have recently replicated this finding on a group of clinically depressed subjects (Henriques and Davidson, 1991).

An important question concerning these findings with depressives is the degree to which they are state-dependent. Is the decrease in left frontal activation a marker of the state of depression, or is it a more traitlike characteristic which marks an individual's vulnerability to depression? To obtain initial evidence relevant to this question, Henriques and I (Henriques and Davidson, 1990) compared remitted depressives to healthy controls who were screened for lifetime history of psychopathologic behavior and mental disorders. The remitted depressives all met Research Diagnostic Criteria (RDC; Spitzer, Endicott, and Robins, 1978) for major or minor depression within the past 2 years. All of the remitted were currently normothymic, with no depressive symptomatology and none were currently taking medication for their depression. We examined EEGs during resting baseline conditions. We found that the remitted depressives, like the acutely depressed subjects, had significantly less left frontal activation compared with the healthy controls, in the frontal region. This pattern was found for the anterior electrodes only, again underscoring the specificity of this asymmetry to the anterior cortical regions. Figure 13.4 presents the left and right hemisphere alpha power data from each of the regions from which we recorded, for the remitted depressives and healthy controls.

These results indicate that the decreased left anterior activation which is characteristic of depression remains even when depression is remitted. In turn, these findings suggest that "depressogenic" asymmetry patterns may be a state-independent marker that indexes risk for depression. Clearly, to more comprehensively test this hypothesis, a prospective design is required in which subjects are classified on the basis of asymmetry patterns and followed over time. We would predict that, relative to comparison groups, a higher proportion of subjects who demonstrate decreased left anterior activation would develop subsequent psychopathologic disorders.

In three recent studies in adults (Tomarken et al., 1990; Wheeler et al., 1993), we examined the relation between individual differences in anterior asymmetry and reactivity to emotional film clips in normals. We hypothesized

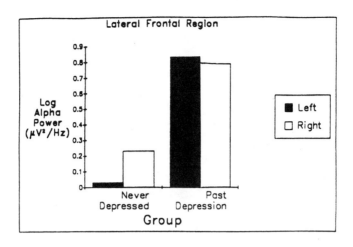

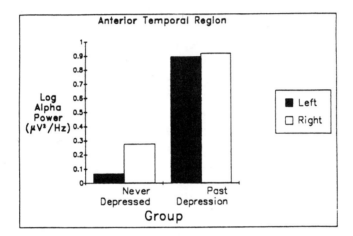

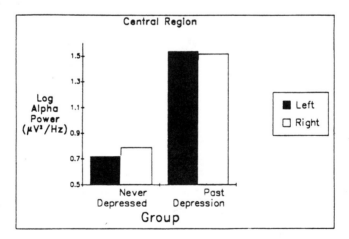

Figure 13.4 Mean log-transformed alpha power in left and right hemisphere sites from the lateral frontal (F7 and F8), midfrontal (F3 and F4), anterior temporal (T3 and T4), posterior temporal (T5 and T6), central (C3 and C4), and parietal (P3 and P4) regions for subjects with a past depression and for those that were never depressed. (From Henriques and Davidson, 1990.)

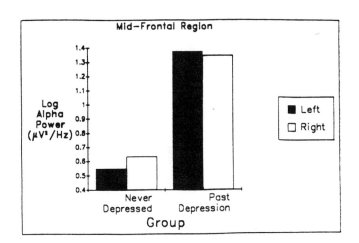

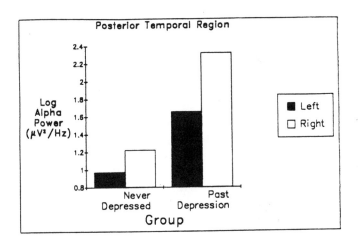

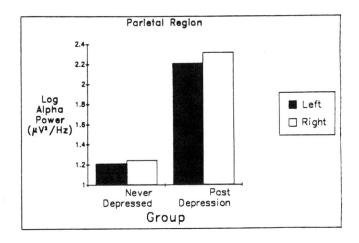

Davidson: Cerebral Asymmetry, Emotion, and Affective Style

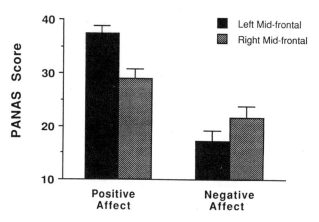

Figure 13.5 Mean Positive and Negative Affect Scale (PANAS) scores for left frontal and right frontal groups. (From Tomarken et al., 1992.)

that subjects with greater right-sided frontal activation at rest would report more intense negative affect in response to film clips designed to elicit fear and disgust. In each of these studies, we found that measures of frontal activation asymmetry recorded prior to the presentation of the film clips accounted for significant variance in subjects' self-reports of negative affect in response to the clips. Subjects with greater relative right-sided frontal activation reported more intense negative affect to the clips. In should be noted that the studies included entirely independent groups of subjects and entirely different film clips. In each of the studies, the correlations between frontal asymmetry and positive affect were in the opposite direction, such that greater relative left-sided frontal activation at rest was associated with increased intensity of reports of positive affect in response to film clips designed to elicit happiness and amusement. It is important to note that all of these effects remained significant even when measures of mood at baseline were statistically partialled out. In other words, frontal asymmetry accounted for significant variance in emotional reactivity to film clip elicitors after the variance accounted for by measures of mood during baseline was statistically removed. This observation strengthens our suggestion that baseline anterior asymmetry is a state-independent measure of affective reactivity, but is itself unrelated to measures of phasic, unprovoked mood. We also examined relations between frontal asymmetry and the overall intensity of emotion reported by subjects irrespective of valence (i.e., positive plus negative emotion). Here, there was no relation between frontal asymmetry and overall affect, suggesting that our effect is one related to a valence-specific bias rather than to overall intensity.

Baseline anterior asymmetry is related to measures of dispositional mood or affective style. Using the Positive and Negative Affect Scale (PANAS; Watson, Clark, and Tellegen, 1988), we found that subjects selected on baseline EEG measures to show extreme and stable left frontal activation report more dispositional positive affect and less dispositional negative affect than their right frontally activated counterparts (Tomarken et al., 1992; see figure

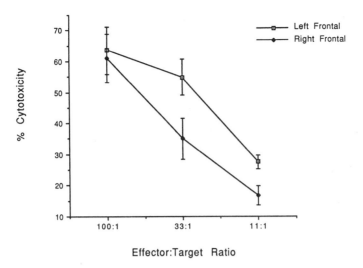

Figure 13.6 Mean natural killer cell activity (percent cytoxicity) for three different effector–target cell ratios in left and right frontal groups. (From Kang et al., 1991.)

13.5). We have also found that the right frontal subjects are immunosuppressed relative to their left frontal counterparts (figure 13.6). During a baseline state, the right frontal subjects show significantly less natural killer cell activity compared with the left frontal subjects (Kang et al., 1991). In these studies, subjects were selected exclusively on the basis of their baseline frontal EEG asymmetry and then tested on another occasion to obtain measures of dispositional mood and immune function. These studies provide further validity for our suggestion that individual differences in frontal asymmetry reflect important features of affective style.

The studies described above in this section have all concerned the association between individual differences in anterior activation asymmetries and affective style in adults. We have recently embarked upon a series of studies to explore this relation in infants and young children. Among 10-month-old infants, there is substantial heterogeneity in the response to maternal separation. Some infants become distressed immediately and cry as soon as their mother has departed. Other infants show a very different pattern of response and evince relatively few signs of negative affect. We (Davidson and Fox, 1989) divided 10-month-old infants into two groups on the basis of whether they cried or not in response to maternal separation lasting approximately 60 seconds. We found that about half of our group cried within this time period and half did not. We recorded baseline measures of frontal and parietal activation from the two hemispheres approximately 30 minutes prior to subjecting the infants to the episode of maternal separation. We then examined EEG measures of frontal activation asymmetry during this preceding baseline period, separately for the group of infants that subsequently cried and those that did not cry. We found a large difference in frontal asymmetry that predicted which infants would cry and which would not cry. The criers had greater right-sided and less left-sided frontal activation during the preceding baseline period compared with the noncriers. Parietal asymmetry from the same points in time failed to differentiate between the groups. To establish that the emotional states of the two groups of infants during the baseline period itself (when measures of brain activity were obtained) were comparable, we coded the facial behavior of the infants during this period. There were no differences in the frequency or duration of any facial signs of emotion during the baseline period between the infants that subsequently cried in response to maternal separation and those that did not. This suggests that our measures of regional brain activity were not reflecting phasic state differences between criers and noncriers.

These data were the first to show that in infants, individual differences in frontal asymmetry predict affective reactivity. The direction of the relation is identical to that observed in our studies with adults. Subjects that show greater relative right-sided frontal activation at rest are likely to express more intense negative affect in response to a stressful event compared with their more left frontally activated counterparts. The findings in both adults and infants provided the foundation for a current study in our laboratory on relations between temperament and frontal asymmetry. Kagan, Reznick, and Snidman (1988) have been studying the temperamental construct of behavioral inhibition for the past 10 years. Behavioral inhibition refers to the young child's tendency to withdraw or freeze in situations of novelty or unfamiliarity. Behaviorally inhibited children at $2\frac{1}{2}$ years of age would likely withdraw in response to a novel object, such as a robot. Such a child would also be unlikely to approach a stranger, climb through a toy tunnel, or interact with a same-sex peer. In a novel peer play situation, behaviorally inhibited children spend the majority of their time in close proximity to their mothers, without playing or interacting in any way. While Kagan and his colleagues have studied autonomic differences between inhibited and uninhibited children, there have been no studies on central nervous system differences between these groups. We therefore embarked upon a longitudinal study whose principal aims were to determine if inhibited children showed greater relative right-sided frontal activation compared with uninhibited children, and to examine relations between frontal asymmetry and measures of behavioral inhibition over time. To select groups of inhibited and uninhibited children, we adopted the procedures that Kagan and his colleagues (1988) had developed.

We tested 386 children aged 31 months in a peer play session. The children were randomly selected from birth announcements in the newspaper. Two unfamiliar same-sex peers came to the laboratory with their mothers and were escorted to a large playroom. The mothers were instructed to sit on chairs and fill out an extensive series of questionnaires. They were instructed not to interact with their children. There were age-appropriate toys on the floor in the playroom, including a toy tunnel through which the children could crawl. At minute 10 of the play session, the experimenter brought a remote-controlled robot into the room. The robot began to speak and walk toward each of the children. It was controlled by an experimenter from behind a one-way mirror. After remaining in the room for 3 minutes, the robot said that it was tired and had to go home to take a nap. The experimenter then entered the room and removed the robot. At minute 20, a stranger who had not been seen before by either child entered the room. The stranger was holding a tray on which were placed several very interesting-looking toys. The stranger invited the children to play with the toys. After 3 minutes, the stranger left the tray of toys on the floor for the children to play with and then departed. The play session ended at minute 25. During the entire play session, two observers were positioned behind a one-way mirror to code the behavior of each child. The major measures that were coded included the total time the child was proximal to the mother (within arm's length) and not interacting, the latency to touch the first toy, the latency to speak the first utterance, the latency to approach the robot, the latency to approach the stranger, and the latency to enter the tunnel.

On the basis of these measures, we selected three groups of children for our longitudinal study. The criteria we used were based on the work of Kagan et al. (1988), but were more stringent. The inhibited children were those that spent more than 9.5 minutes (out of a total of 25 minutes) proximal to mother and that also met four of the following five additional criteria: (1) latency of ≥ 3 minutes to touch their first toy; (2) latency of ≥ 3 minutes to speak their first utterance; (3) no approach to the robot; (4) no approach to the stranger; and (5) latency of ≥ 10 minutes to enter the tunnel. The criteria for the uninhibited children were all of the following: (1) total duration of time proximal to mother ≤ 30 seconds; (2) latency of ≤ 30 seconds to touch their first toy; (3) latency of ≤ 60 seconds to speak their first utterance; (4) latency of ≤ 60 seconds to approach the robot; (5) latency of ≤ 60 seconds to approach the stranger; (6) latency of ≤ 60 seconds to take a toy from the stranger; and (7) enter the tunnel at some point during the session. In addition to selecting groups of inhibited and uninhibited children, we also selected a group of middle children who showed values in the midrange for all of the measures described above. We selected approximately 28 subjects in each of the three groups, balanced evenly by sex. The average duration of time spent proximal to mother among children in the inhibited and uninhibited groups underscores the magnitude of the difference between the two extreme groups. The inhibited children remained proximal to their mothers for an average of 1171 seconds (of a total of 1500 seconds [25 minutes] representing 78% of the total time) while the uninhibited children were proximal to their mothers for an average of 9 seconds (representing less than 1% of the total time).

We tested the longitudinal cohort at 38 months of age in a session during which we recorded brain electrical activity at rest and in response to several tasks. To date, we have analyzed the data for the resting baselines. Our major prediction was that inhibited children would show greater relative right-sided frontal activation compared with their uninhibited counterparts. Middle children were hypothesized to fall in between. Figure 13.7 presents the frontal

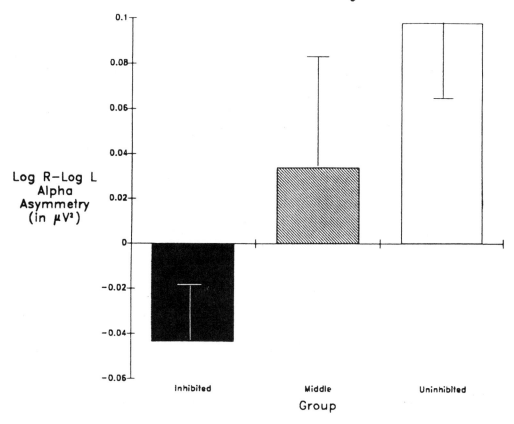

Figure 13.7 Mean asymmetry scores (log-right minus log-left power in the 7- to 10-Hz band—the toddler alpha frequency range) for the midfrontal electrodes (F3 and F4) for inhibited, middle, and uninhibited children. Higher numbers on this metric denote greater relative left-sided activation. (From Davidson, Finman, Straus, Rickman, and Kagan, 1993.)

asymmetry data for the three groups. As in previous figures, negative asymmetry scores indicate greater right frontal activation, and positive scores indicate left frontal activation. As can be seen from the figure, inhibited children show right frontal activation, while the uninhibited children show the opposite pattern. The middle children fall predictably in between the two extreme groups.

For theoretical reasons, it is important to ascertain how the two hemispheres are contributing to this group difference in asymmetry. If the primary difference among the groups is in the withdrawal-related component, we would expect the inhibited children to show *more* right frontal activation compared with the uninhibited children. However, if the fundamental difference between the groups is in the approach-related component, we would expect the inhibited children to show *less* left frontal activation compared with their uninhibited counterparts. This latter pattern would suggest that inhibited

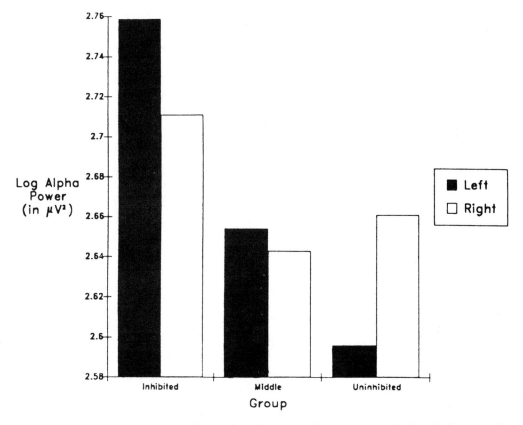

Figure 13.8 Mean log-transformed power in the 7- to 10-Hz band in the left and right midfrontal region (F3 and F4) for inhibited, middle, and uninhibited children. (From Davidson, Finman, Straus, Rickman, and Kagan, 1993.)

children show deficits in approach-related behavior and emotion, rather than accentuated withdrawal-related behavior. Most accounts of behavioral inhibition have implied a strong linkage to fear and anxiety. On this view, the difference among groups should be most pronounced in the right frontal region. Figure 13.8 presents the frontal EEG data for each of the three groups, separately by hemisphere. The Group × Hemisphere interaction was highly significant ($P = .0003$). As can be clearly seen from this figure, the difference among the groups is primarily in the left hemisphere, with the inhibited children showing more power (i.e., less activation) in this region compared with the other two groups. These data clearly indicate that the group difference is in the approach-related system and suggest that it would be most appropriate to characterize the inhibited children as showing deficits in a frontal approach system, rather than hyperactivation in a frontal withdrawal system.

It is instructive to consider the possibility that our sample of inhibited children is more extreme than samples that have been studied previously by

Kagan's group. Certainly, the magnitude of the difference between our extreme groups on the play session variables (e.g., time proximal to mother) is greater than Kagan's group observed in their sample. It is also possible that there are different subtypes of inhibition, with one subtype characterized by approach-related deficits and the other characterized by accentuated withdrawal tendencies. Our grouping procedures may have inadvertently selected for subjects in the former category. A testable prediction which follows from our initial finding is that our sample of inhibited children should not differ from uninhibited children in their propensity to display withdrawal-related negative affect in response to appropriate elicitors. Rather, they should be more prone to sadness and depression-like reactions following situational elicitors of these emotions. We intend to examine these predictions in the course of our future longitudinal work. The pattern of decreased left frontal activation we found among our inhibited children is similar to the pattern we have reported in depressives. It is important to emphasize that this pattern is viewed as a marker of *vulnerability* to emotion and behavior that is associated with deficits in the approach system. Such vulnerability will become expressed psychopathologically only in response to relatively extreme life stresses. Thus, only a small percentage of affected children (i.e., those with the marker) would be expected to actually develop an affective disorder. However, a larger percentage might be expected to have subclinical characteristics such as dysthymic mood, shyness, and decreased dispositional positive affect. It will be of interest to examine these children as they confront increasingly more complex life challenges (e.g., entry into school) to help define what the environmental circumstances are that predispose individuals with decreased left frontal activation to exhibit depression-related symptoms. It will be equally of interest to study the children at the opposite extreme. It is not clear whether the uninhibited children are likely to display impulsive behavior and show an oversensitivity to reward contingencies. We are currently testing some of these hypotheses in our assessment of the children at $4\frac{1}{2}$ years of age.

SUMMARY AND CONCLUSIONS

This chapter has presented an overview of recent research on anterior asymmetries associated with emotion and individual differences in emotional reactivity, psychopathologic states, dispositional mood, and temperament. I proposed that the anterior regions of the two cerebral hemispheres are specialized for approach and withdrawal processes, with the left hemisphere specialized for the former and the right for the latter. Using electrophysiologic measures of regional cortical activation, data were presented which demonstrated that the experimental arousal of approach-related positive affect was associated with left anterior activation, whereas arousal of withdrawal-related negative affect was associated with right anterior activation. In the second half of the chapter, evidence was presented which indicated that individual differences in patterns of anterior asymmetry are stable over time and predict important features of affective style—an individual's dispositional emotional profile including characteristic patterns of emotional reactivity, mood, and temperament.

From the data already available, it is clear that asymmetry in the anterior cortical regions is significantly associated with emotion and emotional reactivity. It will be important for future research to characterize both the proximal and distal causes of this asymmetry. The study of proximal causes will necessarily require the examination of subcortical and neurochemical contributions. Distal causes will inevitably be some combination of heritable and early environmental factors. We have recently developed a primate model of affective lateralization and have found that the benzodiazepine diazepam induces an asymmetric shift in frontal brain electrical activity in rhesus monkeys (Davidson, Kalin, and Shelton, 1992). This implies that there may an asymmetric distribution of benzodiazepine receptors in the frontal cortex. Using PET to examine this question, preliminary evidence appears consistent with this suggestion (Abadie et al., 1991). Many other transmitter systems are represented in frontal cortex and it is likely that several contribute to the regulation of emotion and affective style. For example, it has recently been reported that the asymmetry of serotonin S2 receptors in frontal cortex of depressives differs significantly from controls (D'haenen et al., 1992). Studies such as these offer considerable promise in unifying what up until now have been rather disparate approaches to the study of emotion and affective disorders. We have every reason to think that future research on this topic will be as exciting and revealing as the recent work has been.

ACKNOWLEDGMENTS

The research described in this chapter was supported in part by an NIMH Research Scientist Development Award MH00875, NIMH grants MH40747, MH43454, and P50-MH52354 and a grant from the John D. and Catherine T. MacArthur Foundation.

NOTES

1. While baseline anterior asymmetries are unrelated to measures of unprovoked emotional *state*, they are related to individual differences in dispositional mood or emotional *traits* (Tomarken et al., 1992). This is discussed in a later section.

2. One important variable in evaluating the literature on the effects of unilateral lesions is the time since lesion to assessment. With increased time, there should be an increased likelihood of exposure to negative life events and therefore, a higher probability that the individual would show depressive symptomatology.

3. We typically examine power in all frequency bands. However, the majority of variance in task-related and baseline EEGs is in the alpha band for adult subjects. Moreover, we have demonstrated that asymmetries in alpha power are more consistently related to both cognitive (e.g., Davidson et al., 1990a) and affective (e.g., Davidson et al., 1990b) processes than asymmetries of power in other frequency bands.

REFERENCES

Abadie, P., Bisserbe, J. C., Boulenger, J. P., Travere, J. M., Barre, L., Petit, M. C., Zarifian, E., and Baron, J. C. (1991). Central benzodiazepine receptors: Quantitative positron emission tomography study in healthy subjects and anxious patients. In M. Briley and S. E. File (Eds.), *New concepts in anxiety*. Boca Raton, FL: CRC Press.

Ahern, G. L., and Schwartz, G. E. (1985). Differential lateralization for positive and negative emotion in the human brain: EEG spectral analysis. *Neuropsychologia, 23,* 745–756.

Blom, B. L., and Anneveldt, M. (1982). An electrode cap tested. *Electroencephalography and Clinical Neurophysiology, 54,* 591–594.

Borod, J. C., Koff, E., Perlman, L. M., Lorch, M., and Nicolas, M. (1986). The expression and perception of facial emotion in brain-damaged patients. *Neuropsychologia, 24,* 169–180.

Burke, A., Younkin, D., Kushner, M., Gordon, J., Pistone, L., Shapiro, H., and Reivich, M. (1982). Recovery from acute stroke and changes in cerebral blood flow. *Annals of Neurology, 12,* 84.

Damasio, A. R. (1989). The brain binds entities and events by multiregional activation from convergence zones. *Neural Computation, 1,* 123–132.

Darwin, C. (1872). *The expression of the emotions in man and animals.* Chicago, IL: University of Chicago Press, 1965.

Davidson, R. J. (1984). Affect, cognition and hemispheric specialization. In C. E. Izard, J. Kagan, and R. Zajonc (Eds.), *Emotion, cognition and behavior.* New York, NY: Cambridge University Press.

Davidson, R. J. (1987). Cerebral asymmetry and the nature of emotion: Implications for the study of individual differences and psychopathology. In R. Takahashi, P. Flor-Henry, J. Gruzelier and S. Niwa (Eds.), *Cerebral dynamics, laterality and psychopathology.* New York, NY: Elsevier.

Davidson, R. J. (1988). EEG measures of cerebral asymmetry: Conceptual and methodological issues. *International Journal of Neuroscience, 39,* 71–89.

Davidson, R. J. (1992a). Anterior cerebral asymmetry and the nature of emotion. *Brain and Cognition, 20,* 125–151.

Davidson, R. J. (1992b). Prolegomenon to the structure of emotion: Gleanings from neuropsychology. *Cognition and Emotion, 6,* 245–268.

Davidson, R. J. (1993). Cerebral asymmetry and emotion: Conceptual and methodological conundrums. *Cognition and Emotion, 7,* 115–138.

Davidson, R. J., Chapman, J. P., Chapman, L. P., and Henriques, J. B. (1990a). Asymmetrical brain electrical activity discriminates between psychometrically-matched verbal and spatial cognitive tasks. *Psychophysiology, 27,* 528–543.

Davidson, R. J., Ekman, P., Saron, C. D., Senulis, J. A., and Friesen, W. V. (1990b). Approach/withdrawal and cerebral asymmetry: Emotional expression and brain physiology I. *Journal of Personality and Social Psychology, 58,* 330–341.

Davidson, R. J., Finman, R., Rickman, M. D., Straus, A., and Kagan, J. (1994). Childhood temperament and frontal lobe activity: Patterns of asymmetry differentiate between wary and outgoing children. In preparation.

Davidson, R. J., and Fox, N. A. (1982). Asymmetrical brain activity discriminates between positive versus negative affective stimuli in human infants. *Science, 218,* 1235–1237.

Davidson, R. J. and Fox, N. A. (1989). Frontal brain asymmetry predicts infants' response to maternal separation. *Journal of Abnormal Psychology, 98*, 127–131.

Davidson, R. J., Kalin, N. H., and Shelton, S. E. (1992). Lateralized effects of diazepam on frontal brain electrical asymmetries in rhesus monkeys. *Biological Psychiatry, 32*, 438–451.

Davidson, R. J., Taylor, N., and Saron, C. (1979). Hemisphericity and styles of information processing: Individual differences in EEG asymmetry and their relationship to cognitive performance. *Psychophysiology, 16*, 197.

Davidson, R. J., and Tomarken, A. J. (1989). Laterality and emotion: An electrophysiological approach. In In F. Boller and J. Grafman (Eds.), *Handbook of neuropsychology*, Vol 3 (pp 419–441). Amsterdam: Elsevier.

D'haenen, H., Bossuyt, A., Mertens, J., Bossuyt-Piron, C., Gijsemans, M., and Kaufman, L. (1992). SPECT imaging of serotonin$_2$ receptors in depression. *Psychiatry Research: Neuroimaging, 45*, 227–237.

Duchenne, B. (1862). *Mécanisme de la physionomie humaine ou analyse électrophysiologique de l'expression des passions.* Paris: Baillière.

Ekman, P., Davidson, R. J., and Friesen, W. V. (1990). Duchenne's smile: Emotional expression and brain physiology, II. *Journal of Personality and Social Psychology, 58*, 342–353.

Ekman, P., and Friesen, W. V. (1978). *The Facial Action Coding System: A technique for the measurement of facial movement.* Palo Alto, CA: Consulting Psychologists Press.

Ekman, P., and Friesen, W. V. (1982). Felt, false and miserable smiles. *Journal of Nonverbal Behavior, 6*, 238–252.

Etcoff, N. L. (1986). The neuropsychology of emotional expression. In G. Goldstein and R. E. Tarter (Eds.), *Advances in clinical neuropsychology*, Vol 3. New York, NY: Plenum Press.

Fox, N. A., and Davidson, R. J. (1988). Patterns of brain electrical activity during facial signs of emotion in ten month old infants. *Developmental Psychology, 24*, 230–236.

Gainotti, G. (1972). Emotional behavior and hemispheric side of lesion. *Cortex, 8*, 41–55.

Gainotti, G. (1989). Disorders of emotions and affect in patients with unilateral brain damage. In F. Boller and J. Grafman (Eds.), *Handbook of Neuropsychology*, Vol 3 (pp 345–361). Amsterdam: Elsevier.

Goldstein, K. (1939). *The organism.* New York, NY: American Books.

Henriques, J. B., and Davidson, R. J. (1990). Regional brain electrical asymmetries discriminate between previously depressed and healthy control subjects. *Journal of Abnormal Psychology, 99*, 22–31.

Henriques, J. B., and Davidson, R. J. (1991). Left frontal hypoactivation in depression. *Journal of Abnormal Psychology, 100*, 535–545.

House, A., Dennis, M., Warlow, C., Hawton, K., and Molyneux, A. (1990). Mood disorders after stroke and their relation to lesion location. *Brain, 113*, 1113–1129.

Jackson, J. H. (1878). On the affections of speech from disease of the brain. *Brain, 1*, 304–330.

Jerison, H. J. (1973). *Evolution of the brain and intelligence.* New York, NY: Academic Press.

Kagan, J., Reznick, J. S., and Snidman, N. (1988). Biological bases of childhood shyness. *Science, 240*, 167–171.

Kang, D. H., Davidson, R. J., Coe, C. L., Wheeler, R. W., Tomarken, A. J., and Ershler, W. B. (1991). Frontal brain asymmetry and immune function. *Behavioral Neuroscience, 105*, 860–869.

Kolb, B., and Taylor, L. (1990). Neocortical substrates of emotional behavior. In N. L. Stein, B. Leventhal, and T. Trabasso (Eds.), *Psychological and biological approaches to emotion*. Hillsdale, NJ: Lawrence Erlbaum Associates.

Leventhal, H., and Tomarken, A. J. (1986). Emotion: Today's problems. In M. R. Rosenzweig and L. Y. Porter (Eds.), *Annual review of psychology*, Vol 37 (pp 565–610). Palo Alto, CA: Annual Reviews, Inc.

Levy, J. (1972). Lateral specialization of the human brain: Behavioral manifestation and possible evolutionary basis. In J. A. Kriger (Ed.), *The biology of behavior*. Corvallis, OR: Oregon State University Press.

Luria, A.R. (1973). *The working brain*. New York, NY: Basic Books.

Morris, M., Bradley, M., Bowers, D., Lang, P., and Heilman, K. (1991). Valence-specific hypoarousal following right temporal lobectomy. Paper presented at the Annual Meeting of the International Neuropsychological Society, San Antonio, TX, February 14.

Reiman, E. M., Raichle, M. E., Butler, F. K., Hercovitch, P., and Robins, E. (1984). A focal brain abnormality in panic disorder, a severe form of anxiety. *Nature, 310*, 683–685.

Robinson, R. G., Kubos, K. L., Starr, L. B., Rao, K., and Price, T. R. (1984). Mood disorders in stroke patients: Importance of location of lesion. *Brain, 107*, 81–93.

Sackeim, H. A., Greenberg, M. S., Weiman, A. L., Gur, R., Hungerbuhler, J. P., and Geschwind, N. (1982). Hemispheric asymmetry in the expression of positive and negative emotions. *Archives of Neurology, 39*, 210–218.

Schaffer, C. E., Davidson, R. J., and Saron, C. (1983). Frontal and parietal EEG asymmetries in depressed and non-depressed subjects. *Biological Psychiatry, 18*, 753–762.

Schneirla, T. C. (1959). An evolutionary and developmental theory of biphasic processes underlying approach and withdrawal. In M. R. Jones (Ed.), *Nebraska symposium on motivation*. Lincoln, NE: University of Nebraska Press.

Shagass, C. (1972). Electrical activity of the brain. In N. S. Greenfield and R. A. Sternbach (Eds.), *Handbook of psychophysiology* (pp 263–328). New York, NY: Holt, Rinehart & Winston.

Silberman, E. K., and Weingartner, H. (1986). Hemispheric lateralization of functions related to emotion. *Brain and Cognition, 5*, 322–353.

Sobotka, S., Davidson, R. J., and Senulis, J. (1992). Anterior brain electrical asymmetries in response to reward and punishment. *Electroencephalography and Clinical Neurophysiology, 83*, 236–247.

Spitzer, R. L., Endicott, J., and Robins, E. (1978). Research diagnostic criteria: Rationale and reliability. *Archives of General Psychiatry, 35*, 773–782.

Stellar, J. R., and Stellar, E. (1985). *The neurobiology of motivation and reward*. New York, NY: Springer-Verlag.

Tomarken, A. J., Davidson, R. J., and Henriques, J. B. (1990). Resting frontal brain asymmetry predicts affective responses to films. *Journal of Personality and Social Psychology, 59*, 791–801.

Tomarken, A. J., Davidson, R. J., Wheeler, R. W., and Doss, R. (1992). Individual differences in anterior brain asymmetry and fundamental dimensions of emotion. *Journal of Personality and Social Psychology, 62*, 676–687.

Tomarken, A. J., Davidson, R. J., Wheeler, R. W., and Kinney, L. (1992). Psychometric properties of resting anterior EEG asymmetry: Temporal stability and internal consistency. *Psychophysiology, 29*, 576–592.

Tucker, D. M., Stenslie, C. E., Roth, R. S., and Shearer, S. L. (1981). Right frontal lobe activation and right hemisphere performance decrement during a depressed mood. *Archives of General Psychiatry, 38,* 169–174.

Watson, D., Clark, L. A., and Tellegen, A. (1988). Development and validation of brief measures of positive and negative affect: The PANAS scales. *Journal of Personality and Social Psychology, 54,* 1063–1070.

Wheeler, R. W., Davidson, R. J., and Tomarken, A. J. (1993). Frontal brain asymmetry and emotional reactivity: A biological substrate of affective style. *Psychophysiology, 30,* 82–89.

Young, G., Segalowitz, S. J., Misek, P., Alp, I. E., and Boulet, R. (1983). Is early reaching left-handed? Review of manual specialization research. In G. Young, S. J. Segalowitz, C. M. Corter, and S. E. Trehub (Eds.), *Manual specialization and the developing brain* (pp 13–32). London: Academic Press.

14 Emotion in Asymmetric Corticolimbic Networks

Mario Liotti and Don M. Tucker

The aim of this chapter is to review some of the key evidence on hemispheric specialization for emotion, then speculate on how hemispheric asymmetries of corticolimbic interaction may help explain this evidence. The most fundamental division of corticolimbic architecture is not left/right, but dorsal/ventral. The neocortex evolved from paralimbic cortices along two paths of network differentiation: (1) the dorsal archicortical networks, centered on the hippocampus, and (2) the ventral paleocortical networks, centered on the olfactory cortex with important interconnections with the amygdala (Pandya, Seltzer, and Barbas, 1988). Studies of perceptual and cognitive abilities are demonstrating the functional differentiation between these divisions of the cortex, for example, showing the specialization of the dorsal pathways for spatial memory and of the ventral pathways for object memory (Ungerleider and Mishkin, 1982). Although the motivational and emotional differences between dorsal and ventral networks have not been considered in recent models of emotion in human neuropsychology, the functional differences between these networks are likely to be as profound in the motivational domain as they are in the cognitive domain. In attempting to understand the two hemispheres' differing modes of corticolimbic interaction in emotion, we have considered the possibility that the elaboration of the dorsal and ventral networks has not been equivalent in the two hemispheres. In this chapter, we explore this possibility, specifically that left hemisphere specialization at the cortical level has elaborated the cybernetic characteristics of the ventral cortical networks. In contrast, right hemisphere specialization may have elaborated the self-regulatory and information representation characteristics of the dorsal cortical networks. This hypothesis is most easily evaluated at the cognitive level, and we review relevant evidence from human neuropsychological studies of perception and cognition. However, we propose that corticolimbic interactions apply inherent adaptive constraints in the process of consolidating cortical representations, such that asymmetries of dorsal and ventral elaboration lead to hemispheric asymmetries in the limbic regulation of cognition.

INHERENT MOOD VALENCE ASYMMETRY

Theories of lateralized hemispheric control of emotion have been formulated in two rather different contexts. Observations on mood changes following unilateral brain lesions or unilateral sedation with barbiturates have led to interpretations based on classic neurologic principles. Disinhibited emotional behavior after a cortical lesion would be interpreted to reflect release of normal control exerted over areas of the contralateral hemisphere, or over the ipsilateral subcortical centers.

In contrast, studies in normals using methods of cognitive psychology and experimental neuropsychology have emphasized hemispheric contributions to cognitive skills in emotional communication. We review in turn the key evidence in support of these two approaches.

The first line of research emphasizes differential roles for the two hemispheres in regulating positive and negative emotional orientations. Goldstein (1952) and Gainotti (1969, 1972) found that lesions in the dominant hemisphere were associated with a *catastrophic* reaction (tears, despair, anger) while damage to the minor hemisphere was accompanied by an *indifference* reaction (unawareness, euphoria, lack of concern). Gainotti proposed that mood changes were secondary to expressive difficulties in left hemisphere aphasic patients, and to unawareness and neglect in right hemisphere patients. At about the same time, an Italian group in Genoa reported similar emotional changes during unilateral hemispheric sedation with amobarbital sodium for the assessment of speech dominance (Terzian, 1964; Rossi and Rosadini, 1967). Discounting cognitive or functional factors, they proposed that mood reactions are a direct consequence of cortical damage. The left and right hemispheres were seen to exert opposite influences on emotional tone, with the left hemisphere tending toward positive affect and the right hemisphere biased toward negative affect. This view has been supported by Sackheim et al. (1982). They reviewed the available literature on pathologic, uncontrollable laughing and crying not produced by nuclear brainstem lesions, that is, pseudo-bulbar palsy (Poeck, 1969; Rinn, 1984). Their results confirmed the association of pathologic laughing with right hemisphere lesions, and pathologic crying with left hemisphere lesions. Conversely, a review of the literature on emotional outbursts as ictal components in epilepsy lead to a significant association of pathologic laughing with left-sided epileptic foci. Sackheim et al. (1982) concluded that mood changes following unilateral insult should reflect disinhibition of contralateral regions, and not release of ipsilateral subcortical regions (see below).

The Wada test results from the Italian group raised considerable controversy. A puzzling finding was that the mood changes were found quite late (4–10 minutes after the injection), after the electroencephalographic (EEG) activity on the sedated hemisphere was restored and motor and speech function had recovered. Furthermore, attempts at replicating these findings at the Montreal Neurological Institute met with failures, although dosage differences may have contributed to the discrepancy (e.g., Kolb and Milner, 1981). Recently, however, Lee et al. (1992) have replicated the earlier findings. They videotaped and analyzed facial expressions immediately after injection and found changes congruent with the previous reports. Interestingly, their emotional reactions took place within 30 seconds from the injection, when the hemisphere injected was still clearly sedated.

There are other aspects of hemispheric function that seem to entail the regulation of primitive emotional influences that are also difficult to explain by cognitive mediation. The first area is arousal. Right hemisphere patients have been described as "hypoaroused" (Heilman, Schwartz, and Watson, 1978), with reduced cortical and autonomic responsivity (such as skin conductance or heart rate), particularly to emotionally charged stimuli (Morrow et al., 1981; Zoccolotti et al., 1982). They also display fewer avoidant eye movements to unpleasant visual stimuli (Zoccolotti et al., 1986). The right hemisphere may also be involved in the regulation of sexual arousal, since right hemisphere patients and epileptic patients with right temporal foci show more frequent sexual dysfunction (reviewed by Tucker and Frederick, 1989).

Other evidence that may be difficult to account for in terms of cognitive mediation concerns emotional expression. Normal adults express emotions more intensely on the left side of the face, the lower half of which is innervated prominently by the contralateral right hemisphere (e.g., Borod and Caron, 1980). Patients with right hemisphere damage are less facially expressive than those with left hemisphere lesions (Borod et al., 1985; Borod, 1992). Impairment in expressive behavior in the presence of normal nonemotional facial motility has been associated with right prerolandic lesions (Ross, 1981) and to mediofrontal lesions involving the supplementary motor area and the gyrus cinguli (Tucker and Frederick, 1989).

RIGHT HEMISPHERE COGNITION IN EMOTIONAL COMMUNICATION

Another line of evidence on hemispheric asymmetry for emotion derives from half-field and dichotic studies in normals and research on emotional communication deficits in brain-injured patients. Most of this evidence can be explained by the particular role of the right hemisphere's cognitive skills in emotional communication. Tachistoscopic studies in normals have shown that the right hemisphere is generally faster and more accurate than the left hemisphere in discriminating facial expressions of emotion (e.g., Ley and Bryden, 1979; Strauss and Moscovitch, 1981). Similarly, patients with right hemisphere damage showed greater impairment in recognizing facial expressions of emotion (e.g., Bowers et al., 1985; Kolb and Taylor, 1981). Recognition of emotional tone in speech has also been found to be particularly impaired by right hemisphere damage (Ross, 1981; see Borod, 1992, for a review).

The right hemisphere's superiority in holistic cognitive processing of visual and auditory stimuli seems to be sufficient to explain most of these effects.

The nondominant hemisphere prevails in the analysis of complex visuospatial configurations, such as faces, particularly when holistic organization is required. This type of processing is demanded with low spatial-frequency stimuli as opposed to the focus on detail required to process high spatial-frequency stimuli (e.g., De Renzi and Spinnler, 1966; Rizzolatti, Umiltá, and Berlucchi, 1971; Kitterlie, Hellige, and Christman, 1992). Even for the recognition of emotional tone in auditory information, such as speech prosody, a similar account has been proposed. The right hemisphere may be specialized in processing the acoustic stimuli in which the emotional message is embedded, rather than the emotional stimuli per se. Low temporal-frequency stimuli are processed more efficiently by the minor hemisphere, while high temporal-frequency information seems to be analyzed preferentially by the dominant hemisphere (Ivry, 1991). Sidtis (1980) and Ivry (1991) suggested that *low* temporal frequency is the critical acoustic parameter characterizing emotional prosody. The right hemisphere role in emotional prosody would depend on its superiority in processing low temporal-frequency sounds.

The right hemisphere appears to mediate emotional processing even with certain forms of linguistic materials. This may consist in an advantage in accessing meanings or knowledge about emotional events or facts in long-term memory, i.e., emotional lexical representations. Emotional words have been found to be processed more efficiently in the left visual field (Ley and Bryden, 1983; Graves et al., 1981). Aphasic patients have been found to read preferentially emotional compared to nonemotional words (Landis, Graves, and Goodglass, 1982). Wechsler (1973) reported that right hemisphere patients show more difficulty in recalling emotional than nonemotional stories. The idea of a right lateralized emotional lexicon is also supported by recent evidence of the role of the nondominant hemisphere in the integration of contextual cues, such as those necessary to appreciate verbal or pictorial humor, metaphor, and connotative meaning. Right hemihere patients are prone to literal interpretations and inappropriate affective responses (Gardner et al., 1975, 1983).

In an effort to single out perceptual from lexical effects in emotional processing, Etcoff (1984) found that right hemisphere patients were impaired in a task in which they were asked similarity judgments of photographs of facial expressions, whereas they behaved normally when the similarity judgments involved emotional words, suggesting a perceptual rather than a symbolic or verbal defect in emotion processing.

In spite of considerable evidence in favor of a cognitive mediation of right hemisphere emotional processing in recognition tasks, the results of some studies seem to show that the right hemisphere superiority cannot be explained solely by cognitive variables. Dissociations between recognition of facial expression and face recognition have been obtained in patients with bilateral temporo-occipital lesions, although ceiling effects due to different task difficulty may have contributed to these differences (Tranel and Damasio, 1987; Etcoff, 1986; Wexler, 1973). In addition, the results of some half-field studies in normals showed that, even though the right hemisphere was superior in both face identification and recognition of emotional expressions, a right hemisphere superiority was still evident when the effect of face identity was partialled out (e.g., Strauss and Moscovitch, 1981). Other studies have shown that extraction of emotional information may be dissociated from recognition of the identity of familiar faces. Prosopagnotic patients show normal autonomic responses (galvanic skin response) to the presentation of familiar faces they are unable to recognize. Conversely, patients with orbito-frontal lesions—especially on the right—showed normal recognition of familiar faces but flattened emotional response to them (Tranel and Damasio, 1985, 1987). This latter result may be a consequence of a difficulty in extracting emotional information as well as a deficit in controlling emotional responses to the same stimuli. Altogether, this evidence suggests parallel processing between cognitive and emotional aspects of emotional stimuli.

It has been recently proposed that the right hemisphere may store and access purely *emotional* nonverbal representations. These specialized representations would encode the facial, prosodic, and gestural configuration of specific nonverbal signs involved in social communication (Blonder, Bowers, and Heilman, 1991). Blonder et al. found that right hemisphere patients that had deficits in the recognition of facial expression and prosody were also unable to extract the meaning of facial, prosodic, and gestural expressions when these displays were described using verbal language. At the same time these patients performed comparably to left hemisphere patients in a task of comprehension of emotional sentences. To interpret their results Blonder et al. (1991) proposed a two-stage hierarchic model similar to the one applied to visual agnosias. At the perceptual level, right hemisphere patients may fail to recognize emotional stimuli because of difficulties in processing the visuospatial or acoustic information conveyed in them. At a more abstract level, the right hemisphere may contain category-specific lexical representations of nonverbal expressions. As in the associative agnosias, either storage deterioration or impaired access may result in right hemisphere patients displaying impaired recognition of emotional stimuli.

A related finding may be that of Bowers et al. (1990), who found that right hemisphere lesions impair the ability to generate and use visual images of emotional expressions, paralleling the effect of left posterior lesions on the ability to generate images of visual objects (Bowers et al., 1990).

Cognitive Neuropsychology and Vertical Integration of Neural Systems

Much of the evidence on right hemisphere specialization for emotion can thus be explained in terms of right hemisphere specialization for the cognitive processes, such as the holistic integration of percepts and the representation of analogical information that are required for successful nonverbal emotional communication (Tucker, 1986). Perhaps because neuropsychology has been based on the study of perceptual and cognitive functions, explanations of emotional asymmetries have emphasized the cognitive implications of hemispheric specialization, from frustration with the impairment of verbal expressive ability in anterior left hemisphere lesions (Gainotti, 1972) to the specific deficits in nonverbal affect lexicon with right hemisphere lesions (Blonder, Bowers, and Heilman, 1991). As research continues to elucidate the cognitive differences between the left and right hemispheres, there will be additional ways to understand how lateralized cognitive processes may contribute to emotional asymmetries.

However, it may be important to proceed beyond a view of each hemisphere as a cognitive module. The physiologic circuitry subserving emotional behavior encompasses multiple levels in a highly integrated vertical hierarchy, reflecting the successive evolution of new forms of information representation and organismic self-regulation, traversing the brainstem, midbrain, limbic, and cortical levels (Derryberry and Tucker, 1991; Jackson, 1879; MacLean, 1958). Anterior and posterior cortical regions seem to exert different degrees of regulatory control over the vertical hierarchy of subcortical centers (Robinson et al., 1984; Starkstein, Boston, and Robinson, 1988) In addition, there is substantial evidence of hemispheric asymmetry of the brainstem neuromodulator projection systems that are critical to the regulation of emotion and arousal (Tucker and Liotti, 1989). An important unanswered question is therefore whether the two hemispheres differ in their relations with subcortical emotional control circuits.

A More Paralimbic Organization of the Right Hemisphere?

With the initial recognition of the importance of the right hemisphere to emotional communication, researchers speculated that its global conceptual skills may be important to combining information from both interoceptive and exteroceptive sources to achieve the integration of emotional experience (Safer and Leventhal, 1977). Tucker (1981) proposed that the right hemisphere supports a more primitive, syncretic form of conceptualization which is both holistic and affectively immediate. Buck (1985) suggested that this syncretic cognition allows the right hemisphere to have a special access to the internal feelings that monitor the internal state.

These speculations were made largely at the cognitive level. A continuing question has been whether there is any anatomic basis for the right hemisphere's emotional role, such as a greater degree of connection to limbic circuits (Borod, 1992; Tucker, 1981). One way of approaching this issue begins with the evidence that there is greater interconnection between regions in the right hemisphere than the left (Tucker, 1991). The initial evidence and interpretation were provided by Semmes (1968). She observed that a focal left hemisphere lesion produced discrete somatosensory and cognitive deficits, whereas an equally focal right hemisphere lesion produced more diffuse deficits in both somatosensory and cognitive domains. Reasoning from these observations to consider the differing structures of mental representation implied for the two hemispheres, Semmes proposed that the right hemisphere's unique psychological skills were consistent with its more diffuse representational format, allowing a dynamic and holistic integration across sensory modalities. EEG studies of signal coherence across scalp locations have been consistent with the Semmes hypothesis, showing greater coherence among right hemisphere regions for both children (Thatcher, Krause, and Rhybyk, 1986) and adults (Tucker, Roth, and Bair, 1986).

A cortical network pattern of dense interconnection between regions is characteristic of paralimbic cortex. Studies of cortical anatomy in the monkey by Pandya and associates (1988) have shown that for both the archicortical (dorsal) and paleocortical (ventral) pathways, the most highly differentiated networks (koniocortex) of the sensory modalities are connected only to the adjacent levels of the pathway. However, with increasing proximity to paralimbic cortex along the pathway, the connections to and from other divisions of the cortex, including dorsal-ventral connections, increase. The greatest density of interregional connection is thus achieved by paralimbic cortex.

To the extent that connection density reflects functional integration, the brain's function integration would not be achieved, therefore, by the "association" cortex of the parietal or frontal lobes (which is typically of intermediate architectonic differentiation, i.e., between primitive paralimbic and articulated sensory and motor koniocortex), but by the paralimbic cortex (Tucker, 1991). Each hemisphere may be specialized for a different form of network architecture, the left hemisphere's greater development of discrete modality-specific cortex (Goldberg and Costa, 1981) reflecting the greater network elaboration of coherent or "like" elements, and the right hemisphere's greater development of interregional connections supporting its more holistic representation of a "supramodal space" (Semmes, 1968). Almost by necessity, given that cortical network architecture is organized around its limbic roots, greater connection density in the right hemisphere implies that its representations will be formed with greater constraints from paralimbic influences.

OTHER FACTORS AFFECTING EMOTIONAL BEHAVIOR

The Anteroposterior Dimension

The early studies on lateralization of emotional behavior suggested differential roles for the two hemispheres. However, other variables, such as the lesion location within the hemispheres, were not taken into account. Traditional observations on the effect of frontal lobe lesions and psychosurgery on behavior strongly implied that the frontal regions are involved in the regulation of emotional behavior (Nauta, 1971; Stuss and Benson, 1984). With improved anatomic specification of lesions, it has become apparent that the *anteroposterior* dimension is an important factor in predicting the occurrence of emotional changes following unilateral lesions. Robinson and Szetela (1981) found that poststroke depression was more frequent in the case of anterior lesions of the left hemisphere, and its severity correlated with the distance from the frontal pole. Robinson et al. (1984) also reported that for right hemisphere lesions, anterior lesions were associated with inappropriate cheerfulness and apathy, while posterior lesions involving the parietal lobe were more frequently associated with depression. Starkstein and Robinson (1988) found that poststroke mania was significantly associated with damage to right anterior regions. Importantly, the relation between poststroke depression and left anterior locus of lesion held when patients with aphasic symptoms were excluded, or the effect of aphasia was partialled out (Starkstein and Robinson, 1988).

The Cortical-Subcortical Dimension

Another important variable not considered in earlier mood studies was the extent of damage to *subcortical* structures. Watson and Heilman (1982) predicted that a left subcortical lesion would *fail* to induce depression because it would not interrupt hemispheric processing of positive emotions and would not "release" the depression-prone right hemisphere. By disrupting the left corticoreticular system, a left subcortical lesion would, rather, affect the patient's arousal level, leading to unawareness, but not to depression.

However, several metabolic studies in primary unipolar depression have shown abnormalities of blood flow and glucose utilization in subcortical structures, such as the caudate nucleus (Baxter et al., 1985; Buchsbaum et al., 1986). Basal ganglia dysfunction has been implicated in the pathogenesis of depression in Parkinson's disease and Hungtington's chorea. Contrary to Heilman and Watson's prediction, left anterior *subcortical* lesions (body and head of the caudate, anterior limb of the internal capsule) were found to be significantly associated with major depression, the severity of which correlated with the distance from the frontal pole, as it does for cortical lesions (Starkstein, Robinson, and Price, 1987). Furthermore, in Parkinson's disease patients with exclusively or primarily unilateral symptoms, Starkstein et al. (1990) reported more depression in patients with prevalent right-sided as opposed to left-sided symptoms, consistent with the earlier findings that left caudate lesions are associated with greater depression.

Poststroke patients with major depression have been found to show more subcortical atrophy, indexed by higher values of ventricular-brain ratio on computed tomography (CT) scans, than nondepressed stroke patients matched for lesion size and location (Starkstein and Robinson, 1988). Starkstein et al. (1988) also described secondary mania patients with lesions confined to right subcortical structures, such as the thalamus and anterior caudate.

Asymmetries of Subcortical Release

The previous section reviewed evidence that subcortical structures, in particular the basal ganglia, are involved in the genesis of affective disorders. This section provides further evidence that changes in emotional behavior cannot be satisfactorily explained by release of contralateral cortical regions (e.g., Sackheim et al., 1982).

An alternative position that can account for the above findings maintains that the lateralized changes result from release of ipsilateral subcortical centers within the vertical hierarchy of emotional control (e.g., Tucker, 1981; Tucker and Frederick, 1989). Extensive reviews on pathologic emotional outbursts in the absence of brainstem lesions—pseudobulbar palsy—by Poeck (1969) and Rinn (1984) found involvement of subcortical structures (basal ganglia and the internal capsule) in virtually all the cases studied. In this condition, mood is often reported to be unaffected; at other times it is unrelated or even opposite to the displayed emotion. Earlier, Stern and Brown (1957) proposed that disinhibition of *cortical* centers may lead to the experience of euphoric mood during laughing outbursts, whereas outbursts not accompanied by mood change may involve release only of subcortical centers. Consistent with this view is the observation that anencephalic newborns show normal facial expressions of emotion, suggesting that brainstem centers may be sufficient for emotional display (Buck, 1988). Studying the effect of lesion location on emotional behavior, Kleist (1931) and Blumer and Benson (1975) proposed a vertical model in which lesions including the frontal convexity—both dorsolateral and dorsomedial prefrontal regions—are associated with slowness, indifference, apathy, and lack of initiative—"pseudodepression." In contrast, lesions of the orbitofrontal cortex may lead to disinhibition, lack of social constraint, hyperactivity, grandiose thinking and euphoria—a "pseudopsychopathic" syndrome. Starkstein and colleagues (Starkstein, Robinson, and Price, 1987; Starkstein and Robinson 1988) systematically analyzed the relation between poststroke mania and lesion location. They confirmed that secondary mania was significantly associated with cortical paralimbic (both orbitofrontal and basal temporal) damage, especially in the right hemisphere. However, mania was also more frequent for right than for left *subcortical* lesions (thalamus and basal ganglia).

Discussing their findings, Starkstein and Robinson (1988) mention that many manic symptoms, such as euphoria, hyperactivity, and insomnia, may be explained by a disruption of the control exerted by the orbitofrontal cortex over septal, hypothalamic, and mesencephalic regions (Nauta, 1971). In agreement with a vertical model of ipsilateral release, mania may be triggered by disinhibition of intact subcortical centers as a result of cortical dysfunction. These findings in human mania have a correlate in lesion effects observed in rats, where right but not left hemisphere lesions, especially lesions centered in the frontal lobe, were followed by hyperactivity (Robinson, 1979; Pearlson and Robinson, 1981). Similar qualitative effects, although interpreted as a decrease in anxiety rather than disinhibition, were seen in the psychosurgery literature with orbitofrontal or anterior cingulate ablations (see Tucker and Derryberry, 1991).

A closer look at the Wada test procedure suggests additional arguments for the ipsilateral release hypothesis. If the injection is carried out rapidly as a single bolus, the unilateral inactivation primarily affects the territory of the ipsilateral middle cerebral artery, which includes the cortical mantle of the dorsal and lateral surface of the brain (Terzian, 1964; Rossi and Rosadini, 1967). The anterior and posterior cerebral arteries communicate with the branches of the opposite side. They provide blood to the medial surface of the brain and to the occipital lobes, and to most of the subcortical structures, including the basal ganglia and most of the hippocampus. Therefore the unilateral sedation will involve the dorsal cortical mantle to a much greater extent than the ventromedial paralimbic cortical and subcortical structures. Therefore unilateral sedation may result not only from disinhibition of the opposite hemisphere but also from a release of ipsilateral paralimbic and subcortical limbic structures.

A last piece of evidence comes from a recent positron emission tomography (PET) study. Drevets et al. (1992) found that primary depressed patients showed evidence of *increased* blood flow in orbitofrontal cortex and parts of the cingulate gyrus, especially on the left side, concomitant with *reduced* metabolism in temporal and parieto-occipital regions. A similar activation of left ventrolateral prefrontal cortex was reported in a PET study in which normal subjects were asked to contemplate sad thoughts or memories (Pardo, Pardo, and Reichle, 1991). The posterior hypometabolism in Drevets's study is in line with the increased orbital-hemisphere ratio found by Baxter et al. (1987) and possibly the increased frontal-occipital ratio reported by Buchsbaum et al. (1986) in unipolar depression patients. An inverse relation between frontal and posterior activation has been seen in normal EEG studies (Davidson, 1984; Davidson, Chapman, and Chapman, 1987; Tucker et al., 1981) and may be important to the posterior right hemisphere deficits seen in depressed patients (reviewed by Tucker and Liotti, 1989). Drevets et al. (1992) speculate that in major depression the neural systems involved in the processing of sensory, exteroceptive information are inhibited in favor of systems involved in the processing of internal information, emotion, and negative thoughts, relying upon limbic-paralimbic representations (Nauta, 1971). This unbalance of activity, with paralimbic and limbic regions more active than neocortical areas during the experience of intense emotional states, may be interpreted as a functional "release" of limbic regions involved in emotional processing.

It is worth noting that other PET studies in depressed patients did not find increased, but instead decreased metabolism in the orbitofrontal cortex and other paralimbic areas (see Mayberg, 1992).

CORTICAL-SUBCORTICAL CIRCUITS IN DEPRESSION

Corticostriatothalamic Loops

In considering how basal ganglia dysfunction may lead to depression in Parkinson's disease, it has been proposed that it is the disruption of frontal cortical function that leads to depression. The caudate shares common pathways with frontal cortical structures, either directly or through the dorsomedial nucleus or the thalamus. Alexander, DeLong, and Strick (1986) described five functionally segregated parallel frontal corticostriathalamic loops, two of which are purely motor, while the remaining three, nonmotor, have variable degrees of limbic input. Each loop would represent a functional unit including the target prefrontal region. Among the nonmotor loops, a dorsolateral prefrontal network would support temporary storage in working memory of spatial locations (Goldman-Rakic, 1987) or rules for stimulus-response contingencies (Fuster, 1992). A lateral orbitofrontal circuit, projecting from the orbitofrontal cortex, connecting to a different sector of the caudate and the pallidus, would project to the thalamus and to the orbitofrontal cortex again. This circuit may be involved in the control of inhibitory responses during learning and recognition tasks requiring frequent shifts of set. This interpretation explains the pronounced perseverations consequent to orbitofrontal damage. An anterior cingulate circuit would include ventral striatum, nucleus accumbens, and mediodorsal nucleus of the thalamus. Hippocampus and entorhinal cortex would send inputs in this circuit, integrating information from paralimbic association cortex. The nucleus accumbens is also the target of dopaminergic terminals from the midbrain ventrotegmental area (VTA). The functions of this network are less established, but may include the integration of emotional cues and the individual's response to the hedonic quality of a stimulus.

In an attempt to prove a functional dissociation of these corticostriathalamic loops related to depression, Mayberg et al. (1988) carried out a PET study in basal ganglia stroke patients divided into two groups: (1) those having lesions of motor loop nuclei (putamen alone, putamen plus posterior internal capsule), and (2) those with lesions of nonmotor loop nuclei (head of the caudate alone, caudate plus anterior limb of the internal capsule, anterior and dorsomedial thalamus). While patients with putamen lesions and motor symptoms had widespread ipsilateral cortical and thalamic hypometabolism, caudate strokes in patients with only cognitive symptoms resulted in focal ipsilateral hypometabolism involving localized regions within frontal, temporal, or cingulate cortex. In a following study, patients with stroke in the head of the caudate were subdivided into euthymic, depressive, and manic patients. Compared to the euthymic patients, all the patients with mood change showed hypometabolism in orbital inferior frontal cortex, anterior temporal cortex, and cingulate cortex (Mayberg, 1992).

Ascending Neurotransmitter Pathways and Their Asymmetry

While dysfunction in frontostriathalamic loops has been emphasized by some authors, other interpretations have emphasized asymmetries in ascending neurotransmitter pathways. For example, Robinson and colleagues (1988) consider how laterality of emotion may be linked to primitive emotional influences. Some ascending neurotransmitter systems, in particular the norepinephrine (NE) and 5-hyrdroxytryptamine (5-HT) pathways thought to be disordered in depression and targeted by antidepressants may be inherently lateralized to the right hemisphere (see review in Tucker and Liotti, 1989). This possibility is supported by findings in the rat showing that right, but not left, anterior cortical ischemic lesions lead to depletion of brain and locus caeruleus NE bilaterally, with the more anterior the lesion the greater the depletion (Robinson, 1985), and to a greater concentration of plasma NE and resulting blood pressure increases (Hachinski et al., 1992). Lesions in the frontal cortex or basal ganglia (anterior brain) may interrupt the relevant fibers, since they run through the basal ganglia, then ascend to the frontal pole, before arching posteriorly around the corpus callosum to reach the deep layers of cortex.

A recent PET study (Mayberg et al., 1988) showed that patients with right hemisphere strokes had significantly higher ratios of ipsilateral to contralateral binding for S2 (serotonin or 5-HT) receptors than patients with left hemisphere strokes. The upregulation of S2 receptors took place in noninjured temporal and parietal cortex. In addition, in the left hemisphere stroke group, the S2 binding ratio significantly correlated with depression severity, with lower binding corresponding to higher depression. To account for greater depression in left frontal and basal ganglia lesions, yet more ipsilateral S2 upregulation for right-sided lesions, Mayberg et al. (1988) resorted to the following explanation. Animal and human evidence show right lateralization of 5-HT and NE cortical terminals (see Tucker and Liotti, 1989). As a result, a right hemisphere stroke would produce higher compensatory receptor upregulation in the intact ipsilateral tissue than corresponding left hemisphere lesions. Therefore a left lesion would produce a relative S2 and NE depletion not accompanied by an adequate upregulation of ipsilateral receptors. This may be sufficient to yield to depression. The hemispheric differences in S2 binding after unilateral cortical lesions have also been replicated in rats (Mayberg, Moran, and Robinson, 1990).

The long-term receptor upregulation, however, does not seem adequate to explain the rapid mood changes taking place after unilateral hemispheric sedation in the Wada procedure.

There is some evidence that disordered NE modulation may also be associated with human mania. Right hemisphere lesions involving limbic regions may result in secondary mania (Starkstein et al., 1991; Robinson et al., 1988). In rats, infarcts due to ligation of the right middle cerebral artery result in hyperactivity more frequently than do homologous left lesions (Robinson, 1985).

Dopaminergic (DA) pathways have been involved in the pathogenesis of depression in Parkinson's disease. DA terminals specifically target corticolimbic and limbic regions, i.e., prefrontal and cingulate cortex, nucleus accumbens, and amygdala. Most of these fibers originate in the midbrain VTA. A marked loss of DA neurons in the VTA has been found in a group of patients with Parkinson's disease dementia and depression (Torack and Morris, 1988). A dysfunction in the mesolimbic DA system may also play a role in the production of deficits in "frontal-lobe" tasks among Parkinson's disease patients with major depression. It is not clear, however, if these mechanisms play a role in primary major depression as well.

Recent research in rats undergoing experimental stress suggests that emotional states may entail asymmetric activation of ascending DA pathways. Stressors such as electric foot shock, conditioned fear, food deprivation, and restraint have been found to increase the DA metabolism in the terminal regions of the mesocortical (prefrontal cortex) or mesolimbic (nucleus accumbens) systems in the rat (Thierry et al., 1976; Lavielle et al., 1979). It has been recently shown that stress-induced prefrontal DA metabolic changes show hemispheric differences that are dependent on the time of exposure to the stressor. Prolonged, uncontrollable foot-shock stress, or long-lasting restraint (60 minutes), are both effective in leading to learned helplessness, an animal model of depression. These procedures resulted in greater activation of prefrontal DA on the *right* side of the brain (Fitzgerald et al., 1989; Carlson et al., 1991; Carlson and Glick, 1991). Conversely, brief food deprivation (24 hours) or brief restraint stress (15 minutes) resulted in greater activation of DA prefrontal metabolism on the *left* side of the brain (Carlson and Glick, 1991; Carlson et al., 1991). The increased prefrontal DA metabolism in an animal model of depression and stress may be relevant to the finding of increased frontal activation of the EEG (alpha desyncronization) in depressed patients (Perris et al., 1979), and in state and trait depression in normal students (Tucker et al., 1981; Davidson, 1984; Davidson et al., 1987). It may also bear on the notion of an increased frontal inhibitory influence in depression (Tucker et al., 1981).

Asymmetric Cybernetics of Tonic Activation and Phasic Arousal

The inherent asymmetry of neuromodulator projections provides important clues for integrating the neuropsychological evidence on hemispheric specialization for emotion with the biological psychiatry evidence on neuromodulator dysfunction in psychopathologic disorders. It seems clear that the explanatory framework that will be necessary for both these bodies of evidence will need to encompass the regulatory circuits through which brainstem, midbrain, basal ganglia, and limbic structures exert elementary influences on cortical function. The idea that a "hemisphere" has monolithic emotional qualities may be heuristic, but only to a point. Similarly, the idea that a psychiatric disorder can be traced to a neurochemical abnormality is simplistic, and may lead to a functional understanding only as the neuromodulator systems are seen within the context of the parts they play in the brain's multileveled motivational circuitry.

Lacking an explicit model of subcortical mechanisms, Tucker and Williamson (1984) speculated on the primitive attentional controls that may emerge from asymmetric neuromodulator projections. Drawing from Pribram and McGuinness's (1975) theorizing on neural systems for activation and arousal,

Tucker and Williamson proposed that a *tonic activation* system, supporting motor readiness, applies a primitive cybernetic influence on ongoing information processing, a *redundancy bias*. This influence, relying on controls from the mesolimbic and possibly striatal DA projections, maintains not only motor readiness but a focal form of attention. Tucker and Williamson suggested that this control mode is inherent to states of anxiety and hostility. Furthermore, consistent with the greater left lateralization of DA projections, this primitive control mode of the redundancy bias may underlie the focal attention and analytic cognition shown by the left hemisphere.

In contrast, a qualitatively different control bias is seen as emerging from the NE projections which support a *phasic arousal* system. This system applies a *habituation bias* to attention that is integral to the orienting response to novelty, and to perceptual orienting processes generally. Consistent with the catecholamine hypothesis of depression, increased NE activity in mania is seen as leading to a shortened attention span and stimulus seeking, both of which are produced by the habituation bias of a strongly engaged phasic arousal system. This system is hypothesized to have both attentional influences and affective qualities, with high phasic arousal associated with mania and low phasic arousal associated with depression. The inherent right lateralization of the phasic arousal system is proposed to be integral to the right hemisphere's mediation of elementary attentional orienting, as seen in the evidence on neglect and arousal, and to many of the affective functions of the right hemisphere, as shown by its responsiveness to mood variations (Liotti et al., 1991; Liotti and Tucker, 1992; Tucker and Liotti, 1989).

This theorizing attempted to forge links between elementary neural controls from neuromodulator systems and more complex cognitive and attentional systems as appear to be reflected by hemispheric specialization. In more recent theorizing, an important recognition has been that brain lateralization is unlikely to have evolved as orthogonal to the fundamental division of the cortex between dorsal and ventral networks (Derryberry and Tucker, 1991; Tucker, 1991). In the following sections, we continue this line of reasoning. We begin with evidence of differing forms of corticolimbic interactions for the two hemispheres. These interactions are clearly relevant to questions of self-regulation at the emotion and personality level, but they may also be relevant to hemispheric differences in the control of cognitive processes. We then review the anatomy of dorsal and ventral limbic circuits that underlies the division between the dorsal and ventral cortical networks. We emphasize the evolutionary interpretation that helps explain the origins and functional significance of this major feature of cortical architecture. Finally, we review evidence that hemispheric specialization for cognitive functions has involved left hemisphere elaboration of the object identification functions of the ventral cortical pathway as well as right hemisphere elaboration of the spatial orienting functions of the dorsal cortical pathway. Although the human evidence on emotional functions of the dorsal and ventral networks is limited, we attempt with the cognitive and perceptual evidence to build an initial theoretical framework which may serve as a basis for further work toward a general model of adaptive self-regulation of cortical systems.

LATERALIZED MODES OF CORTICOLIMBIC REGULATION

In the initial controversy over whether mood valence effects of unilateral lesions reflect release of ipsilateral or contralateral emotional tendencies (Sackeim et al., 1982; Tucker, 1981), a key piece of evidence was the observations on differences in emotional changes in unilateral epilepsy (Tucker, 1981). The research by Bear and Fedio (1977) found that patients with left temporal lobe epilepsy showed both clinical symptoms and a psychometric profile that indicated an *ideative* exaggeration in their cognitive function. These patients became preoccupied with moral ideals or religious concerns, often writing extensive treatises on these topics. The changes observed in patients with right temporal lobe epilepsy, on the other hand, suggested an exaggeration of emotional processes, with greater mood lability suggesting impaired affective self-regulation. These differences suggested to Bear and Fedio that the epileptic process resulted in a functional hyperconnection of cortical with limbic structures.

In addition, each patient group showed a characteristic bias in self-description in the psychometric procedures. Bear and Fedio compared the patients' self-ratings with ratings of their behavior and characteristics made by observers. The left temporal epilepsy group tended to emphasize their negative characteristics, while the right temporal epilepsy group tended to deny problems and emphasize their positive traits.

These results were interpreted by Tucker (1981) as consistent with the ipsilateral release interpretation of the brain lesion effects. The apparent functional hyperconnection of cortical and limbic structures in the left hemisphere leads to an exaggerated significance of ideational concerns, and with a more negative, critical affective orientation. This combination seems reminiscent of anxious, obsessive, and paranoid personality styles which also include highly analytic cognitive styles (Shapiro, 1965). The exaggeration of limbic contributions to right hemisphere cognition leads not only to more emotionality but to the denial and Pollyannaish optimism characteristic of hysterical, histrionic, and hypomanic personality styles (American Psychiatric Association, 1987), who also show holistic, unanalytic, and impressionistic cognitive styles (Shapiro, 1965).

Although the literature on personality changes with temporal lobe epilepsy has been controversial, the major findings of Bear and Fedio (1977) have been replicated by more recent research (Fedio, 1986; Fedio and Martin, 1983). In theorizing on the limbic mechanisms that may be important to the differential hemispheric emotional characteristics, Bear (1983) took up the issue of how lateralization may interact with the functional differentiation between dorsal and ventral cortical pathways. He proposed that right hemisphere specialization for the spatial functions of the dorsal cortical pathway may be relevant to both the attentional deficits (neglect) and the emotional deficits (denial, indifference) observed following right hemisphere damage. The right hemisphere may be responsible for "emotional surveillance," so that when this capacity is diminished following a lesion the patient fails to recognize the significance of emotionally important information. In this view, denial and indifference represent a kind of emotional neglect.

Tucker and Derryberry (Tucker, 1991; Tucker and Derryberry, 1991) developed a complementary formulation, suggesting that the left hemisphere's affective characteristics may have evolved in line with its elaboration of the motivational and cognitive functions of the ventral limbic circuitry. The affective characteristics of anxiety and hostility, mediated by the amygdala and ventral paralimbic cortex including orbital frontal regions, may be particularly important to regulating the left hemisphere's operations, so that the hyperconnection of limbic with cortical functions observed in the left temporal lobe epilepsy patients would result in a more negative, critical affective bias.

Although there have been few solid findings relating individual differences in cognitive and emotional style to brain lateralization, Swenson and Tucker (1983) found that subjects reporting a more analytic cognitive style were more self-critical in their self-report bias compared to subjects reporting a more holistic cognitive style, whose self-report bias was more positive. A related finding may be that observed by Levy and associates (1983) in a study relating individual differences to how subjects evaluate their performance in the left and right visual fields. All subjects were accurate in judging their performance in the right visual field. For performance in the left visual field, subjects showed biases that may be related to characteristic patterns of hemispheric activation or cognitive style. Subjects who showed a strong right visual field effect on a syllable identification task, perhaps reflecting an emphasis on left hemisphere cognition, showed a negative bias in judging their left field's performance. Subjects not showing the strong right field effect, perhaps reflecting more of a right hemisphere cognitive style, showed a positive bias in rating their left visual field performance. Thus the evidence on both normal and abnormal patterns of cognitive style suggests there may be important links between the two hemispheres' cognitive capacities, and differing styles of affective self-regulation.

Although it is difficult to research, the relation between limbic and cortical systems seems to hold important clues to cognitive-affective interactions at the personality level. In order to provide a background for this question, and research that may clarify it, we review some of the fundamentals of corticolimbic architecture and the evidence suggesting that right and left hemisphere specialization has involved differential elaboration of the information-processing capacities of the dorsal and ventral cortical regions, respectively.

Two Cortical Visual Pathways

Ungerleider and Mishkin (1982) proposed a model of cortical visual processing based on two parallel visual systems, one directed ventrally to the inferotemporal cortex, and one directed dorsally to the inferior parietal lobe. The original model was derived from lesion studies in monkeys. Lesions of the inferior temporal cortex produce severe deficits in performance in a variety of visual discrimination learning tasks but not in visuospatial tasks. By contrast, posterior parietal lesions cause marked impairments in visuospatial performance, such as in visually guided reaching and in judging which of two objects is located closer to a visual landmark, but these lesions spare visual discrimination performance (Ungerleider and Mishkin, 1982). Within each pathway the multiple visual areas form processing hierarchies, since virtually all connections between successive areas are reciprocal. Importantly, the functional segregation of the two visual pathways is not limited to corticocortical connections, since it can be traced downstream to the retina ganglion cells (Desimone and Ungerleider, 1990). Many psychophysical studies have identified "sustained" and "transient" channels subserving, respectively, pattern recognition in foveal vision, and flicker, motion, and depth perception in peripheral vision (e.g., Breitmeyer and Ganz, 1977). Both systems originate in specialized retinal ganglion cells whose axons terminate in different layers of the lateral geniculate nucleus (LGN). These LGN neurons in turn send projections to different regions of the striate cortex, with unique histologic and functional properties (Hubel and Livingstone, 1987). These striate modules are then connected to specific regions of the secondary visual areas V2–V4 and MT.

Ventral Pathway for Object Recognition   The ventral visual pathway terminates in the inferior temporal lobe (area IT or TE). Neurons in area TE have large, often bilateral receptive fields, thought to mediate perceptual equivalence of objects over translation in retinal position. A small proportion of cells respond selectively to high-order complex stimuli, such as faces or hands. Most of the neurons, however, respond selectively on the basis of object features, such as color, shape, and texture rather than specific objects. It seems likely therefore that cells in IT, instead of each representing different visual objects, constitute a distributed network for the representation of general object features. Mishkin, Malamut, and Bachevalier (1984) found that lesions of IT cause loss of perceptual constancies and profound loss of visual memories. Memories of visual inputs would be restricted to a "habit" learning system involving the basal ganglia (Mishkin et al., 1984). Mishkin proposes that IT contains the "central representations" for visual objects, and that the loss of IT leads to an inability to form new memories as well as to the loss of old memories. Neurophysiologic evidence that IT could actually be a site of memory storage (Fuster and Jervey, 1981) is available but not definitive. Limbic lesions, especially when restricted to the hippocampus, have been found to impair memory storage only temporarily. Amnesic patients have difficulty recalling the recent past but can recall remote events as well as normal subjects (Squire, 1987, 1992).

Dorsal Visual Pathway for Spatial Orienting   This system provides the basis for peripheral vision, motion perception, stereopsis, perception of three-dimensionality of objects based on perspective and shading, and most of the gestalt phenomena of "linking operations" (Livingstone and Hubel, 1987). Through several intermediary areas, the dorsal pathway terminates in area PG of the inferior parietal lobule and in the intraparietal sulcus. In the monkey, a proportion of cells in area PG fire when the animal fixates interesting objects in particular regions of space (Mountcastle, 1978). These cells may be involved in mediating the so-called ambient vision (Motter and Mountcastle, 1981; Trevarthen, 1968). Importantly, some cells show an increase in firing rate when the animal is expecting a stimulus in a specific region of the visual field ("enhancement effect"; e.g., Robinson, Goldberg, and Stanton, 1978). In monkeys and humans, the posterior parietal cortex is one of the structures involved in the control of spatial attention. Lesions centered in this region impair the ability to orient attention to the contralateral side upon presentation of "invalid" directional cues (Posner and Cohen, 1984; Posner et al., 1987).

The two visual networks outlined above are parallel hierarchies of sequential neocortical—cognitive—representations, from those of low input to more complex and abstract ones. The following sections review anatomic, physiologic, and developmental evidence that the two visual systems are not exclusively neocortical. The ventral system has direct reciprocal projections to the amygdala and to the orbitofrontal cortex. The dorsal system projects heavily to the cingulate gyrus, the hippocampus, and surrounding limbic areas. These regions participate in the perceptual and mnemonic functions of the two visual streams, most likely providing the integration of emotional, motivational, and interoceptive qualities of visual percepts. Particularly relevant to the notion of integrated corticolimbic visual pathways are developmental studies showing that neocortical visual areas—like areas PG and TE—have evolved through consecutive cytoarchitectonic trends from two distinct limbic moieties—the olfactory cortex and the hippocampus. This suggests that the role of limbic representations within the dorsal and ventral systems goes well beyond anatomic and functional connections to neocortical pathways. In origin, the two visual pathways may have been entirely limbic.

Limbic Connections of the Ventral System

The neural circuit subserving visual object recognition includes connections to two structures belonging to the limbic system: the amygdala and the orbitofrontal cortex (Van Hoesen and Pandya, 1975). Bilateral damage to both TE and amygdaloid complex produce severe and long-lasting recognition loss (Miskhin, 1978; Zola-Morgan, Squire, and Mishkin, 1982).

Amygdala   Lesions involving neocortical temporal areas produce disturbances in visual discrimination learning. In contrast, lesions of the temporal pole and amygdaloid nuclei generate the emotional changes characteristic of the Klüver-Bucy syndrome (Ledoux, 1987; see also Zola-Morgan et al., 1991). This has led to two lines of research, one concerned with the role of the temporal lobe in visual processing, and the other dealing with the role of the amygdala in emotion. The two lines have converged in studies suggesting that the affective components are added to visual stimuli by connections between neocortical aspects of the temporal lobe and amygdala.

Downer (1961) and Geschwind (1965) proposed that lesions of the temporal lobe disconnect the visual system from reinforcement mechanisms located in the amygdala. They argued that the formation of associations between limbic and nonlimbic stimuli was a key aspect of the behavioral tasks used to implicate the temporal lobe and amygdala in visual learning. In the absence of these connections, it would be impossible to associate reward conditions with visual stimuli. When monkeys receive selective lesions confined to the amygdala, they exhibit deficits indicating impairment of stimulus-reinforcement association. In single-cell studies in the monkey, amygdala neurons showed differential responses to visual stimuli signaling food and shock (Fuster and Uyeda, 1971), or edible or inedible objects (Ono et al., 1983). In man, electrical stimulation of the amygdala is sufficient to elicit the complex combination of perceptual, mnemonic, and affective features present in the "experiential" phenomena of temporal lobe epilepsy (Gloor, 1990). This suggests that the amygdala may have a critical role not only in combining emotional cues to perceptual stimuli but also in integrating perceptual and affective memories into a subjective experience (Gloor, 1990; Ledoux, 1987).

New research on the amygdala's role in emotional processing suggests that peripheral information reaches the amygdala not only through a polysynaptic corticoamydaloid circuit. A direct monosynaptic connection between thalamus and amygdala has been demonstrated in the rabbit (Ledoux, 1987). Ledoux speculates that it would provide the amygdala with rapid, primitive representations of the peripheral stimulus, in contrast to the more precise and processed inputs from the neocortex. The role of the thalamoamygdala projection could be to prepare the amygdala for the subsequent reception of highly processed information from the cortex. Alternatively, the two systems may function independently. The thalamoamygdala system may mediate more primitive emotional reactions, more loosely coupled to the stimulus, and not requiring object recognition. Inputs to the amygdala from polymodal association areas can be involved in evaluation of object information integrated from different sensory modalities (Ledoux, 1987).

Orbitofrontal Cortex   The orbital region is often described as the neocortical representation of the limbic system (Nauta, 1971). This region has direct reciprocal connections to the temporal pole and the amygdala, and is considered by some as the direct frontal extension of the ventral visual pathway. Severe impairments in visual object learning have been reported in monkeys with orbitofrontal lesions (Thorpe, Rolls, and Maddison, 1983). The role of the orbital region in visual object memory may be in establishing associations between stimuli and rewards, especially when the task requires the frequent making and breaking of stimulus-reward associations (see Ledoux, 1987; Derryberry and Tucker, 1992). In the absence of orbitofrontal neurons, the brain continues to respond to stimuli no longer rewarded. This may contribute to the perseverative behavior shown by monkeys and humans with orbitofrontal damage (Sandson and Albert, 1984). Learning and unlearning the emotional significance of sensory events would require a close interaction between the amygdala and orbital region.

We mentioned previously evidence of disinhibited emotional behavior following orbitofrontal lesions. The orbitofrontal region exerts control over septal, hypothalamic, and mesencephalic regions (Nauta, 1971). Mania and inappropriate social behavior may be triggered by disinhibition of intact subcortical centers as a result of orbitofrontal dysfunction. Right-sided lesions are particularly implicated in these release phenomena, both in humans (Starkstein et al., 1998) and in rats (Robinson, 1979).

Damasio and Tranel (1988) suggest a "cognitive" interpretation for the behavioral effects of orbitofrontal lesions. According to them, disinhibited emotional behavior may be conceived as a category-specific memory impairment. The ventromedial frontal cortex would store complex specialized representations about social events, such that lesions of this portion of the frontal lobe would result in an "acquired sociopathy." The orbitofrontal cortex would be one of the highest-order convergence zones, where complex conjunctions of spatial and temporal features identifying social events would be stored and accessed for later recall (Damasio, 1989). Undoubtedly intriguing, this interpretation clearly shows the current fascination of neuroscientists for "cognitive" models of emotion, leading sometimes to frankly excessive "cortical chauvinism."

Limbic Connections of the Dorsal Pathway

Massive inputs to the posterior parietal lobe derive from limbic areas, including the cingulate gyrus, the retrosplenial area, and the cholinergic nucleus basalis. The last input is quite nonspecific, since ascending projections are distributed to virtually all other cortical areas, thus possibly influencing the state of the entire cortical mantle. However, the cingulate and retrosplenial projections are more selective and may be related to more complex and learned aspects of motivation. The convergence of limbic input from the cingulate-retrosplenial cortex with the extensively preprocessed sensory information may allow parietal neurons to recognize motivational relevance in complex sensory events (Mesulam, 1985).

Cingulate Cortex Monkeys with unilateral cingulotomy display contralateral inattention in visual and somatosensory modalities (Watson et al.,

1973). Single-cell recordings show increases of firing rates when the animal pays attention to a meaningful object in a particular location of the visual space. In humans, both right parietal or medial frontal infarcts including the cingulate cortex give rise to typical unilateral neglect for the left hemispace (Heilman et al., 1983), and a marked inability to deal with spatial memory in that half of the world (Mesulam, 1985). Patients lose the ability to navigate and appreciate space. Large bilateral cingulate lesions result in a profound inertia to initiate voluntary responses to sensory stimulation, culminating in the "lock-in" syndrome or coma vigil. Smaller lesions can result in lack of appreciation of pain. Pain has little saliency for the patients, causing anterior cingulotomy to be used for the relief of chronic pain. Pandya and Yeteran (1985) propose that the inattention due to cingulotomy may be failure to appreciate the significance of stimuli. The indifference to interoceptive and exteroceptive stimulation may stem from the inability to attach significance to that stimulation. The cingulate gyrus may mediate adaptively significant attention, as opposed to the more spatially oriented attention subserved by the posterior parietal region.

In discussing the possible circuits for the formation of spatial memories, Pandya and Yeteran (1985) describe two pathways. The first, connecting area 7 and the cingulate gyrus to the hippocampus via the presubiculum, may be a rapidly acting memory circuit for *significant* objects located in space. The second circuit, connecting area 7 and the cingulate gyrus to the hippocampus and amygdala via the parahippocampal gyrus, may be a slower system, more attuned to the formation of complex spatial memories. In support of this distinction, the authors mention that bilateral cingulate infarcts in humans produce an akinetic state and attentional dysfunction, whereas bilateral para-hippocampal damage results in a deficit in the discrimination of complex geometric forms and faces. The first implies a role in spatial behavior that has immediate *survival* value. The latter implies a role in dealing with spatial relationships that pertain to the construction of complex images such as faces. Selective lesions to the hippocampal formation in monkeys have been shown to produce an enduring deficit in the ability to memorize the location of objects in space (Parkinson and Miskhin, 1982).

Evolution of the Ventral and Dorsal Visual Systems

An interesting perspective on cortical visual areas and corticocortical connections derives from studies on the evolutionary development of the cortex. Sanides (1970, 1972) proposed that the architectonic differentiation of the mammalian cerebral cortex may be explained in terms of evolutionary development. The various isocortical areas are elements in a sequence of different trends, each of which begins in proisocortex and shows increasing laminar differentiation as it grows more distant from its origin from the two primordial moieties in the limbic core, the hippocampus (archicortex) and the olfactory cortex (paleocortex). The archicortical moiety is the precursor of the isocortex on the medial and dorsal cortical surface, whereas the paleocortical moiety gives rise to the isocortex of the lateral and ventral surfaces.

Pandya et al. (1988) applied Sanides' evolutionary concepts, according to an architectonic-connectional schema, to explain the development of the ventral and dorsal visual system. The ventral cortical system specialized for object recognition in central vision evolves from the primordial paleocortical moiety of the temporal pole and olfactory cortex, through different stages of cytoarchitectonic differentiation, to reach the six-layered isocortical stage of the primary visual cortex. Conversely, the dorsal cortical system for spatial perception and memory in peripheral vision evolves through subsequent stages from the archicortical moiety of the hippocampus. Each of these intermediary cortices persists in the human brain.

A very important part of the model of Pandya et al. is that the cortical pathways are not unidirectional. The view that the dual visual system leads away from the primary sensory cortices toward association areas and limbic areas—viewed as a route whereby incoming sensory information is processed sequentially through adjoining areas before reaching the limbic system—is challenged by the finding that all intrinsic corticocortical connections are in fact reciprocal. "Backward," that is, from limbic to cortical, projections are particularly important, since they link areas of increasing laminar differentiation, and their functional value has to be considered with respect to the fact that they parallel the stages of architectonic development. This opposite pathway, leading away from proisocortex, may be viewed as a feedback system whereby limbic information on the internal state of the organism is relayed to cytoarchitectonically more differentiated areas. This reverted direction may provide critical clues to the way in which motivational and emotional states mediated by limbic regions exert regulatory and adaptive functions—determining which representations will dominate the information processing and behavior of the whole brain (Derryberry and Tucker, 1991; Tucker, 1991).

Neuropsychological Evidence in Humans

Some findings in humans suggest that hemispheric lateralization has differentially elaborated the cognitive functions subserved by the dorsal and ventral corticolimbic pathways.

Right Hemisphere and the Dorsal System   As early as the 1880s a dissociation between impairment in recognizing things and impairment in apprehending spatial relationships was noted, and the distinction was thus drawn between object agnosia and "spatial agnosia" (De Renzi, 1982).

There is a large body of evidence that supports the primary role of the right hemisphere in visuospatial behavior in humans. Although the most severe deficits of visuospatial behavior occur with large bilateral parieto-occipital lesions (Balint's syndrome), more focal lesions encroaching upon the right posterior regions and including the parietal lobe seem to be sufficient to disrupt several aspects of visuospatial behavior, such as visual judgments of line orientation (Benton, Varney, and Hamsher, 1978a), visually guided stylus maze performance (De Renzi, Faglioni, and Villa, 1977), and the ability to identify objects presented from an unusual visual perspective (Warrington, 1982). Constructional apraxia, dressing dyspraxia, and prosopagnosia were associated with right posterior damage in some of the earliest experimental neuropsychology studies (Hécaen and Angelergues, 1962; Arrigoni and De Renzi, 1964). Although not studied as extensively, memory processes show hemispheric asymmetry along the same lines (Milner, 1974). In tachistoscopic experiments in normal subjects, it has been found repeatedly that there is a left visual field/right hemisphere superiority for depth perception (Kimura, 1961), spatial localization (De Renzi, 1982), and the identification of complex geometrical shapes (Umiltá, Bagnara, and Simion, 1978). Some evidence points to a right hemisphere superiority during tasks requiring the programming of exploratory eye movements (Sava, Liotti, and Rizzolatti, 1988). Finally, the left hand is more accurate in judging the orientation of a rod by palpation (Benton, Varney, and Hamsher, 1978b).

The neglect syndrome, an inability to attend to stimuli presented in the contralesional hemispace in the absence of primary sensory or motor deficits, is more frequent, severe, and long-lasting following right than left inferior parietal lobe lesions (De Renzi, 1982). Mesulam (1981) proposed that the right hemisphere contains the neural machinery for attending to both sides of the extrapersonal space, whereas the left hemisphere contains only the machinery for attending to the contralateral right hemispace.

The network of cortical and subcortical regions subserving visual orienting in monkeys and humans (Heilman, 1979; Mesulam, 1981) involves areas that are functionally part of the dorsal visual system, or that are highly connected to it, i.e., the posterior parietal region, the cingulate cortex, the dorsolateral frontal cortex, the pulvinar, and the inferior colliculus.

Recently, cognitive psychologists have tried to explain the nature of right hemisphere representations and to relate them to the function of the dorsal visual system. Kosslyn (1987) developed a model according to which the right hemisphere bases its computations on high-order coordinate, metric representations of spatial locations. The right hemisphere stores and manipulates coordinate representations of visual objects. These representations would be necessary to explore and navigate in the environment, and to position attention at specific locations where specific objects are to be found. These representations would be necessary in the processing of complex multipart objects, requiring the coding of complex spatial relations.

A related, but not completely overlapping interpretation is that the right hemisphere stores global configurations or gestalts of visual objects in contrast to local features or details of objects. These are not necessarily high-order representations. The right hemisphere is faster in processing global than local features of objects, and there is evidence that this global level is coded faster than the local level (global precedence effect), which suggests that these representations may be of lower order in the hierarchy of visual processing. Right hemiphere patients are impaired at the global level, showing preserved categorization of local features (Nebes, 1978).

Left Hemisphere and the Ventral Pathway for Object Recognition
While the evidence in favor of a right lateralization for the neural computations supported by the dorsal visual system is strong, the evidence in favor of a greater elaboration of the ventral visual pathway in the left hemisphere is less established. Recent data from clinical neuropsychology suggest that a lesion restricted to the left occipitotemporal area may be sufficient to produce visual object agnosia (McCarthy and Warrington, 1990). The identification of objects shown with unusual perspectives, however, seems to require the right hemisphere (Warrington, 1982). Therefore, visual object recognition seems to be left-lateralized for objects shown in canonical views. It is also important to point out that another type of object recognition, i.e., the identification of familiar faces, shows evidence of being right-lateralized. A recent PET study in normals showed unilateral left activation of temporo-occipital areas in an object identification task in which subjects had to categorize the stimulus as natural or man-made, whereas a more bilateral and right hemisphere activation accompanied a task of face-gender categorization and face identity (Sergent, Ohta, and MacDonald, 1992). It seems reasonable that it is not object identification per se that is lateralized, but the particular strategy employed to process the visual object. Objects with unusual perspectives may be more easily coded in terms of spatial relations, or as configurations or gestalts, the type of representations that the right hemisphere, and within it, the dorsal pathway, is able to process. The same holds true for the recognition of faces.

It has been proposed that the left hemisphere contains the long-term semantic representations—the lexicon—to be retrieved in order to identify or categorize a visual object. However, when a visual object is processed in terms of its general physical configuration or on the basis of the spatial relationship between parts, this would require access to long-term representations stored in the right hemisphere. This interpretation is in line with several recent findings. Judgments of line orientation are known to be largely a function of the right posterior regions (Benton et al., 1978b). In normal subjects, however, it was found that the left hemisphere can encode line orientation better than the right hemisphere when vertical, horizontal, or 45-degree diagonal orientations were used, whereas the right hemisphere was better than the left when nonstandard oblique orientations were used (Umiltá et al., 1974).

Recently, a similar pattern of hemispheric lateralization has been found in the case of more abstract visual representations. Levine, Warach, and Farah (1985) reported two patients with a double dissociation between processing of identity ("what?") or spatial relations ("where?") on visual internal representations. Bisiach and Luzzatti (1978) reported the case of a right parietal patient, a native of Milan, Italy, with contralateral neglect in perception, who

exhibited, in addition, a difficulty in exploring the left side of a *mental represen-*
tation of the main city square, the Piazza del Duomo. Conversely, temporo-
occipital lesions of the *left* hemisphere have been associated with a deficit in
the *generation* of images of visual objects (Farah, 1984; Kosslyn, 1987). Patients
would fail in assembling the parts of a visual image into a unified ensemble
according to spatial and temporal relations, such as above-below, right-left;
these categories may be stored preferentially in the left hemisphere (Grossi et
al., 1986; Kosslyn, 1987).

In summary, one account for the left hemisphere specialization for object
recognition in perception and, perhaps, representation emphasizes the advantage of the left hemisphere for the access and long-term storage of categorical,
propositional, or semantic knowledge concerning the object. According to
Kosslyn (1987), this asymmetry may have developed as a consequence of left
hemisphere dominance for language processes.

A rather different possibility, however, is that the left hemisphere superiority for object recognition derives from its advantage in the sequential analysis
of information that is parsed in "object-like" units. Patients with left hemisphere damage are more likely to have difficulty with the analysis of "local"
levels of a visual scene, while patients with right hemisphere lesions are more
impaired with information on a "global" level. This performance asymmetry
occurs whether the dependent measure is errors in reconstruction or recognition, subjective judgments, or reaction time (Robertson and Lamb, 1991;
Lamb, Robertson, and Knight, 1990). In most of these studies the local features
are single letters or single elements of a scene that are unlikely to require
naming. Furthermore, sequential analysis of local information—high spatial
frequency—in the auditory modality is also performed more efficiently by the
left hemisphere (Ivry, 1991). It is possible that left hemisphere processing of
language comprehension may have followed its preference for sequential processing of parsed object-like units (Kimura, 1961).

Interestingly, Broca's area 44 is both cytoarchitectonically and functionally
part of prefrontal area 6, which animal and human evidence shows to be
critical for the programming of learned motor sequences. The execution of
complex motor sequences—such as those involved in sign language or ideo-
motor praxis—is also dependent on the integrity of the left hemisphere
(Heilman and Vallenstein, 1985). The symbolic aspects of these activities may
require access to linguistic information stored preferentially in the dominant
hemisphere. However, a superiority of the left hemisphere in voluntary
learned motor sequences can be demonstrated even in the presence of minimal
or absent processing of symbolic information, as during nonautomatic
finger-tapping (Kimura and Archibald, 1974; Rizzolatti et al., 1979) or during
the pantomime of manual gestures (Heilman and Valenstein, 1985). Interestingly, the lateral premotor region in the frontal cortex of the monkey
is thought to develop phylogenetically from the cortex of the olfactory
paleopallium, which is also the limbic core of the ventral visual pathway
(Goldberg, 1985). Therefore, even this aspect of left hemisphere sequential

motor processing may have capitalized on the cybernetics of the ventral corticolimbic system.

INTEGRATED ASYMMETRIC CORTICOLIMBIC SYSTEMS

In this rather superficial review of several diverse literatures, we have attempted to suggest that hemispheric specialization for cognitive and perceptual processes has very likely involved differential elaboration of the dorsal and ventral cortical networks. The dynamic patterns of intracortical network relations must be understood, then, in terms of balances not only between left vs. right, and anterior vs. posterior, but dorsal vs. ventral within each of these more traditional neuropsychological subdivisions. A specialization pattern that emphasizes an alignment of one of these dimensions with the other, e.g., right hemisphere elaboration of the dorsal pathway's spatial functions, must raise questions of the complementarity of the secondary network, e.g., the complementary role of the ventral cortical pathways for object identification in the right hemisphere.

As these issues are sorted out, it may be important to avoid the tendency to separate cognitive processes from emotional processes as topics for neuropsychological research. The dynamic interactions among cortical systems are likely to be understood not only in terms of the *representative* functions of the networks, the ability to form cognitive representations of the environment, but the *regulatory* functions as well, the control operations that determine which representations will dominate the information processing and behavior of the whole brain. These regulatory operations are motivational, adaptive processes that are critically dependent on the integrated functioning of the multiple levels of the vertically evolved neural hierarchy. Corticolimbic interactions are positioned at the crossroads of the essential regulatory functions of the subcortex and the flexible representative functions of the massive cortical networks.

For example, the right hemisphere's elaboration of the spatial orienting functions of the dorsal pathway are likely to be important to its role in emotional processes, such as through the coordination of spatial with hedonic processes (Mesulam, 1981), the facilitation of attention to emotionally significant events (Bear, 1983), and the integration of elementary arousal mechanisms with holistic attention (Tucker and Williamson, 1984). However, if this is so, the question becomes the complementary role of the ventral pathway. The cases of mania following brain damage described by Starkstein et al. (1988) and Cummings and Mendez (1984) have shown a clear association of this pathologic positive affect with lesions disrupting cortical-subcortical circuits on the right side. The cortical lesions producing this effect are those of the anterior ventral (orbital, temporal) regions of the right hemisphere. The ventral limbic circuits of the right hemisphere thus appear to have a particularly important role in regulating, apparently inhibiting, the neural circuitry of positive affective arousal (elation). This circuitry almost certainly involves brainstem neuromodulator projection systems, and a primary candidate is the dorsal noradrenergic system, which itself appears to be right-lateralized (Tucker and Williamson, 1984).

Thus an understanding of the lateralized control of emotional processes requires an appreciation of how hemispheric specialization has developed themes of both regulation and representation across multiple levels of the brain's control hierarchy. Analyzing the complex relations among vertically integrated circuits, and interpreting their function in relation to human emotional behavior, is likely to be a difficult and controversial process. It may seem that research on the neural systems of emotion suffers, therefore, from the particular problem of having to decipher the complex puzzle of vertebrate neural evolution in order to specify the primary functional mechanisms. While this problem is real, it is no less real for research on the brain's cognitive self-regulation. And it may be expressed in the positive sense. As we come to understand the evidence on neural mechanisms of emotion and emotional disorders, we must clarify the evolutionary basis of human psychological processes.

REFERENCES

Alexander, G. E., DeLong, M. R., and Strick, P. L. (1986). Parallel organization of functionally segregated circuits linking basal ganglia and cortex. *Annual Review of Neuroscience, 9,* 357–381.

American Psychiatric Association (1987). *Diagnostic and statistical manual of mental disorders,* ed 3, revised. Washington, DC: American Psychiatric Association.

Arrigoni, G., and De Renzi, E. (1964). Constructional apraxia and hemispheric locus of lesion. *Cortex, 1,* 170–197.

Baxter, L. R., Phelps, M. E., Mazziotta, J. G., Schwartz, J. M., Gerner, R. H., Selin, C. E., and Sumida, R. M. (1985). Cerebral metabolic rates for glucose in mood disorders: Studies with positron emission tomography and fluorodeoxiglucose F18. *Archives of General Psychiatry, 42,* 441–447.

Bear, D. M. (1983). Hemispheric specialization and the neurology of emotion. *Archives of Neurology, 40,* 195–202.

Bear, D. M., and Fedio, P. (1977). Quantitative analysis of interictal behavior in temporal lobe epilepsy. *Archives of Neurology, 34,* 454–467.

Benton, A. L., Varney, N. R., and Hamsher, K. de S. (1978a). Lateral differences in tactile directional perception. *Neuropsychologia, 16,* 109–114.

Benton, A. L., Varney, N. R., and Hamsher, K. de S. (1978b). Visuospatial judgement. *Archives of Neurology, 35,* 364–367.

Bisiach, E., and Luzzatti, C. (1978). Unilateral neglect of representational space. *Cortex, 14,* 129–133.

Blonder, L. X., Bowers, D., and Heilman, K. M. (1991). The role of the right hemisphere in emotional communication. *Brain, 114,* 1115–1127.

Borod, J. C. (1992). Interhemispheric and intrahemispheric control of emotion: A focus on unilateral brain damage. *Journal of Consulting and Clinical Psychology, 60,* 339–348.

Borod, J. C., and Caron, H. (1980). Facedness and emotion related to lateral dominance, sex, and expression type. *Neuropsychologia, 18,* 237–241.

Borod, J. C., Koff, E., Lorch, M. P., and Nicholas, M. (1985). The expression and perception of facial emotion in brain-damaged patients. *Neuropsychologia, 24,* 169–180.

Bowers, D., Bauers, D. M., Coslett, H. B., and Heilman, K. M. (1985). Processing of faces by patients with unilateral hemispheric lesions. I. Dissociation between judgements of facial affect and facial identity. *Brain and Cognition, 4,* 258–272.

Breitmeyer, B. G., and Ganz, L. (1977). Temporal studies with flashed gratings: Inferences about human transient and sustained channels. *Vision Research, 17,* 861–865.

Buchsbaum, M. S., Wu, J., DeLisi, L. E., Holcomb, H., Kessler, R., Johnson, J., King, A. C., Hazlett, E., Langston, K., and Post, R. M. (1986). Frontal cortex and basal ganglia metabolic rates assessed by positron emission tomography with [18F]2-deoxiglucose in affective illness. *Journal of Affective Disorders, 10,* 137–152.

Buck, R. (1985). Prime theory: An integrated view of motivation and emotion. *Psychological Review, 92,* 389–413.

Buck, R. (1988). *Human motivation and emotion.* New York, NY: John Wiley & Sons.

Carlson, J. N., Fitzgerald, L. W., Keller Jr., R. W., and Glick, S. D. (1991). Side and region dependent changes in dopamine activation with various durations of restraint stress. *Brain Research, 550,* 313–318.

Carlson, J. N., and Glick, S. D. (1991). Brain laterality as a determinant of susceptibility to depression in an animal model. *Brain Research, 550*(2), 324–328.

Cummings, J. L., and Mendez, M. F. (1984). Secondary mania with focal cerebrovascular lesions. *American Journal of Psychiatry, 141,* 1084–1087.

Damasio, A. R. (1989). Time-locked regional retroactivation: A systems level proposal for the neural substrate of recall and recognition. *Cognition, 33,* 25–62.

Damasio, A. R., and Tranel, D. (1988). Domain-specific amnesia for social knowledge. *Society for Neuroscience, 14,* 1289.

Davidson, R. J. (1984). Affect, cognition and hemispheric specialization. In C. E. Izard, J. Kagan, and R. Zajonc (Eds.), *Emotion, cognition and behavior.* New York, NY: Cambridge University Press.

Davidson, R. J., Chapman, J. P., and Chapman, L. J. (1987). Task-dependent EEG asymmetry discriminates between depressed and non-depressed subjects. Paper presented at the Society for Psychophysiologic Research, Amsterdam, 1987.

De Renzi, E. (1982). *Disorders of space exploration and cognition.* Chichister, England: John Wiley & Sons.

De Renzi, E., Faglioni, P., and Villa, P. (1977). Topographical amnesia. *Journal of Neurology, Neurosurgery and Psychiatry, 40,* 498–505.

De Renzi, E., and Spinnler, H. (1966). Visual recognition in patients with unilateral cerebral disease. *Journal of Nervous and Mental Disease, 142,* 515–525.

Derryberry, D., and Tucker, D. M. (1991). The adaptive base of the neural hierarchy: Elementary motivational controls on network function. In R. Dienstbier (Ed.), *Nebraska symposium on motivation.* Lincoln, NE: University of Nebraska Press.

Desimone, R., and Ungerleider, L.G. (1990). Neural mechanisms of visual processing in monkeys. In F. Boller, and J. Grafman (Eds.), *Handbook of Neuropsychology,* Vol 2 (pp 267–299). Amsterdam: Elsevier.

Downer, D. C. (1961). Changes in visual gnostic function and emotional behavior following unilateral temporal lobe damage in the split-brain monkey. *Nature, 191,* 50–51.

Drevets, W. C., Videen, T. O., Price, J. L., Preskorn, S. H., Carmichael, S. T., and Raichle, M. E. (1992). A functional anatomical study of unipolar depression. *The Journal of Neuroscience, 12,* 3628–3641.

Etcoff, N. L. (1986). The neuropsychology of emotional expression. In G. Goldstein and R. E. Tarter, (Eds.), *Advances in clinical neuropsychology,* Vol 3. New York, NY: Plenum Press.

Farah, M. J. (1984). The neurological basis of mental imagery: A componential analysis. *Cognition, 18,* 245–272.

Fedio, P. (1986). Behavioral characteristics of patients with temporal lobe epilepsy. *Psychiatric Clinics of North America, 9,* 267–281.

Fedio, P., and Martin, A. (1983). Ideative-emotive behavioral characteristics of patients following left or right temporal lobectomy. *Epilepsia, 24,* 117–130.

Fitzgerald, L. W., Keller, R. W., Glick, S. D., and Carlson, J. N. (1989). The effects of stressor controllability on regional changes in mesocorticolimbic dopamine activity. *Society for Neuroscience Abstracts, 15,* 1316.

Fuster, J. M. (1992). Neurophysiology of neocortical memory in the primate. Presented at the annual meeting of the International Neuropsychological Society, San Diego, CA, February 1992.

Fuster, J. M., and Jervey, J. P. (1981). Inferotemporal neurons distinguish and retain behaviorally relevant features of visual stimuli. *Science, 212,* 952–954.

Fuster, J. M., and Uyeda, A. A. (1971). Reactivity of limbic neurons of the monkey to appetitive and aversive signals. *Electroencephalograph and Clinical Neurophysiology, 30,* 281–293.

Gainotti, G. (1969). Réactions "catastrophiques" et manifestations d'indifférence au cours des atteintes cérébrales. *Neuropsychologia, 7,* 195–204.

Gainotti, G. (1972). Emotional behavior and hemispheric side of lesion. *Cortex, 8,* 41–55.

Geschwind, N. (1965). The disconnection syndromes in animals and men. *Brain, 88,* 237–254.

Gloor, P. (1990). Experiential phenomena of temporal lobe epilepsy. Facts and hypotheses. *Brain, 113,* 1673–1694.

Goldberg, E., and Costa, L. D. (1981). Hemisphere differences in the acquisition and use of descriptive systems. *Brain and Language, 14,* 144–173.

Goldberg, G. (1985). Supplementary motor area structure and function: Review and hypothesis. *Behavioral and Brain Science, 8,* 567–616.

Goldman-Rakic, P. S. (1987). Circuitry of the primate prefrontal cortex and regulation of behavior by representational memory. In F. Plum (Ed.), *Handbook of physiology. The nervous system,* Vol 5. *Higher cortical functions* (pp 373–417). Bethesda, MD: American Physiological Society.

Goldstein, K. (1952). The effect of brain damage on the personality. *Psychiatry, 15,* 245–260.

Graves, R., Landis, T., and Goodglass, H. (1981). Laterality and sex differences for visual recognition of emotional and non-emotional words. *Neuropsychologia, 19,* 95–102.

Grossi, D., Orsini, A., Modafferi, A., and Liotti, M. (1986). Visuoimaginal constructional apraxia: On a case of selective deficit of imagery. *Brain and Cognition, 5,* 255–266.

Hachinski, V. C., Oppenheimer, S. M., Wilson, J. X., Guiraudon, C., and Cechetto, D. F. (1992). Asymmetry of sympathetic consequences of experimental stroke. *Archives of Neurology, 49,* 697–702.

Hécaen, H., and Angelergues, R. (1962). Agnosia for faces (prosopoagnosia). *Archives of Neurology*, 7, 92–100.

Heilman, K. M., Schwartz, H. D., and Watson, R. T. (1978). Hypoarousal in patients with the neglect syndrome and emotional indifference. *Neurology*, 28, 229–232.

Heilman, K. M., and Valenstein, E. (1985). *Clinical neuropsychology*. New York, NY: Oxford University Press.

Heilman, K. M., Watson, R. T., Valenstein, E., and Damasio, A. R. (1983). Localization of lesions in neglect. In A. Kertesz (Ed.), *Localization in neuropsychology* (pp 445–470). New York, NY: Academic Press.

Hubel, D. H., and Livingstone, M. S. (1987). Segregation of form, color and stereopsis in primate area 18. *Journal of Neuroscience*, 7, 3378–3415.

Ivry, R. (1991). High versus low temporal frequency analysis of auditory information in the cerebral hemispheres: An account of hemispheric asymmetries. Paper presented at the annual meeting of the American Psychonomic Society, San Francisco, CA.

Jackson, J. H. (1879). On affections of speech from diseases of the brain. *Brain*, 2, 203–222.

Kimura, D. (1961). Cerebral dominance and the perception of verbal stimuli. *Canadian Journal of Psychology*, 15, 166–171.

Kimura, D., and Archibald, Y. (1974). Motor functions of the left hemisphere. *Brain*, 97, 337–350.

Kolb, B., and Milner, B. (1981). Observations on spontaneous facial expression after focal cerebral excisions and after intracarotid injection of sodium amytal. *Neuropsychologia*, 19(4), 505–514.

Kolb, B., and Taylor, L. (1981). Affective behavior in patients with localized cortical excisions: role of lesion site and side. *Science*, 214, 89–90.

Kosslyn, S. M. (1987). Seeing and imagining in the cerebral hemispheres: A computational approach. *Psychological Review*, 2, 148–175.

Ledoux, J. E. (1987). Emotion. In F. Plum (Ed.), *Handbook of physiology. The nervous system.* Vol 5. *Higher cortical functions* (pp 419–459). Bethesda, MD: American Physiological Society.

Lee, G. P., Laing, D. W., Dehl, J. L., and Meador, K. J. (1992). Hemispheric specialization for emotion: An examination of the transcallosal inhibition hypothesis. Presented at the annual meeting of the International Neuropsychological Society, San Diego, CA, February 1992.

Levine, D. N., Warach J., and Farah, M. (1985). Two visual systems in mental imagery: dissociation of 'what' and 'where' in imagery disorders due to bilateral posterior cerebral lesions. *Neurology*, 35, 1010–1018.

Levy, J., Heller, W., Banich, M. T., and Burton, L. A. (1983). Are variations among right-handed individuals in perceptual asymmetries caused by characteristic arousal differences between hemispheres? *Journal of Experimental Psychology: Human Perception and Performance*, 9, 329–358.

Ley, R. G., and Bryden, M. P. (1979). Hemispheric difference in processing emotions and faces. *Brain and Language*, 7, 127–138.

Ley, R. G., and Bryden, M. P. (1983). Right hemisphere involvement in imagery and affect. In E. Perecman (Ed.), *Cognitive processing in the right hemisphere* (pp 111–123). New York, NY: Academic Press.

Levine, D. N., Warach, J., and Farah, M. J. (1985). Two visual systems in mental imagery: Dissociation of "what" and "where" in imagery disorders due to bilateral posterior cerebral lesions. *Neurology*, 35, 101–108.

Liotti. M., Sava, D., Rizzolatti, G., and Caffarra, P. (1991). Differential hemispheric asymmetries in depression and anxiety: A reaction time study. *Biological Psychiatry, 29*(9), 887–899.

Liotti, M., and Tucker, D. M. (1992). Right hemisphere sensitivity to arousal and depression. *Brain and Cognition, 18,* 138–151.

Livingstone, M. S., and Hubel, D. H. (1987). Psychophysical evidence for separate channels for the perception of form, color, movement and depth. *Journal of Neuroscience, 7,* 3416–3468.

MacLean, P. D. (1958). Contrasting functions of limbic and neocortical systems of the brain and their relation to psychophysiological aspects of medicine. *American Journal of Medicine, 25,* 611–626.

Mayberg, H. S. (1992). Neuroimaging studies of depression in neurological disease. In S. E. Sterkstein and R. G. Robinson (Eds.), *Depression in neurologic disease.* Baltimore, MD: Johns Hopkins University Press.

Mayberg, H. S., Moran, T. H., and Robinson, R. G. (1990). Remote lateralized changes in cortical [³H]spiperone binding following focal frontal cortex lesions in the rat. *Brain Research, 516,* 127–131.

Mayberg, H. S., Robinson, R. G., Wong, D. W., Parikh, R., Bolduc, P., Starkstein, S. E., Price, T., Dannals, R. F., Links, J. M., Wilson, A. A., Ravert, H. T., and Wagner, H. N. (1988). PET imaging of cortical S2 serotonin receptors after stroke: lateralized changes and relationship to depression. *American Journal of Psychiatry, 145,* 937–943.

McCarthy, R. A., and Warrington, E. K. (1990). Object Recognition. In R. A. McCarthy and E. K. Warrington, (Eds.), *Cognitive neuropsychology: A clinical introduction* (pp 22–55). New York, NY: Academic Press.

Mesulam, M. M. (1981). A cortical network for directed attention and unilateral neglect. *Annals of Neurology, 10,* 309–325.

Mesulam, M. M. (1985). Attention, confusional states and neglect. In M. M. Mesulam (Ed.), *Principles of behavioral neurology* (pp 125–168). Philadelphia, PA: F. A. Davis Co.

Milner, B. (1974). Hemispheric specialization: scope and limits. In F. O. Schmidt, and F. G. Warden (Eds.), *The neuroscience: Third study program* (pp 75–89). Cambridge, MA: MIT Press.

Mishkin, M. (1978). Memory in monkeys severely impaired by combined but not separate removal of amygdala and hippocampus. *Nature, 273,* 297–298.

Mishkin, M., Malamut, B., and Bachevalier, J. (1984). Memories and habits: Two neural systems. In G. Lynch, J. L. McGaugh, and N. M. Weinberger (Eds.), *Neurobiology of learning and memory* (pp 65–77). New York, NY: Guilford Press.

Morrow, L., Urtunski, P. B., Kim, Y., and Boller, F. (1981). Arousal responses to emotional stimuli and laterality of lesion. *Neuropsychologia, 19,* 65–71.

Motter, B. C., and Mountcastle, V. B. (1981). The functional properties of the light-sensitive neurons of the posterior parietal cortex studied in waking monkeys: foveal sparing and opponent vector organization. *Journal of Neuroscience, 1,* 3–26.

Mountcastle, V. B. (1978). Brain mechanisms for directed attention. *Journal of the Royal Society of Medicine, 71,* 14–28.

Nauta, W. J. H. (1971). The problem of the frontal lobe: a reinterpretation. *Journal of Psychiatric Research, 8,* 167–187.

Nebes, R. D. (1978). Direct examination of cognitive function in the left and right hemispheres. In M. Kinsbourne (Ed.), *Asymmetrical function of the brain* (pp 99–140). New York, NY: Cambridge University Press.

Ono, T., Fukuda, M., Nishino, H., Sasaki, K., and Muramoto, K.L. (1983). Amygdaloid neuronal response to complex visual stimuli in an operant feeding situation in the monkey. *Brain Research Bulletin, 11,* 515–518.

Pandya, D. N., Seltzer, B., and Barbas, H. (1988). Input-output organization of the primate cerebral cortex. In *Comparative primate biology,* Vol 4. *Neurosciences* (pp 39–80). New York, NY: Allen Ardlis, Inc.

Pandya, D. N., and Yeteran, E. H. (1985). Proposed neural circuitry for spatial memory in the primate brain. *Neuropsychologia, 22(2),* 109–122.

Pardo, J. V., Pardo, P. J., and Raichle, M. E. (1991). Human brain activation during dysphoria. *Society for Neuroscience Abstracts, 17,* 664.

Parkinson, J. K., and Mishkin, M. A. (1982). A selective mnemonic role for the hippocampus in monkeys: memory for the location of objects. *Society for Neuroscience Abstracts, 8,* 23.

Pearlson, G. D., and Robinson, R. G. (1981). Suction lesions of the frontal cerebral cortex in the rat induce asymmetrical behavioral and catecholaminergic responses. *Brain Research, 218,* 233–242.

Poeck, K. (1969). Pathophysiology of emotional disorders associated with brain damage. In P. J. Vinken and G. W. Bruyn (Eds.), *Handbook of Clinical Neurology,* Vol 3 (pp 343–376). New York, NY: Elsevier.

Posner, M. I., and Cohen, Y. (1984). Components of visual orienting. In H. Bouma and D. G. Bouwhuis (Eds.), *Attention and performance X: Control of language processes.* Hillsdale, NJ: Lawrence Erlbaum Associates.

Posner, M. I., Inhoff, A. W., Friedrich, F. J., and Cohen, A. (1987). Isolating attentional systems: A cognitive-anatomical analysis. *Psychobiology, 15,* 107–121.

Pribram, K. H., and McGuinness, D. (1975). Arousal, activation, and effort in the control of attention. *Psychological Review, 82,* 116–149.

Rinn, W. E. (1984). The neuropsychology of facial expression: A review of the neurological and psychological mechanisms for producing facial expressions. *Psychological Bulletin, 95,* 52–77.

Rizzolatti, G., Umiltá, C., and Berlucchi, G. (1971). Opposite superiorities of the right and left cerebral hemispheres in discriminative reaction time to physiognomical and alphabetical material. *Brain, 94,* 431–442.

Robinson, D. L., Goldberg, M. E., and Stanton, G. B. (1978). Parietal association cortex in the primate: sensory mechanisms and behavioral modulations. *Journal of Neurophysiology, 50,* 1415–1432.

Robinson, R. G. (1985). Lateralized behavioral and neurochemical consequences of unilateral brain injury in rats. In *Cerebral lateralization in nonhuman species* (pp 135–156). New York, NY: Academic Press.

Robinson, R. G., Boston, J. D., Starkstein, S. E., and Price, T. R. (1988). Comparison of mania and depression after brain damage: Causal factors. *American Journal of Psychiatry, 145(2),* 142–148.

Robinson, R. G., Kubos, K. L., Starr, L. B., Rao, K., and Price, T. R. (1984). Mood disorders in stroke patients: importance of location of lesion. *Brain, 107,* 81–93.

Ross, E. D. (1981). The aprosodias: functional-anatomical organization of the affective components of language in the right hemisphere. *Archives of Neurology, 38,* 561–569.

Rossi, G. F., and Rosadini, G. (1967). Experimental analysis of cerebral dominance in man. In C. H. Millikan and F. L. Darley (Eds.), *Brain mechanisms underlying speech and language* (pp 167–184). New York, NY: Grune & Stratton, Inc.

Sackeim, H. A., Greenberg, M. S., Weiman, A. L., Gur, R. C., Hungerbuhler, J. P., and Geschwind, M. (1982). Hemispheric asymmetry in the expression of positive and negative emotions: Neurologic evidence. *Archives of Neurology, 39*, 210–218.

Safer, M. A., and Leventhal, H. (1977). Ear differences in evaluating emotional tone of voice and verbal content. *Journal of Experimental Psychology: Human Perception and Performance, 3*, 75–82.

Sanides, F. (1970). Functional architecture of motor and sensory cortices in primates in the light of a new concept of neocortex evolution. In C. R. Noback and W. Montagna (Eds.), *The primate brain: Advances in primatology*, Vol 1. New York, NY: Appleton-Century-Crofts.

Sanides, F. (1972). Representation in the cerebral cortex and its areal lamination pattern. In G. H. Bourne (Ed.), *The structure and function of nervous tissue*, Vol 5. New York, NY: Academic Press.

Sandson, J., and Albert, M. L. (1984). Varieties of perseveration. *Neuropsychologia, 22*(6), 715–732.

Sava, D., Liotti, M., and Rizzolatti, G. (1988). Right hemisphere superiority for programming oculomotion: Evidence from simple reaction time experiments. *Neuropsychologia, 26*, 201–211.

Semmes, J. (1968). Hemispheric specialization: A possible clue to mechanism. *Neuropsychologia, 6*, 11–26.

Sergent, J., Ohta, S., and MacDonald, B. (1992). Functional neuroanatomy of face and object processing. A positron emission tomography study. *Brain, 115*, 15–36.

Shapiro, D. (1965). *Neurotic styles*. New York, NY: Basic Books.

Sidtis, J. J. (1980). On the nature of the cortical function underlying right hemisphere auditory perception. *Neuropsychologia, 18*, 321–330.

Squire, L. R. (1987). *Memory and brain*. New York, NY: Oxford University Press.

Squire, L. R. (1992). Memory and the hippocampus: A synthesis from findings with rats, monkeys, and humans. *Psychological Review, 99*(2), 195–231.

Starkstein, S. E., Boston, J. D., and Robinson, R. G. (1988). Mechanisms of mania after brain injury: 12 case reports and review of the literature. *Journal of Nervous and Mental Disease, 176*(2), 87–100.

Starkstein, S. E., Robinson, R. T. (1988). Comparisons of patients with and without post-stroke major depression matched for size and location of lesion. *Archives of General Psychiatry, 45*(3), 247–252.

Starkstein, S. E., Robinson, R. T., and Price, T. R. (1987). Comparison of cortical and subcortical lesions in the production of post-stroke mood disorders. *Brain, 110*, 1045–1059.

Stern, W. E., and Brown, W. J. (1957). Pathological laughter. *Journal of Neurosurgery, 14*, 129–139.

Strauss, S., and Moscovitch, M. (1981). Perception of facial expressions. *Brain and Language, 13*, 308–332.

Stuss, D. P., and Benson, D. F. (1984). Neuropsychological studies of the frontal lobes. *Psychological Bulletin, 85*, 3–28.

Swenson, R. A., and Tucker, D. M. (1983). Lateralized cognitive style and self-description. *International Journal of Neuroscience, 21*, 91–100.

Terzian, H. (1964). Behavioral and EEG effects of intracarotid sodium amytal injection. *Acta Neurochirurgica, 12,* 230–239.

Thatcher, R. W., Krause, P. J., and Rhybyk, M. (1986). Cortico-cortical associations and EEG coherence: A two-compartmental model. *Electroencephalography and Clinical Neurophysiology, 64,* 123–143.

Thierry, A. M., Tassin, J. P., Blanc, G., and Glowinski, J. (1976). Selective activation of the mesocortical DA system by stress. *Nature, 263,* 242–244.

Thorpe, S. J., Rolls, E. T., and Maddison, S. (1983). The orbitofrontal cortex: neuronal activity in the behaving monkey. *Experimental Brain Research, 490,* 93–115.

Tranel, D., and Damasio, A. R. (1985). Knowledge without awareness: An autonomic index of facial recognition by prosopoagnosics. *Science, 228,* 1453–1454.

Tranel, D., and Damasio, A. R. (1987). Recognition of gender, age, and meaning of facial expression can be dissociated from recognition by prosopoagnosics. Presented at the 39th Annual Meeting of the American Academy of Neurology, New York, NY,

Trevarthen, C. B. (1968). Two mechanisms of vision in primates. *Psychologische Forschung, 31,* 299–337.

Tucker, D. M. (1981). Lateral brain function, emotion, and conceptualization. *Psychological Bulletin, 89,* 19–46.

Tucker, D. M. (1986). Neural control of emotional communication. In P. Blank, R. Buck, and R. Rosenthal (Eds.), *Nonverbal communication in the clinical context.* Cambridge, England: Cambridge University Press.

Tucker, D. M. (1991). Development of emotion and cortical networks. In M. Gunnar and C. Nelson (Eds.), *Minnesota symposium on child development: Developmental neuroscience.* New York, NY: Oxford University Press.

Tucker, D. M., and Derryberry, D. (1991). Motivated attention: Anxiety and the frontal executive functions. *Neuropsychiatry, Neuropsychology, and Behavioral Neurology,*

Tucker, D. M., and Frederick, S. L. (1989). Emotion and brain lateralization. In: H. Wagner and A. Manstead (Eds.). *Handbook of social psychophysiology.*

Tucker, D. M., and Liotti, M. (1989). Neuropsychological mechanisms of anxiety and depression. In F. Boller and J. Grafman (Eds.), *Handbook of neuropsychology.* Amsterdam: Elsevier.

Tucker, D. M., Roth, D. L., and Bair, T. B. (1986). Functional connections among cortical regions: Topography of EEG Coherence. *Electroencephalography and Clinical Neurophysiology, 63,* 242–250.

Tucker, D. M., Stenslie, C. E., Roth, R. S., and Shearer, S. (1981). Right frontal lobe activation and right hemisphere performance decrement during a depressed mood. *Archives of General Psychiatry, 38,* 169–174.

Tucker, D. M., and Williamson, P. A. (1984). Asymmetric neural control systems in human self-regulation. *Psychological Review, 91,* 185–215.

Umiltá, C., Bagnara, S., and Simion, F. (1978). Laterality effects for simple and complex geometrical figures, and nonsense patterns. *Neuropsychologia, 16,* 43–49.

Umiltá, C., Rizzolatti, G., Marzi, C. A., Zamboni, G., Franzini, C., Camarda, R., and Berlucchi, G. (1974). Hemispheric differences in the discrimination of line orientation. *Neuropsychologia, 12,* 165–174.

Ungerleider, L. G., and Mishkin, M. (1982). Two cortical visual systems. In D. J. Ingle, R. J. W. Mansfield, and M. A. Goodale (Eds.), *The analysis of visual behavior* (pp 549–586). Cambridge, MA: MIT Press.

Van Hoesen, G. W., and Pandya, D. N. (1975). Some connections of the entorhinal (area 28) and perirhinal (area 35) cortices in the monkey. *Trends in Neuroscience, 5,* 345–350.

Warrington, E. K. (1982). Neuropsychological studies of object recognition. *Philosophical Transactions of the Royal Society of London, 298,* 15–27.

Watson, R. T., and Heilman, K. M. (1982). Affect in subcortical aphasia. *Neurology, 32,* 102–103.

Watson, R. T., Heilman, K. M., Cauthen, J. C., and King, F. A. (1973). Neglect after cingulectomy. *Neurology, 23,* 1003–1007.

Zoccolotti, P., Caltagirone, C., Benedetti, N., and Gainotti, G. (1986). Perturbation des réponses végétatives aux stimuli émotionels au cours des lésions hémisphériques unilaterales. *L'encéphale, 12,* 263–268.

Zoccolotti, P. G., Scabini, D., and Violani, C. (1982). Electrodermal responses in patients with unilateral brain damage. *Journal of Clinical Neuropsychology, 4,* 143–150.

Zola-Morgan, S., Squire, L. R., Alvarez-Royo, P., and Clower, R. (1991). Independence of memory functions and emotional behavior: Separate contributions of the hippocampal formation and the amygdala. *Hippocampus, 1,* 207–220.

Zola-Morgan, S., Squire, L. R., and Mishkin, M. (1982). The neuroanatomy of amnesia: Amygdala-hippocampus vs temporal stem. *Science, 218,* 1337–1339.

VII Interhemispheric Interaction

15 Interhemispheric Processing: Theoretical Considerations and Empirical Approaches

Marie T. Banich

This chapter presents a model of interhemispheric processing that presumes it to be a complex phenomenon characterized by three major features. The first feature of the model is that it presumes interhemispheric interaction not to be a unitary phenomenon. Rather it views information transfer between the hemispheres as occurring via a series of "channels" of communication that are utilized in a temporally cacophonous manner. This symphony of heterogeneous signals is thought to be carried over separate channels, some of which are contained in the 200 to 800 million nerve fibers that compose the corpus callosum, and some of which are contained in subcortical commissures. The second major feature of the model is that it views the contribution of each hemisphere to its interaction with the other as ranging along a continuum. At one end of the continuum is the case in which the interaction between the hemispheres is dominated completely by one hemisphere, a model often referred to as metacontrol. At the other end of the continuum is the case in which the interaction between the hemispheres shares no characteristics in common with the processing of each individual hemisphere. This latter type of interaction, which can be considered emergent because the whole cannot be deduced from the sum of the parts, is important because it suggests that to understand interhemispheric interaction requires more than understanding the specializations of each hemisphere. The third major feature of the model is that it views interhemispheric interaction as allowing for more complex processing than is afforded by the combination of each hemisphere processing information in isolation, especially under computationally demanding conditions. This advantage is thought to accrue because processing can occur in parallel and be divided over a greater expanse of neural space when interhemispheric processing is required to perform a task as compared to when it is not. In this way, the model specifies the manner in which information-processing capabilities are influenced by interhemispheric processing.

The chapter is divided into five sections. The first section examines the ways in which interhemispheric interaction can be characterized as occurring through separate "channels." In the second section, data are presented to support the idea that there are varieties of interhemispheric interaction, with special emphasis on the evidence that interhemispheric interaction is more than the sum of the workings of each hemisphere in isolation. The third section of the chapter outlines research suggesting that interhemispheric interaction has a role in information processing in that it enhances the capacity of the brain to process complex tasks. The fourth section discusses methodologic issues that are important to consider when examining questions of interhemispheric processing. The final section outlines some of the major unresolved issues currently facing researchers examining interhemispheric interaction.

INTERHEMISPHERIC INTERACTION AS SEPARATE CHANNELS OF PROCESSING

This section attempts to demonstrate that interhemispheric interaction should not be thought of as a unitary mechanism or entity whereby information gets shipped in mass from one hemisphere to another. Rather there are major and minor routes of communication between the hemispheres both in terms of the information carried, the fidelity of the information sent, and the speed at which information is transmitted. Hence, interhemispheric interaction is better thought to consist of channels that have both relative autonomy and some functional specialization. The notion of a channel is discussed in three senses. The first sense of a channel is an anatomic one. There are several commissures that connect the cerebral hemispheres, and each commissure can be considered a channel. For example, the corpus callosum is the largest channel, but there are others as well, for example, the anterior commissure and the hippocampal commissure. The second sense of a channel is a route of information transfer that is dedicated to carrying a specific type of information. For example, it is suggested that visual information is carried over certain regions of the callosum, whereas auditory information is transferred over others. Finally, one can also think of a channel in a temporal sense. Myelinated fibers can be thought of as fast channels and unmyelinated fibers as slow ones. The evidence presented here suggests that these channels are usually separable, although not necessarily totally independent.

Anatomic Channels

Generally, when one discusses interhemispheric processing the assumption often is that one is talking about callosal interaction, but this need not always be the case. It is important to remember that although the callosum is indeed the largest fiber tract connecting the two hemispheres, consisting of between 200 and 800 million nerve fibers, there are other fiber tracts that have a similar function (see Clarke and Zaidel, 1989, for an example of how these different routes may be identified). Hence cortical and subcortical channels are distinguished in the discussion below.

Cortical Channels　One way to determine exactly what type of information can be relayed by the corpus callosum, the major cortical commissure, is to determine which tasks can and cannot be performed by split-brain patients, in whom the cortical but not the subcortical commissures have been severed for the relief of epilepsy. If split-brain patients cannot integrate certain types of information across the hemispheres it is inferred that such integration must be critically dependent on cortical commissures, whereas when information can be integrated by these patients, it is assumed to occur via a subcortical route. The list of researchers who have used this logic is long (e.g., Cronin-Golumb, 1986; Johnson, 1984; Myers and Sperry, 1985; Trevarthen and Sperry, 1973), and other researchers have taken a similar approach with acallosal patients in whom the callosum never formed (e.g., Jeeves, 1979).

Although researchers thought initially that little information presented to opposite hemispheres could be integrated in split-brain patients, more recent studies have suggested that certain types of information can be integrated in the absence of cortical commissures. A series of studies by Sergent (e.g., 1990) is instructive in this regard since she demonstrated that although patients could not determine if items on either side of the visual midline were identical, they could nonetheless make simple binary decisions about whether those same items belonged to similar categories (e.g., whether one digit is larger than the other or if both are equal in value). From these results, Sergent argues that the cortical commissures have the ability to transfer some higher-order information between the hemispheres.

The exact nature of this higher-order information remains unclear. So, for example, in the case of a particular digit, abstract information such as whether it is odd or even, is not transferable. Yet, the information about a face that can be communicated from the right hemisphere to the left is generally about abstract categorical attributes, such as whether the person is old or young, male or female, white or black, and other semantic information, such as the person "not being nice" or "not being an American." In all cases, information that cannot be transferred includes information that uniquely identifies an item, whether it be exactly which digit was viewed, or which person's face was seen. Hence, the cortical commissures appear to be the interhemispheric channel critical for transferring an item's identity or information that allows an item to be uniquely identified. In contrast, it appears that in certain cases, the subcortical commissures are able to support transfer between the hemispheres of information with regard to basic attributes or categories.

Not only does transfer of information about item identity rely critically on the corpus callosum but transfer of detailed information about spatial position appears to do so as well. Without a callosum, spatial localization of items across the midline is, at least in the visual modality, crude at best. Some ability to grossly localize information has been found in cases of cross-comparisons of large moving objects in the periphery (Trevarthen and Sperry, 1973) (which presumably rely on integration of information at the level of the superior colliculus), decisions about relative position (e.g., above and below) (Sergent, 1991), and comparisons when a frame provides multiple cues (Holtzman, 1984). It should be noted that the ability of split-brain patients to integrate information about spatial localization dissociates from the ability to allocate attention in a spatial manner (e.g., Holtzman et al., 1981). This is discussed in more detail in the next section.

Noncortical Channels   There are two broad classes of information that can be integrated without the cerebral commissures: emotional information and aspects of spatial attention. Information about emotional tenor can be communicated via subcortical commissures. For example, Sperry, Zaidel, and Zaidel (1979) report that when information is projected exclusively to the right hemisphere of a split-brain patient, the left hemisphere can interpret the tenor of the right hemisphere's emotional response to a sufficient degree to influence its oral production. For example, when the right hemisphere of one split-brain patient, N.G., was presented with an array of pictures containing three strangers and her son, her left hemisphere was able to receive enough information to enable her to point to her son and verbally report that she felt good about him.

There is also a broad base of work suggesting that attentional information can be integrated across the hemispheres in split-brain patients. This work has been reviewed recently by Gazzaniga (1987) so only highlights are presented here. Elegant work by Holtzman and colleagues (e.g., Holtzman et al., 1981) indicates that for at least some aspects of directing attention, the hemispheres remain unified after commissurotomy. For example, they found that responses to a target were speeded when a cue had been previously presented in the opposite visual field in the analogous location. To demonstrate that the information being integrated was attentional and not spatial, they employed a control condition in which subjects decided if two items, one on each side of the midline, appeared in analogous locations in the visual fields. Because the split-brain patients were unable to perform this control task, Holtzman et al. concluded that the information being integrated was attentional in nature.

It should be noted that not all aspects of visuospatial attention are unified in split-brain patients. Although attention to a specific location in space is integrated between the hemispheres, that aspect of attention required for search of a target in a complex visual array is not. Luck et al. (1989) found that visual search rates of split-brain patients were actually faster than those of neurologically intact subjects because the split-brain patients could search each half of space for a target in parallel whereas normal subjects could not. For subjects with an intact callosum, search rate was identical whether the location of all the items was restricted to one visual field (unilateral condition) or dispersed across both visual fields (bilateral condition). Although for split-brain patients, the search rate for bilateral trials did not differ from that of neurologically intact subjects, their search rate for the unilateral condition was twice as fast. Thus, when attention was not directed to a particular portion of space, but rather needed to be distributed, the hemispheres of the split-brain patient could act independently.

The work reviewed in this section suggests that the cortical commissures are an interhemispheric channel critical for transferring information about item attributes and for the precise localization of information in space. The next section examines in more detail the ways in which the cortical commissures are organized to convey such information.

Specific Information Channels within the Callosum

Within the callosum there are various channels which are differentiated by the specific types of information carried within them. This specificity is most obvious with regard to the segregation of signals in different sensory modalities, and appears to result from the topography of callosal connection. In general, the topography is such that anterior sections of the brain are connected by anterior sections of the callosum and likewise more posterior sections of the brain are connected by more posterior sections of the callosum. Support for this organization comes from studies of patients with partial callosal sections (e.g., Geffen, 1980) as well as patients who have tumors in specific regions of the callosum (e.g., Geschwind and Kaplan, 1962) and studies of callosal degeneration after ischemic infarction (e.g., DeLacoste, Kirkpatrick, and Ross, 1985). In general, it appears that the fibers traversing the most anterior part of the callosum, the genu, connect prefrontal areas. The region of the callosum directly posterior to the genu connects the posterior superior frontal areas, followed by regions of the callosum that connect motor cortex and then, more posteriorly, somatosensory cortex. The caudal part of the body of the callosum connects more posterior regions, especially the temporoparieto-occipital junction. The splenium also connects portions of the temporoparieto-occipital junction, as well as the dorsal parietal and occipital regions.

Although neuroanatomic studies performed on rhesus monkeys (see Pandya and Seltzer, 1986, for a review) suggest that, in general, fibers from a given cortical region tend to occupy a specific place in the callosum and that little overlap exists between fibers from different brain regions, recent work suggests that in humans this segregation may be somewhat less precise than previously thought (Risse et al., 1989). For example, although it is generally assumed that fibers carrying somatosensory information are anterior to those carrying auditory information, it appears that they may be intermixed.

The anatomic findings reviewed above suggesting a specific organization to callosal connectivity have an important functional inference, namely, that different types of information are sent over different sections of the callosum. Confirmatory evidence for such a separability of interhemispheric channels is indeed suggested by behavioral research on persons with an intact callosum. For example, behavioral dissociations suggest that visual and motor channels of information transfer may be separable. In a series of studies Milner and colleagues (Milner and Lines, 1982; Rugg, Lines, and Milner, 1984) examined interhemispheric transfer by comparing two conditions: one in which the hemisphere controlling a motor response also received a visual stimulus (within-hemisphere condition), and one in which although the signal was initially directed to one hemisphere, the response was made by another (across-hemisphere condition). The difference between these two conditions was taken as an estimate of the time needed for interhemispheric transfer. When the dependent measure was vocal reaction time, the advantage observed for within-hemisphere processing increased as the intensity of the stimulus decreased. From this finding it was inferred that the signal being transferred was sensory in nature, since it varied with intensity, a sensory characteristic of the stimulus. In contrast, when a manual rather than a vocal response was required, the within-hemisphere advantage did not vary with stimulus intensity, which is consistent with findings of other researchers (Berlucchi et al., 1971; Clarke and Zaidel, 1989), and has been interpreted as a relay of a motor command. A subsequent study in which estimates of interhemispheric transfer time were derived from electroencephalographic (EEG) measures (Rugg et al., 1984) suggested that these signals were likely to be relayed by different regions of the callosum because estimates of transfer time obtained at occipital lobe leads varied with signal intensity, whereas those obtained at central leads (over motor regions) did not. Further indicating that the visual and motor channels are indeed distinct, the estimates of interhemispheric transfer time calculated from verbal responses of a subject are uncorrelated with estimates calculated from manual responses in that same subject (St. John et al., 1987).

The work described above provides evidence for a conceptualization of the callosum as consisting of separate channels that may have a fair degree of autonomy. The implication is that the callosum should not be thought of as a unitary system for information transfer, but rather may be better conceived of as a collection of commissural systems with the ability to act independently.

Temporal Channels

Another way to conceptualize callosal channels is as an entity in time rather than in space. A temporal channel would be conceptualized as a blocked transfer of information that occurs within a particular temporal window or time frame. Reasons to think that such channels exist come from both the empirical and conceptual domains. Empirically, recent work in the cat has demonstrated that under certain conditions, regions in opposite hemispheres fire synchronously, a phenomenon which is eliminated by callosal deconnection, suggesting its mediation specifically by callosal fibers (Engel et al., 1991). Thus, these synchronously firing neurons may represent a temporal callosal channel.

Variations in the degree of myelinization of callosal fibers also provide the substrate for temporal channels, since myelinization influences transmission time. Relay of information by well-myelinated as compared to unmyelinated fibers could be considered the basis of slow and fast temporal channels. That the notion of fast and slow callosal channels may have some utility in explicating interhemispheric processing is suggested by recent work by Braun et al. (1994), who invoke this idea to explain seemingly discrepant results between a large number of studies that provide estimates of interhemispheric transfer in humans as inferred from simple unimanual reaction time.

Conceptually, one could argue that temporal channels are likely to exist from the time course of information processing. For example, when performing a complex task, it is likely that the transfer of motor commands to produce a final output is preceded, to some degree, by transfer of information between association areas, which in turn may precede transfer between sensory regions. In fact, this temporal sequencing of transfer may be related to the degree of myelinization of callosal fibers because, in both the monkey and in humans, large myelinated callosal axons predominate in portions of the callosum connecting sensory areas relative to regions of the callosum connecting association areas (Lamantia and Rakic, 1990; Aboitiz et al., 1992).

Some researchers, although not conceptualizing the callosum as consisting of temporal channels, have suggested that the timing of callosal transfer may have important implications for information processing. For example, Davidson, Leslie, and Saron (1990) have suggested that even in free vision, callosal transfer from one hemisphere to the other provides a source of redundant information that is useful in information processing. However, they have hypothesized that such redundant information may be useful only if it arrives within a narrow time window; otherwise its effect is to disrupt the flow of information processing by causing interference. As this short reviews indicates, there is not much research that has attempted to address the issue of temporal channels in interhemispheric transfer. Nonetheless, there are both theoretical considerations and experimental findings that suggest further exploration of this concept is likely to be fruitful.

VARIETIES OF INTERHEMISPHERIC PROCESSING

The findings discussed in the section above suggest that the hemispheres can communicate with each other across many different channels and in many different manners. This section examines the variety of interactions between the hemispheres, some of which can be predicted quite easily from the processing performed by each hemisphere alone and some of which cannot be predicted at all. Hence, one can conceptualize the varieties of interaction as being along a continuum with one end of the continuum representing interaction that is dominated totally by a single hemisphere, to another end in which the interaction is emergent, that is, the whole is greater than the sum of the parts.

At one end of the continuum is the notion of interhemispheric processing as occurring via metacontrol, which is the idea that when information is presented to both hemispheres, one hemisphere takes control of processing. In this case the interaction of the hemispheres is one in which there is a leader and a follower, and the interaction is essentially governed by one hemisphere. The idea of metacontrol was originally derived from observations of patients in whom the callosum had been sectioned. In such patients, one hemisphere appeared to dominate responding even when both were given information, and surprisingly, the hemisphere that dominated was not always the hemisphere specialized for the task (e.g., Levy and Trevarthen, 1976). The concept of metacontrol was later applied to explain certain aspects of interhemispheric interaction in normal subjects as well (e.g., Hellige, Jonsson, and Michimata, 1988; Hellige, Taylor, and Eng, 1989).

The paradigm typically employed by Hellige and colleagues is one in which performance on unilateral trials is compared to performance on bilateral trials in which identical information is directed to each hemisphere. Under these conditions, Hellige and colleagues have found that on bilateral trials, the pattern of performance observed is usually similar to that observed on unilateral trials directed to one hemisphere but not the other. Furthermore, the pattern observed does not always reflect processing of the superior hemisphere. For example, using a consonant-vowel-consonant (CVC) task, Hellige and colleagues (1989) observed that the type of errors made on bilateral trials were qualitatively similar to those on left visual field (LVF) trials, but dissimilar to those observed on right visual field (RVF) trials. Thus, Hellige's data appear to support the idea of metacontrol because the performance on bilateral trials seemed to be dominated by right hemisphere rather than left hemisphere processing.

An intermediate variety of interhemispheric interaction is one in which neither hemisphere dominates performance but rather one aspect of processing mimics the style of one hemisphere, while another aspect of processing mimics the style of the other hemisphere. Thus, although each aspect of bihemispheric performance can be said to mimic a single hemisphere, the overall pattern cannot. Recently, we have obtained evidence in our laboratory for such a variety of interhemispheric processing (Banich, Nicholas, and Karol, 1994).

The paradigm we used was similar to that employed by Hellige and colleagues, in that we compared performance on unilateral and bilateral trials. However, our design differed from theirs in two important ways. First, our unilateral trials always contained two items, unlike the single unilateral item utilized by Hellige et al.. Second, on their bilateral trials, identical information was always presented to each hemisphere, whereas in ours that was not the case. A detailed description of the paradigm follows below.

In our paradigm, on every trial a target number appeared at the center of a computer screen for 1 second. After a 1-second delay, two probe numbers appeared on the screen for 200 ms and the subject pressed a "yes" response key if *either* number was smaller in value than the previously presented target number, or a "no" response key if both were equal to or greater in value than the target number. Half the trials required a "yes" response and half a "no" response, which was evenly divided across all the other factors in the design to be discussed next. On one third of the 144 trials, both numbers were presented in the RVF, on another third both numbers were presented in the LVF, and on the final third, which were bilateral visual field trials (BVF), one number was presented to each visual field.

RVF, LVF, and BVF trials were divided further into distinct trial types, two of which are of most importance for the present discussion. On some trials, known as Same-Digit/Same-Decision trials, the probe digits were identical (e.g., target: 12; stimuli: 17 and 17). On other trials, known as Different-Digit/Same-Decision trials, the digits were distinct, yet both had the same relationship to the target (i.e., they were either both smaller or bigger) (e.g., target: 12; stimuli: 17 and 14).

Thus, we can examine bihemispheric performance relative to unihemispheric performance with regard to two manipulations in the design: the type of decision required ("yes" vs. "no"), and the type of trial (Same-Digit/Same-Decision vs. Different-Digit/Different-Decision). What is of interest is that the pattern observed for BVF trials mimicked the left hemisphere with regard to the former variable, but the right hemisphere with regard to the latter variable.

More specifically, we found for LVF trials that reaction time (RT) to trials requiring a "yes" response were not significantly faster than to those requiring a "no" response, whereas for RVF trials the difference was significant. On this aspect of processing, the pattern observed on BVF trials mimicked that on RVF trials because "yes" responses were significantly faster than "no" responses. On the other hand, for trial type, performance on BVF trials was dissimilar to RVF trials, but similar to LVF trials. For RVF trials, responses to Same-Digit/Same-Decision trials were much faster than to Different-Digit/Same-Decision trials ($P < .0001$), whereas this difference just reached significance for LVF trials and was marginally significant for BVF trials.

In considering this pattern of results it is important to remember that in the design of the study, the type of decision ("yes" or "no") and the type of trial (Same-Digit/Same-Decision vs. Different-Digit/Different Decision) were entirely crossed to produce four distinct sets of trials (i.e., "yes" Same-Digit/Same-Decision, "no" Same-Digit/Same-Decision, "yes" Different-Digit/Same-Decision, and "no" Different-Digit/Same-Decision) that were randomly intermixed. Because the type of stimulus to appear on any given trial was random and could not be predicted, it is highly unlikely that different strategies could be employed for different trial types. Rather, the pattern of responding on any given trial seemed to have reflected a combination of processes. For example, on BVF Different-Digit/Same-Decision trials requiring a "yes" decision, the speed of response seems to the reflect two processes. The first process is one that results in slower responding to Different-Digit/Same-Decision trials than to Same-Digit/Same-Decision trials, which is similar to what is observed for LVF trials, but not for RVF trials. The second process is one that yields faster responding to "yes" trials than to "no" trials, which is similar to what is observed on RVF trials, but not on LVF trials. Hence, performance on BVF trials cannot be said, overall, to be similar to that of either the right hemisphere or the left. Rather, performance on BVF trials appears to reflect the effects of two factors, each of which mimics the processing of a different hemisphere.

At the other end of the continuum is a variety of interhemispheric processing in which the hemispheres act in a manner that cannot be predicted at all from processing on unilateral trials. Evidence for this variety of interhemispheric interaction comes from a series of five studies, only two of which will be discussed here (Banich and Karol, 1992, Experiments 4 and 5). The experimental paradigm was similar to that for the digit experiment described above, except that in this task, subjects made a rhyme decision rather than a digit value decision, determining whether any laterally presented probes rhymed with the previous presented centrally projected target word. In the first of the two relevant experiments, we observed that for RVF trials, responses to Same-Word/Same-Decision trials were faster than to Different-Word/Same-Decision trials by 179 ms. This difference was significantly greater than the 63-ms difference observed for BVF trials, which in turn differed from a nonsignificant 15-ms difference for LVF trials.

On the basis of these results, one might argue that the pattern observed on BVF trials was a blend of that observed on unilateral trials because the difference in speed of response between Same-Word/Same-Decision and Different-Word/Same-Decision BVF trials is intermediate (63 ms) between that observed for RVF (179 ms) and LVF trials (15 ms). To investigate this possibility and for reasons beyond the scope of this chapter, we ran the identical experiment except that this time the two words on each trial were presented in a different font and case (e.g., one word in Chicago font in uppercase and one word in Los Angeles font in lowercase). The results clearly indicated that BVF trials were processed differently than unilateral ones and could not be characterized as a blend of performance on unilateral trials. For both RVF and LVF trials, the font and case manipulation had no effect on performance. Once again, for RVF trials a large advantage for Same-Word/Same-Decision trials over Different-Word/Same-Decision trials was observed, whereas there was no significant difference between these two trial types for LVF trials. Of most importance, however, is the fact that the manipulation of Font/Case completely changed the pattern for BVF trials. Now, unlike the previous experiment, no difference between Same-Word/Same-Decision and Different-Word/Same-Decision trials was observed. Thus, although the font and case manipulation had no effect on unilateral trials, it did affect bilateral trials. These results make clear that processing of the hemispheres in relative isolation cannot be used to predict the interaction of the two hemispheres since a variable (i.e., the Font/Case manipulation) that had no effect on the performance of either hemisphere nonetheless affected the interaction of the hemispheres.

The pattern of results observed in this experiment is an example of interhemispheric processing that is emergent, meaning it cannot be deduced from the sum of the parts. These results suggest that although the interaction of the hemispheres is surely influenced by the relative specialization of each hemisphere, it is not necessarily constrained by them. Likewise, although knowledge of cerebral specialization can guide our investigations of interhemispheric interaction, it cannot always be used to deduce the nature of interhemispheric processing.

The evidence reviewed above supports the contention that the interaction between the hemispheres can take many different forms. The question then becomes under which conditions is each of these variations observed. One speculation is that metacontrol is most likely to occur when the task can be successfully performed on the basis of information received by a single hemisphere even though both are receiving information (Hellige, personal communication, 1991). In the Hellige et al. studies, the information presented to each hemisphere was always identical, so that it was not imperative on BVF trials that information presented to both hemispheres be processed completely for a decision to be reached. In contrast, in our studies the information presented to each hemisphere was often not redundant. Hence, in our experiments, metacontrol might be a maladaptive strategy. The speculation that metacontrol characterizes processing when decisions are made on the basis of information directed to only one hemisphere is consonant with work by Sergent. She notes that in many of the studies with split-brain patients, metacontrol was observed when the hemispheres were given competing information so that it would be near to impossible to base a response on information presented to both hemispheres unless two responses rather than one were emitted (e.g., Levy and Trevarthen, 1976). In contrast, when split-brain patients were instructed to integrate information across the visual fields to make a whole, a larger degree of integration could occur.

It is not yet clear which factors differentiate between those conditions in which interhemispheric interaction can be characterized as somewhat similar rather than totally dissimilar to processing by a single hemisphere. There are a number of differences between the digit and rhyme tasks we have used that may have contributed to the difference in the pattern of results obtained. The digit task yields a right hemisphere advantage, can be processed by both hemispheres, and is relatively easy. The rhyme task yields a left hemisphere advantage, relies exclusively on one hemisphere for the end result of processing (e.g., the phonemic comparison), and is more difficult, as evidenced by reaction time and error rates. Which of these factors, if any, is important for the obtained pattern of results awaits further inquiry. In sum, different varieties of interhemispheric interaction have been demonstrated. The next challenge is to determine the factors that differentiate the conditions under which each is observed.

THE INFLUENCE OF INTERHEMISPHERIC INTERACTION ON INFORMATION PROCESSING

The third major attribute of the model of interhemispheric processing presented in this chapter is that interhemispheric interaction is conceptualized as more than a mechanism by which one hemisphere photocopies experiences and feelings for its partner. Instead, in a series of studies conducted by Aysenil Belger and myself (Banich and Belger, 1990; Belger and Banich, 1992; Belger, 1993) we found that interhemispheric processing is particularly useful when tasks are computationally demanding. Because difficult tasks require multiple steps in processing, a division of processing between the hemispheres aids task performance by allowing the hemispheres to work in parallel or to perform two distinct operations simultaneously (see Liederman, Merola and Martinez, 1985, for a somewhat similar interpretation of the effects of dividing perceptual inputs between the hemispheres).

To test this hypothesis, we performed a series of studies in which computational complexity was manipulated by varying the number of computations required for a decision (Banich and Belger, 1990). In a relatively easy task, subjects decided if two letters were physically identical (e.g., A A). In the more difficult task, subjects decided if two letters had the same name (e.g., A a). Whereas the former task can be performed solely on the basis of physical characteristics of the stimulus, the latter task is more complex because it requires not only that the items be physically identified but in addition, that a name be attached to the physical form.

For the physical identity task, responses were faster and more accurate when matching items were directed to only one hemisphere (within-hemisphere trials) as compared to different hemispheres (across-hemisphere trials). However, the opposite was true for the name-identity task: across-hemisphere trials were processed more quickly and accurately. The within-hemisphere advantage on the physical-identity task is not specific to the stimuli employed (i.e., letters), since it is also obtained when digits are used.

To determine whether across-hemisphere processing is also advantageous in other situations in which the decision process requires more steps than a simple comparison of physical features, we devised two additional tasks, both of which used digits as stimuli: a summation task and an ordinal task. In the summation task, subjects determined whether the sum of two items equaled 10 or more. In half of the match trials, the two items equalling 10 or more were in the same visual field, and for the other half they were in opposite visual fields. In the ordinal task, subjects decided if one number was smaller than another. In some cases the smaller number was positioned in the same visual field as the larger one, and in other cases it was positioned in the opposite visual field. Consistent with our prediction, an across-field advantage was obtained for both of these difficult tasks (Banich and Belger, 1990). Furthermore, we demonstrated an across-hemisphere advantage for another task that was more computationally difficult than a physical-identity task. In this task subjects heard a three-letter word. One second later, they saw a display and had to decide if two letters in particular spatial positions were the second and third letters of the word they had just heard. This task also yielded an across-hemisphere advantage (Banich et al., 1990).

All these studies yielded evidence that difficult tasks are performed more easily when they are divided between the hemispheres, but in all these experiments we had manipulated task difficulty by varying the complexity of decision, while holding the nature of the input constant. What we wished to investigate, therefore, was whether other manipulations of complexity would also reveal interhemispheric interaction to be beneficial to task performance. To do so, we varied the number of items to be recognized and compared before a decision could be reached. In our previous experiments, three items (i.e., letters or digits) had been displayed on all trials, arranged in the spatial layout of an inverted triangle. Subjects decided if the bottom item matched either of the top two (or in the case of the Banich et al. (1990) study, whether the bottom letter and one of the top two were the second and third letters of the previously presented word). In our next study, we had three conditions: a three-item physical-identity task with letters, identical to that we had used previously; a five-item physical-identity task; and a five-item name-identity task (Belger and Banich, 1992). In the five-item tasks, one item was presented in the bottom position and the subject had to decide if it matched any of four items presented above. A comparison of the three-item and five-item physical-identity tasks allowed us to determine whether interhemispheric processing aided performance when complexity was increased by manipulating the number of items to be recognized and compared before a decision could be reached. If so, then on the five-item physical-identity task, we should observe a shift away from the within-hemisphere advantage found in our previous studies for the three-item physical-identity task. Furthermore, if complexity as manipulated by the number of items to be recognized and compared is separable from complexity as manipulated by the decision process, then the across-hemisphere advantage should be greater on the five-item name-identity task, which is complex both in the number of items and the nature of the decision, than on the five-item physical-identity task, which is complex only in the number of items.

Our results revealed the expected pattern of results. For the three-item physical-identity task, we obtained a marginally significant within-hemisphere advantage (which did not differ significantly from our previous results with this task). In contrast, the five-item physical-identity task yielded an across-hemisphere advantage that was significantly different from the pattern observed on the three-item physical-identity task. Furthermore, the across-hemisphere advantage on the five-item name-identity task was significantly larger than that observed on the five-item physical-identity task, suggesting that interhemispheric interaction was influenced by both types of complexity. This latter finding indicates that the effects of complexity as manipulated by the number of items to be recognized and compared are separable from the effects of complexity as manipulated by increasing the number of steps required to reach a decision.

We have speculated on the basis of the above findings that interhemispheric interaction is useful under computationally complex conditions because it allows for a division of processing across the hemispheres. Recently, Belger (1993) provided more evidence that indeed it is the division or separability of processing that is quite important in obtaining an across-hemisphere advantage. In a paradigm similar to those we have employed previously, Belger created a rhyme decision task. Since phonetic discrimination is a task that can be performed by only the left hemisphere in the vast majority of right-handers (Rayman and Zaidel, 1991), the final stages of processing (i.e., those required for the rhyme decision as compared to those involved in identifying the letters of a word) can *only* be performed by the left hemisphere. In such a case, Belger reasoned, the usual across-hemisphere task should not be observed because a large division of processing is not possible. Consistent with Belger's hypothesis, when given the rhyme task, subjects do not exhibit an across-hemisphere advantage.

The lack of an across-hemisphere advantage in this study is compelling for two reasons. First, the rhyme task was as taxing for subjects as the other tasks that have yielded an across-hemisphere advantage, as evidenced by equally long reaction times and similar error rates. Thus, a lack of computational complexity cannot be argued as the basis for not obtaining an across-hemisphere advantage. Second, the same subjects that did not exhibit an across-hemisphere advantage on the rhyme task did in fact exhibit an across-hemisphere advantage for other computationally complex tasks (e.g., name-identity tasks). Hence, the lack of a significant across-hemisphere advantage on the rhyme task can also not be attributed to some anomaly in the subject population tested. Thus, all the evidence reviewed suggests that interhemispheric processing can increase the processing capacity of the brain by allowing for a dispersal of processing load across the hemispheres, and that such a dispersal is especially useful when tasks are difficult.

How do these findings stand in relation to work done by other researchers in the field? Our findings are quite consonant with those of Liederman, Merola, and Martinez (1985) who suggest that interhemispheric processing is most beneficial to task performance when the hemispheres are engaged in the processing of mutually exclusive operations, such that these conflicting operations are insulated from one another. Our results support the general idea that interhemispheric interaction provides for parallel or separable processing, although the details of our findings suggest that the notion of mutual exclusivity is not a requirement for such an advantage to accrue (see Banich and Belger, 1990, and Banich and Karol, 1992, for a longer discussion of this issue).

METHODS FOR STUDYING INTERHEMISPHERIC PROCESSING

One of the issues regarding interhemispheric processing is knowing how to demonstrate that an effect is indeed due to an interaction between the hemispheres and not some other factor. This section considers some issues in this area and provides highlights of methodologic issues that have been discussed in more detail elsewhere (Banich and Shenker, 1994). In particular it focuses on two major issues. First, it examines what conditions must be met to ensure that an observed behavioral phenomenon does indeed arise from the interaction of the hemispheres and not some other aspect of information processing. Second, it considers what is required to link behavioral aspects of interhemispheric processing to specific aspects of neural structure and function.

Requirements for Indicating that a Finding Is Related to Interhemispheric Processing

To ensure that a phenomenon is due specifically to interhemispheric interaction, two basic contrasting conditions are required: (1) interhemispheric processing or bihemispheric stimulation, and (2) a control condition requiring, at least initially, only within-hemisphere processing. Furthermore, it is essential when illustrating an effect of interhemispheric processing that an interaction occur between some manipulation and processing on within- as compared to across-hemisphere trials. This is akin to the hemisphere-by-task interaction that Hellige (1983) has argued is critical to making inferences in studies of lateralization.

Without the interaction between within- and across-hemisphere trials and some task manipulation, unequivocal interpretation of the data is not possible. Consider a paper in which the authors purported to provide evidence that females have better interhemispheric transfer than males (Potter and Graves, 1988) based on the finding that females were better than males at determining whether material presented to the left and right palms was the same, and determining whether two nonverbalizable shapes presented on either side of the midline were the same. As pointed out by Burton, Pepperrell, and Stredwick (1991), the conclusion of Potter and Graves may be erroneous because these trials only constitute the across-hemisphere condition, without a suitable control. Burton et al. speculate that superior tactile performance of females might have occurred because they have more sensitive palms (possibly because of fewer calluses), and hence would have exhibited better performance on this task regardless of whether or not the test required interhemispheric integration. As for the visual matching task, Burton et al. speculate that the superior accuracy of females may have been generated by a speed-accuracy tradeoff with females making their decisions more accurately but also more slowly than males. Only by employing a within-hemisphere control, such as trials in which the two shapes appeared in the same visual field, could one evaluate whether interhemispheric processing in females is superior to than in males.

In some investigations of interhemispheric processing, a portion of the task can only be performed by one hemisphere and these studies require extra consideration in designing a within-hemisphere control. An example is an investigation of interhemispheric interaction in which verbal output, which can only be produced only by the left hemisphere in right-handers, is used as a dependent measure (e.g., Dimond et al., 1979). In such studies it is assumed that if a subject must produce the name for either a word presented to the LVF or an unseen object placed in the left hand, the verbal response requires that information be relayed from the right hemisphere to the left, and as such requires interhemispheric processing. The within-hemisphere control used in such cases is usually a condition in which the item is presented in the RVF or palpated by the right hand because such information is received directly, at least initially, by the left hemisphere, and hence no interhemispheric integration is required to perform the task. Differences between these two types of conditions, however, are not enough to infer that a disruption in interhemispheric processing has occurred. One must first demonstrate that the ability of each hemisphere to recognize the items is equivalent. If such a control is not performed, differences in hemispheric competence could be misinterpreted as an interhemispheric effect.

Consider the following hypothetical case. Without the knowledge of the researcher, the left hemisphere is better able in the tactile modality to recognize a class of objects than is the right. The researcher, in an attempt to investigate interhemispheric interaction, designs a purported within-hemisphere condition, in which the subject must *name* an object placed in the right hand, and a purported across-hemisphere condition, in which the subject must name an object placed in the left hand. The researcher finds that the naming of right hand objects is better than the naming of left hand objects and concludes, erroneously, that poor interhemispheric relay of information from the right hemisphere to the left explains the results. In fact, the differences between right and left hand performance do not reflect interhemispheric processing but rather differences in hemispheric competence, and would have been obtained under conditions in which no interhemispheric interaction was required (e.g., recognition, rather than naming, of items placed in the right as compared to the left hand). Hence, to conclude that a disruption in interhemispheric processing exists would require demonstrating that the deficit on left hand performance was greater in a naming condition than in a recognition condition.

Linking Interhemispheric Processing to Other Aspects of Neural Structure and Function

This section considers what is required to link behavioral aspects of interhemispheric processing to specific aspects of neural structure and function. Three issues are considered: (1) linking behavioral aspects of interhemispheric processing to particular commissural systems or channels, (2) linking the efficiency of interhemispheric communication to individual anatomic variations, and (3) linking deficits in interhemispheric processing to particular neurologic syndromes.

Linking Behavior to Particular Commissural Channels   To suggest that a phenomenon is specific to callosal integration as compared to interhemispheric integration in general requires very careful selection of the task. If the researcher is interested in behavioral aspects of interhemispheric integration, she or he may not care whether such integration occurs at the cortical or subcortical level. In other cases, however, the researcher may be particularly interested in whether there is evidence of specific callosal involvement. For example, if one is attempting to make linkages between individual variation in the anatomic structure of the callosum and the behavioral functions that the callosum supports, it would be imperative to choose a behavioral task that *requires* the callosum to be intact. For example, one might wish to assess integrity of callosal relay of motor signals, and in such a case might utilize a task of bimanual motor control that Preilowski (1975) demonstrated could not be performed by split-brain patients.

If one is interested in investigating callosal function in general, it is important to consider that the callosum is made up of many different channels, as was discussed earlier. Hence, to investigate callosal function thoroughly, one must assess the integrity of each channel by assembling a battery of tests. This approach was taken recently by Braun and Ethier (1989), who examined the possibility of callosal disconnection after closed head injury by giving subjects a variety of tasks designed to assess callosal integration in different sensory modalities as well as in the motor domain.

Linking Behavior to Individual Variations in Anatomy   A large question prevalent in recent research on interhemispheric processing is how anatomic variation in the callosum is related to functional variation (e.g., Hines et al., 1992). Research in this area requires consideration of many issues in order to design studies that will yield rich results. First, one needs to consider what the size of the callosum means. At present, it is equivocal whether a larger callosum is indeed indicative of more nerve fibers. For example, in rats the splenium of males and females is the same size, but on average the female callosum contains a greater number of fibers than the male (Juraska and Kopcik, 1988). A lack of correlation between callosal size and number of fibers has also been reported for the rhesus monkey (Lamantia and Rakic, 1990), and the results from humans are ambiguous (Aboitiz et al., 1992). Thus, one cannot assume that just because one group, such as left-handed males, appears to have a larger isthmus of the callosum than non-left-handed males (Witelson, 1989), that the former have more nerve fibers in their callosa than the latter.

Second, the relationship between the size of the callosum and function is not clear. In different populations, size has been hypothesized to have converse relations to function. For example, it has been suggested that left-handers may have better interhemispheric integration because they have a larger callosum than right-handers. Yet there is also a subpopulation of patients with schizophrenia that have a larger-than-normal callosum, but at least some behavioral studies suggest that schizophrenic patients may have impaired interhemispheric processing (see Coger and Serafetinides, 1990, for a review of these findings). Hence, the only way to relate size to function is to specifically test that relationship. At present, indirect evidence provides little support for a clear relationship between size and function. For example, handedness, which has been related to callosal size, does not appear to be related to functional aspects of interhemispheric processing in the vast majority of studies that have examined this issue (e.g., Banich et al., 1990; Belger, 1993; Beaumont and Dimond, 1973, 1975; Dimond and Beaumont, 1972, 1974; Liederman, 1989; Piccirilli, Finali, and Sciarma, 1989).

Does this doom all studies which attempt to link anatomic variation in callosal size to behavior? The answer is no. First, increased knowledge derived from fine-grained analysis of callosal structure in humans will aid future interpretations of behavioral and anatomic studies. Second, one may examine a population of subjects in whom interpretation of the size of the callosum is somewhat less ambiguous. A case in point are patients with multiple sclerosis. We know that multiple sclerosis is a demyelinating disease, and although other pathologic processes are no doubt occurring, reduced density in the callosum, especially when measured longitudinally, can be reasonably interpreted as the lack of myelin. In this way, the reduced mass of the callosum can be attributed mainly to a reduction in myelin, not necessarily the number of nerve fibers. One can then correlate the size of the callosum with performance on particular behavioral tasks. When such tasks have both within- and across-hemisphere conditions, one can determine the degree to which the thinning predicts specific deficit in callosal function as compared to intrahemispheric decreases in function. A recent example of such an approach is an experiment by Pelletier et al. (submitted for publication).

Linking Deficits in Interhemispheric Processing to Particular Syndromes It has been hypothesized that there may be a disruption of interhemispheric processing in a surprisingly large variety of syndromes, including alexithymia (Dewaraja and Sasaki, 1990), pedophilia (Flor-Henry et al., 1991), dyslexia (Davidson, Leslie, and Saron, 1990), schizophrenia (Doty, 1989), multiple sclerosis (Lindeboom and Horst, 1988), and attention-deficit disorder (e.g., Hynd et al., 1991). What is critical, however, is to understand the role that disrupted interhemispheric processing plays in the disease state. There are numerous possible ways in which interhemispheric interaction could be linked to particular syndromes, each of which will be discussed in turn. For illustrative purposes, a hypothetical situation which illustrates the various types of relationships will be provided. First, disrupted interhemispheric interaction could actually cause the syndrome. So, for example, dyslexia might actually result from poor interhemispheric processing because information about graphic forms of letters, which are analyzed by the right hemisphere, cannot be linked to phonologic processing of that information by the left. Second, it may be that disrupted interhemispheric integration is just a single manifestation of a larger and more ubiquitous deficit in neural processing. For example, some authors have suggested that schizophrenia is a disease typified by neural disorganization (Doty, 1989). In such a case, disrupted interhemispheric processing may be but one of many manifestations of neural disorganization without being the causative factor in the cognitive and emotional dysfunction observed in schizophrenia. Third, poor interhemispheric integration could be merely a marker for the syndrome. For example, because interhemispheric processing has been found to be related to information processing under demanding conditions (e.g., Banich and Belger, 1990; Belger and Banich, 1992), perhaps attention-deficit disorder results in disrupted interhemispheric processing. In this case, it is not necessarily the disruption in interhemispheric processing that might cause attention-deficit disorder, because even if you could improve interhemispheric processing the attention-deficit disorder would remain. Rather, the attention difficulties inherent in the disorder might lead to poor interhemispheric processing, which therefore would act as a powerful marker for the syndrome. This relationship differs from that suggested as possible for schizophrenia. In schizophrenia there is massive neural disorganization so it was suggested that disrupted interhemispheric interaction might be just one of many manifestations of that disorganization. In contrast, in attention-deficit disorder it might be that interhemispheric processing is selectively affected. Finally, the correlation between callosal function and some syndrome may be mediated by other variables whose identity remains obscure. For example, acallosal persons often have other anomalies, such as low intelligence. The developmental malformation that leads to the co-occurrence of callosal agenesis and low intelligence remains unknown.

Distinguishing between these possibilities is of paramount importance. Although dyslexia will now be used as an example, the logic entailed could apply to an attempt to link callosal functioning to any of the syndromes described above. Studies of dyslexic children suggest that they may have disrupted interhemispheric interaction. Some of this evidence has been evinced from data on bihemispheric motor control (e.g., Gladstone, Best, and Davidson, 1989). However, dyslexia is a specific reading disability. On the surface, at least, it is not a learning disability that appears to be related to motor function. So what are we to make of the findings of interhemispheric disruptions of motor coordination in dyslexia? There are many possible interpretations. First, since the deficits in interhemispheric interaction related to dyslexia are specific to the motor regions of the brain and the central part of the callosum that connects them, the findings of motor dysfunction may be totally unrelated to dyslexia per se, since dyslexia is a syndrome that is specific to reading, not motor control. Second, it may well be that dyslexia is characterized by a general problem in interhemispheric processing, in which case interhemispheric disregulation is more likely to fall into the category of a marker for dyslexia rather than a causative mechanism. Given that dyslexia is a specific reading disability, if one wishes to demonstrate interhemispheric interaction as causative in the disease state, it would seem most prudent to assess functioning of those regions of the callosum that a priori appear to be very important for reading (e.g., the isthmus and splenium). Distinguishing between these various possibilities will be important for researchers as they attempt to understand the implications of interhemispheric interaction for a wide variety of syndromes.

ISSUES FOR THE FUTURE

Compared to our knowledge about lateralization of function, our information about interhemispheric interaction is scant. Hence, there is a broad research agenda in this domain that needs to be addressed. This section examines some of the issues that require further examination and which also seem, at present, amenable to analysis.

Two of the issues that are likely to receive much attention in the near future have already been discussed. First, there is a large need to link aspects of callosal anatomy to callosal function. The tools required for this endeavor, including histologic techniques, brain-imaging techniques, and behavioral methods of investigating interhemispheric interaction, are for the most part available. What is required, however, is a clear theoretical and logical path for investigating these issues. The other promising area of research will be to investigate the degree to which disruptions in interhemispheric processing occur in particular disease states. It will be useful not only to demonstrate that a disruption in interhemispheric processing accompanies the disease state but also that the disruption is in some way important or specific.

A third avenue for future research likely to be quite fruitful is the investigation of the degree to which lateralization of function is linked to interhemispheric processing. This question can be examined at two levels, the individual level and the population level. Some research in our laboratory illustrates the ways in which these issues may be investigated. On the individual level, we have found that, for the most part, the direction and size of a within- and across-hemisphere advantage exhibited by an individual subject on a task is unrelated to the direction and degree of lateralization for that task (e.g., Banich and Belger, 1990; Banich et al., 1990; Belger, 1993). Furthermore, we (Banich et al., 1990; Belger, 1993) have not yet observed any differences in interhemispheric processing between populations that have suggested differences in lateralization of function, such as differences between right-handers and left-handers, or between men and women. Whether these findings generalize to most types of interhemispheric interaction or are relatively specific to the types of paradigms and materials previously employed remains to be seen.

Interhemispheric integration obviously occurs between hemispheres that are specialized for different functions. Yet to the degree that certain aspects of interhemispheric integration turn out to be independent of lateralization of function, a fairly uncharted research endeavor awaits us. For example, a portion of our results (e.g., Banich and Karol, 1992) suggests that the factors affecting interhemispheric processing can be separate from those affecting the processing of each hemisphere in relative isolation. To the extent that this pattern characterizes interhemispheric processing, we will be forced to come up with a different set of theoretical heuristics to explain the nature of interaction between the hemispheres than those used to explain lateralization of function. Heuristics, such as the analytic/holistic distinction and other dichotomies, even with all their inexactness, were quite helpful in guiding research on lateralization of function. I suspect that a similar process awaits researchers investigating integration of function between the cerebral hemispheres.

ACKNOWLEDGMENTS

My students Aysenil Belger, Erika Noll, and Joel Shenker helped my thinking on the issues presented in this chapter both through the experimental work we have done together and through their insightful comments on drafts of this manuscript. I also thank Mary Greenpool and Wendy Heller for making comments on the manuscript.

REFERENCES

Aboitiz, F., Scheibel, A. B., Fisher, R. S., and Zaidel, E. (1992). Individual differences in brain asymmetries and fiber composition in the human corpus callosum. *Brain Research, 598*, 154–161.

Banich, M. T., and Belger, A. (1990). Interhemispheric interaction: How do the hemispheres divide and conquer a task? *Cortex, 26*, 77–94.

Banich, M. T., Goering, S., Stolar, N., and Belger, A. (1990). Interhemispheric processing in left- and right-handers. *International Journal of Neuroscience, 54*, 197–208.

Banich, M. T., and Karol, D. L. (1992). The sum of the parts does not equal the whole: Evidence from bihemispheric processing. *Journal of Experimental Psychology: Human Perception and Performance, 18*, 763–784.

Banich, M. T., Nicholas, M., and Karol, D. L. (1994). Interhemispheric interaction: Variations along a spectrum. Paper presented at the Annual Meeting of the International Neuropsychological Society, Cincinnati, Ohio, February, 1994.

Banich, M. T., and Shenker, J. I. (1994). Investigations of interhemispheric processing: Methodological considerations, *Neuropsychology, 7*, 325–342.

Beaumont, J. G., and Dimond, S. J. (1973). Transfer between the cerebral hemispheres in human learning. *Acta Psychologica, 37*, 87–91.

Beaumont, J. G., and Dimond, S. J. (1975). Interhemispheric transfer of figural information in right and non-right-handed subjects. *Acta Psychologica, 39*, 97–104.

Belger, A. (1993). Influences of hemispheric specialization and interaction on task performance Dissertation, University of Illinois at Urbana-Champaign.

Belger, A., and Banich, M. T. (1992). Interhemispheric interaction affected by computational complexity. *Neuropsychologia, 30*, 923–931.

Berlucchi, G., Heron, W., Hyman, R., Rizzolatti, G., and Umiltá, C. (1971). Simple reaction times of ipsilateral and contralateral hand to lateralized visual stimuli. *Brain, 94*, 419–430.

Braun, C. M. J., and Ethier, J. M. C. B. M. (1989). Interhemispheric transfer after spontaneous recovery in 43 cases of severe closed head injury. *Neuropsychology, 3*, 91–102.

Braun, C. M. J., Sapin-Leduc, A. S., Picard, D., Bonnefant, E., Achim, A., and Daigneault, S. (1994). Zaidel's model of interhemispheric dynamics: Empirical tests, a critical appraisal, and a proposed revision. *Brain and Cognition, 24*, 57–86.

Burton, A., Pepperrell, S., and Stredwick, J. (1991). Interhemisphere transfer in males and females. *Cortex, 27*, 425–429.

Clarke, J. M., and Zaidel, E. (1989). Simple reaction times to lateralized light flashes: Varieties of interhemispheric communication routes. *Brain, 112*, 849–870.

Coger, R. W., and Serafetinides, E. A. (1990). Schizophrenia, corpus callosum, and interhemispheric communication: A review. *Psychiatry Research, 34*, 163–184.

Cronin-Golumb, A. (1986). Subcortical transfer of cognitive information in subjects with complete forebrain commissurotomy. *Cortex, 22*, 499–519.

Davidson, R. J., Leslie, S. C., and Saron, C. (1990). Reaction time measures of interhemispheric transfer time in reading disabled and normal children. *Neuropsychologia, 28*, 471–485.

DeLacoste, M. C., Kirkpatrick, J. B., and Ross, E. D. (1985). Topography of the human corpus callosum. *Journal of Neuropathology and Experimental Neurology, 44*, 578–591.

Dewaraja, R., and Sasaki, Y. (1990). A left to right hemisphere callosal transfer deficit of nonlinguistic information in alexithymia. *Psychotherapy and Psychosomatics, 54*, 201–207.

Dimond, S. J., and Beaumont, J. G. (1972). Hemisphere function and color naming. *Journal of Experimental Psychology, 96*, 87–91.

Dimond, S. J., and Beaumont, J. G. (1974). Hemisphere function and paired-associate learning. *British Journal of Psychology, 65*, 275–278.

Dimond, S. J., Scammell, R. E., Pruce, I. G., Huws, D., and Gray, C. (1979). Callosal transfer and left-hand anomia in schizophrenia. *Biological Psychiatry, 14*, 735–739.

Doty, R. W. (1989). Schizophrenia: a disease of interhemispheric processes at forebrain and brainstem levels? *Behavioral and Brain Research, 34*, 1–33.

Engel, A. K., Konig, P., Kreuter, A. K., and Singer, W. (1991). Interhemispheric synchronization of oscillatory neuronal responses in cat visual cortex. *Science, 252*, 1177–1179.

Flor-Henry, P., Lang, R. A., Koles, Z. J., and Frenzel, R. R. (1991). Quantitative EEG studies of pedophilia. *International Journal of Psychophysiology, 10*, 253–258.

Gazzaniga, M. S. (1987). Perceptual and attentional processes following callosal section in humans. *Neuropsychologia, 25*, 119–133.

Geffen, F. (1980). Phonological fusion after partial section of the corpus callosum. *Neuropsychologia, 18*, 613–620.

Geschwind, N., and Kaplan, E. (1962). A human cerebral disconnection syndrome. *Neurology, 12*, 675–685.

Gladstone, M., Best, C. T., and Davidson, R. J. (1989). Anomalous bimanual coordination among dyslexic boys. *Developmental Psychology, 25*, 236–246.

Hellige, J. B. (1983). Hemisphere by task interaction. In J. B. Hellige (Ed.), *Cerebral hemisphere asymmetry: Method, theory and application.* New York, NY: Praeger Publishers.

Hellige, J. B., Jonsson, J. E., and Michimata, C. (1988). Processing from LVF, RVF, and BILATERAL presentations: Examination of metacontrol and interhemispheric interaction. *Brain and Cognition, 7*, 39–53.

Hellige, J. B., Taylor, A. K., and Eng, T. L. (1989). Interhemispheric interaction when both hemispheres have access to the same stimulus information. *Journal of Experimental Psychology: Human Perception and Performance, 15,* 711–722.

Hines, M., Chui, L., McAdams, L. A., Bentler, P. M., and Lipcamon, J. (1992). Cognition and the corpus callosum: Verbal fluency, visuospatial ability, and language lateralization related to midsaggital surface areas of callosal subregions. *Behavioral Neuroscience, 106,* 3–14.

Holtzman, J. D. (1984). Interactions between cortical and subcortical visual areas: evidence from human commissurotomy patients. *Vision Research, 24,* 801–813.

Holtzman, J. D., Sidtis, J. J., Volpe, B. T., Wilson, D. H., and Gazzaniga, M. S. (1981). Dissociation of spatial information for stimulus localization and the control of attention. *Brain, 104,* 861–872.

Hynd, G. W., Semrud-Clikeman, M., Lorys, A. R., Novey, A. R., Eliopulos, D., and Lyytinen, H. (1991). Corpus callosum morphology in attention deficit-hyperactivity disorder: Morphometric analysis of MRI. *Journal of Learning Disabilities, 24,* 141–146.

Jeeves, M. A. (1979). Some limits to interhemispheric integration in cases of callosal agenesis and partial commissurotomy. In I. S. Russell, M. W. van Hoff, and G. Berlucchi (Eds.), *Structure and function of the cerebral commissures* (pp 449–474). New York, NY: Macmillan Publishing Co.

Johnson, L. E. (1984). Bilateral visual cross-integration by human forebrain commissurotomy subjects. *Neuropsychologia, 22,* 167–175.

Juraska, J. M., and Kopcik, J. R. (1988). Sex and environmental influences on the size and ultrastructure of the rat corpus callosum. *Brain Research, 450,* 1–8.

Lamantia, A. S., and Rakic, P. (1990). Cytological and quantitative characteristics of four cerebral commissures in the rhesus monkey. *Journal of Comparative Neurology, 291,* 353–366.

Levy, J., and Trevarthen, C. (1976) Metacontrol of hemispheric function in human split-brain patients. *Journal of Experimental Psychology: Human Perception and Performance, 2,* 299–312.

Liederman, J. (1989). The advantage of between-hemisphere division on inputs: Generalizability across handedness, populations and procedural variations. *Journal of Clinical and Experimental Neuropsychology, 11,* 37.

Liederman, J., Merola, J., and Martinez, S. (1985). Interhemispheric collaboration in response to simultaneous bilateral input. *Neuropsychologia, 23,* 673–683.

Lindeboom, J., and Horst, R. T. (1988). Interhemispheric disconnection effects in multiple sclerosis. *Journal of Neurology, Neurosurgery and Psychiatry, 51,* 1445–1447.

Luck, S. J., Hillyard, S. A., Mangun, G. R., and Gazzaniga, M. S. (1989). Independent hemispheric attentional systems mediate visual search in split-brain patients. *Nature, 342,* 543–545.

Milner, A. D., and Lines, C. R. (1982). Interhemispheric pathways in simple reaction time to lateralized light flash. *Neuropsychologia, 20,* 171–179.

Myers, J. J., and Sperry, R. W. (1985). Interhemispheric communication after section of the forebrain commissures. *Cortex, 21,* 249–260.

Pandya, D. N., and Seltzer, B. (1986). The topography of commissural fibers. In F. Lepore, M. Ptito, and H. Jasper (Eds.), *Two hemispheres—one brain: Functions of the corpus callosum* (pp 47–73). New York, NY: Alan R. Liss, Inc.

Pelletier, J., Habib, M., Lyon-Caen, O., Salamon, G., Poncet, M., and Khalil, R. (submitted for publication). Functional and MRI correlates of callosal involvement in multiple sclerosis.

Piccirilli, M., Finali, G., and Sciarma, T. (1989). Negative evidence of difference between right- and left-handers in interhemispheric transfer of information. *Neuropsychologia, 27,* 1023–1026.

Potter, S. M., and Graves, R. E. (1988). Is interhemispheric transfer related to handedness and gender? *Neuropsychologia, 26*, 319–325.

Preilowski, B. (1975). Bilateral motor interaction: Perceptual motor performance of partial and complete "split-brain" Patients. In K. J. Zulch, O. Cretuzfeldt, and G. C., Galbraith (Eds.), *Cerebral localization* (pp 115–132). Berlin: Springer-Verlag.

Rayman, J., and Zaidel, E. (1991) Rhyming and the right hemisphere. *Brain and Language, 40*, 89–105.

Risse, G. L., Gates, J., Lund, G., Maxwell, R., and Rubens, A. (1989). Interhemispheric transfer in patients with incomplete section of the corpus callosum: Anatomical verification with magnetic resonance imaging. *Archives of Neurology, 46*, 437–443.

Rugg, M. D., Lines, C. R., and Milner, A. D. (1984). Visual evoked potentials to lateralized visual stimuli and the measurement of interhemispheric transmission time. *Neuropsychologia, 22*, 215–225.

St. John, R., Shields, C., Krahn, P., and Tinney, B. (1987). The reliability of estimates of interhemispheric transfer times derived from unimanual and verbal response latencies. *Human Neurobiology, 6*, 195–202.

Sergent, J. (1990). Furtive incursions into bicameral minds. *Brain, 113*, 537–568.

Sergent, J. (1991). Processing of spatial relations within and between the disconnected cerebral hemispheres. *Brain, 114*, 1025–1043.

Sperry, R. W., Zaidel, E., and Zaidel, D. (1979). Self recognition and social awareness in the deconnected minor hemisphere. *Neuropsychologia, 17*, 153–166.

Trevarthen, C., and Sperry, R. W. (1973). Perceptual unity of the ambient visual field in human commissurotomy patients. *Brain, 96*, 547–570.

Witelson, S. F. (1989). Hand and sex differences in the isthmus and genu of the human corpus callosum. *Brain, 112*, 799–835.

16 A Reinterpretation of the Split-Brain Syndrome: Implications for the Function of Corticocortical Fibers

Jacqueline Liederman

The purpose of this chapter is to examine the function of corticocortical association pathways.[1] Traditionally, it has been assumed that the primary role of these pathways is to "transfer" information, and that lesions of these pathways result in disconnection syndromes where information restricted to one region is unavailable to a second part of the brain. The paradigmatic disconnection syndrome is said to occur in split-brain patients, within whom the corticocortical pathways connecting the hemispheres have been surgically severed and the "only" means of interhemispheric integration that remains is subcortical. The symptoms of split-brain patients have traditionally been viewed as illustrating that the two hemispheres operate in isolation from each other and that information projected to only one hemisphere is unavailable to the opposite hemisphere. This view of the split-brain syndrome has been codified into the very terms that we use for testing function in the commissurotomized patient: We refer to these paradigms as "transfer" paradigms. This chapter argues that these assumptions need to be challenged.

The first section of this chapter focuses on the disconnection syndrome in split-brain patients and challenges this traditional view. The claim is made that after sectioning of the interhemispheric corticocortical pathways, subcortical pathways still enable one hemisphere to have access to input restricted to the opposite hemisphere, but that access is on an "implicit" (unconscious) but not "explicit" (conscious) level. The implicit/explicit distinction was first made in the memory literature and refers to the mechanism by which information is retrieved rather than stored (cf. Schacter, 1987, for a review). Thus, in commissurotomized patients, when only one hemisphere is presented with a stimulus, the opposite hemisphere can access information about that stimulus on an implicit level, and can use that information to guide certain kinds of response selection, but the nonviewing hemisphere cannot mediate conscious awareness of the stimulus.

The second section examines several explanations for how and why the subcortical routes that are available after sectioning of the corticocortical pathways provide only limited access to information presented to the opposite hemisphere. Three hypotheses are considered as to why information presented to one hemisphere cannot be consciously accessed by the opposite hemisphere even though the two hemispheres can cooperate to initiate an integrated response. The first considers the low specificity of information transferred subcortically, the second considers the desynchronized process by which information is integrated without the synchronizing influence of the commissures, and the third examines the underactivated state of the non-viewing hemisphere which causes it to neglect inputs to it from other parts of the brain. These hypotheses are by no means mutually exclusive; indeed, the underactivated state of the nonviewing hemisphere is probably secondary to the loss of reciprocal activation that would have occurred had the commissures been intact to mediate synchronization of the hemispheres.

In the third section I make the argument that the corticocortical pathways that connect regions *within* a hemisphere have the same structural and functional characteristics as those that connect regions *between* hemispheres. Thus, it is argued that at least some of the *intra*hemispheric disconnection syndromes can be reinterpreted as a disruption of explicit but not implicit access to information which was restricted to the disconnected region.

In the next section, I address the following question: If intra- and inter-corticocortical pathways are structurally and functionally similar, why is interhemispheric integration inferior to intrahemispheric integration, even in the commissure-intact individual? Evidence of this inferiority, as well as structural and dynamic explanations for it, are examined. The argument is then made that there are two exceptional circumstances within which interhemispheric integration is as good as intrahemispheric integration: when information can be accessed without conscious awareness, and when information can be cross-compared on a superordinate rather than a subordinate level.

I point out that there is a remarkable similarity between commissure-sectioned and commissure-intact persons in terms of the exceptional circumstances for which interhemispheric integration is equivalent to intra-hemispheric integration. The degree of parallelism in the interhemispheric integration profiles of persons with and without cerebral commissures permits two conclusions to be drawn: the first implication is that, to a greater extent than has generally been assumed, subcortical interhemispheric pathways, even in the intact brain, may mediate interhemispheric integration during tasks that can be adequately performed on either a categorical level or by means of implicit, as opposed to explicit, access; the second is that information about the perceptual identity of an item is more vulnerable to disruptions in synchronization and equilibration of arousal than categorical information or information that can be processed automatically, and that even in the intact brain such disruptions occur more between than within hemispheres.

Finally, I reexamine the entire issue of interregional integration of information in the cerebral cortex. Three sorts of integration are described. The first is referred to as *direct transfer*. The products of processing of one area are transferred to a second region where they are integrated with that region's processing and stored. This results in duplication of information across the two regions. It has historically been assumed that this is the major function of the corticocortical pathways, and that there is a loss of detail when direct integration is attempted by subcortical means. This view is challenged. The second kind of integration is referred to here as *third-party convergence*. Here, the two regions feed the products of their processing to a third convergence area, but they do not share information directly with one another. In this second kind of integration, the primary role of the corticocortical pathways is to synchronize the outputs of these two regions to the third convergence area. The third kind of intercortical integration is referred to as *nonconvergent temporal integration*. In nonconvergent temporal integration, the role of the corticocortical pathways is to synchronize the outputs of these two regions and enable them to feed forward, independently, but synchronously, to a variety of other areas. Output from these two regions initiates a synchronized distribution of patterned activation. This forward march of patterned activation can influence relatively independent systems for the control of behavior in a parallel, but synchronized, way. Therefore, in nonconvergent synchronization there is only temporal integration. There is no grandfather convergence zone and no region where traces of the two regions of activity are stored as a compound, single engram.

I argue that this nonconvergent temporal integration is far more common than is currently appreciated, and that it is the most dependent upon corticocortical fibers. Thus the dissociative behavior that occurs after corticocortical pathway section is largely the consequence of desynchronization of the two regions and the imbalances in activation which may be secondary to that desynchronization, rather than the structural limitations of the use of subcortical pathways per se.

INFORMATION RECEIVED BY ONE HEMISPHERE IS NOT REALLY UNAVAILABLE TO THE OTHER HEMISPHERE AFTER SECTION OF THE CEREBRAL COMMISSURES

The Traditional View Is that Interhemispheric Deficits Are Due to "Lack of Transfer" of All but the Crudest or Most Abstract Information

The traditional view of the role of corticocortical association pathways is that they permit information from one region or hemisphere to be "transferred" to a second region or hemisphere. Sectioning of these fibers is said to result in a "disconnection" syndrome, such that only the crudest, least specific information can be transferred from one hemisphere to the other. Indeed, in a state-of-the-art review of the literature on patients with sections of the cerebral commissures, Gazzaniga (1987) claims that "interhemispheric transfer is limited to . . . crude spatial information" (p. 124).

The fact that abstract and categorical information, but not item-specific physical information, could be shared interhemispherically after commissurotomy was suggested by the contrasting results of two experiments by Cronin-Golomb (1986). She presented a sample picture stimulus to one hemisphere and a three-choice picture array to the other hemisphere. The task was to pick which of the pictures in the array was most closely related to the sample picture. The pictures could relate to one another on an abstract or concrete level. Abstract pairs included a guitar and an artist's palette, or a letter and a telephone. The concrete pairs were coordinates or members of the same category such as fish and duck or shoe and sock. Commissurotomized patients were able to perform this task as well between as within hemispheres. However, in a second experiment, subjects were asked to find the best match when the match might include the item itself. Commissurotomized patients could not make the match on the basis of two identical pictures of the same item. It was concluded that they could transfer conceptual and situational information associated with the object represented in the picture, but they could not transfer the physical image of the picture. Indeed, the patients seemed unaware that matching pictures were ever presented.

The View Being Proposed Is that Information Is Accessible to the Nonviewing Hemisphere in Considerable Detail but Only on an Implicit (Unconscious), Not an Explicit (Conscious), Level

Provocative data have been reported by Sergent (1986, 1987, 1990, 1991) which indicate that information of considerable specificity *can* be interhemispherically integrated. In Sergent's (1987) study, the commissurotomized subjects were presented with two distinct stimuli, one to each visual field, and subjects had to make a decision about the relationship between the two stimuli. There were eight tasks. The commissurotomized patients were able to decide if two lines would form a straight or broken line, whether the angle that two arrows made was larger or smaller than 90 degrees, whether the total number of dots displayed summed to an odd or even number, whether the sum of a pair of digits was larger or smaller than 10, and finally whether a four-letter string consisting of two letters to each visual field formed a word. In contrast, these same patients were unable to describe the arrows on the screen, or to name the letters presented to the left visual fields. Thus, decisions were being made in this task on the basis of information that was accessible to a response mechanism but seemed inaccessible to consciousness. Note that the elements of the display did not have to be explicitly individually identified for decisions to be made about their conjoint meaning.

The results from Sergent's (1987) Task 8 are perhaps the most astounding because subject L.B. can perform this task whereas he failed a very similar task in a previous experiment (Sergent, 1986, Task 3). The main difference between the tasks was the extent to which the elements had to be consciously cross-compared. In Sergent's (1987) study, a decision was required as to whether two colors presented to separate hemispheres were the same. Only four colors were used in that experiment: two shades of red and two shades of green. L.B.'s performance was random irrespective of whether stimulus pairs consisted of two identical colors, two shades of the same color, or opposite colors (red and green). On the other hand (Sergent, 1987), a decision was required as to whether a display consisted of a combination of one of two colors (i.e., green vs. blue) with one of two symbols (i.e., an X vs. a circle). Four specific combinations of these colors and symbols were considered targets and four combinations were considered nontargets. These combinations were counterbalanced. Therefore, it was not possible for each hemisphere to simply complete its half of the task independently, since, for example, a blue patch on the right was equally likely to be an element of a correct or an incorrect pairing. Hence, the only way to accomplish this task was for the color and shape information to be considered conjointly, the very thing that L.B. failed to do in the color comparison paradigm.

Another example of lack of conscious access to information which is adequate to guide decision making is the paradigm in which Sergent (1990, Task 8) presents a picture of a face to the left visual field/right hemisphere. She then interviews the patient with a series of yes/no questions about the person in the picture. The subject's verbal responses are presumed to reflect the left hemisphere's knowledge of the picture, because it is the hemisphere which controls speech. The patient can accurately answer yes/no questions about the age, sex, occupation, and personality of the person in the picture, but cannot name the face. The left hemisphere even volunteers extra information about the person in the picture. For example, when referring to the Queen of England, one patient remarks that the person in the picture is rich even though she does not work. Immediately after showing the picture to the right hemisphere, Sergent presented the *same* picture to the patient's left hemisphere. The patient's left hemisphere could name the person in the picture instantly, but consistently denied having been shown the picture before! The fact that the right hemisphere had just been shown the same picture was not accessible consciously to the left hemisphere.

Sergent's (1991) most recent experiments demonstrate that the specificity of spatial information that can be integrated between the hemispheres varies dramatically with instructional set. There was a series of tasks which involved presentation of two different stimuli, one to each hemisphere. Subjects were required to cross-compare these stimuli to make judgments of spatial relation and size. When the task was to indicate which of two circles was bigger, the circles could be cross-compared interhemispherically by two of the three split-brain patients. When the task was to indicate which of two oblique lines was closer to the vertical, the lines could be cross-compared interhemispherically by one of two split-brain patients tested. When an identity match had to be made in terms of both orientation of the line and size of the circle within which the line was an arc, none of the split-brain patients performed above chance.

In contrast, when subjects were instructed to indicate which side was displaying the larger circle and to refrain from responding if the two circles were the same size, the subjects responded accurately even though under the previous set of instructions they were not able to accurately indicate with a button press that the circles were equal. In a second series of tasks the subjects had to decide about the spatial relationship between two dots presented to separate hemispheres. For example, they needed to indicate which dot was on top. They performed this cross-comparison with a precision that could be obtained only if the location of the dots on the two dimensions had been encoded and put in relation to one another by the two hemispheres.

Conclusion

We concur with Sergent (1991): "There was, therefore, more information accessible from the contralateral hemisphere than a direct comparison between informational contents explicitly held by each hemisphere would suggest" (p. 1041).

We now consider three explanations for *why* sectioning of the commissures disrupts the nonviewing hemisphere from being consciously aware of information presented to the opposite hemisphere.

HYPOTHESES AS TO WHY INFORMATION PRESENTED TO ONE HEMISPHERE CANNOT BE CONSCIOUSLY ACCESSED BY THE OPPOSITE HEMISPHERE DESPITE OFTEN BEING ADEQUATE TO GUIDE DECISION MAKING

There is one set of data that is hard to reconcile with the notion that in commissurotomized patients the nonviewing hemisphere has implicit but not explicit access to information restricted to the opposite hemisphere. In Sergent (1990) two numbers were flashed, one to each hemisphere, and the commissurotomized patients were asked to cross-compare them. The command to cross-compare them makes this task explicit.

The patients were able to successfully compare the numbers in terms of single features or dimensions of the stimuli. So, for example, they could indicate (a) on which side the number with the larger value appeared, (b) whether the sum of the numbers was an odd or even number, and (c) whether the sum was greater than or less than 10. In each of these cases, subjects needed to cross-compare the meaning of the number. However, patients *were not able* to cross-compare the numbers in terms of their physical appearance. When asked simply whether the two numbers were the same, performance was at chance levels.

Several explanations for these data spring to mind. The first is that only low-resolution, coded, or categorical data can be conveyed interhemispherically, and that the physical appearance of the numbers is beyond the resolution of subcortical pathways. The second is that there is a decontextualization and fragmentation of information transmission when the synchronizing influence of the commissures is removed. Thus, various aspects of a stimulus can be inferred by the nonviewing hemisphere, but the stimulus itself cannot be reconstructed into a whole, including the idiosyncratic markers that place it within an autobiographic time line. The third possibility is that the integration deficit is a consequence of the underactivated state of the nonviewing hemisphere, which cannot operate upon the desynchronized signals that arrive to it to fuse them into a distinct percept.

Thus three hypotheses will be considered for why certain aspects of information presented to one hemisphere cannot be consciously accessed by the other hemisphere even though the two hemispheres can cooperate to initiate an integrated response. The first has to do with the poor quality of information transferred subcortically, the second considers the desynchronized process by which information is transmitted subcortically without the synchronizing influence of the commissures, and the third considers the underactivated state of the hemisphere receiving the subcortically "transferred" information which causes it to neglect inputs to it from other parts of the brain. These hypotheses are not mutually exclusive; indeed hypotheses 2 and 3 both have to do with the loss of callosal facilitory signals on interhemispheric interaction.

Hypothesis 1: The Poor Quality of Information Available to the Nonviewing Hemisphere Disrupts Explicit Access

This is Sergent's (1987) hypothesis. It has as its premise that subcortical transfer permits only low-resolution, coded, or categorical information to be transferred from the viewing to the nonviewing hemisphere, and that such poor quality information is insufficient for conscious inferences to be made about item identity. Sergent (1987) argues that subcortical pathways may only be capable of transmitting information about the outcome of cortical operations, resulting in reduction and impoverishment of information. Sergent (1987) argues that one reason that such poor-quality information may be transferred by subcortical structures is the relatively smaller amount of area for representation available subcortically as compared to on a cortical level. Thus, Sergent argues transfer will involve a many-to-one rather than a one-to-many mapping of the information. As sensible as these tenets may be, the data are ambiguous in terms of whether the quality of information accessible to the disconnected hemisphere is limited to being categorical or low-resolution.

First, evidence is reviewed which supports the notion that only poor-quality information is *consciously* available to the speaking (left) hemisphere when inputs are restricted to the right hemisphere. Then the question is examined as to whether this fuzziness or coarseness is restricted to the explicit (conscious) level of information access, or whether fuzziness occurs even at the implicit (subconscious) level. Finally, an experimental strategy for reconciling this controversy is outlined.

Evidence that Transferred Information Is Fuzzy on a Conscious Level
In an elegant series of experiments with two commissurotomized patients, Holtzman (1984) demonstrated that information about spatial location on one

side of space could facilitate eye movements to the other side of space. However, when he manipulated the spatial cue so that it provided information not only about a side of space but also about specific location within a side of space (down to 0.25 degrees), there was no longer an advantage to the pre-cue. One patient (J.W.) made an interesting observation. When the target matrix was presented to his left hemisphere (which controls speech) he reported that he could "see" the matrix clearly. But when the matrix was presented to his right hemisphere, (i.e., the mute hemisphere) he reported that the matrix looked like a "shadowy blob." J.W.'s phenomenologic report seems like definitive proof that only "crude" spatial information can be "transferred" from the right hemisphere to the left hemisphere, which controls the verbal report. However, the verbal report reveals only what the subject is conscious of explicitly. Implicitly, the matrix projected to the right hemisphere might be clear. Indeed, even the eye movement task was explicit and volitional: when the subject heard a tone he was expected to deliberately move his eyes to the corresponding position in the opposite visual field. So it is possible that, under different circumstances, the task could be structured so that attention would be automatically oriented to the cued position, without the subject's conscious participation.

The notion that the level of detail available implicitly may be far greater than what is available explicitly can be applied to the data from Sergent (1987) for the lexical decision task. On one trial, the letters RU were presented to one visual field and NK to the other visual field. On a different trial the letter string was BU NK . The words and nonwords were carefully constructed so that no inferences about the beginning of the word could be made on the basis of just reading the end of the word, which was projected to the right visual field. The split-brain patients are able to make an interhemispheric lexical decision but they are not able to actually identify the word. Sergent argues that the way that the input is coded and then transferred subcortically to enable the unified response is too low-resolution to enable naming. This does not follow: if the "transfer" were blurry you would expect the subject to name words that are visually similar, but you would not expect the subject to report no information at all, which was what occurred. Moreover, how fuzzy could the united percept be when to distinguish between RUNK and BUNK the only difference is the horizontal completion of the bottom of the R into a B by means of a tiny line fragment? If that discrimination can be made for the unified response, it does not make sense that the "transfer" process, per se, is too low-resolution. For at least implicit access, the right hemisphere material seems available to the left hemisphere with considerable fidelity.

Similar conclusions can be drawn from a reexamination of the tasks that the commissurotomized patient L.B. passed and failed. As you may recall, L.B. successfully performed a task which required identification of displays with a certain shape in one field and color in the other field (Sergent, 1990). L.B. failed a task that required that two colors be matched between the visual fields. Thus, the information was available in sufficient detail to permit a blue-dot combination to be selected, but not to allow a red-red combination to be selected! Once again, this does not seem to be a difference in the grain of detail required to complete the task, but instead seems to depend upon the mode of inquiry.

Proposed Research which Would Help to Determine whether Information Accessed Implicitly Is as Low-resolution as Information Accessed Explicitly   The question is the extent to which information presented to one hemisphere in the commissurotomized patient is implicitly vs. explicitly available to the other hemisphere. There are at least two ways to think about the findings that have been reported in the literature. One view is that high-resolution, item-specific information does not transfer, and that in those instances when patients seem to have transferred something it must have been coded, or abstracted, in some way. In future research, it would be important to make the to-be-transferred material extremely difficult to package or reduce into a simple code. This should reveal the true limits of transfer.

The alternative view is that more detail is available to the nonviewing hemisphere than can ever be gleaned by tasks that require explicit, conscious access to the information made available by subcortical pathways. The notion that implicit transfer is much finer-grained than explicit transfer could be examined by means of *within- vs. between-hemisphere priming tasks*. In the between-hemisphere condition, information projected to one hemisphere would contain information which could facilitate a search task presented afterward to the opposite hemisphere. For the implicit version of the task, the experiment would be run so that the instructions did not orient patients to the prime so that savings that are due to the prime are unconscious and implicit. Then the experiment would be repeated, with exactly the same materials, but the task would be to compare consciously and *explicitly* the prime in the first display to the target in the second display, even though they were projected to separate hemispheres. Each of these experiments would be conducted in commissurotomized patients as well as in controls that were commissure-intact.

It is expected that tasks that only require implicit access to information to be integrated interhemispherically will probably be successfully completed by commissurotomized patients, whereas those requiring explicit access to the information will be failed. However, it is likely that even implicit interhemispheric integration will be more limited in these patients than in normals. How much detail can be communicated interhemispherically, even on an implicit level, may depend on the number of dimensions that need to be computed simultaneously. The experiments could be varied in terms of task difficulty so as to identify the limits of performance.

However, irrespective of the structural limits of subcortical interhemispheric integration, it will be argued that, in addition, there are some *dynamic* aspects of interhemispheric interaction that probably affect whether material made available to the nonviewing hemisphere can be consciously perceived. These dynamic factors are reviewed as hypotheses 2 and 3.

Hypothesis 2: Commissurotomy Causes the Two Hemispheres to be Desynchronized; This Desynchronization Prevents Stimuli Experienced by One Hemisphere from Being Accessed by the Opposite Hemisphere along with the Contextual Features that Bind It into an Explicit Event Memory

The argument being made here has three components. The first component is that interregional synchronization is critical for binding the dimensions of an object into a single, idiosyncratic, event memory. Physiologic data are reviewed which support certain aspects of this notion. The second component is that commissurotomy causes the two hemispheres to be desynchronized. For this, there is considerable evidence, as is documented below. The third component of the argument is that interhemispheric desynchronization prevents stimuli experienced by one hemisphere from being accessed by the opposite hemisphere along with the contextual features that bind it into an explicit event memory. The last argument is purely speculative; its defense will ultimately require experimental validation.

Evidence that Interregional Synchronization Is Critical for Binding the Occurrence of an Object and Its Context into a Single, Idiosyncratic, Event Memory   Temporal synchronization of activity among distributed neuronal cell assemblies permits the binding or integration into a single event memory of various physical dimensions of an object, such as location, shape, direction of movement, color, texture, and sound. This concept has been supported by the work in the laboratories of Singer (Gray et al., 1989; Gray and Singer, 1989; Engel et al., 1991) and Poppel (Poppel, 1988; Poppel, Schill, and von Steinbuchel, 1990). For example, Poppel et al. (1990) argue that intersensory, within-hemisphere integration occurs by means of a synchronization mechanism which essentially temporally integrates distributed activity approximately every 20 to 40 ms. Thus, information from these different senses is grouped within the same temporal window, despite considerable differences in transduction time at the receptor level. Each of the independent populations of cell assemblies oscillate at about 40 Hz. *Oscillations* can be defined as recurrent synchronous bursting of neuronal groups; the oscillations enable cell groups which are connected by means of reciprocal pathways to fall into synchrony. The oscillations do not represent or code information directly.

Some of these ideas have been incorporated into a recent theoretical piece by Damasio (1989). Damasio argues that regions of the brain integrate their activity via "binding" rather than information "transfer." Thus, the integration of multiple aspects of experience, both within each modality and across modalities, depends on the time-locked coactivation of geographically separate sites of neural activity within sensory and motor cortices, *rather than on neural transfer* and integration of different representations toward rostral integration sites (Damasio, 1989, p. 39, emphasis added).

According to Damasio (1989), feed-forward signals indicate the location of records of activity earlier (upstream) in the network; feedback signals reactivate these earlier (downstream) records. Damasio (1989) points out repeatedly that "no representations of reality as we experience it are ever transferred in the system; that is, no concrete contents and no psychological information move about in the system" (p. 57). Indeed, feedback and feed-forward signals "do not transport a moveable representation being entered or reentered" (p. 57). For these distributed networks of information to be unified into a conscious percept, they must be simultaneously coactivated and "bound" by a temporary attentional enhancement quite like Crick's (1984) attentional spotlight.

It is easy to see why the physical dimensions of an object need to be bound into a single percept. What is being argued here is that explicit access to a memory requires that the regions that processed the physical dimensions of the object be reactivated along with the regions that processed the observer's idiosyncratic emotional and cognitive reactions to the stimulus. Without reactivation of this contextual surround, retrieval of the memory is apt to be fragmented, and restricted to a single region coding for a single physical dimension of the stimulus, or overgeneralized, and restricted to an abstraction.

Evidence that Commissurotomy Causes the Two Hemispheres to be Desynchronized   It has been demonstrated in cats that the corpus callosum is necessary for the interhemispheric synchronization of two populations of cells in area 17, each of which shows a local pattern of oscillation at a rate of about 40 Hz (Engel et al., 1991). Engel et al. hypothesize that this synchronization permits temporal integration or "binding" of populations of cells which are tuned to different dimensions of a single visual stimulus which is positioned so that it overlaps the midline. What is critical is that Engel et al. (1991) have shown that after callosal transections, there is no longer interhemispheric synchronization of homologous neuronal populations in the two hemispheres in response to a single object which overlaps the midline.

This team of scientists has also been able to demonstrate within-hemisphere synchronization between regions in areas 17, 18, and 19, at intercortical distances as great as 7 mm. The authors conclude that this binding is a corticocortical phenomenon that is not secondary to some kind of subcortical pacemaker, or simply conjoint input from the thalamus (see Engel et al., 1992, for a review).

Interhemispheric Desynchronization Prevents the Nonviewing Hemisphere from Being Able to Reactivate the Diverse Regions Involved in Processing the Event and Its Contextual Surround so as to Reconstitute an Episodic Memory   What is now being proposed is that the synchronization of neural activity between the two hemispheres is a major function of the corpus callosum. As reviewed above, so far the callosum has only been demonstrated to be involved in the interhemispheric integration of a single object that crosses the vertical meridian. However, the behavioral data reviewed at the beginning of this chapter indicate callosal section disrupts explicit cross-comparison of stimuli that simultaneously appear on opposite sides of space, even though neither of them crosses the vertical meridian. Since the corpus callosum connects only those area 17 cells whose receptive fields include the vertical meridian (Berlucchi and Antonini, 1990), cross-comparison of two stimuli lateralized in the periphery must occur by means of callosal connections between higher-order visual areas. What is being proposed is that this cross-comparison is mediated by an analogous process of interhemispheric synchronization.

Regions that are jointly activated can conjointly feed forward to regions that receive inputs from the two areas. Thus, the purpose of the callosum may be to permit neuronal assemblies within disparate associational areas of the two cortices to be simultaneously active so that their outputs, by virtue of their temporal synchronicity, may be "bound" into a single percept, or cross-compared and revealed as separate entities. The reciprocal pathways of the corpus callosum would allow activity in these disparate areas to become synchronized and would enable them to be temporally organized into a single episodic event memory. Thus, the role of the callosum may be to provide a parallel wave of activation within each of the two hemispheres so that widespread activity that occurs at the time of encoding the stimulus can be integrated into a single event perception which would be fed forward independently by each hemisphere to a wide variety of regions positioned to receive their conjoint output.

What is being proposed is that without the reciprocal connections of the callosum, which permit opposite regions of the two hemispheres to self-synchronize, information from a wide variety of cortical sites in one hemisphere can be channeled through a variety of subcortical sites to the opposite hemisphere. However, this transmission will be fragmented and asynchronized and will not permit the various dimensions of stimulus encoding to be transmitted together as a single event. Therefore, the available memory will not have been tagged with the idiosyncratic markers of emotion, timing, history, and so forth. that make it retrievable as a singular, episodic, experience bathed in its contextual surround. What is new in this proposal is that the absence of this joint mobilization of activity results in a very special kind of interhemispheric transmission loss—a loss of conscious experience of the otherwise available information. Elements, pieces, and even abstractions of the experience are conveyed, but they are retrievable only by the "semantic" or context-independent system, and do not permit conscious retrieval of the initial idiosyncratic and specific event that caused the memory.

This possibility is best exemplified by the amnesia that the patients had when the left hemisphere was confronted with a picture that had just been shown to the right hemisphere (Sergent, 1990). Sergent (1990) explains this effect by saying that only information about the picture which is categorical rather than perceptual is transferred subcortically. On the basis of just this categorical transfer, the patient is thought to be unable to tell whether the new picture is the same as the old. However, one would think that if what transferred was low-resolution or coded, the patients would say: "The previous picture was similar to the current picture." Or if only categorical information got across, one would think they would say: "I saw a queen but I do not know if it was this particular queen." Or they might volunteer that they had just seen a picture of some other rich person. What is unusual is that there is not even a memory of the categorical information that was available to the disconnected hemispheres moments before. The fragmented information was not properly indexed or tagged with those unique temporal and autobiographic elements which enable it to be retrieved as an episodic memory. What is being proposed is that the process by which events are episodically encoded is the very heart of the mechanism of consciousness.

It should be noted that the notion that the corpus callosum primarily synchronizes the activity between the two hemispheres so that thereafter they may conjointly influence other brain structures is consistent with callosal anatomy. The majority of fibers in the corpus callosum which connect associational areas are fine-caliber or unmyelinated. LaMantia and Rakiç (1990) have commented that such fibers seem best suited to convey tonic impulses between assemblies of neurons located in opposite hemispheres.

However, callosal anatomy also indicates that the fibers are of different sizes and degree of myelination, which means that conduction times will differ greatly (LaMantia and Rakiç, 1990). One would expect this to be incompatible with the posited role of the callosum in interhemispheric synchronization. But Somplinsky, Golumb, and Kleinfeld (1990) demonstrate by means of neural modeling that coupled oscillators can be reliably synchronized even if the conduction delays show a broad distribution and are not homogeneous across the network.

If one accepts the notion that the corpus callosum serves to synchronize the hemispheres, it suggests that certain evoked potential data have been misinterpreted. In commissure-intact persons, when a visual stimulus is restricted to one visual field, there is first a contralateral evoked potential in the contralateral hemisphere, and then there is a later, evoked potential in the hemisphere ipsilateral to the stimulus. The difference in time between the contralateral and ipsilateral evoked potentials has historically been taken to indicate the time that it takes for information to cross the callosum (the interhemispheric transmission time, IHTT).[2] It has been demonstrated that patients without a corpus callosum lack a normal ipsilateral visual evoked potential in the nonviewing hemisphere (Mangun et al., 1991; Rugg, Milner, and Lines, 1985). This lack of an ipsilateral response has been taken as proof that without a callosum the information is not transferred interhemispherically.

It can now be suggested that the evoked potential technique is inadequate because of its dependency upon synchronized changes in cell firing. Without the synchronizing influence of the callosum, information may be made available subcortically in a fragmented and desynchronized manner that cannot be picked up by evoked potential technology. The lack of a normal evoked potential may not indicate that the hemisphere ipsilateral to the stimulus lacks any access to the input; it simply may not be activated by that input in a synchronized way. For example, Rugg et al. (1985) point out that some ipsilateral evoked activity did occur in the early N160 component, and that the later ipsilateral potentials were *quite similar* to their contralateral counterparts. Similarly, Ringo, and O'Neill (1993) have shown within monkeys with split commissures and optic chiasm, that at least a few units of the inferomedial temporal cortex of the *isolated* hemisphere fire in a stimulus-specific way in response to a visual stimulus presented to the opposite hemisphere.

Conclusion   Corticocortical association pathways permit disparate regions of the the brain to be simultaneously active and to interact. Dissociations which result from the severing of pathways are due to a desynchronization of this attentional binding process rather than a lack of transfer of information in the traditional sense.

Hypothesis 3: The Underactivated State of the Nonviewing Hemisphere Causes a Kind of "Internal Neglect" and Disrupts Explicit Access to Otherwise Adequately Transferred Information

In this subsection it is argued that lack of explicit awareness of information that is implicitly available to the nonviewing hemisphere is not due (solely) to the quality of information made available to the nonviewing hemisphere, or to the fact that without the cerebral commissures, it is made available in a desynchronized way. The nonviewing hemisphere's lack of explicit access to information presented to the opposite hemisphere is also due to its underactivated state. This argument has several elements. The corpus callosum is part of a system that equilibrates the level of activation of the two hemispheres. Thus, after callosal lesions, the nonviewing hemisphere becomes underactivated and behaves in a manner which is analogous to the unilateral neglect syndrome. Therefore, "lack of explicit awareness," as a result of commissural section, is not due to the fact that subcortical structures can only process or "transfer" implicit information; lack of explicit awareness is due to an arousal imbalance which prevents the underactivated hemisphere from further operating upon inputs it receives. It cannot, so to speak, "attend" to the inputs which are available to it from other regions. As a result, the underactivated hemisphere cannot fuse the disparate elements made available asynchronously from diverse subcortical regions into a unified percept embedded in a rich episodic contextual surround. In the final portion of this subsection, it is argued that other symptoms of commissurotomy (such as mutism) can be explained in terms of arousal imbalance as well.

A Model of How the Corticocortical Commissures Are Important for Equilibration and Distribution of Activation between the Hemispheres

There have been a series of theorists who propose that the main function of the cerebral commissures is equilibration of activation between the hemispheres as opposed to transfer of information (cf. Kinsbourne, 1987a, 1988; Levy, 1985, 1990).[3] However, the most complete treatment of how an arousal imbalance, as a result of callosal transection produces disconnection symptomology was given by Guiard (1980) and Guiard and Requin (1978). Their explanation relied heavily upon the reasoning of Kinsbourne (1970, 1974) and Trevarthen (1974b).

In their 1978 paper, Guiard and Requin hypothesize that a unitary "attention-distribution center" (p. 393), located in a subcortical structure (e.g., the reticular formation) distributes attention between the two cortices, which are compared to peripheral computers. According to this model, the commissures serve a stabilizing function. Guiard (1980), following Kinsbourne (1974), assumes that the corpus callosum conveys primarily excitatory signals. This has since been demonstrated electrophysiologically by Lassonde (1986). These excitatory signals enable cortical modules in one hemisphere to "alert" homotopic modules in the other hemisphere. Without this alerting signal, one hemisphere is apt to be more aroused than the other, with the less aroused hemisphere being functionally asleep. Thus, Guiard argues, transfer of information occurs by means of brainstem routes, while the commissural system is the necessary mediator for the coordinated mobilization of the neuronal circuits located on opposite sides of the cortex (Guiard, 1980). Guiard then argues that many experiments which had previously been interpreted as demonstrating lack of information transfer can be reinterpreted as the effects of loss of callosal arousal. If, for example, the corpus callosum and optic chiasm of an animal are cut prior to unilateral training of one hemisphere, when subsequent testing reveals that the untrained hemisphere failed to learn the task, it is unclear whether it was because (a) the specific information had not been transferred across the corpus callosum or (b) the untrained hemisphere was not provided with a callosal alerting stimulus during the training. If the relevant portion of contralateral cortex had been, in effect, "asleep" during the training, then it may well be that any information sent to it by any route would not have been recorded there.

There is certainly good evidence that the corpus callosum (and probably the other forebrain commissures) are involved in the equilibration of arousal between the hemispheres. An increase in arousal in the hemisphere contralateral to a stimulus is typically accompanied by an inhibition of arousal in the opposite hemisphere, mediated at least in part by reciprocal inhibitory connections through the brainstem. For example, animal studies suggest that unilateral sensory stimulation not only produces facilitation of dopamine release in the contralateral substantia nigra (and ipsilateral caudate nucleus) but also inhibition of dopamine release in the ipsilateral substantia nigra (and contralateral caudate nucleus; Leviel et al. 1981). Evidence that suggests that, in rats, these neurochemical asymmetries are modulated by the corpus callosum has been provided by Glick et al. (1975). They have shown that this striatal dopamine asymmetry (and the orientational biases associated with them) were significantly exaggerated after anterior callosal sections. In addition to doubling the dopaminergic asymmetry, an asymmetry of striatal acetylcholine was induced. Overall levels of dopamine and acetylcholine were not changed. This suggests that the amount of central nervous system asymmetry is exaggerated when the modifying influence of the callosum is removed.

Sergent (1986) attempts to refute Guiard (1980) by arguing that in commissurotomized patients the hemisphere ipsilateral to the input is not really asleep. Sergent (1986) points to her experiments in which patients are able to integrate information from two distinct stimuli presented simultaneously, one to each hemisphere. She argues persuasively that there is no tendency for the information from one side of space to be "perceptually erased" or truly extinguished.

However, a careful reading of Guiard (1980) reveals that he is not only talking about neglect of external events, *he is referring to neglect of events projected to the underactive hemisphere by other regions of the brain*. In order to make the distinction clear, we will refer to this second kind of neglect as *internal neglect* to distinguish it from neglect of a side of space, which we will refer to as *sensory neglect*. In the following paragraphs it is argued that at least one form of the classic syndrome of unilateral neglect (caused by a lesion of the parietal lobe) is also a form of internal, not sensory, neglect, where inputs are ineffectively processed at some point after sensory reception.

Callosal Lesions Disrupt the Attentional Capacity of the Underactivated Hemisphere in a Manner Analogous to the Unilateral Neglect Syndrome: There Is "Internal Neglect" of Inputs after Sensory Reception

Our understanding of the classic syndrome of hemispatial neglect has undergone a very recent revision. One of the most popular theories as to the mechanism underlying hemispatial neglect was that there was a lack of intake of information from the leftmost side of space. The best representative for this view was Kinsbourne (1987b) who claimed that a right parietal lobe lesion disinhibited the left hemisphere which strongly pulled attention to the contralateral (right) side of space. This pull to the right resulted in lack of orientation and sensory pickup of materials on the left side of space. Kinsbourne made the critical contribution of indicating that neglect was a product of a disrupted equilibrium.

However, the emerging view of neglect is that it is an abnormality of processing of input *after* sensory reception: there is now evidence that inputs to the neglected field actually "get into" the central nervous system. It now seems that sensory inputs are underprocessed, as opposed to being occluded or truly neglected. Evidence that the neglected stimulus actually "gets into" the system is illustrated by Marshall and Halligan (1988). Patients were shown two pictures which were identical except for an unpleasant detail in the left corner. For example, two houses were presented which were identical except that the left side of one of the houses was on fire. When asked to explicitly compare the two houses, patients reported that the two pictures were identical. But when they were tested implicitly by asking which house they would prefer to live in, they reliably rejected the burning house even though they were unaware of the fire!

Other evidence that neglected material is actually processed is provided by McGlinchey-Berroth et al. (1993). They have shown that pictures presented to the left visual field were "neglected" as indicated by (a) the patient's report of unawareness of a stimulus, and (b) the patient's chance performance when asked to discriminate between new and old pictures. Yet these pictures must have been processed at a semantic level since they "primed" lexical decisions with reference to a word presented centrally after the picture presentation. Thus, patients shown a picture of a cat were unaware of having seen it, yet presentation facilitated a subsequent decision that a centrally presented letter string (e.g., "d-o-g") was in fact a word.

Another set of behavioral data suggests, once again, that neglected input actually "gets into" the system normally, but it is how the system operates upon it that is abnormal. Prather and colleagues (1992) have demonstrated that right parietal lobe lesions result in a deficit in integration, not detection. The neglect patients had no difficulty directing attention to single-feature targets. They had specific difficulty searching for conjunctions among distractors consisting of the two elements which together would constitute the conjunctive stimulus. Thus neglect did not seem to affect automatic detection of features. Instead, the patients were deficient in conjoining or integrating information after attention had been focused on the features. They lacked the ability to use "selective attention" as the glue to bind these features.

In what sense do callosal lesions induce a kind of internal neglect? The most dramatic example of internal neglect in commissurotomized patients was the beautiful experiment by Levy, Trevarthen, and Sperry (1972), which used chimeric stimuli of faces and objects. Split-brain patients never noticed that the left and right sides of the figures differed. They reported either the right or the left side of the picture depending upon whether their answer was in words (right side reported) or by means of pointing (left side reported). The question that Levy et al. addressed was whether the patients had ignored the input from the other side or were unaware of it, even though on some level the patients had registered the other half of the stimulus. To test this, they interrupted the patient on a few trials before a pointing response could occur, removed the array, and asked unexpectedly for a verbal description. It was thought that this procedure would direct attention to information held in the left hemisphere, and indeed patients then supplied a description of the face projected to the left hemisphere. When the array was replaced and the patients were asked to pick a matching choice, the face projected to the right hemisphere was picked (and vice versa for other combinations). Thus, both stimuli were encoded, and the neglect occurred some time after sensory reception such that only one of the two percepts was available to consciousness at any one moment.

Similarly, Reuter-Lorenz, Nazawa, and Hughes (1991) presented bilaterally redundant stimuli to split-brain patients and asked them to indicate whether they detected one vs. two targets. There was a significant tendency for the patients to neglect left-sided targets. Targets which were neglected during double trials nonetheless facilitated reaction times. What was surprising about their finding was that the split-brain patients benefited from the redundancy of the signals presented to separate hemispheres even more than did normal subjects.

In fact, it is now becoming clear that unilateral neglect is a common sequela of callosectomy. In the past, gross symptoms of neglect after callosal surgery were underestimated. They were thought to be restricted to the early postoperative period and were assumed to be a temporary sequela of surgical compression of the right medial frontal and medial parietal lobes (Joynt, 1977; Plourde and Sperry, 1984; Wilson et al., 1977). However, there are now several reports of persistent unilateral neglect after partial callosal lesions due to bleeding or ischemia (Goldenberg, 1986; Heilman, Bowers, and Watson, 1984).

Beyond evidence that callosal lesions can induce neglect, there is now considerable evidence that sectioning of the callosum can *reinstate* neglect. This has been shown in animals and humans who had previously recovered from a lesion which had induced neglect (rats: Crowne et al., 1988; monkeys: Watson et al., 1984; man after sectioning of the entire forebrain commissures: Novelly and Lifrak, 1985). Indeed, I recently saw a case of a young man who suffered a right parietal hematoma in infancy and had a callosectomy in adolescence. One of his most persistent postsurgical symptoms was an unawareness of a soccer ball when it approached from the left side. He got hit by the ball so often that they had him manage the team rather than play.

Thus, what is being argued is that, after callosal section, the underactivated hemisphere is rendered inattentive in a manner similar to that which occurs after a right parietal lesion. From this perspective, the corpus callosum is critical for regulating the distribution of activation between the hemispheres.

It should be noted that there are other symptoms associated with commissurotomy that can be explained by an arousal imbalance causing one hemisphere to be underactivated. This suggests that the underactivation can account for a wide range of symptoms. These symptoms are now reviewed.

Other Disconnection Symptoms that Occur in Callosectomized Patients as a Result of an Underactivation of One Hemisphere There are a variety of symptoms seen in split-brain patients that can also be accounted for in terms of one hemisphere being underactivated. For example, split-brain patients have an exceptionally sluggish mental set; one hemisphere becomes aroused through some stimulus condition and it is very hard, sometimes impossible, for the inactive hemisphere to be made active. For example, Sperry (1962) mentioned that "occasionally the commissurotomized patient may become so absorbed in a right-hemisphere task that speech and left-hemisphere functions are temporarily depressed to the extent that one questions whether *consciousness may not be shifted entirely to the working hemisphere*" (p. 105, emphasis added).

Indeed, mutism after callosal section may be the most extreme example of an arousal imbalance that disrupts performance. Sullivan and McKeever (1985) point out that one variable which predicts whether a patient will be mute after callosal surgery is whether the hemisphere which controls speech differs from the hemisphere which controls the preferred hand. There were three cases for which the hemisphere which controlled speech and the preferred hand were discordant. Two patients were left-handed and left hemisphere–dominant for speech; one patient was right-handed and right hemisphere–dominant for speech. These discordant cases had either a severe (n = 2) or a substantial loss (n = 1) of spontaneous speech. In contrast, the three cases that were concordant for speech and handedness had normal speech post surgery. Postsurgical loss of speech in patients discordant for speech control and hand preference was also reported in two cases of complete callosal section by Wilson's method (Censori et al., 1989). Both patients were left-handed and were presumed to have left hemisphere speech; both were akinetic and mute after surgery. A somewhat similar finding was reported by Sussman et al. (1983) in which akinesia and mutism were found to be correlated with mixed hand dominance. At least in the cases reported by Sullivan and McKeever, one can be sure that the mutism was not secondary to damage of the frontal regions during surgery. Their cases were all two-stage surgeries. The mutism only occurred after the second stage, which was transection of the posterior portion of the callosum.

What especially points to an arousal imbalance explanation for the mutism is that an attentional manipulation ameliorated the speech problem. Sullivan and McKeever (1985) reported that when the patient palpated an object with the hand contralateral to the hemisphere that controls speech, speech was improved. An alternative interpretation of these data is that these discordant patients really had bihemispheric speech control, and that without a corpus callosum some kind of interhemispheric coordination of the output process was disrupted. However, Sullivan and McKeever (1985) concluded that none of their discordant patients had bihemispheric control of speech on the basis of interfield differences in visual and tactile testing. Nonetheless, even if the mutism was a case of conflict between two speech centers, the fact that using the nondominant hand improved speech suggests that the disruption was fundamentally attributable to an arousal imbalance.

Another example of a symptom which can be explained as underactivation of a hemisphere was reported by Trevarthen (1974a,b) about one commissurotomy patient (N.G.). An object situated in the right visual field was reported as having disappeared as soon as N.G. oriented leftward to move her left hand over to the object to mark it. This perceptual erasure may have been due to conflict between the side of space the object was on and the need to move the opposite hand. This would be analogous to the conflict which occurred in the commissurotomy patients between hand preference and speech control.

The final symptom that can also be explained as underactivation of a hemisphere is the change that occurs in left ear extinction of commissurotomized patients during dichotic listening in response to changes in task demands. Peschstedt (1986) demonstrated that as task difficulty is increased (by increasing the number of digits to be remembered), there is increased suppression of verbal material presented to the left ear. A dynamic explanation of this effect is that the verbal left hemisphere is even further aroused by the increased verbal demand and that there is reciprocal inhibition of right hemisphere processing at the level of the brainstem.

Conclusion Commissurotomized patients display a form of internal neglect that is marked by an abnormality of processing of input after sensory reception, in which the less active hemisphere tends not to effectively process inputs to it (a) directly from the contralateral side of space or (b) indirectly from the opposite hemisphere. These underprocessed inputs are not consciously perceived. Hence, the nonviewing hemisphere has only implicit but not explicit access to information restricted to the viewing hemisphere.

CORTICOCORTICAL PATHWAYS THAT CONNECT REGIONS WITHIN A HEMISPHERE HAVE THE SAME STRUCTURAL AND FUNCTIONAL CHARACTERISTICS AS THOSE THAT CONNECT REGIONS BETWEEN HEMISPHERES

Why It Is Anatomically Reasonable to Propose that Corticocortical Pathways All Have a Similar Function Irrespective of whether They Are between or within Hemispheres

Intra- and interhemispheric corticocortical pathways have similar developmental origins. Indeed, Innocenti (1986) points out that the neurons whose projections form the corpus callosum are the same as those that form intracortical fiber pathways. Trevarthen (1990) notes that during the late stages of fetal development, the two populations of fiber pathways are differentiated from the same basic stem association cells through selective loss of either their between-hemisphere collaterals or their within-hemisphere collaterals. In fact, there are some neurons which retain both between- and within-hemisphere collaterals. These are the so-called heterotopic callosal neurons which often take the form of collaterals of within-hemisphere connections (Hedreen and

Yin, 1981). (Wherever the within-hemisphere fiber terminates, the callosal collateral terminates in the homologous region of the opposite hemisphere. This assures that the unilateral region of origin communicates bilaterally with the region of termination. Cook [1986] refers to these connections as "symmetrical heterotopic connections.")

Inter- and intrahemispheric projections also have largely the same regional distribution. Fleschig, whose work was popularized by the writing of Geschwind (1965), pointed out that corticocortical connections occur between association areas, which, according to Barbas (1986), are areas that have cytoarchitectonically relatively undifferentiated layering. The primary sensory and motor areas are largely without corticocortical projections.

Conclusion   The intra- and intercortical pathways are so similar in origin and structure that they should have similar functions.

Is a Loss of Explicit but Not Implicit Access to Information a Symptom of Intra- as well as Interhemispheric Corticocortical Pathway Section?

It was argued earlier that the interhemispheric commissures are critical for equilibrating activation levels between two regions or synchronizing activity, or both, thereby permitting outputs to be "bound" into a single event memory (see above). The next step is to propose that the within-hemisphere corticocortical pathways have the same equilibrating and synchronizing functions. Indeed, Kinsbourne (1987a) has recently argued that all disconnection phenomenology can be viewed as secondary to an imbalance in activation rather than the absence of transfer of information.

There is at least one "within-hemisphere" syndrome which is often caused by corticocortical fiber damage and is somewhat reminiscent of the disconnection symptomology manifested by commissurotomized patients. The syndrome is conduction aphasia which is thought to result from damage to the arcuate fasciculus, a corticocortical pathway from Wernicke's area to Broca's area. Whether conduction aphasia requires arcuate fasciculus damage is controversial (cf. Mendez and Benson, 1985, for a discussion), but it is clear that a small lesion that is confined to the arcuate fasciculus is sufficient to cause conduction aphasia (Tanabe et al., 1987). The cardinal symptom of conduction aphasia is the inability to repeat what is heard, even though language production is relatively fluent and without dysarthria, and aural comprehension is fundamentally intact (Benson, 1979). Geschwind (1965) argued that damage to the fiber tract prevented the auditory information analyzed in Wernicke's area from being "transferred" to Broca's area for repetition.

A moment's reflection reveals that the syndrome is odd. Patients can paraphrase what has been said to them and converse normally in response to auditory input. This leads to the suggestion that detailed information about what was heard may be available on an implicit but not explicit level. The inability to repeat what has just been said may be due to a situation-specific underactivation of Broca's area by Wernicke's area (due to the lack of activation along the arcuate fasciculus), rather than lack of transfer per se.

Measures of metabolic activity in conduction aphasia suggest just such a situation-specific underactivation of Broca's area. Demeurisse and Capon (1991) found that during a naming task, ten patients with conduction aphasia showed less of an increase of blood flow to Broca's area than normal patients. This was a task-specific lack of activation of Broca's area, and computed tomography (CT) scans revealed that Broca's area was physically intact. In contrast, Broca's region is not invariably underaroused when metabolism is assessed in conduction aphasia patients at rest, in a nonlinguistic context (Kempler et al., 1988). Thus, under conditions when the subject initiates his or her own speech, there is sufficient activation of Broca's area to subserve fluent output. But under conditions when the patient's speech is an attempt to echo that which was just heard, Broca's area is insufficiently activated by Wernicke's area to permit word-by-word repetition. The activation is sufficient to permit general themes to be repeated. This interpretation of conduction aphasia would be supported if conduction aphasic patients both failed the following recognition task and succeeded at the following priming task. Patients would hear a sentence and then would be asked to pick which one of two written sentences match it verbatim; the two sentences would convey the same meaning, only differing in word selection. In contrast, if these patients could prime implicitly to a word that they did not recognize, one could conclude that they had lost explicit access to the information but retained access to it both on a categorical level and on an implicit level.

Conclusion   The intra- and intercortical pathways probably have the same synchronizing and equilibrating functions.

IF INTRA- AND INTERCORTICOCORTICAL PATHWAYS ARE SO SIMILAR, WHY IS INTERHEMISPHERIC INTEGRATION DIFFICULT, EVEN WHEN THE COMMISSURES ARE INTACT?

In the Commissure-intact Brain, Interhemispheric Integration Is Inferior to Intrahemispheric Integration

In the intact brain, when both commissural and subcortical mechanisms are operating, interhemispheric integration is nonetheless deficient compared to intrahemispheric performance. Thus performance when information needs to be integrated between the hemispheres is generally inferior to when information is restricted to either the left or the right hemisphere, even when one considers the average of the peformances during the two unihemispheric conditions. For example, recognition of complex random shapes or words is harder when the sample and target are successively presented to different hemispheres than when they are successively presented to a single hemisphere (Lordahl et al., 1965; Banich and Shenker, in press; Dimond, Gibson, and Gazzaniga, 1972; Leiber, 1982; and Coney and MacDonald, 1988).

A relative inferiority of the between-hemisphere condition is also seen for transfer of training tasks. In transfer of training tasks, one hemisphere is trained at a task and the other (untrained) hemisphere is tested for savings. Bilateral "engrams" are inferred if the untrained hemisphere benefits from the indirect experience. Bogen (1990) reviews a handful of studies that have demonstrated unilateral engrams localized to the hemisphere that was directly trained. But as a rule, bilateral engrams are inferred (Butler, 1968; Doty, Ringo, and Lewine, 1986; Doty, Lewine, and Ringo, 1985; Hamilton, 1977), although they are almost invariably asymmetric with the "better" engram on the side that was directly trained. (Cf. Ringo and O'Neill, 1993, for a series of experiments which induce a unihemispheric reversible amnesia by means of tetanization of the medial temporal lobe in monkeys. Ringo combines unilateral stimulation with lesions of the optic tract and the commissures to make inferences about the locus of memories and their strength.)

The notion that a symmetric "carbon-copy" engram is not made in the nonviewing hemisphere is reminiscent of Sperry's (1962) notion that the function of the callosum is to enable each hemisphere to provide "supplementary" and "complementary" information about events in the opposite hemisphere. Sperry does not comment on how interhemispheric connections, which primarily connect homotopic areas, could be involved in creating such asymmetric engrams.

There Are Exceptional Circumstances under which Interhemispheric Is as Good as Intrahemispheric Integration

When Information Can Be Accessed without Conscious Awareness
For most interhemispheric tasks, the subject is either explicitly told to cross-compare information projected to separate hemispheres or the behavior which must be executed requires a specific recollection of some prior event. But there is another class of studies where interhemispheric integration can be inferred on the basis of times when subjects inadvertently and erroneously use information projected to one hemisphere to make decisions about information projected to the other hemisphere. For example, we have devised a within- vs. between-hemisphere version of the Stroop task. A color is presented to one side of space at the same time as a word that refers to a different color name is presented to either the same or the opposite side of space. The task is to name the color as quickly as possible; the Stroop effect is the slowing of naming which occurs during those trials when an interfering word is presented. The surprising result is that in commissure-intact subjects, the Stroop effect is as strong when the color and the discordant word are presented in separate hemispheres as when they are presented to the same hemisphere (Liederman, 1986b; N. Weekes and E. Zaidel, personal communication, July 12, 1992). Similarly, in a different task, subjects were shown a tachistoscopic

display of four trigrams and their task was to name the words. The four words were either presented to a single hemisphere or they were distributed so that each hemisphere received two words. Occasionally subjects named words which were an inadvertent interfield integration of separate words on a screen. These were "blends" such as the words *fat* and *dog* being inadvertently blended to create the word *fog*; blends were made from elements presented to separate fields as often as they were made from elements presented to the same field (Liederman, 1986a). Once again, when information between the hemispheres is shared inadvertently, unconsciously and implicitly there is no interhemispheric integration deficit.

An exception to this exception might be Banich and Belger's (1991) experiment which they interpret as a demonstration that interhemispheric access to implicit memory *is* deficient as compared to intrahemispheric access. Their finding was that independent estimates of line length, without feedback as to their accuracy, are more stable when the line is repeatedly projected to the same hemisphere than when the judgments are made alternately by either hemisphere (Banich and Belger, 1991). Banich and Belger have argued that this demonstrates that even implicit interhemispheric access is disrupted. They are quick to point out that the instability of the interhemispheric estimates is not due to one hemisphere being biased or more accurate than the other. This study would have been more satisfying as a demonstration of implicit memory or learning if some evidence of actual learning had been provided, for example, if the opportunity to make repeated estimates made the later estimates more accurate than the earlier estimates.

When Comparisons Can Be Made on a Superordinate rather than Subordinate Level   When information can be cross-compared on a superordinate rather than subordinate level inter- and intrahemispheric performances are roughly equivalent. By means of a delayed recognition paradigm Kleinman and Little (1973) found two different patterns of interhemispheric performance depending upon the kind of trigram they presented to the hemispheres for cross-comparison. When trigrams with low association values were used, those presented to separate hemispheres were recognized less frequently than trigrams presented serially to the same hemisphere. However, when trigrams with high association values were used (and therefore could be compared on a more abstract level) inter- and intrahemispheric performances were equivalent. Similarly, Liederman, Merola, and Martinez (1985) demonstrated that decisions as to whether two words were in the same *category* were performed as well between as within hemispheres.

Structural and Dynamic Factors Can Account for the Relative Interhemispheric Deficit

A Structural Factor: The Paucity of Interhemispheric Connections
Despite the similarities between inter- and intrahemispheric corticocortical

pathways, there is one important structural difference that may make inter-hemispheric integration more difficult than intrahemispheric integration. There is a relative paucity of inter- as compared to intrahemispheric cortical connections despite the great size of the corpus callosum. Bogen (1990) has pointed out that there are at least 10 billion neurons within a hemisphere and each has connections with at least 100 other neurons. He estimates that only 800 million of these connections are with the other side of the brain via the corpus callosum (and his estimate is probably on the high side). Based on somewhat similar estimates, Ringo et al. (1992) conclude that only 2% of the connections within a hemisphere are interhemispheric projections to the opposite hemisphere.[4]

Cook (1986) argues that if we accept Szentagothai's (1978) notion that medium- and long-range fibers make point-to-point connections which are between *columns* of 50-μm width, rather than between specific neurons, then there are sufficient callosal fibers in man to permit one afferent and one efferent connection between pairs of homotopic columns in each hemisphere. Cook (1986) estimates that each of these "functional" columns would contain 100 to 1000 cortical neurons. Thus, there is simply less intercortical connectivity between than within hemispheres and this could render interhemispheric integration more difficult.

A Dynamic Factor: The Vulnerability of Interhemispheric Processing to Asymmetric Fluctuations in Arousal   One of the consequences of the paucity of connections is that even in the intact brain, the two hemispheres can sustain somewhat more independent arousal levels than adjacent regions within a single hemisphere. Very large disparaties in arousal should not occur with the callosum intact except under special circumstances. These special circumstances consist of stimulus conditions which render the untrained or nonviewing hemisphere either too busy or too minimally alert to adequately subserve interhemispheric integration. The final circumstance is when the two hemispheres are activated by somewhat different emotions.

The importance of the state of the untrained hemisphere was demonstrated by Hicks, Frank, and Kinsbourne (1982). Subjects learned a sequence of finger movements with one hand/hemisphere while the other hand/hemisphere was either occupied (the hand was gripping a table leg) or idle (the hand was resting). A moderate interhemispheric savings effect was seen when the contralateral hand was resting, but no savings effect was found when the hand was occupied. In a similar vein, Lepore and colleagues (1982) argue that the excellent interhemispheric savings effects seen in most artificial laboratory tests involve procedures which induce deafferentiation of the nonviewing hemisphere (in animals by means of section of the optic chiasm and patching of the eye ipsilateral to the stimulus; in humans by means of unilateral tachistoscopic stimulation). These relatively deafferent cells of the nonviewing hemisphere may be extremely receptive to any stimulation from the opposite hemisphere. In contrast, the authors argue, in the normal state, input from the callosum must compete with direct thalamocortical input which will be dominant and occasionally even incompatible.

There is a second set of circumstances during which interhemispheric processing is vulnerable to asymmetric fluctuations in hemispheric arousal, i.e., when one hemisphere is favored for processing or otherwise maintained at a high level of arousal for an extended time. Under such circumstances, there is an activation imbalance, and the underutilized hemisphere becomes refractory. For example, when subjects repeatedly performed a task during a session that selectively matched the processing style of only one hemisphere, normal, commissure-intact subjects showed disconnection symptomology when attempting to direct a response from the underaroused, nonperforming hemisphere. Landis, Assal, and Perret (1979) and Landis, Graves, and Goodglass (1981) required subjects to perform tasks associated with either a left or right hemisphere advantage. Subjects indicated their decisions by pressing a button. Sometimes subjects tried to verbally correct their button-pressing errors. The investigators noted that verbal (left hemisphere–controlled) self-corrections of a task requiring primarily left hemisphere processing were accurate. However, verbal self-corrections of a task requiring primarily right hemisphere processing were random. Two questions spring to mind: Is verbal self-monitoring at chance levels even at the beginning of the right hemisphere task before the left hemisphere has had a protracted period of underactivation? Similarly, if the two types of tasks, verbal and nonverbal, were alternated between trials (thereby preventing the induction of a strong hemispheric bias) would verbal self-monitoring of the right hemisphere task be accurate?

There is a third context within which interhemispheric integration may be diminished due to asymmetric fluctuations in hemispheric arousal or emotional state. In the intact brain, the amygdaloid nuclei lack any major interhemispheric commissural connections (Demeter, Rosene, and Van Hoesen, 1990). Thus, the aspects of emotionality that are mediated by the amygdaloid nuclei may occur in the two hemispheres somewhat independently. If the two hemispheres are then differentially aroused, this could form the basis of memories which are stored in somewhat different emotional surrounds. These state-dependent memories would result in interhemispheric deficits in access to stored material whenever the two hemispheres were momentarily in different emotional states. Such state-dependent incompatibilities would be less likely between regions within a single hemisphere than between hemispheres.

Conclusions In both commissurotomized and commissure-intact subjects, inter- is inferior to intrahemispheric integration, except for tasks that can be performed without conscious awareness, or on an abstract or categorical level. For there to be so much similarity between the interhemispheric integration profiles of persons with or without cerebral commissures implies that the inferiority of interhemispheric integraton is largely due to extracommissural factors (i.e., dynamic and systems-level factors). Even more important, as is discussed in the next section, it suggests that the interhemispheric systems that commissure-sectioned and commissure-intact subjects have in common (i.e., subcortical pathways) may govern more of the normal interhemispheric integration that can be done on an automatic level than is generally assumed.

THREE MECHANISMS OF INTEGRATION OF INFORMATION BETWEEN REMOTE CORTICAL REGIONS

In this section the entire issue of how information is integrated between remote cortical regions is reexamined. As stated in introductory paragraphs, three sorts of integration will be described: direct transfer, third-party convergence, and nonconvergent temporal integration.

Direct Transfer

Direct transfer assumes that the products of processing of one area are transferred directly to a second region where they are integrated with that region's processing and stored. This results in duplication of information across the two regions. It has historically been assumed that this is the major function of the corticocortical pathways.

As was mentioned above, Ringo and O'Neill (1993) have provided evidence that when input is restricted to one hemisphere, the second hemisphere has its own store of that memory. He demonstrated this in monkeys by restricting input to one hemisphere (say the left) and then testing the opposite (right) hemisphere for knowledge of that input while the left hemisphere was temporally out of commission owing to medial temporal lobe tetatinization. Although the nonviewing hemisphere's performance was inferior to the viewing hemisphere's performance, it was above chance. After the commissures were sectioned, performance fell to chance levels. Ringo seems to assume that this task was shared interhemispherically by means of the process that is being referred to as direct transfer.

Third-party Convergence

"Third-party" (Goldman-Rakiç, 1988) convergence assumes that two or more regions feed forward the products of their processing to a third convergence area, but they do not share information directly with one another. In this second kind of integration, the role of the corticocortical pathways is to synchronize the outputs of these two regions to the third convergence area. For example, the parietal, prefrontal, limbic, and temporal areas are unified by a joint projection to the medial pulvinar nucleus (Balaydier and Mauguiere, 1987). This may be a feed-forward integration area for these disparate cortical regions. A somewhat different kind of integration may involve the claustrum. Tigges and Tigges (1985) review data from their work with squirrel monkeys. They note that the claustrum has reciprocal projections to areas 17, 18, 19, and MT. Although individual neurons connect with only one visual area, claustral cells projecting to different visual areas are intermingled (Norita, 1983). Thus, at the level of the claustrum, there may be local interactions between back-projections from disparate visual regions of the cortex. According to Tigges and Tigges (1985), the fact that claustrocortical fibers terminate in layer IV suggests that the claustrum projection participates in the early processing of visual information, perhaps after it has been influenced by these "higher" areas. Similarly, Goldman-Rakiç (1988) reviews her own data in which she has found, by means of double-labeling techniques in monkeys, that the principal sulcus of the frontal lobe and the posterior parietal cortex are mutually interconnected with as many as *15 other cortical areas*, and most of these projections are reciprocal.

All of the aforementioned examples are of intrahemispheric convergence to a third-party subcortical or cortical zone. In terms of third-party interhemispheric convergence it is reasonable to suppose that such zones occur in the brainstem to which the two hemispheres could each project.

Nonconvergent Temporal Integration

In nonconvergent temporal integration, the role of the corticocortical pathways is to synchronize the outputs of two or more remote regions and enable them to feed forward, independently, but synchronously, to a variety of other areas. Output from these two regions initiates a synchronized distribution of patterned activation. This forward march of patterned activation can influence relatively independent systems for the control of behavior in a parallel, but synchronized way. Therefore, in nonconvergent synchronization there is only temporal integration. There is no grandfather convergence zone and no region where traces of the two regions of activity are stored as a compound, single engram.

As an example of two regions that might operate primarily by means of nonconvergent temporal integration one can point to the dorsal and ventral visual systems. The relative independence of the dorsal and ventral streams of processing within the visual system has been pointed out repeatedly; there are few connections between these two systems (Livingstone and Hubel, 1988). What is being proposed is that for many behaviors, these two systems may not need to communicate directly. This is not to say that the two systems do not operate at all in terms of third-party convergence, for this must occur. For example, both project to the frontal lobes, and it is possible that they interact with one another at that level by means of local circuits. This interaction would be to affect some kind of output process rather than to create an "integrated" representation for storage or further "processing" by other brain regions.

What is being argued is that they may quite often operate by means of nonconvergent temporal integration, simply by influencing relatively independent behaviors. Indeed, Goodale and Milner (1992) have put forth the provocative notion that the dorsal and ventral streams of visual information processing subserve entirely different action systems. They suggest that "the set of object descriptions that permit identification and recognition may be computed independently of the set of descriptions that allow an observer to shape the hand appropriately to pick up an object" (p. 20). The ventral stream of projections to the inferotemporal cortex is the neural substrate for visual perception, whereas the dorsal stream to the posterior parietal region mediates the sensorimotor processing which underlies visually guided movements directed at such objects. To support their view they point to a patient with Balint's syndrome (Jakobson et al., 1991). Balint's syndrome disrupts the dorsal system since it is caused by bilateral damage to the parietal cortex. The patient had adequate object perception but had an impairment in the ability to use information about size, shape, and orientiation of an object to control the hand and fingers during a grasping movement. Therefore, information that is available for object identification and description was unavailable to direct movement. In contrast, a visual agnostic patient, with somewhat diffuse damage including ventral stream regions, showed accurate guidance of hand and finger movements directed toward objects even though the patient could not recognize the objects. In summary, in the normal brain, the dorsal and ventral systems are capable of controlling behavior relatively independently, and need not converge. They may need to be synchronized but they do not necessarily need to be integrated at a single point of convergence. This is not to say that that the two systems do not interact, for there are many points of interconnection between components of the system (Goodale and Milner, 1992), and these are likely to be involved in the synchronization process. But it seems unlikely that a region will be discovered that consists of a map "where" the object is superimposed on "what" the object is. Synchronization may be the best way to get independent maps to cohere.

This general point is made by Kinsbourne (1987a):

The experience of the moment (the event) is represented by a distributed but specifically configured pattern of neuronal excitation across wide areas of cortex. It would be the pattern as a whole, rather than some bystanding area that observes it, that generates the experience and initiates the decisions. The neurons that fire in concert during specifically patterned activation need not be conceived to be interconnected while doing so. Instead, they might fire in parallel to yield an output the stochastic characteristics of which exert the required control over some component of behavior (p. 425).

Indeed, Kinsbourne (1987a) challenges the notion that intersensory integration occurs in association zones. He points to cerebral blood flow data by Lassen and Roland (1983). In that work, regions of cortical activation were observed when a subject successively attended to a stimulus via one of three modalities, and this compared to the distribution of activation when the subject attended to the stimulus through all three modalities simultaneously. Kinsbourne points out that the same regions were activated under both circumstances, and there was no additional activation in so-called convergence or association regions (such as the supramarginal gyrus) when the subject had the polysensory experience.

Interhemispheric Integration of Categorical Information or Item-specific Information That Can be Accessed Only Implicitly May be Mediated by Subcortical Systems to a Greater Extent Than is Generally Assumed

What has been argued throughout this chapter is that subcortical pathways are adequate for the interhemispheric integration of (a) categorical information or (b) context-independent, fragmented information which can be accessed only implicitly. This can be accomplished either by third-party convergence, where the convergence zone is subcortical, or by direct transfer where the transfer is multi- rather than monosynaptic. Third-party convergence will not be normal, however, because information from the two hemispheres will not be synchronously forwarded to the convergence zone. Direct transfer will not be normal because of the relatively smaller ratio of subcortical to cortical fibers, and because such routes are multisynaptic and this would slow processing and might lead to information distortion.

One should not overemphasize, however, the inadequacy of subcortical interhemispheric integration. First, Cook (1986) points out that convergence is the rule in sensory systems, and that it does not necessarily imply a loss of topographic information. Cook reminds us that "the retina is known to have approximately 126 million rods and cones, the optic tract carries all of its information along a tract of only 3 million fibers. At striate cortex, this information is again expanded over a cortical region estimated to have upwards of 20 million cortical columns" (p. 72). Hence the visual system involves considerable convergence of information. In addition, just because the direction of information flow is from cortex to a subcortical area does not mean that it is a "many-to-one" mapping. As Sjenowski and Churchland (1990) point out, there are ten times as many projections from visual cortex back to lateral geniculate nucleus as there are forward projections.

Second, with reference to the issue of slowness, it should be noted that many callosal fibers are unmyelinated, and according to Ringo et al. (1992) could have transmission times as slow as 300 ms. It is conceivable that myelinated fibers that travel subcortically could be faster than that.

Indeed, Guiard (1980) claims that there has been entirely too much emphasis on "horizontalist" (corticocortical) pathways and that instead most integration is apt to occur "vertically" via subcortical mechanisms. Many theorists agree. Perhaps the most prominent is Karl Pribram, who wrote: "The hierarchical aspects of visual processing can be as readily attributed to systems of cortical-subcortical loops as to the operations of a transcortical mechanism." (Pribram, 1986, p. 534). Pribram's (1986) claim stems from the following paradox: lesions of inferotemporal cortex have lasting effects on visual discrimination, whereas complete removals of the prestriate cortex do not (Pribram, Spinnelli, and Reitz, 1969). Pribram (1986) argues that since there are no known direct inputs to the inferotemporal cortex from primary visual cortex, if information processing is by stages, along a corticocortical route from 17 to 18 to 19 to 37, how does the inferotemporal cortex receive the visual input, when the go-between stage of processing via prestriate cortex has been eliminated? Pribram suggests that the input is subcortical: either the lateral geniculate nucleus sends collaterals directly to the inferotemporal cortex, or input from the geniculate reaches the inferotemporal cortex via the pulvinar nucleus. Pribram reminds us that each of these pathways would still be more direct than the multisynaptic route from 17 to 18 to 19 to 37. Indeed, Pribram points out that despite extensive prestriate and inferotemporal resections, callosectomy, and chiasm and visual tract sections (in one combination or another), there are always some monkeys that recover the ability to make visual discriminations! Pribram concludes that there is a hierarchy of *precortical* visual mechanisms, and that the cortex adds finer grain and enables "reflective awareness of the resultants of the process."

Kornhuber back in 1974 also criticized the historically popular notion that corticocortical pathways mediate an intracortical reflex arc analogous to spinal reflexes, with cortical sensory areas inducing movements via projections to motor areas. Perhaps the most famous champion of the corticocortical reflex was Geschwind (1965) who explained various "disconnection syndromes," such as the repetition deficit of conduction aphasia, as a lack of transfer of auditory signals from Wernicke's area to Broca's area due to damage of a corticocortical pathway (the arcuate fasciculus). Kornhuber cautions that both Broca's and Wernicke's areas have direct access to the basal ganglia and (via the pons) to the cerebellum, and that each of these structures has been implicated in movement and speech disorders. Thus, Kornhuber advocates for a cortical-subcortical loop, in which cortical activity is transformed into spatiotemporal motor patterns by subcortical generators, such as the basal ganglia and the cerebellum (cf. Glickstein [1990] for an updated version of this viewpoint).

Similarly, Penfield back in 1950 remarked on how cortical removals could be made with impunity around Broca's and Wernicke's areas, suggesting to him that the mechanism that is responsible for the coordination of these highly specialized centers must utilize subcortical projection pathways rather than transcortical association paths.

Interhemispheric Integration of Item-specific Information which Needs to be Accessible on an Explicit (Conscious) Level Seems Uniquely Dependent on Commissural Pathways

It seems likely that item-specific information is not transferred from one hemisphere to the other, but is instead integrated by synchronization (i.e., nonconvergent temporal integration). It is being argued that subcortical systems cannot adequately mediate the required synchronization. This was shown in cats, in which sectioning of the corpus callosum was sufficient to desynchronize the two V1 areas, indicating that subcortical inputs to the two hemispheres were not sufficient for the establishment of synchronization (Engel et al., 1991).

Even within a Single Hemisphere, the Ventral System May Rely More on Synchronization than the Dorsal System, and This May Explain why Item-specific Information Requires Synchronization

It has been argued throughout this chapter that the aspect of interhemispheric integration that is disrupted after commissurotomy is that which involves sharing item-specific identity. It is interesting to speculate that the ventral visual system, which processes identity information, may rely more heavily upon interhemispheric synchronization than the portions of the visual system dealing with nonidentity information (e.g., localization). Identity information may require integration across broader regions within a hemisphere *before* it can be integrated between hemispheres. As has been argued earlier, in order to remember a stimulus in its full contextual surround, the dimensions of the stimulus must be bound into an "object perception" and this object perception must be linked with emotional and temporal cues to place it in an autobiographic frame. This complex, spatiotemporal pattern of activation requires multiregional synchronization of activation within the hemisphere that receives the stimulus. Then this entire multiregional spatiotemporal pattern must be integrated with the opposite hemisphere. It is being suggested that it is this kind of integration which is uniquely dependent upon the synchronizing influence of the cerebral hemispheres. Indeed, this would match Goodale and Milner's (1992) recent conjecture that an intact ventral system is a prerequisite to conscious awareness. Thus, it is being suggested that without commissural fibers to integrate the two ventral systems, identity information conveyed to one hemisphere may be accessible only on an unconscious level. What will be available consciously will only be general or categorical information about the stimulus, not detailed identity information.

In contrast, activity associated with stimulus localization, which is computed primarily by the dorsal system, may be readily integrated interhemispherically by asynchronous subcortical mechanisms, and may be able to adequately govern behavior even though the identity of the object being localized is not conscious. Goodale and Milner (1992) have pointed out that brain-damaged individuals, such as those with blindsight, can perform stimulus localization tasks without any conscious awareness of the stimulus to which they are responding. Similarly, split-brain patients are able to respond with one hemisphere/output system to information restricted to the other hemisphere, without the nonviewing hemisphere being fully conscious of the exact identity of the stimulus to which it is responding.

CONCLUSIONS

Split-brain symptomology is not simply due to a lack of transfer of information from one hemisphere to the other. Stimulation restricted to one hemisphere is accessible to the other hemisphere, but its *identity* seems to be accessible only on an implicit (unconscious), not explicit (conscious), level.

What is available consciously is only general, categorical, so-called semantic information about the stimulus, not detailed identity information.

Within and between hemispheres, corticocortical pathways may function to synchronize activity across remote cortical regions, thereby permitting these regions' activity to be bound into a single event memory. This synchronization also has the effect of equilibrating activation between those regions. Thus, disconnection symptoms, such as those that are seen in split-brain patients, can be accounted for mainly by two factors: the desynchronized and fragmented manner by which subcortical pathways permit interhemispheric integration, and the diminished arousal state of the nonviewing hemisphere without the synchronizing influence of the cerebral commissures. The underactivated hemisphere displays an "internal neglect" that is marked by an abnormality of processing of input after sensory reception; it does not effectively process inputs to it (a) directly from the contralateral side of space or (b) indirectly from the opposite hemisphere. These underprocessed inputs are not consciously perceived though they are reacted to on an implicit level.

Despite the structural and functional similarity of the corticocortical pathways, it was pointed out that between-hemisphere processing is generally inferior to within-hemisphere processing, especially for comparison of identity information, even in the intact brain. The inferiority of between-hemisphere processing was attributed to the relative paucity of between- as compared to within-hemisphere fibers and the vulnerability of the separate hemispheres to asymmetries in activation, even when the commissures are intact.

It was noted that there are two kinds of integration tasks for which between-hemisphere performance is not inferior to within-hemisphere performance: when integration can be done on an abstract level, or when the integration can be done automatically, on an implicit level. These are the very kinds of integration tasks that survive commissural section. This could suggest that even in the intact brain some of this sort of integration is relegated to subcortical pathways. Conversely, the fact that identity information is harder to compare inter- than intrahemispherically, even in the intact brain, and is essentially impossible to consciously compare interhemispherically in the split brain, suggests that identity information is very vulnerable to regional differences in arousal or emotional state, which are greater inter- than intrahemispherically.

Two kinds of interhemispheric integration of cortical activity have been identified besides direct transfer. These are third-party convergence and nonconvergent temporal integration. In nonconvergent temporal integration, the role of the commissural pathways is to synchronize the outputs of two or more remote regions and enable them to feed forward, independently but synchronously, to a variety of other areas. Therefore, in nonconvergent synchronization there is only temporal integration. There is no grandfather convergence zone and no region where traces of the two regions of activity are stored as a compound, single engram.

To a greater extent than has been assumed, even in the intact brain, subcortical pathways are adequate for the interhemispheric integration of (a) categorical information or (b) context-independent, fragmented information which can be accessed only implicitly. This can be accomplished either by third-party convergence, where the convergence zone is subcortical, or by direct transfer, where the transfer is multi- rather than monosynaptic. In contrast, interhemispheric integration of item-specific information so that it is accessible on an explicit, conscious level seems uniquely dependent upon commissural pathways.

ACKNOWLEDGMENTS

This work was supported by an NIH Biomedical Seed Grant administered via Boston University. This chapter has benefited from conversations with the following students, colleagues, and friends: Mary Bodwell, Lauren J. Harris, Lisa Jones, Richard Kaplan, Les Kaufman, Kathy Mansley, Alex Marek, Gordon Moe, Daniel Palomo, Young-Sook Park, Erin Pitts, James Ringo, Robert Sokolove, and Nicole Weekes.

NOTES

1. The term *corticocortical pathways* is being used to refer to reciprocal pathways that connect regions of the cortex. Between-hemisphere corticocortical pathways are called commissures. In this chapter, when a patient is said to have a split brain it will imply that at least the corpus callosum and the anterior commissure were surgically sectioned; no assumptions are made about the extent to which the hippocampal commissure was included. When commissurotomy was limited to the corpus callosum, this is specifically stated.

2. Even within commissure-intact persons there is a problem with this index. Interhemispheric transfer times are often found to be negative (indicating that the ipsilateral component appears earlier than the contralateral component (e.g., Saron and Davidson, 1989). This is a problem for the notion that information is first received by the contralateral hemisphere and then transferred to the nonviewing hemisphere. Interestingly, negative IHTTs are also found to occur when behavioral estimates of IHTT are made (cf. Bashore, 1981, for a review).

3. It is not my purpose here to argue that the "only" role of the cerebral commissures is equilibration of activation or that the "only" interhemispheric interactions that occur at the level of the brainstem are inhibitory. Clearly, a pathway which contains millions of different kinds of fibers, which release a variety of kinds of neurotransmitters onto a variety of kinds of receptors, cannot be said to serve only one function. The purpose of this chapter is to focus on how important an equilibratory role can be, and to demonstrate that aberrations in equilibration can account for a great variety of interhemispheric phenomena in split-brain man.

4. Of course, not all of the intrahemispheric connections between neurons are long-distance corticocortical projection fibers. Thus, the specific difference in number of fibers between inter- and intrahemispheric commissures is not represented in this calculation.

REFERENCES

Balaydier, C., and Mauguiere, F. (1987). Network organization of the connectivity between parietal area 7, posterior cingulate cortex and medial pulvinar nucleus: a double fluorescent tracer study in monkey. *Experimental Brain Research, 66,* 385–393.

Banich, M., and Belger, A. (1991). Inter- versus intrahemishpheric concordance of judgments in a non-explicit memory task. *Brain and Cognition, 15,* 131–137.

Banich, M., and Shenker, J. (in press). Systematic and random information loss during interhemispheric transfer.

Barbas, H. (1986). Pattern in the laminar origin of corticocortical connections. *Journal of Comparative Neurology, 252,* 415–422.

Bashore, T. (1981). Vocal and manual reaction time estimates of interhemispheric transfer time. *Psychological Bulletin, 89*(2), 352–368.

Benson, D. (1979). *Aphasia, alexia, agraphia.* New York, NY: Churchill Livingstone Inc.

Berlucchi, G., and Antonini, A. (1990). The role of the corpus callosum in the representation of the visual field in cortical areas. In C. Trevarthen (Ed), *Brain circuits and functions of the mind.* New York, NY: Cambridge University Press.

Bogen, J. (1990). Partial hemispheric independence with the neocommissures intact. In C. Trevarthen (Ed.), *Brain circuits and functions of the mind* (pp 215–230). Cambridge, England: Cambridge University Press.

Butler, C. (1968). A memory record for visual discrimination habits produced in both cerebral hemispheres of monkey when only one hemisphere has received direct visual information. *Brain Research, 10,* 152–167.

Censori, B., Provinciali, L., Quattrini, A., Mancini, S., Papo, I. (1989). Functions of the corpus callosum: Observations from callosotomy performed for intractable epilepsy. *Bollettino Scocieta Italiana De Biologia Sperimentala, 65,* 53–59.

Coney, J., and MacDonald, S. (1988). The effect of retention interval upon hemispheric processes in recognition memory. *Neuropsychologia, 26*(2), 287–295.

Cook, N. (1986). *The brain code—Mechanisms of interhemispheric transfer and the role of the corpus callosum.* London: Methuen.

Crick, F. (1984). Function of the thalamic reticular complex: the searchlight hypothesis. *Proceedings of the National Academy of Sciences of the United States of America, 81,* 4586–4590.

Cronin-Golomb, A. (1986). Subcortical transfer of cognitive information in subjects with complete forebrain commissurotomy. *Cortex, 22,* 499–519.

Crowne, D., Adelstein, A., Dawson, K., and Richardson. (1988). Some effects of commissurotomy on the reinstatement and potentiation of lesion deficits. *Behavioral Brain Research, 29,* 135–146.

Damasio (1989). Time-locked multi-regional retroactivation: a systems level proposal for the neural substrates of recall and recognition. *Cognition, 33,* 25–62.

Demeter, S., Rosene, D., and Van Hoesen, G. (1990). Fields of origin and pathways of the interhemispheric commissures in the temporal lobe of Macaques. *Journal of Comparative Neurology, 302,* 29–53.

Demeurisse, G., and Capon, A. (1991). Brain activation during a linguistic task in conduction aphasia. *Cortex, 27,* 285–294.

Dimond, S., Gibson, A., and Gazzaniga, M. (1972). Cross-field and within-field integration of visual information. *Neuropsychologia, 10,* 379–381.

Doty, R., Lewine, J., and Ringo, J. (1985). Mnemonic interaction between and within cerebral hemispheres in macaques. In D. L. Alkon and C. D. Woody (Eds.), *Neural mechanisms of conditioning* (pp 223–231). New York, NY: Plenum Press.

Doty, R., Ringo, J., and Lewine, J. (1986). Interhemispheric mnemonic transfer in Macaques. In F. Lepore, M. Ptito, and H. H. Jasper (Eds.), *Two hemispheres—one brain: Functions of the corpus callosum* (pp 261–279). New York, NY: Alan R. Liss, Inc.

Engel, A., Konig, P., Kreiter, A., Schillen, T., and Singer, W. (1992). Temporal coding in the visual cortex: New vistas on integration in the nervous system. *Trends in Neurosciences, 15*, 218–226.

Engel, A., Konig, P., Kreiter, A., and Singer, W. (1991). Interhemispheric synchronization of oscillatory neuronal responses in cat visual cortex. *Science, 252*, 1177–1179.

Gazzaniga, M. (1987). Perceptual and attentional processes following callosal section in humans. *Neuropsychologia, 25*(1A), 119–133.

Geschwind, N. (1965). Disconnexion syndromes in animals and man. *Brain, 88*, 237–294.

Glick, S., Crane, A., Jerussi, T., Fleisher, L., and Green, J. (1975). Functional and neurochemical correlates of potentiation of striatal asymmetry by callosal section. *Nature, 254*, 616–617.

Glickstein, M. (1990). Brain pathways in the visual guidance of movement and the behavioral functions of the cerebellum. In C. Trevarthen (Ed.), *Brain circuits and functions of the mind.* Cambridge, England: Cambridge University Press.

Goldenberg, G. (1986). Neglect in a patient with partial callosal disconnection. *Neuropsychologia, 24*(3), 397–403.

Goldman-Rakic, P. (1988). Topography of cognition: Parallel distributed networks in primate association cortex. *Annual Review of Neuroscience, 11*, 137–156.

Goodale, M., and Milner, A. (1992). Separate visual pathways for perception and action. *Trends in Neurosciences, 15*(1), 20–25.

Gray, C., Konig, P., Engel, A., and Singer, W. (1989). Oscillatory responses in cat visual cortex exhibit intercolumnar synchronization which reflects global stimulus properties. *Nature, 338*, 334–337.

Gray, C., and Singer, W. (1989). Stimulus-specific neuronal oscillations in orientation columns of cat visual cortex. *Proceedings of the National Academy of Sciences of the United States of America, 86*, 1698–1702.

Guiard, Y. (1980). Cerebral hemispheres and selective attention. *Acta Psychologica, 46*, 41–61.

Guiard, Y., and Requin, J. (1978). Between-hand vs. within-hand choice: A single channel reduced capacity in the split-brain monkey. In J. Requin (Ed.), *Attention and performance VII* (pp 391–410). Hillsdale, NJ: Lawrence Erlbaum Associates.

Hamilton, C. R. (1977). Investigations of perceptual and mnemonic lateralization in monkeys. In R. W. Doty, L. Goldstein, J. Jaynes, and G. Kravthavmer, (Eds.), *Lateralization in the nervous system* (pp 45–62). New York, NY: Academic Press.

Hedreen, J., and Yin, T. (1981). Homotopic and heterotopic callosal afferents of caudal inferior parietal lobule in *Macaca mulatta. Journal of Comparative Neurology, 197*, 605–621.

Heilman, K., Bowers, D., and Watson, R. (1984). Pseudoneglect in a patient with partial callosal disconnection. *Brain, 107*, 519–523.

Hicks, R., Frank, J., and Kinsbourne, M. (1982). The locus of bimanual skill transfer. *Journal of General Psychology, 107*: 277–281.

Holtzman, J. (1984). Interactions between cortical and subcortical visual areas: evidence from human commissurotomy patients. *Vision Research, 24*, 801–813.

Innocenti, G. M. (1986). General organization of callosal connections in the cerebral cortex. In E. G. Jones and A. Peters (Eds.), *Cerebral Cortex, volume 5* (pp 291–353). New York, NY: Plenum Press.

Jakobson, L., Archibald, Y., Carey, D., and Goodale, M. (1991). A kinematic analysis of reaching and grasping movements in a patient recovering from optic ataxia. *Neuropsychologia, 29,* 803–809.

Joynt, R. (1977). Inattention syndromes in split-brain main. In E. A. Weinstein and R. P. Friedland (Eds.), *Hemi-inattention and hemisphere specialization* (pp 41–50). New York, NY: Raven Press.

Kempler, D., Metter, E., Jackson, C., Hanson, W., Riege, W. Mazziotta, J., and Phelps, M. (1988). Disconnection and cerebral metabolism. The case of conduction aphasia. *Archives of Neurology, 45,* 275–279.

Kinsbourne, M. (1970). The cerebral basis of lateral asymmetries in attention. *Acta Psychologica, 33,* 193–201.

Kinsbourne, M. (1974). Lateral interactions in the brain. In M. Kinsbourne and W. L. Smith (Eds.), *Hemispheric disconnection and cerebral function* (pp 239–259). Springfield, IL: Charles C Thomas.

Kinsbourne, M. (1987a). The material basis of mind. In L. Vaina (Ed.), *Matters of Intelligence: Conceptual structures in cognitive neuroscience* (pp 407–427). Boston: D. Reidel Publishing Co.

Kinsbourne, M. (1987b). Mechanisms of unilateral neglect. In M. Jeannerod (Ed.), *Neurophysiological and neuropsychological aspects of spatial neglect* (pp 69–86). Amsterdam: Elsevier Science Publishers.

Kinsbourne, M. (1988). Integrated field theory of consciousness. In A. Marcel and E. Bisiach (Eds.), *Consciousness in contemporary science* (pp 230–256). Oxford, England: Clarendon Press.

Kleinman, K., and Little, R. (1973). Inter-hemispheric transfer of meaningful visual information in normal human subjects. *Nature, 241,* 55–57.

Kornhuber, H. (1974). Cerebral cortex, cerebellum, and basal ganglia: An introduction to their motor functions. In F. Schmitt and F. Worden (Eds.), *The neurosciences: Third study program* (pp 267–280). Cambridge, MA: MIT Press.

LaMantia, A., and Rakic, P. (1990). Cytological and quantitative characteristics of four cerebral commissures in the rhesus monkey. *Journal of Comparative Neurology, 291,* 520–537.

Landis, T., Assal, G., and Perret, E. (1979). Opposite cerebral hemishpheric superiorities for visual associative processing of emotional facial expressions and objects. *Nature, 278,* 739–740.

Landis, T., Graves, R., and Goodglass, H. (1981). Dissociated awareness of manual performance on two different visual associative tasks: A "split-brain" phenomenon in normal subjects. *Cortex, 17,* 435–440.

Lassen, N., and Roland, P. (1983). Localization of cognitive function with cerebral blood flow. In A. Kertez (Ed.), *Localization in neuropsychology,* New York, NY: Academic Press.

Lassonde, M. (1986). The facilitatory influence of the corpus callosum on intrahemispheric processing. In F. Lepore, M. Ptito, and H. H. Jasper (Eds.), *Two hemispheres—one brain: Functions of the corpus callosum* (pp 385–401). New York, NY: Alan R. Liss, Inc.

Leiber, L. (1982). Interhemispheric effects in short-term recognition memory for single words. *Cortex, 18,* 113–124.

Lepore, F., Phaneuf, J., Samson, A., and Guillemot, J. (1982). Interhemispheric transfer of visual pattern discriminations: Evidence for a bilateral storage of the engram. *Behavioral Brain Research*, 5, 359–374.

Leviel. V., Chesselet, M., Glowinski, J., and Cheramy, A. (1981). Involvement of the thalamus in the asymmetric effects of unilateral sensory stimuli on the two nigrostriatal dopaminergic pathways of the cat. *Brain Research*, 223, 257–272.

Levy, J. (1985). Interhemispheric collaboration: single-mindedness in the asymmetric brain. In C. Best (Ed.), *Hemispheric function and collaboration in the child* (pp 11–31). New York, NY: Academic Press.

Levy, J. (1990). Regulation and generation of perception in the asymmetric brain. In C. Trevarthen (Ed.), *Brain circuits and functions of the mind* (pp 231–248). New York, NY: Cambridge University Press.

Levy, J., Trevarthen, C., and Sperry, R. (1972). Perception of bilateral chimeric fiqures following hemispheric deconnexion. *Brain*, 95, 61–78.

Liederman, J. (1986a). Interhemispheric interference during word naming. *International Journal of Neuroscience*, 30, 43–56.

Liederman, J. (1986b). The Stroop effect is as strong between as within hemispheres. Unpublished manuscript, Boston University.

Liederman, J., Merola, J., and Martinez, S. (1985). Inter-hemispheric collaboration in response to simultaneous bilateral input. *Neuropsychologia*, 23(5), 673–683.

Livingstone, M., and Hubel, D. (1988). Segregation of form, color, movement and depth: Anatomy, physiology and perception. *Science*, 240, 740–750.

Lordahl, D., Kleinman, K., Levy, B., Massoth, N., Pessin, M., Storandt, M., Tucker, R., and Vanderplas, J. (1965). Deficits in recognition of random shapes with changed visual fields. *Journal of the Psychonomic Society*, 3, 245–256.

Mangun, G., Luck, S., Gazzaniga, M., and Hillyard, S. (1991). Electrophysiological measures of interhemispheric transfer of visual information: Studies in split-brain patients. Presented at the meeting of the Society for Neuroscience, New Orleans, November 1991.

Marshall, J., and Halligan, P. (1988). Blindsight and insight in visuospatial neglect. *Nature*, 336, 766–767.

McGlinchey-Berroth, R., Milberg, W., Verfaellie, M., Alexander, M., and Kilduff, P. (1993). Semantic processing in the neglected visual field: evidence from a lexical decision task. *Cognitive Neuropsychology*, 10, 79–108.

Mendez, M., and Benson, D. (1985). Atypical conduction aphasia: A disconnection syndrome. *Archives of Neurology*, 42, 886–891.

Norita, M. (1983). Claustral neurons projecting to the visual cortical areas in the CAT: a retrograde double-labeling study. *Neuroscience Letters*, 36, 33–36.

Novelly, R., and Lifrak, M. (1985). Forebrain commissurotomy reinstates effects of preexisting hemisphere lesions: An examination of the hypothesis. In A. G. Reeves (Ed.), *Epilepsy and the corpus callosum* (pp 467–500). New York, NY: Plenum Press.

Penfield, W. (1950). *The cerebral cortex of man: A study of localization of function*. New York, NY: Springer-Verlag.

Peschstedt, P. (1986). Suppression of ipsalateral auditory pathways increases with increasing task load in commissurotomy subjects. *Bulletin of Clinical Neurosciences*, 51, 73–76.

Plourde, G., and Sperry, R. (1984). Left hemisphere involvement in left spatial neglect from right sided lesions—a commissurotomy study. *Brain, 107,* 95–106.

Poppel, E. (1988). *Mindworks. Time and conscious experience.* Boston, MA: Harcourt Brace Jovanovich.

Poppel, E., Schill, K., and von Steinbuchel, N. (1990). Sensory integration within temporally neutral system states: A Hypothesis. *Naturwissenschaften, 77,* 89–91.

Prather, P., Jarmulowicz, L., Brownell, H., and Gardner, H. (1992). Selective attention and the right hemisphere: a failure in integration, not detection. Presented at the International Neuropsychology Society Meeting, San Diego, CA, February 1992.

Pribram, K. (1986). The role of cortico-cortical connections. In F. Lepore, M. Ptito, and H. H. Jasper (Eds.), *Two hemispheres—one brain: Functions of the corpus callosum* (pp 523–540). New York, NY: Alan R. Liss, Inc.

Pribram, K., Spinnelli, D. N., Reitz, S. L. (1969). Effects of radical disconnexion of occipital and temporal cortex on visual behavior of monkeys. *Brain, 92,* 301–312.

Reuter-Lorenz, P., Nazawa, G., and Hughes, H. (1991). The fate of neglected targets in the callosotomized brain: A chronometric analysis. Paper presented to the Psychonomics Society, San Francisco, CA, November 1991.

Ringo, J. (in press, b). The medial temporal lobe in encoding, retention, retrieval and interhemispheric transfer of visual memory in primates. *Experimental Brain Research.*

Ringo, J., Doty, R., Demeter, S., and Simard, P. (submitted for publication, 1992). Time is of the essence: A conjecture that hemispheric specialization arises from interhemispheric conduction delay.

Ringo, J., and O'Neill, S. (1993). Indirect inputs to ventral temporal cortex of monkey: The influence on unit activity of alerting auditory input, interhemispheric subcortical visual input, reward, and the behavioral response. *Journal of Neurophysiology, 70,* 2215–2225.

Rugg, M., Milner, A., and Lines, C. (1985). Visual evoked potentials to lateralized stimuli in two cases of callosal agenesis. *Journal of Neurology, Neurosurgery and Psychiatry, 48,* 367–373.

Saron, C., and Davidson, R. (1989). Visual evoked potential measures of interhemispheric transfer time in humans. *Behavioral Neuroscience, 103*(5), 1115–1138.

Schacter, D. (1987). Implicit memory: History and current status. *Journal of Experimental Psychology: Learning, Memory and Cognition, 13,* 501–518.

Sergent, J. (1986). Subcortical coordination of hemisphere activity in commissurotomized patients. *Brain, 109,* 357–369.

Sergent, J. (1987). A new look at the human split brain. *Brain, 110,* 1375–1392.

Sergent, J. (1990). Furtive incursions into bicameral minds: Integrative and coordinating role of subcortical structures. *Brain, 113,* 537–568.

Sergent, J. (1991). Processing of spatial relations within and between the disconnected cerebral hemispheres. *Brain, 114,* 1025–1043.

Sjenowski, T., and Churchland, P. (1990). Brain and cognition. In M. Posner (Ed.), *Foundations of cognitive science* (pp 301–356). Cambridge, MA: MIT Press.

Somplinsky, H., Golumb, D., and Kleinfeld, D. (1990). Global processing of visual stimuli in a neural network of coupled oscillators. *Proceedings of the National Academy of Sciences of the United States of America, 87,* 7200–7204.

Sperry, R. (1962). Some general aspects of interhemispheric integration. In V. B. Mountcastle (Ed.), *Interhemispheric relations and cerebral dominance* (pp 43–49). Baltimore, MD: Johns Hopkins Press.

Sullivan, K., and McKeever, W. (1985). Loss of fluent speech in callosotomy: Patients who are discordant for speech and motor control dominances. Presented at the 13th Annual Meeting of the International Neuropsychological Society, February 1985 San Diego, CA.

Sussman, N. M., Gur, R. C., Gur, R. E., O'Connor, M. J. (1983). Mutism as a consequence of callosotomy. *Journal of Neurosurgery, 59,* 514–519.

Szentagothai, J. (1978). The neuron network of the cerebral cortex: a functional interpretation. *Proceedings of the Royal Society of London. Series B, 201,* 219–248.

Tanabe, H., Sawada, T., Inoue, N., Ogawa, M., Kuriyama, Y., and Shiraishi, J. (1987). Conduction aphasia and arcuate fascicus. *Acta Neurologica Scandinavica, 76,* 422–427.

Tigges, J., and Tigges, M. (1985). Subcortical sources of direct projections to visual cortex. In A. Peters and E. G. Jones (Eds.), *Cerebral cortex.* Vol. 3. *Visual cortex* (pp 351–378). New York, NY: Plenum Press.

Trevarthen, C. (1974a). Analysis of cerebral activities that generate and regulate consciousness in commissurotomy patients. In S. J. Dimond and J. G. Beaumont (Eds.), *Hemisphere function in the brain* (pp 235–263). London: Elek Science.

Trevarthen, C. (1974b). Functional relations of disconnected hemispheres with the brain stem and with each other: Monkey and man. In M. Kinsbourne and W. L. Smith (Eds.), *Hemispheric disconnection and cerebral function* (pp 187–207). Springfield, IL: Charles C Thomas.

Trevarthen, C. (1990). Growth and eduction in the hemispheres. In C. Trevarthen (Ed), *Brain Circuits and functions of the mind* (pp 334–363). Cambridge, England: Cambridge University Press.

Watson, R., Valenstein, E., Day, A., and Heilman, K. (1984). The effect of corpus callosum lesions on unilateral neglect in monkeys. *Neurology, 34,* 812–815.

Wilson, D., Reeves, M., Gazzaniga, M., and Culver, C. (1977). Cerebral commissurotomy for control of intractable seizures. *Neurology, 27,* 708–715.

17 Interhemispheric Transfer in the Split Brain: Long-term Status Following Complete Cerebral Commissurotomy

Eran Zaidel

HEMISPHERIC FUNCTION AND INTERACTION IN THE NORMAL AND SPLIT BRAIN

Dynamic Hemispheric Independence

Hemispheric function and interaction in the normal brain can be viewed as a model system for modularity and intermodular communication in the mind/brain in general. In this view, each hemisphere constitutes an independent cognitive system, with its own sensations, perceptions, cognitions, memory, language, attention, and consciousness, and each can operate independently and in parallel with the other. Sometimes one hemisphere dominates processing, which includes inhibition of responses or utilization of information from the other side. At other times they compute in parallel, and at yet other times they share the intermediate results of their independent computations. This requires mechanisms of control that maintain functional independence, initiate and stop exchange of information through the corpus callosum, resolve conflict, and establish priority (E. Zaidel and Rayman, in press). The exchange of information between the two hemispheres is dynamic and can occur selectively at any stage in the information-processing sequence. But the mechanisms that implement selective transfer are still unknown.

Central to this approach to intermodular communication is the assumption that the structure of the brain determines the structure of the mind so that neurophysiologic, neuroanatomic, and neurochemical techniques can reveal facts relevant to behavior. In particular, the structure and function of the corpus callosum are critical for understanding normal interhemispheric interaction. One way to understand the function of the corpus callosum is to ask what forms of interhemispheric exchange can survive its transection in complete cerebral commissurotomy. In this chapter I investigate residual explicit (e.g., verbalizable) and implicit transfer of visual information at different stages of processing in the split brain.

Another assumption we make is that there is continuity between normal function and cognitive deficit following brain damage. In particular, we believe that the normal brain is often temporarily functionally disconnected and that it is possible to induce experimentally some disconnection symptoms and to measure the cost of callosal transfer through behavioral laterality effects in tasks that lateralize stimuli or responses, or both, to one hemisphere. The split brain remains the paradigmatic case for such experiments by operationalizing the concepts of hemispheric competence, hemispheric specialization, hemispheric dominance, and hemispheric independence. Using the split-brain model we interpret behavioral laterality effects in anatomic terms, and this contrasts with attentional models. A priori, we would expect the pattern of hemispheric independence in individual split-brain patients to be the same as the group mean in the normal brain. In this view, individual normal subjects may deviate from the group pattern because the laterality measures we use are noisy and provide somewhat indirect measures of hemispheric independence. The split brain, on the other hand, provides a much more direct, robust, and reliable measure of the same underlying hemispheric competencies.

The anatomic model of behavioral laterality effects distinguishes three categories of tasks: (1) "callosal relay" tasks that are exclusively specialized to one hemisphere and require callosal relay of stimuli projected to the wrong hemisphere before processing can take place, (2) "direct access" tasks that can be processed independently, if differently, in either hemisphere, and (3) tasks that require interhemispheric interaction. Surprisingly many lateralized tasks are direct access, and one common index of hemispheric independence is a statistical interaction ("processing dissociation") between some independent stimulus variable (e.g., Wordness [words, nonwords] in a lexical decision task or Decision [global, local] in a hierarchic perception task) and visual hemifield of stimulus presentation (E. Zaidel, 1983; E. Zaidel et al., 1990a). Of course, tasks can change their status from callosal relay to direct access across individuals or in the same individual with increasing experience. Indeed, there is evidence that control can change from direct access to callosal relay and back from trial to trial as a function of item difficulty (E. Zaidel et al., 1988). All the tasks described in this chapter show evidence of direct access in the normal brain and of bilateral competence in the split brain.

Callosal Channels

Behavioral-anatomic-physiologic correlations, both in clinical and normal populations, now converge on the view that the human corpus callosum consists largely of a set of modality-, material-, or function-specific channels that interconnect homotopic cortical regions in the two cerebral hemispheres (E. Zaidel et al., 1990a). The anteroposterior arrangement of those channels respects the anteroposterior arrangement of the corresponding cortical regions: going in a caudal-rostral direction, the splenium interconnects visual cortices, the isthmus probably interconnects auditory cortices and superior temporal lobes, the posterior midbody interconnects somatosensory cortices, the anterior mid-

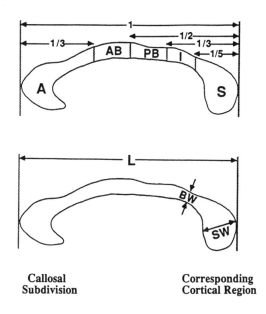

	Callosal Subdivision	Corresponding Cortical Region
A	Anterior third (rostrum, genu, & anterior body)	Prefrontal, premotor, supplementary motor, possibly anterior inferior parietal
AB	Anterior midbody	Precentral, postcentral, possibly midtemporal
PB	Posterior midbody	Postcentral, posterior parietal, possibly midtemporal
I	Isthmus	Posterior parietal, superior temporal
S	Splenium	Occipital, inferior temporal, ventral temporal, superior parietal

Figure 17.1 A schematic representation of the regions of the human corpus callosum and the presumed cortical structures they interconnect. L, total anterior-posterior callosum length; BW, minimum body width; SW, maximum splenial width.

body interconnects motor cortices, and the genu may transfer control signals (including inhibitory ones) between frontal cortices (figure 17.1).

Stabilized Disconnection

Within a few months after the operation, patients who had complete cerebral commissurotomy, including the corpus callosum, anterior commissure, and hippocampal commissure, appear largely unchanged in personality and social reactions, and on routine neurologic examination (Bogen, 1993), with the possible exception of memory (D. Zaidel and Sperry, 1974; D. W. Zaidel, 1990) and pragmatics (E. Zaidel, 1990). But sensory stimuli restricted to one hemisphere remain unavailable to the other, so that each hemisphere has separate learning and memory. Right-handed patients (with left-hemisphere [LH] speech) can generally not make reliable same/different judgments about two visual stimuli, one flashed to each hemifield simultaneously, and they cannot name shapes or words flashed briefly to the left visual hemifield (LVF). When different but acoustically similar auditory stimuli are presented simultaneously to the two ears (dichotic listening), patients cannot name the left ear stimuli, which normally reach the LH via the isthmus of the corpus callosum. Lack of interhemispheric somatosensory transfer occurs for touch, pressure, and proprioception. Patients can generally not make reliable same/different judgments about objects palpated out of view by each hand simultaneously, and they cannot name objects palpated out of view by the left hand. Hand postures impressed on one (unseen) hand by the examiner cannot be mimicked in the opposite hand and a brief flash of a hand form to one visual hemifield cannot be copied by the contralateral hand. After complete cerebral commissurotomy there is partial loss of intermanual point localization, that is, loss of the ability to identify exact points stimulated on the other side of the body, especially of distal parts, such as the fingertips. In all these cases intrahemispheric comparisons are intact. Finally, the chronic disconnection syndrome shows failure to coordinate new interdependent bimanual movements, and there is persisting mild to moderate left hand apraxia to verbal command in spite of good imitation and adequate auditory language comprehension in the disconnected right hemisphere (RH) (D. W. Zaidel and Sperry, 1977).

Partial Disconnection

Interruption of specific callosal channels can result in selective deficits of interhemispheric transfer. This has been demonstrated following partial surgical sections, partial lesions, callosal thinning from multiple sclerosis, and callosal thinning following closed head injury (see review in Bogen, 1993). For example, Risse et al. (1990) found that if only the tip of the splenium was spared, there was good visual transfer together with a unilateral left anomia, a unilateral left apraxia, deficits in both tactile and kinesthetic transfer, and a large right ear advantage on dichotic listening. When the entire splenium and some isthmus were spared there was essentially no anomia, no apraxia (even acutely), nor a kinesthetic deficit. When more (the posterior one third) of the body was spared along with the splenium, there was no deficit in intermanual point localization, but there was still a partial auditory transfer deficit. This last, noted by Risse et al., is surprising because it is inconsistent with anatomic evidence that superior temporal lobe fibers cross through the callosum posterior to parietal fibers. Still unexplored is the distribution of fibers less specified for sensory modality. Thus, precise specification of callosal channels is still missing.

Even more challenging to the channel doctrine is the striking paucity of interhemispheric transfer deficits following interruption of only the anterior half of the corpus callosum. Indeed, even complete disconnection sparing the splenium reveals little or no behavioral disconnection effects (Gordon, Bogen, and Sperry, 1971; see also Bogen, 1993; cf. "the genu enigma" in Bogen,

1993). Further, naturally occurring anterior callosal lesions can cause deficits, such as unilateral left hand apraxia, not observed following surgical section of the same callosal regions. Likely explanations are the plasticity of callosal channels, and extracallosal damage caused by natural lesions, such as ischemia in the anterior cerebral artery.

Another unsolved problem is the role of the anterior commissure. Most of the syndrome seen after a complete cerebral commissurotomy is also seen after a callosotomy sparing the anterior and hippocampal commissures (e.g., McKeever et al., 1982).

EXPLICIT TRANSFER

Occasionally, split-brain patients can name stimuli shown in the LVF or palpated with the left hand (Lh) (Butler and Norsell, 1968; Levy et al., 1971; Teng and Sperry, 1973; Johnson, 1984a; Myers, 1984; D. W. Zaidel, 1988). This could be a result of: (1) improper lateralization of stimuli; (2) ipsilateral projection of sensory information from the LVF or Lh to the LH where verbalization occurs; (3) subcortical transfer of cognitive information sufficient to identify the stimulus to the LH following recognition by the RH; (4) cross-cueing from the RH to the LH, using shared perceptual space (e.g., the RH may fixate on a related item in the room, thus identifying it to the LH, or it may trace the shape of the object in question with the head so the movement can be "read off" by the LH) (Bogen, 1987); or (5) RH speech (e.g., patient P.S. of Gazzaniga et al., 1979). Only when all other alternatives are ruled out can RH speech be considered seriously, given the weight of evidence so far. For example, it was never investigated whether LVF or Lh stimuli could be named at the same time that nonverbal right hand (Rh) identification of these stimuli failed. To date, there is no compelling evidence for RH speech in any of the patients in the California series (cf. Myers, 1984).

Verbalization of left hemifield stimuli resulting from ipsilateral sensory projection is limited to simple sensory features and to items uniquely identified by them. Trevarthen and Sperry (1973) found that ipsilateral visual features are restricted to rate of motion and relative displacement of peripheral stimuli. They believe that the ipsilateral visual system is extrageniculostriate, mediated by the superior colliculus and responsible for "ambient" as opposed to "focal" (described by them as attentional, conscious) vision, which is geniculostriate. At the other end, there is subcortical transfer of abstract semantic features of the stimulus, generally without making identification possible. Those features include affective and connotative information (e.g. happy, sad) (E. Zaidel, 1976; Sperry, Zaidel, and Zaidel, 1979); associative features, both perceptual and semantic (Myers and Sperry, 1985); categorical information (e.g., "animals that go in the water" where one picture is shown to each visual field [VF] simultaneously); functional features (e.g., "shoe-sock"); or abstract semantic relations (communication: envelope-telephone) (Cronin-Golomb, 1986).

Sergent (1987) found that split-brain patients could determine whether arrows in opposite fields were aligned, whether the sum of bilateral dot patterns was odd or even, and whether four-letter strings straddling the midline were words or not. Corballis and Trudel (1993), however, pointed out that a simple guessing strategy suffices to achieve high scores on the parity (odd or even) task, and they failed to replicate the lexical decision findings. In general, the patients use sophisticated cross-cueing strategies and in order to neutralize them, tasks need to employ large and novel stimulus sets. Binary choice tasks are especially susceptible to cross-cueing because only one bit of information need transfer to permit interhemispheric integration. For example, Sergent's parity task need only have a single bit signaling the LVF parity transfer to the LH to be able to perform the task. It is important to note that neither naming of LVF stimuli alone nor cross-matching alone is sufficient to establish complete disconnection. For example, cross-matching may fail because of a tendency to neglect one hemifield with bilateral presentation, even while accurate verbalizing of LVF stimuli is preserved. Conversely, verbalizing of LVF stimuli may fail while cross-matching is present because the transferred code may be so degraded as to be sufficient only for visual pattern matching but not for stimulus identification.

In this section I review two experiments on explicit matching of visual stimuli across the two visual hemifields in split-brain patients. The first requires matching of shape information when no other codes are presumably available for matching. The second experiment contrasts comparing letter shapes and, in turn, letter names between the two visual hemifields. The question is whether more abstract codes (names) may transfer subcallosally when more sensory codes (shapes) do not. A third experiment involving color matching across the two VFs and naming of LVF color patches serves as the control condition for Experiment 6 on the Stroop effect under Implicit Transfer below.

Visual Transfer: Matching Nonsense Shapes within and between the Hemispheres

Interfield matching of meaningful shapes may succeed because of the availability of semantic or other codes associated with the original shapes. This is least likely to occur with hard-to-verbalize nonsense geometric shapes. The stimuli in this experiment (figure 17.2) were chosen to provide minimal associative value and consisted of complex Vanderplas figures (Vanderplas and Garvin, 1959). Further, there was a relatively large stimulus set (N = 20) so that the stimuli could not be learned and associated with new codes. When such shapes are compared across the vertical meridian in normal persons, the visual information most probably transfers across the splenium of the corpus callosum. The splenium interconnects representations of a strip around the vertical meridian in area 18 (de Lacoste, Kirkpatrick, and Ross, 1985; Pandya and Seltzer, 1986; Witteridge, 1965) and has been implicated in interhemispheric

r

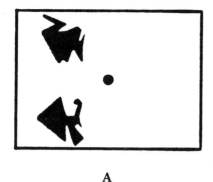 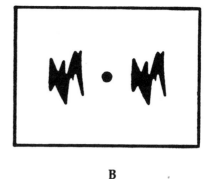

A   **B**

Figure 17.2   Examples of pairs of Vanderplas figures presented *(A)* to the left visual field, and *(B)* bilaterally.

transfer of visual information in humans (Damasio et al., 1980; Gordon, Bogen, and Sperry, 1971; Risse et al., 1989).

Three right-handed split-brain patients from the California series were tested: L.B., N.G., and A.A. (Clarke, 1990; Clarke and Zaidel, in preparation). All had section of the splenium as part of a complete cerebral commissurotomy for treatment of intractable epilepsy. The surgical procedures were performed between 1963 and 1966 by Drs. P. J. Vogel and J. B. Bogen at the White Memorial Hospital in Los Angeles. In each case, the entire corpus callosum, anterior commissure, and hippocampal commissure were divided in a single operation. The subjects differed in sex, IQ, age at testing, age at surgery, and age of onset of epileptic symptoms. Magnetic resonance images (MRIs) taken in 1987 showed complete sections of the neocortical commissures (Bogen, Schultz, and Vogel, 1988). None of these patients showed evidence of massive cerebral damage that would lead to functional reorganization of higher hemispheric functions (E. Zaidel, D. W. Zaidel, and Bogen, 1990b). All showed some evidence for right hemisphere language (E. Zaidel, 1990) and for complementary hemispheric specialization (E. Zaidel, 1978). For further clinical details about the case histories, see Bogen and Vogel (1975).

Patients had to decide whether two visually presented geometric figures were the same or different. The stimuli consisted of pairs from a set of 12- to 16-point Vanderplas figures, half same pairs and half different pairs. Same pairs were identical in shape, size, and orientation. All pairs were presented in each of three VF conditions—LVF, RVF, or bilateral (BVF)—with one member of the pair in each VF. For unilateral presentations, the figures were positioned one above the other, and for bilateral presentations the figures were positioned along the horizontal meridian. Stimuli were projected for 150 ms on a back-projection screen using a slide projector. "Same" and "different" responses were made on a toggle switch positioned at midline. The test was repeated twice, once with each hand responding.

There was no effect of response hand so the data were collapsed over this variable. Patient A.A. could only perform the task above chance in his LVF

(69.4% correct). Patient L.B. had significantly different scores in the three VF conditions. Both LVF and RVF scores were above chance but the score in the bilateral condition was not significantly above chance. RVF score (79.5%) was higher than LVF score (70%), but the difference was not significant ($\chi^2(1) = .94$). Patient N.G. also scored above chance in the LVF (85%) and in the RVF (72.5%). Surprisingly, she also scored above chance in the bilateral condition (89.7%). Although the performance in her three VF conditions was not significantly different, N.G.'s BVF scores were the highest!

In order to confirm N.G.'s surprising ability to match these nonsense shapes across the vertical meridian, the test was repeated on four other occasions. In one session her left eye was patched to eliminate possible leakage of information to the wrong VF by divergent focus. In another session the stimulus exposure was reduced to 50 ms to prevent possible quick saccades to the lateralized stimulus. These manipulations had no effect on N.G.'s bilateral performance, which was above chance in all four tests. Her average performance across all five tests (totalling 600 acceptable trials) showed a significant difference between the VFs; the LVF and BVF conditions did not differ, whereas each was significantly higher than the RVF score.

Thus, there is strong evidence that each disconnected hemisphere can perform the task, although two experimentally sophisticated subjects, L.B. and A.A., could not reliably match the shapes between the two hemispheres, confirming the classic visual disconnection symptom. However, N.G. did show evidence of visual transfer. Moreover, the similarity between the LVF and BVF scores and their superiority to the RVF score suggest that N.G.'s bilateral score resulted from subcortical visual transfer from the LH to the RH.

Previous studies (Johnson, 1984b; Myers and Sperry, 1985) concluded that N.G. is unique among the California patients with complete commissurotomy in being able to match visual stimuli across the vertical meridian. But those studies were limited to small stimulus set sizes and to easily verbalized stimuli that permit cross-cueing or subcortical transfer of a more abstract code. How does N.G. do this? One explanation is that her successful visual matching in the absence of verbal identification results from a transferred code sufficient for low-level template matching but not for high-level identification. N.G. may have a particularly efficient superior collicular system for projecting RVF stimuli to the RH. This extrageniculostriate system appears to be sensitive to simple visual features, such as movement, position, and orientation, as well as to simple high-contrast patterns (Weiskrantz, 1986). Indeed the Vanderplas figures consist of high-contrast patterns with distinct edges of varying orientation. Alternatively, the dissociation suggests some intrahemispheric disconnection within N.G.'s LH between separate modules for early visual processing and for visual verbal identification.

Matching Letter Shapes and Letter Names

Many previous studies have shown that patients with complete cerebral commissurotomy fail to transfer visual stimuli between the two hemispheres, with the exception of crude sensory information about shape and motion, and yet they succeed in transferring more abstract codes associated with the meaning of the stimulus (e.g., E. Zaidel, 1976; Sperry et al., 1979; Cronin-Golomb, 1986; Myers and Sperry, 1985; Sergent, 1986, 1987, 1990, 1991). Can this dissociation be demonstrated in a same/different matching task that uses the same stimuli but different decision criteria? In this experiment we used the Posner-Mitchell paradigm: subjects saw pairs of upper- or lowercase letters within or between the hemispheres and had to match them for physical identity (e.g., AA = same, Aa = different) or for name identity (Aa = same, Ab = different) (Eviatar and Zaidel, 1994). The "higher code transfer" hypothesis would predict (1) successful matching in either shape or name within each disconnected hemisphere, (2) unsuccessful matching of shape between the hemispheres, but perhaps (3) successful matching of name between the hemispheres.

The stimuli in this experiment were letter pairs drawn from the set A, B, D, E, F, G, H, I, J, L, M, N, Q, R, T, and Y in upper- and lowercase. These stimuli were chosen because their upper- and lowercases do not have the same shape. Pairs of letters were flashed either in the same VF or in opposite fields. Each subject had four blocks, one block for each decision type (shape or name) by response hand (left, right) condition. In each block, a third of the trials appeared in each VF condition (LVF, RVF, BVF), and half of the stimuli were same and half were different. All same stimuli in name decisions consisted of an upper- and lowercase pair of the same letter (e.g., "Aa"). Different stimuli in shape decisions were equally likely to be the same letter (e.g., Aa) or different letters (e.g., AG,Ab, aj). The experiment required two-choice unimanual responses.

Recall that for a split-brain patient, the LVF-Lh condition most closely represents RH processing, whereas RVF-Rh most closely represents LH processing. All patients could perform both shape and name matches in either hemisphere with the exception of name matches in the LH of A.A. All patients showed RH superiority on shape matches and L.B. and N.G. showed LH superiority for name matches. By contrast, none of the patients could compare names between the hemispheres (bilateral condition). L.B. and A.A. could also not match shapes across the VFs but, again, NG was above chance in bilateral shape matches, and her performance showed no bias (preference for same or different responses). This confirms Clarke's (1990) finding of good matching of nonsense shapes across the VFs in N.G. but not in the other patients (see above).

N.G.'s ability to cross-compare shapes and not names is remarkable. It suggests that visual information can transfer subcallosally and be available for the Shape task but not for the Name task. This could suggest modularity or even intrahemispheric disconnection between the processors of shape comparisons and those of name comparisons in the LH. Alternatively, it is possible that the transferred visual information is limited to the level of initial representations, or Marr's primal sketch, allowing figure-ground and contour discrimination without specifying the identity of the stimulus. Indeed, N.G.'s responses to different bilateral shapes did not reveal a congruity effect (slower rejection of Same-Name/Different-Shape pairs [Aa] than of Different-Name/Different-Shape pairs [Ag]). This suggests that nominal identity was not processed, and so did not affect responses.

Reaction time (RT) showed that for name matches L.B. and N.G. had a significant LH advantage (LHA) and A.A. had a nonsignificant LHA. L.B. and A.A. had an RH advantage (RHA) for shape matches and N.G. had a nonsignificant LHA.

Normal subjects can classify identical stimuli as "same" faster than they can classify nonidentical stimuli as "different" (the "fast-same effect"). We analyzed RTs to same and different trials in "pure hemisphere" (VF and hand on the same side) and bilateral conditions that showed above-chance performance by the patients and we found that responses to different pairs were generally faster than responses to same pairs. This suggests that the patients are using a different strategy than normal subjects and perhaps that the fast-same effect reflects some form of cross-callosal interaction.

Normal subjects also respond more slowly to the shape of different stimuli that have the same name (e.g., Aa) than to different stimuli that have different names (e.g., Ag) (the "congruity effect"). We analyzed the congruity effect in the pure hemisphere and bilateral conditions and found none. Again, it may be that the congruity effect is interhemispheric and occurs only within a narrow range of relative timing of the different processes.

The two experiments together show that N.G. can match shapes but not names across the two VFs. In contrast, L.B., who sometimes readily names LVF objects, can do neither. Experiment 5 below shows, in addition, that N.G. is barely able to match colors across the two VFs but that she cannot name LVF colors. By contrast, L.B. cannot match colors across the two VFs but he can name LVF color patches (cf. table 17.1). Thus, N.G. and L.B. show selective subcallosal, transfer, suggesting that the two patients differ from each other in the channels that are available for transfer.

IMPLICIT TRANSFER

We may say that interhemispheric transfer in the split brain is implicit if both verbalization of LVF stimuli and cross-matching on demand fail, but there is nonetheless some automatic influence of the (unattended) stimulus in one VF on a decision in the other. In an attempt to demonstrate implicit transfer in the split brain, E. Zaidel (1982, 1989) and Clarke (1990) used a lexical decision task with lateralized targets and lateralized associated primes. When tested with associative priming, normal subjects showed no effect of VF of prime but a significant effect of VF of target, with greater associative priming in the LVF. Split-brain patients showed no priming between the hemispheres. Unfortunately, they also showed no priming within either hemisphere. Similarly, Reuter-Lorenz and Baynes (1992) found no evidence for letter priming across the disconnected VFs. They asked patients to decide whether a target upper-

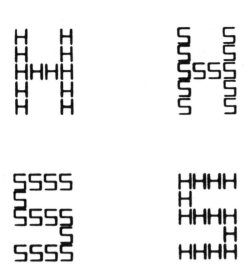

CONSISTENT **INCONSISTENT**

Figure 17.3   The stimuli used in the hierarchic perception experiment.

case letter was an H or a T and found no priming by a preceding lowercase h
or t in the opposite VF. Given the small target set, a positive finding would
not have been convincing because of possible cross-cueing or transfer. On the
other hand, Lambert (1991, 1993) showed presumed negative priming of an
RVF target by an LVF prime in a lexical categorization task (cf. Experiment 6
below). Similarly, Holtzman (1984) showed presumed implicit spatial priming
across the disconnected hemispheres (cf. Experiment 4 below).

In the following series of five experiments, I survey different priming paradigms, adapted to bilateral presentations, ranging from attention to perception and language. The question is whether any of these priming paradigms
shows priming effects across the two VFs in the split brain.

Hierarchic Perception

When large H's or S's made up of little H's or S's (figure 17.3) are presented
peripherally to normal subjects who are required to identify the large (global)
or small (local) letter (H or S), they exhibit two effects. First, they identify
more quickly the global targets. Second, they identify local targets that are
embedded in different global letters (inconsistent: an H made out of S's or an S
made out of H's) more slowly than local targets that are embedded in the
same global letters (consistent: an H made out of H's, an S made out of S's).
This is called "the consistency effect" (figure 17.4). Some find RVF specialization for identifying local targets and, less frequently, LVF specialization for
global targets (van Kleek, 1989). Lamb and Robertson (1988) argued that the
global advantage and the consistency effect in local decision are independent

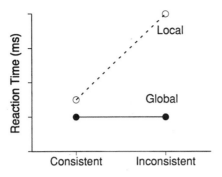

Figure 17.4 The "canonical" effects in Navon's hierarchic perception task.

of each other. Further, based on findings in patients with unilateral temporoparietal lesions (Robertson, Lamb, and Knight, 1988), the authors speculate that the consistency effect is mediated by the corpus callosum. This predicts that the effect should be absent in patients with complete cerebral commissurotomy (Robertson and Lamb, 1991).

Experiment 1 In order to analyze the role of the corpus callosum in the consistency effect of local decisions, it was important to include trials with LVF targets, RVF targets, and identical bilateral copies, one in each VF (BVF). This version was first administered to 16 normal subjects and then to three patients with complete cerebral commissurotomy (Robertson, Lamb, and Zaidel, 1993).

The stimuli (called "hierarchical patterns") consisted of large H's and S's made up of small H's and S's. Each trial contained either unilateral or bilateral presentation of one of the four patterns. One third of the trials were bilateral presentations, one third were unilateral RVFs, and one third were unilateral LVFs. The hierarchic patterns appeared for 100 ms. Response hand was varied across blocks with patients using their right index and middle fingers to respond on half the blocks and their left index and middle fingers to respond to the other half.

Normal Subjects Latency results with 16 right-handed subjects showed the usual global advantage and a Level (global, local) × Consistency (consistent, inconsistent) interaction showing a consistency effect in local but not in global decisions. There was no Level × Consistency × VF (LVF, RVF, BVF) interaction, indicating that the consistency effect was the same in the bilateral condition and in each of the two VFs (figure 17.5). There was a Level × VF (L, R) interaction showing an RVF advantage (RVFA) for local decisions and an LVF advantage (LVFA) for global decisions. Further, bilateral presentations paralleled the RVF for local decisions, but the LVF for global decisions, horserace fashion. Finally, there was no correlation between the consistency effect and the global advantage.

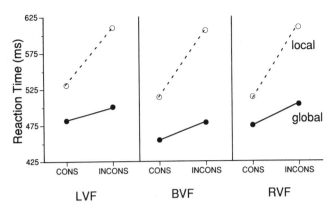

Figure 17.5 Performance of 16 normal subjects on the first hierarchic perception exeriment. CONS, consistent; INCONS, inconsistent; LVF, left visual field trials; BVF, bilateral trials; RVF, right visual field trials. (From Robertson, Lamb, and E. Zaidel, 1993.)

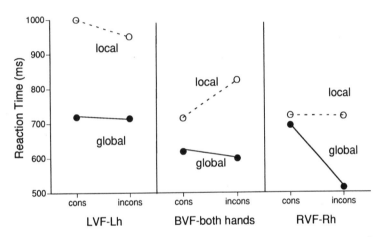

Figure 17.6 Performance of commissurotomy patient L.B. on the first hierarchic perception experiment. *LVF-Lh* = left visual field trials with left hand responses, etc.

L.B. L.B. had a 5.9% error rate overall. His RTs for correct responses were analyzed with trials as the random variable and with response hand (Lh, Rh), Level (global, local), VF (LVF, RVF, BVF), and Consistency (consistent, inconsistent) as between-trial variables. The ANOVA (analysis of variance) disclosed an overall RHA, a global advantage, and an LVF deficit compared to RVF and BVF presentations. BVF and RVF RTs did not differ. There was no main effect of consistency and no Level × Consistency interaction. A separate analysis of the bilateral trials showed an overall global advantage but no other main effects or interactions (figure 17.6). A separate analysis comparing LVF-Lh and RVF-Rh trials, i.e., those reflecting "pure hemisphere" or independent processing by the RH and LH, respectively, showed the usual global advantage, an RVFA, and a Level × VF interaction. As expected, there was a larger

Zaidel: Interhemispheric Transfer in the Split Brain

global advantage with LVF-Lh than with RVF-Rh trials. There were no other significant effects. Thus, L.B. confirms the prediction of no consistency effect.

How does L.B.'s bilateral performance compare to his "pure hemisphere" scores? Inspection of figure 17.5 shows three different patterns: (1) a bilateral advantage, evident in consistent global targets; (2) a "race," or "best condition" pattern evident in inconsistent local targets; and (3) an "average" pattern, as in consistent local and inconsistent global targets. This shows that complex patterns of interhemispheric interaction in general, and of sharing in particular, can occur in the absence of the neocortical commissures, even though the interference effects are normally mediated by the commissures.

N.G. The pure hemisphere conditions (LVF-Lh, RVF-Rh) showed a global advantage and a significant Level × VF (LVF, RVF) interaction. There was an LVFA for global decisions and an RVFA for local decisions. N.G. also showed an RVFA overall. The Level × Consistency interaction was not significant. N.G.'s bilateral RTs are generally averages of her pure hemisphere RTs.

A.A. There was chance performance (53%) with local decisions in LVF presentations. Global decisions yielded an LVFA and a competition (horserace) in the bilateral condition. Bilateral presentations had an overall error rate of 11% and RTs of correct responses showed an overall consistency effect, but there was no Level × Consistency interaction.

Thus, the commissurotomy patients confirm that each hemisphere can perform both global and local decisions and that the LH may be specialized for local decisions, whereas the RH may be specialized for global decisions. Had the consistency effect depended on the global advantage we would expect to find it, especially in the LVF-Lh and BVF conditions. Our general failure to observe a consistency effect supports the callosal hypothesis of its origin as predicted by Robertson and Lamb (1991).

Experiment 2 The hierarchic perception experiment was repeated with 40 right-handed male and female UCLA undergraduates in order to analyze the effect of individual differences in hemispheric specialization or in callosal connectivity on the consistency effect (Carusi, 1992; Carusi, and Zaidel, in preparation). In particular, we compared the performance of subjects who have different degrees of sexual attribution (masculinity and femininity on the Bem scale; cf. Bem, 1974) and who show differences in hemispheric arousal (Levy et al., 1983). We also correlated the consistency effect with measures of hemispheric specialization for local and global decisions and with measures of callosal connectivity (the bilateral advantage). The stimuli and procedures were similar to Experiment 1.

Normal Subjects The results showed the usual global advantage, consistency effect, and Level × Consistency interaction (greater consistency effect for local than global decisions). This time there was a consistency effect for

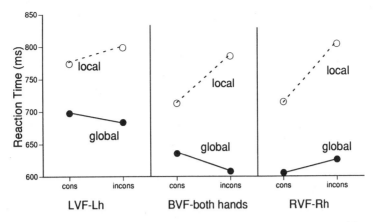

Figure 17.7 Performance of commissurotomy patient L.B. on the second hierarchic perception experiment.

global decisions as well. There was also a VF × Consistency interaction with a weaker consistency effect in the LVF and similar effects in the RVF and BVF.

We also found a significant Sex × Masculine level × Feminine level × Consistency interaction showing that both phenotypical sex and "spectral" sex (Bem scores) affected the consistency effect. At the same time there was a Masculine level × VF interaction showing that only spectral sex affected the laterality effect. Finally, a multiple stepwise regression of the consistency effect in local decisions selected two variables: first, Local RVF/Global LVF, with a multiple partial correlation of .5679 which accounted for 32.25% of the variance; second, the bilateral advantage for local decisions, with a step 2 multiple correlation of .6534 which accounted for 10.5% of the remaining variance. Together, the two variables accounted for 42.7% of the total variance and this supports the interhemispheric model of the consistency effect in local decisions.

L.B. The combined results from two testing sessions were submitted to an ANOVA with trial as the random variable (Weekes, Carusi, and Zaidel, in preparation). There were three between-trial variables: Level (global, local), Consistency (consistent, inconsistent), and VF-hand (LVF-Lh, RVF-Rh, BVF–both hands). This time, there was an overall global advantage, an overall consistency effect and a Level × Consistency interaction showing a consistency effect in local but not in global decisions. There was a VF-hand effect, showing that the LVF-Lh condition (740 ms) was slower than both the RVF-Rh condition (683 ms) and the BVF condition (686 ms), which did not differ from each other (figure 17.7). Considering the LVF-Lh condition alone, there was no consistency effect or Level × Consistency interaction. On the other hand, the RVF-Rh condition had a significant consistency effect; the Level × Consistency interaction did not reach significance. Further, the critical bilateral condition showed both a consistency effect and a significant Level ×

Consistency interaction. The same pattern was observed in BVF-Rh and BVF-Lh responses.

Thus, in the critical BVF condition of this experiment, L.B. did show evidence of both standard effects: he had a significant consistency effect in local but not in global decisions. Consequently, if the consistency effect is indeed interhemispheric, it can be mediated either by the neocortical commissures or by subcortical routes. In that case, subcortical mediation appears to be labile and to vary across similar experimental conditions.

N.G. The ANOVA disclosed a main effect of VF (RVF fastest, LVF slowest, and BVF intermediate). There was also an overall consistency effect and the Consistency × VF interaction approached significance. In the LVF-Lh condition there was no consistency effect in either local or global decisions. In the RVF-Rh condition, there was an overall consistency effect and a significant but unusual Level × Consistency interaction. This was due to a consistency effect for global decisions and not for local decisions. In the critical BVF condition, there was an overall consistency effect and no Level × Consistency interaction. Both local and global decisions showed a consistency effect. The same pattern occurred in BVF with Rh responses and with Lh responses.

Thus, N.G. shows evidence of a classic consistency effect for local decisions although not of the usual Level × Consistency interaction (greater consistency effect for local than global decisions). Her RVF-Rh condition showed an opposite Level × Consistency interaction, where there was a consistency effect for global rather than local decisions. It should be noted that other repetitions of the experiments yielded generally similar results, but on one occasion the LVF-Lh condition showed the same pattern observed in the RVF-Rh condition here, and on another the RVF-Rh condition showed no consistency effects.

Does the bilateral condition differ from the pure hemisphere conditions? Such a difference would suggest interhemispheric interaction in the absence of the neocortical commissures. ANOVAs with trials as a random variable and with Condition (LVF-Lh, RVF-Rh, BVF-Rh, BVF-Lh), Level (global, local), and Consistency (consistent, inconsistent) as between-trial variables did not show a significant three-way interaction in either L.B. or N.G. Neither were the following pairwise comparisons between conditions significant: Condition (BVF-Rh, RVF-Rh) × Level × Consistency or Condition (BVF-Lh, LVF-Lh) × Level × Consistency. Thus, there is no evidence from redundant bilateral presentations of the hierarchic stimuli for any implicit interhemispheric transfer.

The data obtained in Experiment 2 dramatically qualify the conclusions suggested by Experiment 1. The "pure hemisphere" conditions in the split-brain patients did not exhibit the expected specialization effects and they did exhibit consistency effects and Level × Consistency interactions, at least sometimes. Similarly, the bilateral condition exhibits stable consistency effects and can exhibit a classic Level × Consistency interaction (L.B.). Therefore the neocortical commissures are not necessary for the consistency effect.

Covert Orienting of Spatial Attention

The thesis of hemispheric independence in the normal brain suggests that each hemisphere has its own attentional system to coordinate its independent cognitive activities. But there must also be some shared attentional system that coordinates interhemispheric interaction and achieves unified behavior. There are many components of attention and different operationalizations of them. Here we consider covert orienting of spatial attention as operationalized by the Posner paradigm (cf. Posner, 1980). The spatial orienting system is believed to be localized in the posterior parietal lobe and to be specialized in the RH. In the Posner cueing paradigm one shifts selective attention without eye movement by using mostly informative peripheral cues and measuring the benefits that accrue to simple target detection by valid cues and the costs that accrue by invalid ones, relative to neutral cues. The costs and benefits are larger with automatic peripheral cues than with central symbolic or controlled cues and some have argued that informative central cues (controlled) and uninformative peripheral cues (automatic) direct different attentional systems (Briand and Klein, 1987).

Suppose each hemisphere has a separate covert orienting system. Then we may expect some discontinuities in the cost of invalid cues when crossing the vertical meridian in normals. For example, if each hemisphere controls orienting of attention only in the opposite hemifield, then invalid cues that cross the midline should be irrelevant and cost less than invalid cues within the same hemifield as the target. Alternatively, the invalidity cost across the midline may be larger because of the need to engage another attentional system. But then the specific location of the invalid cue within the visual half-field may be irrelevant. The data do not support such strong forms of independence. Some experiments report an increase in the cost of invalid cues when crossing the vertical meridian, though this is more likely to be observed with central than with peripheral cues (see review in Klein and Pontefract, in press). The increase is sometimes attributed to motor programming effects of orienting rather than to hemispheric differences in attention. In this view, covert spatial orienting is accompanied by programming (though not executing) the corresponding eye movements, and attentional shifts across the vertical meridian are more costly because they involve programming a different set of muscles (Umiltá, 1988).

Again, if each hemisphere orients attention in the opposite visual hemifield, then information about the invalid cue across the vertical meridian should be irrelevant and consequently the blocking of such transfer by visual disconnection through callosal (splenial) section should also be irrelevant. This would predict no differences in spatial orienting between the normal and the disconnected hemispheres; both should show the same discontinuities across the vertical meridian. If, on the other hand, there is a unified attentional system in one hemisphere, say the right, that controls both visual hemifields, then information about a cue or a target in the RVF needs to be conveyed first to the RH through the corpus callosum. This shortens the effective stimulus onset asynchrony (SOA) between cue and target and may dilute the cost of invalid cues crossing the midline. It also predicts a smaller invalidity effect in the disconnected than in the normal brain.

Holtzman et al. (1981) showed that two patients (J.W. and P.S.) with section of the corpus callosum but not of the anterior commissure could cue the relative position in a 3- × 3-grid across the vertical meridian, without being able to explicitly compare these positions (at least for J.W.). Since the interstimulus interval (ISI) between cue and target was 1500 ms, cueing was probably controlled rather than automatic and some high-level code could have transferred extracallosally. More recently, Reuter-Lorenz and Fendrich (1990) used a peripheral cueing Posner paradigm with four locations along the horizontal meridian, two on each side of fixation. They found a greater valid-invalid difference when crossing the vertical meridian than within a VF in two callosotomy patients (J.W. and V.P.) but not in normal controls or in a patient with partial section restricted to the anterior two thirds of the corpus callosum (S.C.). The experiment does not include a neutral condition; the ISI is a long 500 ms (long enough to have generated inhibition of return and to permit peripheral eye movements) and the data for the valid and invalid response latencies in each VF are not provided.

In the following experiment we employed a Posner-type paradigm for covert orienting of spatial attention along the four corners of a square centered at the fixation point (Passarotti, Rayman, and Zaidel, in preparation). We included a neutral condition and used a relatively short ISI (150 ms) as well as peripheral arrow cues. We predicted (1) a different pattern of cost and benefit in each VF, both in normal and in split-brain subjects; (2) some discontinuity in invalidity costs when crossing the midline both in normal and in split-brain subjects, and (3) a different degree of discontinuity in normal and in split-brain subjects. Any invalidity effect across the vertical meridian in the split brain is presumably mediated by an attentional system that represents both VFs, a system that has access either to ipsilateral visual cue information or to subcallosal interhemispheric cue information.

Figure 17.8 depicts a strong theoretical prediction of covert orienting within and between the two visual hemifields in normal subjects and in split-brain patients. We assume that (1) the RH has an attentional map that includes both VFs, (2) the LH has an attentional map that includes only the RVF, (3) the LH controls attention for RVF targets and the RH controls attention for LVF targets, (4) the two attentional systems do not communicate with each other even while visual information can transfer across the hemispheres through the corpus callosum, (5) the RH reveals greater costs from invalid cues and greater benefits from valid cues than the LH, and (6) callosal transfer of an RVF cue to the RH will shorten the delay between cue and target and will enhance the invalidity cost. Then an invalid LVF cue preceding an RVF target is ineffective, equivalent to a neutral cue. And this is just as true for a normal subject as for a split-brain patient. On the other hand, an invalid cue preceding an LVF target is costly in the normal brain, though not in the split brain.

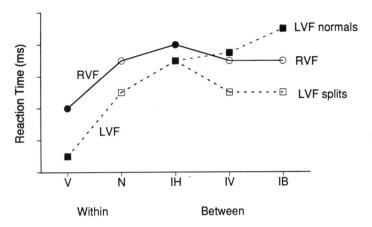

Figure 17.8 Theoretical predictions of covert orienting of spatial attention within and between the two hemifields in normal subjects and in split-brain patients. V, valid cues; N, neutral cues; IH, invalid cues crossing the horizontal meridian; IV, invalid cues crossing the vertical meridian; IB, invalid cues crossing both meridians. Filled symbols, significantly different from the neutral condition.

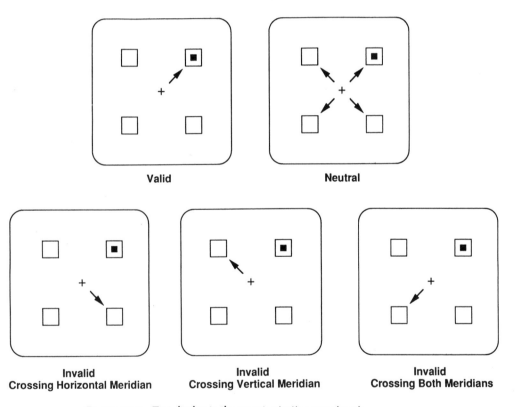

Figure 17.9 Test display in the covert orienting experiment.

Target locations were marked by four square boxes, positioned at the four corners of an imaginary square, displayed on an IBM-PC-compatible computer screen (figure 17.9). Peripheral arrow cues were flashed for 150 ms followed usually by 50-ms target light flashes in one of the boxes. The cues were valid on 80% of the cued trials, or 44% of total trials; they were invalid on 20% of the cued trials, or 11% of total trials; and they were neutral, with four arrows pointing simultaneously at the four boxes, on 22% of the total trials. There were also 23% catch trials where a cue appeared but no target was presented.

Normal Subjects The results with 21 normal right-handed undergraduates are shown in figure 17.10. Subjects responded bimanually in a go–no go paradigm. An ANOVA was carried out on the latency data, with two within-subject factors: Condition (valid, neutral, invalid crossing the horizontal meridian [IH], invalid crossing the vertical meridian [IV], invalid crossing both meridians [IB]) and VF of target (left, right). There was a main effect of Condition and a significant interaction between Condition and Target VF. Both VFs showed faster RTs to valid than to neutral or invalid trials. Invalid trials were slower than valid ones only in the LVF and only for trials crossing the horizontal or both meridians. Indeed, in the LVF, IV targets were faster than IH and IB targets. Thus, the data show (1) a different cost-benefit pattern in each VF, where the LVF shows both cost (invalid slower than neutral) and benefit (valid faster than neutral) while the RVF shows only a benefit, and (2) a discontinuity in priming across the vertical meridian, consistent with some mirror-symmetric priming.

Our predictions (see figure 17.8) that (1) there is an overall LVFA for cueing within a visual hemifield, (2) that there is a greater validity effect in the LVF, (3) that there is significant cost to invalid cues within the RVF (RVF-IH), and (4) that there is significant cost to LVF targets with invalid cues crossing the vertical meridian, were not uniformly and unambiguously confirmed. The absence of cost for RVF-IH targets makes ambiguous the interpretation of no cost in RVF-IV and RVF-IB. If RVF-IV and RVF-IB are equal to RVF-neutral

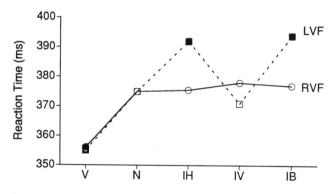

Figure 17.10 Average reaction times of 21 normal subjects by condition and visual field of target. Notation as in figure 17.8.

(RVF-N), then an important prediction is confirmed. On the other hand, RVF-IV and RVF-IB may just be equal to RVF-IH.

L.B. An ANOVA with trials as a random factor showed a main effect of Condition . Valid trials were faster than neutral trials for both the LVF and the RVF. There was also a Condition × VF interaction. RTs to invalid targets were significantly slower than to neutral trials only in the LVF. Thus, like the normals, L.B. shows both cost and benefit in the LVF but only a benefit in the RVF (figure 17.11). L.B. also showed a discontinuity across the vertical meridian but it was opposite to the normals. Whereas they showed a selective gain for IV, he showed a selective cost for those mirror-symmetric invalid trials. In addition, RVF variance was larger than LVF variance.

Together, the data from L.B. and from the normal subjects suggest that there is an asymmetric, callosally mediated mirror image facilitation from the RVF to the LVF, as well as a subcallosally mediated mirror image inhibition in the same direction. In the normal brain, callosal facilitation dominates, whereas the split brain unmasks, subcallosal inhibition.

N.G. ANOVAs with trials or blocks as random factors revealed similar results. The analysis by trials showed a main effect of Condition, a main effect of target VF, and a significant Condition × VF interaction. Like the normals and like L.B., only targets in the LVF show both cost and benefit and a discontinuity across the vertical meridian (figure 17.12). RVF targets show a benefit but no invalidity effect. Thus, valid trials were faster than neutrals in both VFs. There was no cost or invalidity effect in the RVF, but in the LVF IB targets were slower than neutral. Thus, in N.G. IB targets were slower than IV targets (which were equal to neutrals), whereas in L.B. IV targets were slower than IB targets (which were equal to neutrals). In both cases, however, cue information in the RVF affected target detection in the LVF, showing some form of information transfer from the RVF or from the LH to the RH and

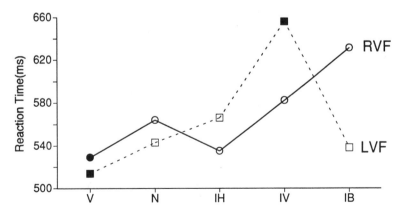

Figure 17.11 Average reaction times of L.B. by condition and visual field of target. Notation as in figure 17.8.

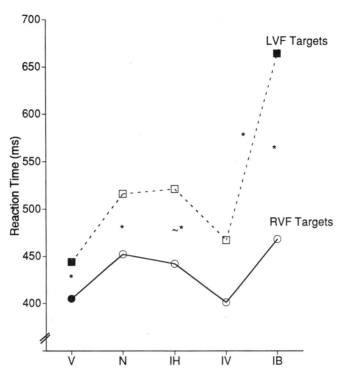

Figure 17.12 N.G.'s performance on the covert orienting experiment. Notation as in figure 17.8.

demonstrating that the attentional map in the disconnected RH includes a representation of both VFs.

Results from both normal subjects and split-brain patients converge on the conclusion that the two VFs show different patterns of cost and benefit. Both fields show benefits by valid cues but the LVF is more likely to show costs by invalid cues. This is consistent with the existence of two different attentional systems in the two hemispheres, or at least with differential access to a unified attentional system for information from the two VFs. The attentional system in the RH, i.e., the one controlling responses to LVF targets, has a representation of both fields and its access to RVF information has both callosally and extracallosally mediated components. One extracallosal pathway that allows RH access to RVF information is an extrageniculostriate system mediated by the right superior colliculus (cf. Trevarthen and Sperry, 1973).

In information-processing terms, we may say that attention is disengaged more easily (from an invalid cue) when the target occurs in the RVF. In other words, novelty is more likely to orient the attentional system in the LVF, but there is faster return to normal in the RVF. Perhaps the RVF is monitored by attentional systems in both hemispheres whereas the LVF is monitored by the RH alone, thus making attentional shifts to the LVF less efficient and particularly vulnerable to brain damage, such as neglect (cf. Mesulam, 1991).

It should not be surprising that the two disconnected hemispheres have access to a unified attentional system. After all, these patients appear to act normally in everyday situations. They do not bump into objects in the LVF and they behave in a left-right coordinated manner. However, our data suggest that their covert spatial orienting may be abnormal because of the absence of the commissures. It may be surprising that this has not resulted in more noticeable deficits, but more subtle observation and testing in ecologically valid conditions may reveal persistent lacunae in behavior, such as responses to threatening, fast, peripheral stimuli.

The Stroop Effect

It is now generally believed that the LH shows a greater Stroop effect than the RH and that this is due to greater interference by incongruent relative to neutral stimuli, consistent with LH specialization for reading (MacLeod, 1991). Thus, Schmit and Davis (1974) displayed the classic Stroop stimuli to the RVF or LVF of normal subjects using manual responses and found greater slowing of RT with incongruent stimuli in the RVF than in the LVF. This was confirmed by Guiard (1981) for RT of manual responses and by Tsao et al. (1979) for accuracy of standard oral verbal responses, but not by Warren and Marsh (1979) who found overall faster RTs but similar interference for RVF stimuli. Franzon and Hugdahl (1986) found that the increased error rate for incongruent stimuli in the RVF was limited to dextral males, consistent with the assumption that they show greatest LH specialization for language.

Dyer (1973) presented a color patch to one VF and a color name (in black ink) to the other and found reliable and similar facilitation and inhibition when the word was flashed to the RVF and to the LVF. David (1991) used color patches and color words presented not only between but also within the hemispheres and required verbal responses. He found similar combined Stroop effects (facilitation plus inhibition) in the two VFs but a larger effect with bilateral presentations, regardless of whether the name appeared in the LVF or RVF. This surprising effect was exaggerated in an acallosal patient, supporting an interhemispheric interpretation for it. Our experiments also addressed the contribution of hemispheric specialization and of callosal connectivity to the Stroop effect and consequently we used manual responses and separated color patches and color words.

The use of manual as opposed to vocal responses is necessary in order to tap either hemisphere with an unbiased response measure. Unfortunately, manual responses dilute the Stroop effect. Although still significant, interference (but perhaps not facilitation) is reduced when response modality is switched from oral to manual (MacLeod, 1991, p. 183). In turn, if the to-be-named color patch and the to-be-ignored color word are presented in separate spatial location, interference will be reduced (but not eliminated) relative to the standard, integrated version of the task (MacLeod, 1991, p. 176). Finally, locational uncertainty with respect to the two dimensions of the task increases the interference effect. We have incorporated some locational uncertainty into our experimental paradigm.

Previous studies suggested that interference is maximal in a 100-ms SOA window around simultaneous presentations of color patch and color word (MacLeod, 1991). Pilot testing of the commissurotomy patients following a suggestion by Kornblum (personal communication, August 28, 1992), however, disclosed a greater Stroop effect when the word preceded the patch by an SOA of 150 ms. We used that delay in an attempt to afford the RH maximum opportunity to process the word, so that each hemisphere could show the Stroop effect.

In this chapter we are especially interested in Stroop effects across the vertical meridian in split-brain patients. Such effects could arise from interhemispheric transfer of information along any stage of processing, from sensory registration to response programming. But the effective transfer must occur at or before the locus of the Stroop effect itself. That locus is still in theoretical dispute. It is convenient to distinguish between "late selection" and "early selection" theories. Both the speed of processing (faster process interferes with slower process) and automaticity (more automatic process interferes with less automatic process) models (MacLeod, 1991) are late selection theories where the conflict occurs late in processing, at a response stage. By contrast, the perceptual encoding model is an early selection theory, where the conflict occurs relatively early in processing, at the perceptual encoding stage. Now, noncallosal transfer of sensory visual information early in the processing sequence would be consistent with either early or late selection theories, but noncallosal transfer of a response code without an identification code would only be consistent with late selection theories.

Assume "direct access," i.e., independent processing by each hemisphere of the patch or word stimuli projected to it. The theoretical predictions of the congruity effects in the various unilateral and bilateral conditions are based on the fact that decoding the color word is a slower and less automatic process in the RH than in the LH. Given that each hemisphere shows the Stroop effect, we also suppose that in the bilateral conditions, the hemisphere that "sees" the patch makes the decision while the other hemisphere decodes the color name. Thus, if there should be an interhemispheric effect in the bilateral conditions, it likely occurs later than both the color identification and the name-decoding processes, perhaps at the level of response selection, implicating an abstract cross-callosal code. We assume that callosal transfer of that code does not degrade it and does not significantly affect the congruity effect that it generates.

In this experiment we used a version of the Stroop test in which (1) the color patches and color words were spatially separated; (2) some trials were unilateral, with patch and word occurring in the same VF, while others were bilateral, with patch and word occurring in opposite fields; and (3) responses were unimanual, made by pressing one of three buttons corresponding to one of the three colors, in order to permit each hemisphere maximum independence to respond (Weekes and Zaidel, in preparation).

The stimuli consisted of three color patches, red, green, and blue, and the three vertically aligned color names RED, GREEN, and BLUE in black on a white background. Stimuli could occur in one of four locations centered 4.5 degrees, and 1.5 degrees to the left or right of fixation. A trial would start with a warning beep followed by one of the color names in one of the four locations for 150 ms, followed immediately by one of the color patches in another location for 100 ms. In half of the trials the patch and name occurred in the same VF (within or unilateral trials) and in half they occurred in the opposite VFs (between or bilateral trials). Half of the stimuli were congruent (color patch matching color name) and half were incongruent. Responses were signaled by pressing one of three buttons on the computer keyboard corresponding to the color patch. Split-brain patients repeated the test twice in each session, once with the Lh responding and once with the Rh responding.

There was also a verbal response version of the test, where the patient named the color patch. Two critical predictions were tested in the split-brain patients. First, it was expected that patients N.G. and L.B. would be able to name patches in the RVF, but we did not expect that N.G. could name LVF patches, although L.B. might. Second, it was expected that Stroop effects would occur with unilateral presentations (RVF only in the case of verbal responses) but not with bilateral presentations. Finally, there was a color match version in which the color name was replaced by the corresponding color patch and subjects had to decide whether the two color patches were the same or different. Responses were signaled unimanually by pressing one of two buttons on the computer keyboard. In this control experiment, it was expected that patients with complete disconnection would be able to match patches within either VF but not between the two VFs.

Normal Subjects   The test was administered to ten normal subjects. An ANOVA on latencies of correct responses was carried out with VF (within = LVF patch and LVF word [LL] or RVF patch and word [RR]; between = LVF patch and RVF word [LR] or RVF patch and LVF word [RL]) and Congruity (congruent, incongruent) as within-subject variables. There was a main effect of Congruity and of VF but no Congruity × VF interaction. Planned comparisons motivated by a priori predictions showed that there was a significant congruity (Stroop) effect in both within-VF conditions (LL, RR). However, only one of the two *between* conditions, LR (where the word projected to the LH), showed a significant Stroop effect, whereas the RL condition did not (figure 17.13). Thus, the normal subjects do seem to suggest a unidirectional discontinuity across the midline in their Stroop effect.

L.B.   The latencies of correct unimanual responses to unilateral and bilateral trials were submitted to an ANOVA with trials as a random factor and with VF by response hand (VF-h) Condition and Congruity (congruent, incongruent) as between-trial factors. There were four input VF-h conditions: LL-L (LVF patch, LVF word, Lh response), RR-R, RL-R/L, and LR-L/R. We found a

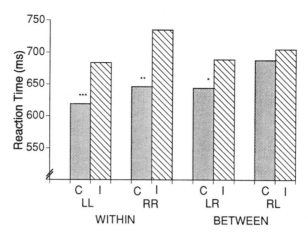

Figure 17.13 The Stroop effects in ten normal subjects with unilateral (within) and bilateral (between) presentations and manual responses. C, Congruent condition, I, Incongruent condition. WITHIN, patch and word within same visual hemifield, BETWEEN, patch and word in opposite visual hemifields. *, significant at $P = .05$; **, significant at $P = .01$; ***, signficant at $P = .001$.

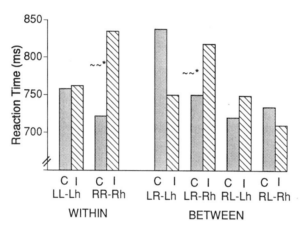

Figure 17.14 L.B.'s latencies of responses in the unilateral/bilateral Stroop experiment with unimanual responses. LL-Lh, LVF color patch, LVF color word, left hand responses; RR-Rh, RVF color patch, RVF color word, right hand responses, etc. $\sim \sim$*, a trend toward a significant Stroop effect ($P < .1$). Other notation as in figure 17.16.

main effect of Condition but no Congruity effect or Condition × Congruity interaction. The congruity effects for all the conditions are depicted in figure 17.14. There was no congruity effect in the RH (LL-L) and only a trend toward one in the LH (RR-R). There was no congruity effect for between conditions with the patch in the RVF (RL-R, RL-L). There was an (insignificant) reversed congruity effect in the bilateral condition with the patch in the LVF and Lh responses (LR-L), but there was a trend toward a significant congruity effect in the bilateral condition with the patch in the LVF and with Rh responses (LR-R).

Thus, if we consider the trends to be meaningful, we conclude that there is a suggestion of a congruity effect in the LH and, critically for this experiment, there is also a suggestion of a congruity effect when the patch occurred in the LVF, the word occurred in the RVF, and the Rh responded. The fact that the trend occurred with Rh responses suggests that performance was under control of the disconnected LH. This could represent transfer of the color information directly from the LVF to the LH. Alternatively, it could represent transfer of color or higher code information from the disconnected RH to the LH. In either case, transfer would be sufficient for manual identification by the LH (Rh) of the identity of color information in the LVF and this process is penetrable (Fodor, 1983) by the results of semantic processing of the color word in the LH.

In the color match control experiment, L.B. could match reliably patches within either the LVF or the RVF but he could not match patches across the two VFs regardless of which hand responded, suggesting that neither hemisphere could perform the bilateral comparison.

In the second control experiment, verbal Stroop, L.B. was required to name the color patch in the classic Stroop paradigm with unilateral and bilateral trials. This time he could reliably name LVF patches in either unilateral or bilateral trials. Indeed, there was a significant congruity effect in accuracy of naming patches in unilateral LVF trials (congruent = 92%, incongruent = 75%, $z = 2.59$). This means that L.B. could name a color patch in the LVF which he could not match with a patch in the RVF, and further that this naming response was affected by the color word in the LVF (the Stroop effect)!

Taken together, the data suggest that in L.B., visual color patch information from the LVF is accessible to components of the linguistic module in the LH that (1) name the color, (2) decode the meaning of a color word in the RVF, and even (3) decode the meaning of a color word in the LVF. But the same visual color patch information from the LVF is not accessible to a same-different color comparison or identification module in the LH that would match the LVF patch with an RVF patch.

N.G. The latencies of N.G.'s unimanual responses in the bilateral/unimanual Stroop experiment were also submitted to an ANOVA with trial as a random variable, and with stimulus VF-h Condition and Congruity (congruent, incongruent) as between-trial factors. There was a main effect of VF-h Condition and a Condition × Congruity interaction. There was no congruity or Stroop effect in either hemisphere alone, i.e., in the unilateral conditions (RR-R, LL-L) or in the bilateral condition with the word in the LVF (RL-R/L). However, there was a significant Stroop effect in the bilateral condition with the word in the RVF (LR-L) (figure 17.15). Accuracies were high in all conditions. Indeed, there was a significant Stroop effect in the LR-L/R conditions in accuracy as well.

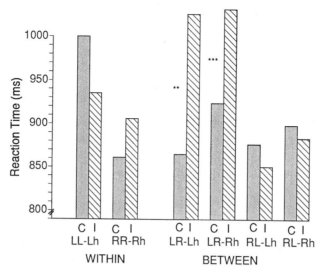

Figure 17.15 N.G.'s latencies of unimanual responses in the unilateral/bilateral Stroop experiment. Notation as in figures 17.13 and 17.14.

N.G. could reliably match colors within each hemisphere but not between the two hemispheres. Her between-field matches with Rh responses show a "same" bias but do not differ from chance. However, her between-field matches with Lh responses almost exceed chance, suggesting some possible color transfer from the RVF or the LH to the RH. At present it appears that color matching by N.G. is essentially as difficult as it is for L.B., contrary to her facile between-field matching of shapes.

N.G.'s accuracy of naming the patch in the verbal Stroop shows the expected accurate naming of RVF patches in either the unilateral or bilateral condition. Not surprisingly, there was also a significant Stroop effect in accuracy when both color and word were in the RVF (RR) but not when the color was in the RVF and the word was in the LVF (RL). In the LR "between" condition, where the color was in the LVF and the word was in the RVF, N.G.'s LH dominated the responses so that she simply read aloud the RVF word. In the unilateral LL condition, N.G. surprisingly named the colors reliably in the incongruent but not in the congruent condition. It is not clear why the color name should affect the noncallosal transfer of the color from the LVF or the RH to the LH.

Using latency as the dependent variable, the normal data suggest that crossing the neocortical commissures dilutes the Stroop effect, and the split-brain data show that the commissures are necessary for maintaining the Stroop effect across the commissures. Thus, there is no example where a significant unilateral Stroop effect was maintained in a bilateral condition. Still, N.G. showed Stroop effects when the patch was in the LVF and the word was in the RVF. Furthermore, accuracy data do suggest occasional congruity effects in both patients in some bilateral conditions with the color patch on either side and with both unimanual and verbal responses. Furthermore, both patients could reliably match color patches within either hemisphere, but neither patient could match colors across the two VFs. This suggests that the information transferred across the meridian and giving rise to the congruity effect in the bilateral condition is not sensory-visual and is accessible to verbal or manual identification but not to perceptual matching.

Lexicality Priming

Consider two consecutive trials in a categorization task where each trial contains two stimuli distinguished by some predesignated perceptual feature (say an arrow) which directs attention to one of them (categorize it, ignore the other). The stimuli in one trial could be related (in terms of the decision category) to those in the next. When two successive *attended* stimuli are related, there is a facilitation in categorizing the second. But the same relationship between the *unattended* stimulus on one trial and the attended stimulus in the next produces inhibition in categorizing the second (e.g., Tipper, 1985; Driver and Tipper, 1989). Both the facilitation and the interference are taken to occur at a response selection stage.

Lambert (1991) argued that these inhibitory effects can also occur between simultaneous stimuli in the same trial, one attended and the other unattended. However, in his design the attended stimulus was flashed for only 35 ms whereas the attended one was flashed for 100 ms so that this may be regarded as a sequential presentation. First, he asked normal subjects to categorize RVF words as living or nonliving and showed that when an unattended LVF word belonged to the same category as the attended RVF word, manual categorization speed was reduced. Lambert then repeated the experiment with split-brain patient L.B. and showed similar inhibition. However, we suspected that this result may have been artifactual because the targets that showed inhibition were different from those that did not. Moreover, there was no independent verification that instructions to attend to the RVF were effective, and that systematic eye gaze shifts did not occur. Further, there were no appropriate control conditions, including neutral unattended stimuli; attended and unattended stimuli within the LVF and, separately, within the RVF; categorizing the attended targets alone in the RVF, and, separately, in the LVF; naming the LVF stimuli; matching the LVF and RVF stimuli, etc.

In the present experiment, we used a lexical decision task to address similar issues. Stimuli were either unilateral or bilateral and consisted of words or pronounceable nonwords, and attention was drawn to the target VF with a peripheral arrow. The critical question is whether lexical decision of a target in the attended VF is affected by the lexical status of the stimulus in the unattended VF. Lambert's account would predict a negative priming effect when the items in both VFs have the same lexical status (both words or both nonwords), whereas a more traditional Stroop-type account would predict a facilitation in the same condition. Whichever effect is found in normals, does it extend to the split brain, especially when the attended target is in the RVF and responses are made with the right hand, i.e., when there is unambiguous and consistent LH control in both the unilateral and bilateral conditions? Here, unilateral presentations can serve as the neutral or control condition.

Consider the "canonical" model, based on the standard account of facilitation/interference (congruity effect) and on a direct access or hemispheric independence model of lateralized presentations. When the target and decoy are both in the same lexical category (words or nonwords) we expect facilitation, and when they are in opposite categories we expect interference. The congruity effect is proportional to the speed and automaticity of processing the decoy relative to the target. We will assume (1) that in the RVF (LH), words are processed faster and more automatically than nonwords so that RVF word decoys should create greater facilitation of and interference with LVF targets than will RVF nonword decoys. We will assume (2) that in the LVF (RH), words are processed about as quickly and automatically as nonwords so that LVF word and nonword decoys create about the same facilitation and interference with RVF targets. We will also assume (3) that words are processed faster and more automatically, and thus create more facilitation/interference as decoys, in the RVF than in the LVF, whereas nonwords are processed about equally quickly and automatically, and thus create equal facilitation/interference, in the two hemispheres. Finally, we will assume that (4) slower processes (LVF targets) are more prone to facilitation/interference than faster processes (RVF targets).

Stimuli in this experiment consisted of three- to six-letter-long strings, half words, and half pronounceable nonwords. Half the trials consisted of unilateral stimuli and half of bilateral stimuli with a word or nonword in the LVF and another word or nonword in the RVF. Each trial included an arrow in one VF next to the fixation mark, which pointed in one direction and signaled the target stimulus the subject had to categorize as word or nonword. The stimuli and arrows were presented for 120 or 165 ms (normals and patients, respectively) on a MacIntosh IIsi computer. Responses were two-choice manual key presses with the index finger responding to words and the middle finger responding to nonwords. Each subject received three blocks: one with Rh responses, one with Lh responses, and one with simultaneous bimanual responses.

Normal Subjects   Two ANOVAs were performed on mean latencies of correct responses with Subject as a random factor (Iacoboni and Zaidel, submitted). The first included, among others, Condition (unilateral, bilateral) and Target Wordness (words, nonwords) as within-subject factors. There were main effects of Condition (unilateral faster than bilateral) and of Wordness (words faster than nonwords). Unilateral trials with RVF targets were faster than the corresponding bilateral trials with either congruent (WW, NN) or incongruent (NW, WN) distractors and so they failed to serve as a neutral control condition. (Here, NW = nonwords in the LVF, words in the RVF, etc.)

The second ANOVA was restricted to bilateral trials and included also Distractor Wordness (words, nonwords) as a within-subject factor. This ANOVA showed a main effect of Wordness, and the significant interactions included a Target Wordness × Distractor Wordness interaction. Further, congruent trials (WW, NN) were faster than incongruent trials (NW, WN). This was true separately for word targets, but not for nonword targets. The Target Wordness x Distractor Wordness interaction was almost significant for RVF targets ($P = .0839$). Here, word targets in the RVF were decided faster when the distractor in the LVF was a word than when it was a nonword. But nonword targets in the RVF were not faster when the LVF distractor was a nonword. Thus, the data support the standard facilitation account rather than the negative priming account.

On the other hand, the data are not consistent with either the speed-of-processing or the automaticity models of the facilitation effect (MacLeod, 1991) because it is generally believed that words are processed faster and more automatically than nonwords so that the facilitation and interference should be greater when the targets are nonwords than when they are words, opposite to our data. Planned comparisons of congruent and incongruent word and nonword targets in the pure hemisphere conditions (LVF-Lh, RVF-Rh) yielded only a trend toward a significant congruity effect for word targets in the LVF-Lh condition ($P = .089$). Could it be that bilateral presentations are processed in a callosal relay (say, exclusively in the LH) rather than a direct access pattern (where each hemisphere processes the targets projected to it)? This is unlikely because bilateral presentations showed a strong Response hand × target VF interaction consistent with strong direct access or hemispheric independence (E. Zaidel, 1983). That means that congruity effects in bilateral conditions really reflect interhemispheric interaction past the visual information-processing stage.

L.B. A conservative test of interhemispheric effects involves analyzing bilateral and unilateral presentations of the pure hemisphere conditions RVF-Rh (RVF target, Rh response = LH) and LVF-Lh (LVF target, Lh response = RH). In L.B., the LVF-Lh yielded an above-chance score only in the unilateral condition (with no decoy in the unattended visual field), precluding an analysis of interhemispheric effects on RH performance. But his RVF-Rh performance was above chance in both the unilateral and bilateral conditions (Iacoboni, Rayman, and Zaidel, in preparation). An ANOVA was performed on L.B.'s bilateral trials with RVF targets, using Target Wordness, Distractor Wordness, and Response Hand as between-trial factors. Results revealed a main effect of Target Wordness (words faster than nonwords), but no effect of Distractor Wordness and no interaction. In particular, congruent targets were not faster than incongruent targets either for words (WW vs. NW) or for nonwords (NN vs. WN) (figure 17.16).

The only significant congruity effect occurred for bimanual responses, which yielded above-chance performance in bilateral presentations with targets

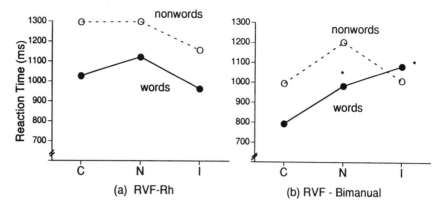

Figure 17.16 The congruity effect of patient L.B. in the lexical decision task. *(a)* Right visual field targets with right hand responses (RVF-Rh). *(b)* Right visual field (RVF) targets with bimanual responses. C, Congruent (Word Word or Nonword Nonword); N, Neutral (—Word, Word—, —Nonword, or Nonword—, where — = empty); I, Incongruent (Nonword Word or Word Nonword); asterisks, Incongruent condition slower than congruent condition.

in either VF. Bimanual bilateral trials showed an almost significant RVFA in latency ($P = .086$), a significant advantage of bilateral presentations and a Word advantage. Most important, there was a Target Wordness × Distractor Wordness interaction. The interaction reflected a significant congruity effect for Word targets. This congruity effect persisted for RVF targets but was not significant for LVF targets. Thus, the only significant congruity effect occurred for RVF word targets with both hands responding, where WW trials were faster than NW trials (see figure 17.16). This *is* evidence for interhemispheric priming but not in the pure LH condition. Indeed, an ANOVA of the latencies of L.B.'s correct responses in the RVF-Rh condition with trial as a random factor and with Target Wordness and Distractor Wordness as between-trial factors revealed only a Target Wordness effect (words faster than nonwords) (see figure 17.16).

N.G. N.G.'s performance was above chance only in the RVF-Rh condition (RVF targets, Rh responses), both with unilateral and bilateral trials. An ANOVA of mean latencies to correct responses, with trial as a random factor and with Condition (unilateral, bilateral) and Target Wordness (words, nonwords) as between-trial variables, showed only a main effect of Target Wordness, with faster processing of words (724 ms) than of nonwords (924 ms). A subsequent ANOVA of bilateral RVF-Rh trials only, with Target Wordness (words, nonwords) and Distractor Wordness (words, nonwords) as between-trial factors, disclosed again a main effect of Target Wordness (words faster) but no effect of Distractor Wordness or interaction between Target Wordness and Distractor Wordness. Mean latencies for the congruent trials (WW, NN) were not different from the incongruent trials (NW, WN). Thus, N.G. shows no evidence of implicit lexicality priming of RVF targets by LVF distractors.

The normal data showed an overall interhemispheric effect which filtered down to word but not to nonword targets. It is noteworthy that this interhemispheric resource sharing occurs even in a condition of maximal hemispheric independence, i.e., with bilateral presentations. The pattern supports a facilitation rather than an interference account of the condition when the target and distractor belong to the same response category. But we have observed congruity effects for word targets and not for nonword targets, arguing against the standard speed-of-processing or automaticity accounts of the effects. The overall congruity effect as well as the Target Wordness × Distractor Wordness interaction for bilateral trials (over all response hand conditions) were significant in the normal subjects and this was also true for RVF targets separately. These effects were not significant in L.B. In the pure hemisphere conditions, the normal data showed at best weak evidence for a congruity effect with LVF word targets. However, this may merely reflect a lack of statistical power owing to relatively few trials in the pure hemisphere conditions. In L.B. and N.G., bilateral trials were above chance only for LH targets. N.G. showed no congruity effect or Target × Distractor interaction in her LH, and L.B. showed it in the LH only for bimanual responses. Perhaps bimanual responses enhance noncallosal interhemispheric interactions in the commissurotomized patient.

CONCLUSIONS

Explicit Transfer

It has been believed for some time that for visual stimuli the chronic complete disconnection syndrome (1) allows interhemispheric transfer or possibly ipsilateral transfer of some simple sensory features, (2) precludes interhemispheric transfer (or ipsilateral projection) of more complex visual information sufficient for object identification in rich displays, and (3) permits interhemispheric transfer of some more abstract semantic features associated with the stimulus. But some individual differences have been observed: N.G. was found to be able to match certain complex visual stimuli across the two VFs even though she could not name the LVF stimuli. On the other hand, L.B. was often able to name LVF stimuli even though unable to match them with RVF stimuli. These past observations in N.G. did not reveal how "deeply processed" the visual signal that transferred must be.

Our data from Experiment 1 show that the signal is relatively "early" in the visual information-processing sequence because it allows matching of nonsense Vanderplas shapes with poor associative value (table 17.1). Experiment 2 confirms that N.G. can match letter shapes but not letter names across the two VFs. Thus, the transferred visual signal has enough features for shape matching but not for letter identification (see table 17.1). Interestingly, N.G.'s ability to match colors across the two VFs (Experiment 5) seems worse than her ability to match shapes (Experiment 1), and in general the transfer appears

Table 17.1 Summary of performance of split-brain patients on tasks that require explicit visual matching within and across the two visual hemifields

Task	Subject	RH	LH	Bi
Nonsense shapes	L.B.	+	+	−
	N.G.	+	+	+
	A.A.	+	−	−
Letter				
Shapes	L.B.	+	+	−
	N.G.	+	+	+
	A.A.	+	+	−
Names	L.B.	+	+	−
	N.G.	+	+	−
	A.A.	+	−	−
Color				
Match	L.B.	+	+	−
	N.G.	+	+	+[a]
Name	L.B.	+[b]	+[c]	+[d]/+[e]
	N.G.	−[b]	+[c]	+[d]/−[e]

[a] Borderline significant with left hand responses
[b] Color patch and color word both in LVF
[c] Color patch and color word both in RVF
[d] Color patch in RVF, color word in LVF
[e] Color patch in LVF, color word in RVF

to be asymmetric, from the RVF or LH to the RH (see table 17.1). If all of N.G.'s visual transfer is unidirectional so that her successful bilateral matches are all done in the disconnected RH, then it would explain her inability to name the stimuli. On this account, her successful matching of bilateral stimuli with either hand responding would reflect effective ipsilateral motor control of the Rh by the RH.

L.B. cannot match nonsense shapes (Experiment 1), letter shapes, or letter names (Experiment 2) or even one of three colors (Experiment 5) across the two VFs. And yet he is able to name LVF colors (see table 17.1). We did not examine his ability to name LVF letters (Experiment 2), but we would expect him to be able to do so if the stimulus set were small and he were given sufficient time, even though he was unable to match bilateral letters for names. Therefore, it is interesting that L.B. is not using a naming strategy to match the bilateral letter names. We do not know yet whether he can be trained to do so, but we have observed a similar failure to use a transitive strategy in his inability to match printed words for rhyming even though he could match printed words with pictures and also match pictures for rhyming names (E. Zaidel and Peters, 1981).

Implicit Transfer

The canonical case for preserved implicit priming in the split brain would consist of the following combination of findings: (0) failure of explicit transfer;

(1) a significant, if unequal, congruity effect in each VF with ipsilateral hand responses, found in both the normal and the split brain; (2) a smaller congruity effect across the two VFs in the normal brain; and (3) a smaller yet, but significant, congruity effect across the two VFs when the responding hand is ipsilateral to the target, in the split brain. This combination of findings did not obtain in any of our experiments! The evidence of implicit transfer that did obtain in each experiment is weak not only because some effects failed to reach statistical significance owing to lack of power but also because the interpretations of some patterns in the data are ambiguous (table 17.2).

Standard models of the congruity effects fail to account for the consistency effect in hierarchic perception just as they fail to account for the hemispheric Stroop effect or for lexicality priming. The priming effects that we observed both in normal subjects and in split-brain patients seem sensitive to both the timing and priorities of the two competing processes. Thus, they cannot be explained by passive parallel races alone and seem to involve active control.

What subcallosal codes mediate the congruity effects across the vertical meridian in the split brain when they do occur? Spatial priming in Experiment 4 may reflect visual transfer through systems that do not preserve or that misalign spatial localization in the attentional maps of the two hemispheres. However, the effect, in which RVF primes (invalid cues) influence LVF targets, may reflect subcallosal LH-to-RH transfer of a more abstract spatial-attentional code. The signal that permitted a bilateral Stroop effect in N.G. in Experiment 5 (with a color patch in the LVF and a color word in the RVF, using either hand for responding) is unlikely to be a sensory color code because the effect occurred in the absence of accurate color matching across the VFs. By the same token, the signal is unlikely to be a verbal code because the effect occurred in the absence of verbal identification of the LVF color. Again, the signal may be "late" and abstract, perhaps a response selection code. Similarly, priming at a response selection stage can account for the results of Experiments 3 and 6. In all these cases, it is noteworthy that the transfer codes are not accessible to consciousness.

In sum, there are considerable individual differences in the interhemispheric pathways that are available to different patients with cerebral commissurotomy. For explicit transfer, N.G. seems to have good subcallosal access to "early" shape but not color information or to "later" identity codes or verbal labels. L.B., on the other hand, does not have subcallosal access to visual information but he does have some access to verbal codes (see table 17.1). For implicit transfer there is also much variability across patients and, in some cases, more surprisingly, across testing sessions as well as across minor variants of the same task. This means that negative data are especially inconclusive. The evidence for implicit transfer in the split brain is also weak because none of the experiments show all the patterns of the canonical case outlined above (cf. table 17.2). And when a planned comparison does reveal significant interhemispheric priming, this is often not accompanied by the appropriate overarching statistical interaction, presumably due to lack of statistical

Table 17.2 Summary of the four experiments on implicit interhemispheric transfer in normal subjects and in split-brain patients

Experiment	Task	Effect	Subject	LVF	RVF	Hemispheric specialization[a]	Interhemispheric effect?[b]
3	Global/Local	Consistency	Normals	+	+	+/−[1]	NA[2]
			NG	−/+[1]	−/+[1]	+/−[1]	NA[2]
			LB	−/+[1]	−/+[1]	+/−[1]	NA[2]
4	Attention	Spatial Priming	Normals	+	+	+	+
			NG	+	+	+	+[3]
			LB	+	+	+	+[3]
5	Stroop	Color name priming	Normals	+	+	+	+[4]
			NG	−	−	−	+[5]
			LB	−	∼∼+	−	∼∼+[6]
6	Lexical Decision	Lexicality Priming	Normals	∼∼+[7,8]	∼∼+[7,9]	+	NA[7]
			NG	−	−	−	NA[7]
			LB	−	+[7,10]	+	NA[7]

[a] Is there a hemispheric specialization in the effect?

[b] Is there a Condition (unilateral, bilateral) × Effect interaction? Or in splits: Is there an effect in the interhemispheric condition?

[1] X/Y = X in Robertson, Lamb, and Zaidel (1993), Y in Carusi and Zaidel (in preparation) and in Weekes, Carusi, and Zaidel (in preparation)

[2] The hypothesis is that the consistency effect is interhemispheric even in unilateral presentations

[3] Only with LVF targets

[4] Planned comparison, no interaction

[5] In LR-Lh/Rh conditions (LVF color, RVF word, either hand responding)

[6] In LR-Rh condition

[7] No unilateral condition. LVF = target in LVF, distractor in RVF; RVF = target in RVF, distractor in LVF

[8] Planned comparison. Only for word targets in LVF with left hand responses

[9] For word targets only

[10] Only for word targets in the RVF condition with bimanual responses

NA = not applicable.

power. Even when an experiment does provide some evidence for probable or likely interhemispheric priming, the priming is sporadic, unreliable, and variable.

The Split Brain vs. the Normal Brain

The anatomically split brain has motivated the functional concept of dynamic hemispheric independence in the normal brain. But the split brain itself reveals an extremely dynamic system with multiple parallel interhemispheric pathways that can modulate hemispheric function, especially at late stages of information processing. This does not mean that all previous research on hemispheric specialization in the split brain is wrong. But it does suggest that the disconnected hemispheres may differ cognitively from the truly isolated hemispheres (as in hemispherectomy) just as they differ from the normal hemispheres. In particular, the normal hemispheres demonstrate consistently greater perceptual and cognitive competence than the disconnected hemispheres, even in conditions that qualify as direct access. Most likely, the normal hemispheres may share resources even while maintaining independent information-processing strategies. Such sharing of resources is possible even in the split brain (E. Zaidel, 1978).

Open Questions

We have barely begun to find out how the hemispheres interact in the normal brain. How does the mind/brain implement independent hemispheric functioning? Hemispheric inhibition? Hemispheric exchange? Is there a single control system? If so, where is it? In particular, how can transfer be made selective for a particular stage of information processing? It is plausible that this is done through dynamic gating of a set of callosal channels, each interconnecting a different cortical region with its own code and each with its own control subchannel. What, then, is the detailed anatomic, electrophysiologic, and neurochemical characterization of these callosal channels? We have already seen some hints for systematic individual differences in how the structure of callosal channels is related to hemispheric specialization (Aboitiz, Scheibel, and Zaidel, 1992; Aboitiz et al., 1992) and this is a promising avenue for more research. Further, the split-brain data demonstrate that there are also subcallosal channels that can convey information between the two hemispheres at arbitrarily late loci of information processing, and we would like to know their role in normal cognitive functioning. Indeed, the role of hemispheric specialization vis-à-vis that of interhemispheric interaction in normal cognition in general is still largely unexplored. If our view is right, that the two normal hemispheres usually maintain dynamic independence, then any task involves some degree of interhemispheric interaction and there can be no general cognitive psychology without a neuropsychology of laterality.

ACKNOWLEDGMENTS

Thanks to Elicia David for assistance and to Alessandra Passarotti, Janice Rayman, Nicole Weekes, and especially Joseph Bogen and Marco Iacoboni for helpful comments on earlier drafts. This work was supported by NIH grant NS20187 and NIH RSA MH00179.

REFERENCES

Aboitiz, F., Scheibel, A. B., Fisher, R. S., and Zaidel, E. (1992). Individual differences in brain asymmetries and fiber composition in the human corpus callosum. *Brain Research, 43,* 154–161.

Aboitiz, F., Scheibel, A. B., and Zaidel, E. (1992). Morphometry of the Sylvian fissure and the corpus callosum, with emphasis on sex differences. *Brain, 115,* 1521–1541.

Bem, S. L. (1974). The measurement of psychological androgyny. *Journal of Counseling and Clinical Psychology, 42,* 155–162.

Bogen, J. E. (1987). Physiological consequences of complete or partial commisural section. In M. L. J. Apuzzo (Ed.), *Surgery of the third ventricle* (pp 175–194). Baltimore, MD: Williams & Wilkins Co.

Bogen, J. E. (1993). The callosal syndrome. In K. M. Heilman and E. Valenstein (Eds.), *Clinical Neuropsychology,* ed 3 (pp 337–407). New York, NY: Oxford University Press.

Bogen, J. E., Schultz, D. H., and Vogel, J. P. (1988). Completeness of callosotomy shown by magnetic resonance imaging in the long term. *Archives of Neurology, 45,* 1203–1205.

Bogen, J. E., and Vogel, P. J. (1975). Neurologic status in the long term following complete cerebral commissurotomy. In F. Michel and B. Schott (Eds.), *Les syndromes de disconnexion calleuse chez l'homme* (pp 227–251). Lyon, France: Hôpital Neurologique.

Briand, K. A., and Klein, R. M. (1987). Is Posner's "beam" the same as Treisman's "glue"?: On the relation between visual orienting and feature integration theory. *Journal of Experimental Psychology: Human Perception and Performance, 13,* 228–241.

Butler, S. R., and Norsell, U. (1968). Vocalization possibly initiated by the minor hemisphere. *Nature, 220,* 793–794.

Carusi, D. A. (1992). The Global/Local consistency effect between and within the hemispheres: Clues from individual differences. Undergraduate Honors Thesis, Department of Psychology, University of California, Los Angeles, CA.

Carusi, D. A., and Zaidel, E. (in preparation). Interhemispheric determinants of the consistency effect in hierarchic perception.

Clarke, J. M. (1990). Interhemispheric functions in humans: Relationships between anatomical measures of the corpus callosum, behavioral laterality effects, and cognitive profiles. Dissertation, Department of Psychology, University of California at Los Angeles, CA.

Clarke, J. M., and Zaidel, E. (in preparation). Matching nonsense shapes within and between the disconnected hemispheres.

Corballis, M. C., and Trudel, C. I. (1993). Role of the forebrain commisures in interhemispheric integration. *Neuropsychology, 7,* 306–324.

Cronin-Golomb, A. (1986). Subcortical transfer of cognitive information in subjects with complete forebrain commissurotomy. *Cortex, 22,* 499–519.

Damasio, A. R., Chui, H. C., Corbett, J., and Kassell, N. (1980). Posterior callosal section in a non-epileptic patient. *Journal of Neurology, Neurosurgery and Psychiatry, 43*, 351–356.

David, A. S. (1991). Stroop effects within and between the cerebral hemispheres: Studies in normals and acallosals. *Neuropsychologia, 30*, 161–175.

de Lacoste, M. C., Kirkpatrick, J. B., and Ross, E. D. (1985). Topography of the human corpus callosum. *Journal of Neuropathology and Experimental Neurology, 44*, 578–591.

Driver, J., and Tipper, S. P. (1989). On the nonselectivity of "selective" seeing: Contrasts between interference and priming in selective attention. *Journal of Experimental Psychology: Human Perception and Performance, 15*, 304–314.

Dyer, F. N. (1973). Interference and facilitation for color naming with separate bilateral presentations of the word and color. *Journal of Experimental Psychology: General, 98*, 102–108.

Eviatar, E., and Zaidel, E. (1994). Letter matching within and between the disconnected hemispheres. *Brain and Cognition, 25*, 128–137.

Fodor, J. A. (1983). *The modularity of mind.* Cambridge, MA: MIT Press.

Franzon, M., and Hugdahl, K. (1986). Visual half-field presentations of incongruent color words: Effects of gender and handedness. *Cortex, 22*, 433–495.

Gazzaniga, M. S., Volpe, B. T., Smylie, C. S., Wilson, D. H., and LeDoux, J. E. (1979). Plasticity in speech organization following commissurotomy. *Brain, 102*, 805–815.

Gordon, H. W., Bogen, J. E., and Sperry, R. W. (1971). Absence of deconnexion syndrome in two patients with partial section of the neocommissures. *Brain, 94*, 327–336.

Guiard, Y. (1981). Effect of processing mode on the degree of motor asymmetry in the manual Stroop test. *Cortex, 17*, 495–501.

Holtzman, J. D. (1984). Interactions between cortical and subcortical visual areas: Evidence from human commisurotomy patients. *Vision Research, 24*, 801–813.

Holtzman, J. D., Sidtis, J. J., Volpe, B. T., Wilson, D. H., and Gazzaniga, M. S. (1981). Dissociation of spatial information for stimulus localizaiton and the control of attention. *Brain, 104*, 861–872.

Iacoboni, M., and Zaidel, E. (submitted). Hemispheric independence in word recognition: Evidence from bilateral presentations.

Iacoboni, M., Rayman, J., and Zaidel, E. (in preparation). Failure of interhemispheric lexicality priming in the split brain.

Johnson, L. E. (1984a). Vocal responses to left visual field stimuli following forebrain commissurotomy. *Neuropsychologia, 22*, 153–166.

Johnson, L. E. (1984b). Bilateral visual cross-integration by human forebrain commissurotomy subjects. *Neuropsychologia, 22*, 167–175.

Klein, R. M., and Pontefract, A. (in press). Does oculmotor readiness mediate cognitive control of visual attention? Revisited! In C. Umiltà and M. Moscovitch (Eds.), *Attention and performance XV: Conscious and nonconscious processes.* Cambridge, MA: MIT Press.

Lamb, M. R., and Robertson, L. C. (1988). The processing of hierarchical stimuli: Effects of retinal locus, locational uncertainty, and stimulus identity. *Perception and Psychophysics, 44*, 172–181.

Lambert, A. J. (1991). Interhemispheric interaction in the split brain. *Neuropsychologia, 29*, 941–948.

Lambert, A. J. (1993). Attentional interaction in the split brain: Evidence from negative priming. *Neuropsychologia, 31*, 313–324.

Levy, J., Heller, W., Banich, M. T., and Burton, L. A. (1983). Are variations among right-handed individuals in perceptual asymmetries caused by characteristic arousal differences between hemispheres? *Journal of Experimental Psychology: Human Perception and Performance, 9*, 329–359.

Levy, J., Nebes, R. D., and Sperry, R. W. (1971). Expressive language in the surgically separated minor hemisphere. *Cortex, 7*, 49–58.

MacLeod, C. M. (1991). Half a century of research on the Stroop effect: An integrative review. *Psychological Bulletin, 109*, 163–203.

McKeever, W. F., Sullivan, K. F., Ferguson, S. M., and Rayport, M. (1982). Right hemisphere speech development in the anterior commissure-spared commissurotomy patient: A second case. *Clinical Neuropsychology, 4*, 17–22.

Mesulam, M. M. (1991). A cortical network for directed attention and unilateral neglect. *Annals of Neurology, 10*, 309–325.

Myers, J. J. (1984). Right hemisphere language: Science or fiction? *American Psychologist, 39*, 315–320.

Myers, J. J., and Sperry, R. W. (1985). Interhemispheric communication after section of the forebrain commissures. *Cortex, 21*, 249–260.

Pandya, D. N., and Seltzer, B. (1986). The topography of commissural fibers. In F. Lepore, M. Ptito, and H. H. Jasper (Eds.), *Two hemispheres—one brain: Functions of the corpus callosum* (pp 47–73). New York, NY: Alan R. Liss, Inc.

Passarotti, A., Rayman, J., and Zaidel, E. (in preparation). Hemispheric contributions to orienting covert visual attention.

Posner, M. I. (1980). Orienting of attention. *Quarterly Journal of Experimental Psychology. A. Human Experimental Psychology, 32*, 3–25.

Reuter-Lorenz, P. A., and Baynes, K. (1992). Modes of lexical access in the callosotomized brain. *Journal of Cognitive Neuroscience, 4*, 155–164.

Reuter-Lorenz, P. A., and Fendrich, R. (1990). Orienting attention across the vertical meridian: Evidence from callosotomy patients. *Journal of Cognitive Neuroscience, 2*, 232–238.

Risse, G., Gates, J., Lund, G., Maxwell, R., and Rubens, A. (1989). Interhemispheric transfer in patients with incomplete section of the corpus callosum. *Archives of Neurology, 46*, 437–443.

Robertson, L. C., and Lamb, M. R. (1991). Neuropsychological contributions to theories of part/whole organization. *Cognitive Psychology, 23*, 299–330.

Robertson, L. C., Lamb, M. R., and Knight, R. T. (1988). Effects of lesions of temporal-parietal junction on perceptual and attentional processing in humans. *Journal of Neuroscience, 8*, 3757–3769.

Robertson, L. C., Lamb, M. R., and Zaidel, E. (1993). Interhemispheric relations in processing hierarchical patterns: Evidence from normal and commissurotomized subjects. *Neuropsychology, 7*, 325–342.

Schmit, V., and Davis, R. (1974). The role of hemispheric specialization in the analysis of Stroop stimuli. *Acta Psychologia, 38*, 149–158.

Sergent, J. (1986). Sub-cortical coordination of hemispheric activity in commissurotomized patients. *Brain, 109*, 357–369.

Sergent, J. (1987). A new look at the human split-brain. *Brain, 110*, 1375–1392.

Sergent, J. (1990). Furtive incursions into bicameral minds: Integrative and coordinating role of subcortical structures. *Brain, 113,* 537–568.

Sergent, J. (1991). Processing of spatial relations within and between the disconnected cerebral hemispheres. *Brain, 114,* 1025–1043.

Sperry, R. W., Zaidel, E., and Zaidel, D. (1979). Self recognition and social awareness in the disconnected minor hemisphere. *Neuropsychologia, 17,* 153–166.

Teng, E. L., and Sperry, R. W. (1973). Interhemispheric interaction during simultaneous bilateral presentation of letters or digits in commissurotomized patients. *Neuropsychologia, 11,* 131–140.

Tipper, S. P. (1985). The negative priming effect: Inhibitory priming by ignored objects. *Quarterly Journal of Experimental Psychology. A. Human Experimental Psychology, 37,* 571–590.

Trevarthen, C., and Sperry, R. W. (1973). Perceptual unity of the ambient visual field in human commissurotomy patients. *Brain, 96,* 547–570.

Weekes, N. Y., Carusi, D. A., and Zaidel, E. (in preparation). Hierarchic perception in commissurotomy patients; A second look.

Weekes, N. Y., and Zaidel, E. (in preparation). Stroop effects within and between the disconnected hemispheres.

Witteridge, D. (1965). Area 18 and the vertical meridian of the visual field. In E. G. Ettlinger, A. V. S. de Reuck, and R. Porter (Eds.), *Functions of the corpus callosum* (pp 115–120). London: Churchill.

Zaidel, D. W. (1990). Memory and spatial cognition following commissurotomy. In F. Boller and J. Grafman (Eds.), *Handbook of neuropsychology,* Vol 4 (pp 151–166). New York, NY: Elsevier.

Zaidel, D., and Sperry, R. W. (1974). Memory impairment after commissurotomy in man. *Brain, 97,* 263–272.

Zaidel, D., and Sperry, R. W. (1977). Some long-term motor effects of cerebral commissurotomy in man. *Neuropsychologia, 11,* 193–204.

Zaidel, E. (1976). Auditory vocabulary of the right hemisphere following brain bisection or hemidecortication. *Cortex, 12,* 191–211.

Zaidel, E. (1978). Concepts of cerebral dominance in the split brain. In P. Buser and. A. Rougeul-Buser (Eds.), *Cerebral correlates of conscious experience* (pp 263–284). Amsterdam: Elsevier.

Zaidel, E. (1982). Reading in the disconnected right hemisphere: An aphasiological perspective. In Y. Zotterman (Ed.), *Dyslexia: Neuronal, cognitive and linguistic aspects* (pp 67–91). Oxford, England: Pergamon Press.

Zaidel, E. (1983). Disconnection syndrome as a model for laterality effects in the normal brain. In J. Hellige (Ed.), *Cerebral hemisphere asymmetry: Method, theory, and application* (pp 95–151). New York, NY: Praeger.

Zaidel, E. (1989). Hemispheric independence and interaction in word recognition. In C. von Euler, I. Lundberg, and G. Lennerstrand (Eds.), *Brain and reading* (pp 77–97). Hampshire, England: Macmillan.

Zaidel, E. (1990). Language functions in the two hemispheres following cerebral commissurotomy and hemispherectomy. In F. Boller and J. Grafman (Eds.), *Handbook of neuropsychology,* Vol 4 (pp 115–150). Amsterdam: Elsevier.

Zaidel, E., Clarke, J., and Suyenobu, B. (1990a). Hemispheric independence: A paradigm case for cognitive neuroscience. In A. B. Scheibel and A. F. Wechsler (Eds.), *Neurobiology of higher cognitive function* (pp 297–362). New York, NY: Guilford Press.

Zaidel, E., and Peters, A. M. (1981). Phonological encoding and ideographic reading by the disconnected right hemisphere: Two case studies. *Brain and Language, 14,* 205–234.

Zaidel, E., and Rayman, J. (in press). Interhemispheric control in the normal brain: Evidence from redundant bilateral presentations. In C. Umiltà and M. Moscovitch (Eds.), *Attention and Performance XV: Conscious and nonconsious processes.* Cambridge, MA: MIT Press.

Zaidel, E., White, H., Sakurai, E., and Banks, W. (1988). Hemispheric locus of lexical congruity effects: Neuropsychological reinterpretation of psycholinguistic results. In C. Chiarello (Ed.), *Right hemisphere contributions to lexical semantics* (pp 71–88). New York, NY: Springer-Verlag.

Zaidel, E., Zaidel, D. W., and Bogen, J. E. (1990b). Testing the commissurotomy patient. In A. A. Boulton, G. B. Baker, and M. Hiscock (Eds.), *Neuromethods: Methods in human neuropsychology,* Vol 15 (pp 147–201). Clifton, NJ: Humana Press.

VIII　Ontogeny and Developmental Disabilities

18 Phylogeny and Ontogeny of Cerebral Lateralization

Merrill Hiscock and Marcel Kinsbourne

Lateralization refers to deviations from complete bisymmetry in the specializations of paired structures in the nervous systems of bisymmetric organisms (Bilateria). Bisymmetry appears to be an adaptation for motility, and therefore applies particularly to the locomotor system, including bones, joints, and muscles, and those parts of the nervous system that control their actions. The relationship between side of body and side of control system is uncrossed in all phyla except Chordata, in which it is crossed (see Kinsbourne, 1978, for a discussion of how this difference might have evolved). This chapter refers to the vertebrates, which constitute the vast majority of Chordata.

Deviations from bisymmetry have attracted interest because they characterize the representation of many higher mental functions, and were first observed in humans. Hemispheric specialization in the adult human has often been regarded as the culmination of phylogenetic and ontogenetic progressions from simple and symmetric to complex and asymmetric nervous systems. Luria (1973) proposed that the more abstract a function is, the more its cerebral basis is asymmetric. This view of cerebral lateralization provides a convenient neural basis for distinguishing between that which is human and that which is nonhuman (subhuman); mature and immature; refined and unrefined. It has led to a narrow view of hemispheric specialization as originating in a characteristically human attribute: upright, bipedal locomotion. The disengaged forelimbs become specialized for complementary functions, i.e., for manipulating tools and for holding things (Bruner, 1968; Lovejoy, 1981). For unknown reasons the right hand generally assumed the manipulating role and the left hand assumed the holding function. Left speech specialization is presumed to have developed from this manual asymmetry, perhaps through the superiority of the left hemisphere for controlling sequences of rapid movements (Kimura and Archibald, 1974), or from an asymmetric gestural communication system in which the right hand played the preeminent role (Hewes, 1973).

The many instances of brain lateralization in infrahuman species do not invalidate these speculations about the origin of lateralization in hominids, but the animal evidence does offer a broader perspective on lateralization. It becomes necessary either to invoke convergent evolution or to attempt a more general formulation of the adaptive pressures that favor the natural selection of lateralized brain function.

Whether an overarching formulation is applicable to the embryogenesis of lateralization is equally uncertain. Using Spemann and Falkenberg's (1919) classic studies of the developing newt embryo as a point of departure, Morgan (1977) and Corballis and Beale (1976) proposed a basic left-to-right developmental gradient as a comprehensive explanation of both peripheral and central laterality. The right hemisphere's specialization is a default option, representing only those functions not preempted by its earlier differentiating counterpart. However, the current evidence on early (infant and even fetal) asymmetries favors the view that, if anything, the right hemisphere has priority in development, and complicates the issue with interacting anteroposterior asynchronies (Best, 1988). It becomes necessary to elucidate each instance of laterality individually, in the context of parallel differentiation of right and left brain.

We begin by summarizing the animal asymmetry literature. We then review studies of the ontogeny of hemispheric specialization in the human. Finally, after having gleaned some general principles from the phylogenetic and ontogenetic findings, we consider possible mechanisms of cerebral lateralization in the adult human.

PHYLOGENETIC ANTECEDENTS

In tracing the origins of structural and functional asymmetries in the human brain, one may begin by looking for similar asymmetries in the brains of nonhuman animals. A few years ago the existence of brain asymmetries in animals, or at least the relevance of such asymmetries to human laterality, was a matter of dispute, but the situation is now radically changed.

Fish, Amphibians, and Reptiles

Striking asymmetries of the habenular nuclei and their afferents from other brain structures have been found in the dorsal diencephalon of sturgeons, cyclophone fish, petromyzons, ammocoetes, frogs, lizards, and other species (Braitenberg and Kemali, 1970; Galaburda, Sherman, and Geschwind, 1985). They favor the left side in some species, the right in others. Initially observed in the nineteenth century and among the first known animal brain asymmetries, their functional significance remains unknown.

Songbirds

The brains of male passerine songbirds—e.g., chaffinches, canaries, white-crowned sparrows—are lateralized for control of song. The left hypostriatum ventrale, pars caudale, has primary control over singing even though the homologous structure in the right brain is anatomically similar. This asymmetric vocalization control is present from the onset of singing (Nottebohm, Stokes, and Leonard, 1976). Once established, singing is instantly and permanently disrupted by a left hypoglossal nerve lesion, which disconnects the left hypostriatum from the syringeal mechanism that effects vocalization. Cutting the left hypoglossal nerve eliminates most of the bird's repertoire of song syllables, whereas cutting the right nerve leaves most in place (Nottebohm, 1977). These asymmetries of song control represent the converse of the habenular asymmetries in fish, amphibians, and reptiles. The habenular nuclei offer a structural asymmetry without obvious functional implications; the hyperstriatum is functionally asymmetric without asymmetric morphology.

Songbird asymmetries become even more intriguing when developmental changes in lesion effects are examined (Nottebohm, 1971; Nottebohm, Manning, and Nottebohm, 1979). Even though sectioning the left hypoglossal nerve produced permanent singing deficits in adult chaffinches, its early sectioning failed to prevent development of normal singing. The right hypostriatum and right syringeal muscles can implement normal song if the homologous structures on the left side are incapacitated prior to maturity. This compensatory capacity of the right side persists throughout the period of motor learning, which ends when the stereotyped adult song is established. The canary shows similar age-related changes in lesion effects except that there is substantial apparent recovery of singing ability in the adult canary following left hypoglossal nerve sectioning (Nottebohm et al., 1979). But this reflects the addition of new syllables to the bird's repertoire rather than the reappearance of syllables that were abolished by the nerve sectioning. The greater plasticity observed in the lesioned adult canary, relative to the chaffinch, may be attributed to song changes that normally take place between the first and second singing seasons.

Parrots

Lateralized vocal control is not a characteristic of all birds or even of all species with highly developed vocalization skill. In parrots (Psittaciformes), cutting the left and the right hypoglossal nerve has approximately the same effect on vocalization (Nottebohm, 1976); vocalization returns to normal within a few days. This difference between passerine birds and parrots reflects a fundamental difference in the connections between brain and syrinx. Whereas innervation of syringeal muscles in passerines is ipsilateral, each side of the parrot brain innervates the syringeal muscles on both sides. Moreover, the vocal control pathways within the parrot brain include bilateral projections. The functional asymmetries of passerine birds occur in the context of largely independent left and right song-control systems, in which the two sides of the syrinx can produce harmonically unrelated sounds simultaneously (Greenewalt, 1968). In contrast, the parrot's left and right syringes function as a unit, and each side of the brain controls both. Evidently this bilateral innervation is not a source of conflicting instructions, a point that becomes relevant when anomalies of lateralization of speech control in humans are considered.

Fowl

Various asymmetries have been demonstrated in domestic chicks. When injected into the brains of 2-day-old chicks, cycloheximide, a protein synthesis inhibitor, and glutamate, a synaptic transmitter, altered attack and copulatory behaviors as well as auditory habituation and visual discrimination learning (Howard, Rogers, and Boura, 1980; Rogers, 1980a,b). However, the specific effects of the agents depended on the side of injection. Visual discrimination learning, for example, was disrupted when glutamate was injected into the left but not the right striatal hemisphere. Convergent evidence for left brain superiority in visual discrimination learning was reported by Andrew, Mench, and Rainey (1982), who found faster learning in chicks when the left eye rather than the right eye was occluded. Because the optic pathways in the chicken are fully decussated (crossed), occluding one eye precludes information from reaching the contralateral side of the brain. Rogers (1982) and Zappia and Rogers (1983) have argued that functional asymmetries in the chick brain depend on the position of the chick embryo in the egg. This positioning determines how much light each eye receives during the final phase of the incubation period.

The domestic chick displays imprinting, i.e., a tendency to follow a moving object to which the chick was exposed soon after hatching, and this may be based on an asymmetric neural substrate (Arnold and Bottjer, 1985). Imprinting has been linked to changes in a dorsal forebrain region, the intermediate medial hyperstriatum ventrale (IMHV). Bradley, Horn, and Bateson (1981), using electron microscopy to examine the IMHV, identified an asymmetric structural change that could be related to the length of exposure to an imprinting stimulus. Synaptic apposition zones were longer in the right IMHV than in the left of chicks that had had little exposure to the imprinting stimulus, but there was no asymmetry in chicks that had had greater exposure. Perhaps the right IMHV is more involved initially in the imprinting process, but the left IMHV plays an increased role the longer the stimulus is exposed. This interpretation is consistent with findings from a two-stage lesion study (Cipolla-Neto, Horn, and McCabe, 1982), in which the combined effects of an early right IMHV lesion and a subsequent left IMHV lesion abolished imprinting, whereas imprinting was maintained following early left and subsequent right IMHV lesions. This shift of control with increasing familiarity or practice is reminiscent of Goldberg and Costa's (1981) formulation of differential hemisphere control in the human: the right hemisphere for initial responses to a novel situation, the left for subsequent responding as an appropriate behavioral schema is developed (see Kinsbourne and Bruce, 1987, for a possible case in point).

Other Birds

Early reports of asymmetries in birds usually involved limbs and ear structure (Galaburda et al., 1985). However, Cobb (1964), who studied owls and other bird species, discovered asymmetries in the volume of the torus, an auditory nucleus embedded within the optic lobe of the brain. The torus-to-optic lobe ratio was larger on the left in some species, especially in the species most dependent on acoustic information.

Rodents

The literature on rodent asymmetries not only includes various instances of morphologic, physiologic, and behavioral asymmetry but extends beyond the description of behavioral asymmetries, to their neuroanatomic and neuro-chemical bases.

Brain morphology Asymmetries of cortex, hippocampus and amygdala in the rat are described by Lewis and Diamond in chapter 2.

Behavior There is considerable evidence of behavioral asymmetry in the rat. Under certain circumstances, left and right hemisphere ablation has differential effects on open-field activity (Denenberg et al., 1978). Ablation of the right hemisphere caused the greater change in activity level, but only among animals who had been handled during the first 20 days of life. The direction of the change in activity level depended on whether the animal had been reared in a standard cage or in an enriched environment. Studies of taste aversion and mouse killing in handled rats with left or right hemisphere ablation indicate that representation of fear is more right hemispheric than left, but the expression of fear may be inhibited by an intact left hemisphere (Denenberg et al., 1980; Garbanati et al., 1983). This model of lateralized emotionality in the rat was supported by another experiment in which mouse killing was enhanced in split-brain rats (Denenberg et al., 1986). It was reasoned that cutting the corpus callosum blocked the inhibitory influence of the left hemisphere.

Denenberg and Yutzey (1985) pointed out that these population-level hemisphere-specific lesion effects on open-field activity may represent a change in spatial behavior as well as in emotionality. Lateralized processing of spatial information could explain why the leftward turning tendency of non-handled male rats with an intact right hemisphere exceeds the rightward turning tendency of rats with an intact left hemisphere (Sherman et al., 1980). This interpretation, however, does not explain why lesion effects vary with sex as well as previous handling (Sherman et al., 1983).

Other rodent asymmetries exist primarily at the level of the individual. Individual animals may show marked behavioral or neurochemical asymmetries even though there is little or no overall asymmetry in the strain, because an equal number of animals show the opposite asymmetry. In some instances, however, an asymmetry at the population level may develop as the animals gain additional practice in performing the task (Castellano et al., 1989).

Spontaneous turning, or circling, is an example of an asymmetry at the level of the individual (see Carlson and Glick, 1989; Glick, Jerussi, and Zimmerberg, 1977; Glick and Shapiro, 1984, 1985). Rats, as well as other mammals, show spontaneous circling under some circumstances (Glick and Shapiro, 1985), some leftward, others to the right. A weak overall tendency for rats to turn more often to the left varies with the animal's strain, sex, and previous handling as well as the testing situation (Camp, Robinson, and Becker, 1984; Denenberg and Yutzey, 1985; Sherman et al., 1980, 1983). Glick and Ross (1981) even observed a significant bias in the opposite direction.

Neurochemistry Though other neural systems also may produce circling (Buckenham and Yeomans, 1993), the nigrostriatal system has been the principle focus of neurochemical studies. Unilateral lesions of the nigrostriatal system (substantia nigra, nigrostriatal bundle, corpus striatum) cause rats to circle at a high rate in a direction ipsilateral to the side of the lesion (e.g., Ungerstedt, 1971). Amphetamine and other dopaminergic drugs potentiate this surgically induced lateralized behavior (Ungerstedt and Arbuthnott, 1970). This suggests that an imbalance in dopamine activity in the left and right nigrostriatal systems causes the animal to turn in a direction opposite to the more activated side (Arbuthnott and Crow, 1971). Both D_1 and D_2 dopamine (DA) receptors appear to contribute to the turning activity (Pazo, Murer, and Segal, 1993).

Since systemic amphetamine induces circling in rats without lesions (Jerussi and Glick, 1974), spontaneous circling in normal rats has been attributed to an endogenous asymmetry in nigrostriatal dopamine levels (Glick et al., 1974; Jerussi and Glick, 1976). There is a higher concentration of dopamine in the striatum contralateral to the preferred direction of rotation (Zimmerberg, Glick, and Jerussi, 1974) and the direction of amphetamine-induced rotation is the same as the direction in which the same animal rotates spontaneously (Glick and Cox, 1978).

More recent data, however, suggest that the link between behavioral and neurochemical asymmetries is less straightforward. Asymmetric dopamine uptake in the striatal region is associated not with contralateral turning, as expected, but with increased turning in either the contralateral or ipsilateral direction (Shapiro, Glick, and Hough, 1986). Some rats rotate contralateral to the side of greater dopaminergic activity and some ipsilateral. In other words, "the net influence of the dopaminergic input could be either excitatory or inhibitory in different rats" (Glick and Shapiro, 1985, p. 168). Several subsequent findings have supported this "two-population hypothesis" (Glick, Hinds, and Baird, 1988; Shapiro, Camarota, and Glick, 1987; Shapiro, Glick, and Camarota, 1987).

Some apparent inconsistencies in the direction of circling may be attributable to different physical arrangements. Wise and Holmes (1986) found that the direction of experimentally induced unilateral circling in rats was determined by the animal's position relative to the wall of the enclosure. Animals that turned in one direction within the enclosure walls turned in the opposite direction when on the outside. From this we conclude that circling is not autonomous motor behavior, but involves biased orientation relative to salient environmental stimuli. The animal turns along the contralesional side of the display in each condition.

Another possible source of contradictions in the literature is a confounding of motor asymmetry with perseverative tendency. Kokkinidis and Anisman (1977) found that dextro-amphetamine induced comparable levels of circling behavior in female Swiss Webster mice whether administered focally (i.e., intraventricularly) or systemically (i.e., intraperitoneally). However, the two modes of amphetamine injection had opposite effects on alternation behavior in a Y-maze: The proportion of alternation responses increased with increasing levels of intraventricular amphetamine and decreased with increasing levels of intraperitoneal amphetamine. From this dissociation of effects, the investigators concluded that systemic injection of dextro-amphetamine produces perseveration rather than an asymmetric circling tendency. Since these two factors are confounded in studies employing a rotometer or circular alleyway (e.g., Jerussi and Glick, 1974), the amphetamine-induced circling observed in those studies may reflect perseverative running rather than potentiation of a preexisting dopaminergic motor asymmetry. This conclusion was supported in a study by Kokkinidis (1987) in which male Swiss mice were tested in a circular alleyway, an open field, and a Y-maze. After comparing the findings from these different paradigms, Kokkinidis concluded that "rotational behavior is indeed complex, and dependent upon a number of factors other than hemispheric imbalances of striatal dopamine" (p. 531). He suggested that direction of turning in an open field constitutes a better measure of rodent laterality than does circling behavior in the circular alleyway.

Another group of studies provides information about neurochemical influences on activity level in rodents. Circumscribed lesions in the left and right hemispheres of the male Sprague-Dawley rat produce strikingly dissimilar effects on spontaneous activity as measured in terms of running wheel revolutions (Robinson, 1985). Right hemisphere lesions produced by ligating the middle cerebral artery (Robinson et al., 1975), suctioning cortical tissue (Moran et al., 1984; Pearlson and Robinson, 1981), or cutting transcortical connections (Kubos and Robinson, 1984) caused as much as a 50% increase in running-wheel activity. Comparable lesions in the left hemisphere did not increase activity level. This behavioral asymmetry was accompanied by asymmetric lesion effects on catecholamine concentrations in the brain. Right hemisphere lesions caused a bilateral depletion of DA and norepinephrine (NE) (Robinson, 1979; Robinson, Shoemaker, and Schlumpf, 1980) as well as a bilateral increase in serotonin S2 receptor binding (Mayberg, Moran, and

Robinson, 1990). No such changes resulted from comparable left hemisphere lesions. When lesions were placed at various points along the anteroposterior dimension (Pearlson, Kubos, and Robinson, 1984), the effects of right hemisphere lesions on activity level and NE concentrations increased the closer they were to the anterior pole.

Neurochemical manipulations have confirmed the role of right hemisphere NE in regulating activity level (Robinson and Bloom, 1977; Robinson and Stitt, 1981). For example, when intracortical injections of 6-hydroxydopamine (6-OHDA) depleted NE in the right hemisphere, the rat became hyperactive. The corresponding injection of the left hemisphere usually had no effect on activity level. But lesions of the right hemisphere that do not deplete catecholamines can also produce hyperactivity (Kubos, Pearlson, and Robinson, 1982; Kubos and Robinson, 1984). Robinson (1985) concluded that depletion of right hemisphere NE is sufficient but not necessary to elicit hyperactivity. He referred the neural asymmetries responsible for this hyperactivity not to the NE pathways within the cerebral cortex but to the efferent pathways post-synaptic to the NE neurons, i.e., in the glutamatergic corticostriatal pathways.

Other Findings A particularly interesting behavioral asymmetry was reported by Ehret (1987), who observed a right ear advantage (REA) in mice for artificial pup calls, i.e., 50-kHz tone bursts or noise bursts with a central frequency of 50 kHz. Lactating primiparous mice, after being positioned in the center of a running board, heard artificial pup calls from a loudspeaker at one end of the board and neutral signals from a loudspeaker at the opposite end. By moving toward the source of the pup calls, the mice showed a significant preference for this category of stimulus. However, pup calls were preferred over neutral stimuli only in binaural and left ear–plugged conditions: When the right ear was plugged, no significant preference for either signal was observed. This was taken as evidence of left hemisphere superiority for the recognition of pup calls. In a subsequent experiment, Ehret (1987) conditioned virgin female mice—which can discriminate pup calls from other sounds but ordinarily show no preference for these calls—to respond preferentially to the calls. When placed in the two-alternative-choice situation, these animals showed a significant preference for the artificial pup calls irrespective of whether they listened with the left, right, or both ears. Ehret concluded that left hemisphere superiority is manifested only when the auditory stimuli possess intraspecific communicative significance.

Cats

Both neuroanatomic and functional asymmetries have been reported in the cat (Webster, 1972, 1981; Webster and Webster, 1975). Individual cats display a paw preference in reaching for food even though no asymmetry seems to exist at the population level (Warren, Abplanalp, and Warren, 1967). Webster (1972) discovered that the paw preference in the individual cat is related to hemispheric asymmetries in visual discrimination. Intact cats were trained to criterion on a variety of pattern and form discrimination tasks, after which the corpus callosum and optic chiasm of each animal were sectioned. Postoperative testing on the same discrimination tasks, which were now presented to an isolated left or right hemisphere, yielded instances of superior performance with the hemisphere ipsilateral to the preferred paw, i.e., the "nondominant" hemisphere. In subsequent work, Webster (Webster, 1981; Webster and Webster, 1975) reported asymmetries in the configuration of sulci in the cerebral cortex of the cat. Since these asymmetries were most frequently found posteriorly, in the visual area, it seemed possible that they were related to functional asymmetries in visual processing. However, there was no relationship between anatomic asymmetry and paw preference.

Dogs

Adams, Molfese, and Betz (1987) reported that collies can discriminate consonants based on voice onset time (VOT). Auditory evoked responses indicate that this relies on right hemisphere specialization. The same group has found similar evoked response patterns for VOT differences in monkeys and humans.

Nonhuman Primates

From a traditional perspective, primates occupy a pivotal position on the phylogenetic scale, between the largely nonlateralized infrahuman vertebrates and the lateralized *Homo sapiens*. The recent discovery of sundry asymmetries in nonprimates demands a new perspective. If there is no overall phylogenetic progression from symmetry to asymmetry, then the primate should no longer be considered the nexus between infrahuman and human with respect to brain lateralization. Primate laterality nonetheless remains of special interest because of the genetic, neurologic, and behavioral similarity between primates and humans. Since lateralization in the human is usually defined in terms of hemispheric specialization for either language or hand control, the nonhuman primate continues to provide valuable insight into the evolution of the neural systems subserving communication and limb movement. Although the literature is not as extensive as that concerning rodent asymmetries, numerous instances of structural and functional asymmetry in monkeys and great apes have been reported.

Brain Morphology   Structural asymmetries are reviewed by Galaburda in chapter 3.

Behavior   The cerebral hemispheres of nonhuman primates may be differentially specialized, but the evidence of performance asymmetries is fragmentary and difficult to interpret. Nowhere is the interpretative ambiguity better exemplified than in the literature on primate handedness.

Although individual animals often show consistent hand preference across repetitions of the same task, the preponderance of evidence suggests that nonhuman primates do not have a hand preference at the population level (see reviews by Corballis, 1983; Hamilton, 1977a; Warren, 1980). More recently, however, various investigators have challenged the conclusion that population-level asymmetries are nonexistent in primates. According to MacNeilage, Studdert-Kennedy, and Lindblom (1987, 1988), the data suggest a left-hand preference for reaching, the strength of which increases from simple to more complex tasks, and a right-hand preference for object manipulation. This claim is supported, in part, by recent evidence that female Old World monkeys show a strong left-hand preference for picking up their babies in an emergency situation (Hatta and Koike, 1991) and that prosimians typically use the left hand when reaching for food under circumstances that require postural adjustments (Ward, 1991).

Fagot and Vauclair (1991) attempted to clarify the issue of manual laterality in primates by distinguishing between low-level tasks, such as reaching for food, and various high-level tasks, which demand more extensive perceptual, motor, and cognitive processing. Fagot and Vauclair summarized evidence that prosimians, monkeys, and apes show left-hand specialization for performing high-level tasks. Recent studies, nonetheless, indicate that rhesus monkeys and chimpanzees may exhibit a right-hand preference for tasks requiring fine motor skill (Hopkins, Washburn, and Rumbaugh, 1989; Morris, Hopkins, and Bolser-Gilmore, 1993).

Other data address the lateralization of cognitive processes in nonhuman primates. Hörster and Ettlinger (1985) reported that the speed with which rhesus monkeys learned to discriminate tactually between cylinders and squares depended on the hand that they chose for performing the task. The 78 animals that performed spontaneously with the left hand outperformed the 77 monkeys that chose to use the right hand. As pointed out by Ettlinger (1987), this result is ambiguous in the absence of information about the animals' performance with their nondominant hand. Interpretation of this finding is further complicated by the 82 animals that showed no consistent hand preference but nevertheless performed the tactile discrimination task better than the monkeys in either of the other two groups. Moreover, studies of commissurotomized (split-brain) monkeys suggest that memory for tactile discriminations is represented bilaterally in the monkey brain (Ebner and Myers, 1962a,b).

Studies of visual processing in split-brain monkeys have yielded a mixture of results, the most common of which is equal performance with the left and right hemispheres (Butler, 1968; Downer, 1962; Hamilton and Gazzaniga, 1964). One approach used by Hamilton (1977a,b) entailed teaching visual discriminations to intact rhesus monkeys and then testing the left and right hemispheres separately following commissurotomy. Not only did this procedure fail to reveal lateralized storage in the intact brain but other studies showed that even when the pattern discrimination information was acquired following partial splitting of the brain, the information was stored bilaterally. For example, if monkeys had either the anterior commissure or the splenium left intact, and the visual patterns were presented to only one hemisphere during training, the discrimination was performed almost as well by the opposite hemisphere following subsequent complete commissurotomy.

The relevance of many primate studies to human lateralization may be questioned because they do not use tasks that would elicit asymmetric processing in humans. But where this has been rectified, the results still do not show any straightforward homology between primate and human laterality. Hamilton (1977a,b), for example, failed to find evidence of hemispheric specialization in the rhesus monkey for learning discriminations based on facial or perspective cues even though similar tasks would be expected to show right hemisphere superiority in humans. Indeed, when asymmetries are found in monkeys, they tend to be opposite to those found in humans. Split-brain rhesus monkeys show left hemisphere superiority for discriminating line orientations (Hamilton, 1983; Hamilton and Vermeire, 1988), a finding that is discrepant with the right hemisphere superiority shown by humans (e.g., Benton, Varney, and Hamsher, 1978). Left hemisphere superiority of monkeys for certain spatial discriminations has been corroborated by other findings (Hamilton, 1983; Hamilton and Lund, 1970; Hamilton, Tieman, and Farrell, 1974; Jason, Cowey, and Weiskrantz, 1984). Jason et al. (1984), for example, reported that monkeys show an asymmetry opposite to that usual in humans for discrimination of dot displacement (Bryden, 1982). The performance of monkeys was more impaired by left than by right occipital lobectomy. Equally at odds with findings for humans is evidence from two recent studies of baboons' performance on matching-to-sample tasks in which the comparison stimuli were presented to either the left or right visual half-field. Hopkins, Fagot, and Vauclair (1993) found that baboons, when performing a task in which the spatial orientation of the comparison stimuli was varied, did better in the right visual half-field for matches between asymmetric stimuli and in the left visual half-field for mirror-image stimuli. Vauclair, Fagot, and Hopkins (1993) reported that baboons showed humanlike performance on a mental rotation task with mirror-image stimuli, but only when the rotated stimuli were presented in the right visual half-field.

Until recently, there was little reason to think that face discrimination is similarly lateralized in monkeys and humans. Hamilton's (1977a,b) negative findings have already been noted. A study of face processing in intact pigtail monkeys and humans (Overman and Doty, 1982) also failed to show any evidence of asymmetric processing in the monkeys even though humans showed the expected asymmetry. In this study, both the human subjects and the monkeys were shown composite photographs consisting of either the left or right half of a human or monkey face joined to the mirror image of the same half-face. The task entailed matching the composite photograph to an unmodified photograph of the same human or monkey. As expected, human subjects usually chose the composite human face that consisted of two right half-faces. This outcome is consistent with an hypothesized tendency to focus attention on the right side of faces (i.e., on the left half of the face as seen by the observer) and thus with right hemisphere superiority for processing physiognomic information. Human subjects failed to show a preference for either half-face of monkeys, and monkeys failed to show a preference for either half-face irrespective of whether it was that of a monkey or a human. However, Morris and Hopkins's (1993) finding of a left half-field advantage for the discrimination of human chimeric facial stimuli by three chimpanzees is more consistent with single cell microelectrode findings of more temporal neurons selectively sensitive to faces on the right than on the left in monkeys (Perrett, Rolls, and Caan, 1982).

With the accumulation of more data on face processing in monkeys, a different picture is emerging. Hamilton and Vermeire (1983, 1988) reported that split-brain monkeys are more adept at distinguishing individual animals and facial expressions with their right than with their left hemispheres. The monkeys were required to distinguish between photographs of two different monkeys displaying the same expression and between photographs of two different facial expressions made by the same animal. Overall, 19 of 27 (70%) split-brain monkeys showed right hemisphere superiority on these tasks (Hamilton and Vermeire, 1991). The same animals, on retesting, yielded a right hemisphere advantage for performing the facial discriminations learned 6 months previously. In addition, by reproducing these findings using new photographs of the same monkeys, Hamilton and Vermeire (1988) were able to show that the lateralized processing involved facial attributes rather than incidental details of the photographs.

Consistent with previous findings, Hamilton and Vermeire's (1988, 1991) split-brain monkeys showed a strong left hemisphere superiority for discrimination of line orientation and no significant laterality for discrimination of geometric patterns. The lack of correlation between laterality for faces and line orientation implies that these manifestations of hemispheric specialization are independent. Even though 70% of the monkeys showed a right hemisphere advantage for face discrimination and 88% showed a left hemisphere advantage for orientation discrimination (Hamilton and Vermeire, 1991), there was no indication of a causal complementarity (see Bryden, 1982; Bryden, Hécaen, and DeAgostini, 1983). Having one hemisphere specialized for face discrimination did not necessitate that the opposite hemisphere be specialized for discrimination of line orientation.

Vermeire and Hamilton (1988) extended the parallel between physiognomic information processing in monkeys and humans by showing that monkeys perform similarly to humans on a task requiring the discrimination of inverted faces. As a group, 16 split-brain monkeys showed the expected right hemisphere superiority for discriminating upright monkey faces but showed no significant laterality when the faces were inverted. This is similar to results obtained with human subjects (e.g., Leehey et al., 1978).

It has been reported that language-trained chimpanzees show lateralized priming effects (Hopkins et al., 1991, 1992). Simple reaction time to a visual cue was accelerated more by a warning signal in the right visual half-field (i.e., left hemisphere) than by a warning signal in the left visual half-field (i.e., right hemisphere), but only when the warning signal was meaningful to the chimpanzee. This lateralized priming resembles verbal priming in humans (e.g., Bowers and Heilman, 1980; Kinsbourne, 1973).

Additional evidence of humanlike hemispheric specialization in nonhuman primates comes from studies of auditory processing in macaques. Dewson (1977) reported that lesions of the left superior temporal gyrus (the primary auditory reception area) disrupted auditory-visual matching, whereas comparable lesions on the right side had no effect. Peterson and his colleagues (Beecher et al., 1979; Peterson et al., 1984), reported that Japanese macaques show an REA for discriminating among the vocalizations of their conspecifics. Other species of Old World monkeys showed no REA for the Japanese macaque calls, even though they appeared to be attending to the same features as were the Japanese macaques. This result not only is reminiscent of Ehret's (1987) findings for mice but also resembles findings from dichotic listening studies in humans: REA appears most reliably when the sounds have communicative significance to the listener (e.g., Spellacy and Blumstein, 1970; Van Lancker and Fromkin, 1977).

Discrimination of macaque calls and left hemisphere functioning were linked by Heffner and Heffner (1984), who found that the capacity of Japanese macaques to discriminate between two similar vocalizations was impaired by removal of the left, but not the right, superior temporal gyrus. These findings also are similar to what one would expect to find in the human (e.g., Kimura, 1961).

Pohl's (1983, 1984) finding of left ear advantage (LEA) in baboons for various acoustic discriminations is not incompatible with the instances of REA in Japanese macaques, nor with findings obtained in dichotic listening studies of humans. Some of the stimuli that Pohl used, such as pure tones and musical chords, might be expected to yield an LEA in humans, whereas stimuli such as vowel sounds and consonant-vowel (CV) syllables, which would be linguistic to the human listener, presumably have no communicative meaning to the baboon.

Hamilton and Vermeire (1982) studied the discrepancy between the asymmetric performance observed with auditory tasks and the lack of asymmetry found at that time with visual tasks. Might it be attributed to a difference between sequential and simultaneous presentation, since visual stimuli are usually presented simultaneously whereas auditory-verbal stimuli are presented sequentially? If so, primates should perform asymmetrically on a visual laterality task that entails sequential presentation of stimuli. However, same-different judgments with sequentially presented stimuli yielded no asymmetry in rhesus monkeys. Hamilton and Vermeire reported a statistically significant correlation of .77 between the cognitive asymmetry score and hand preference for reaching, such that left-handed animals learned the task faster with the right hemisphere and vice versa. This correlation may reflect an attentional bias favoring the cerebral hemisphere that controls the preferred hand (Kinsbourne, 1970). If so, this is another parallel between nonhuman primate and human laterality.

Overview of Animal Laterality

Rather than characterizing the peak of an evolutionary progression, laterality has now been found in mammalian species across a wide range of behavioral specialization. Lateralized control centers do not share any qualitatively similar functional role. If they have anything in common, it is that their functions do not require bilateral representation; that is, they do not involve orienting or acting toward specific points in ambient space. Animal laterality is more likely a product of convergent than of progressive evolution.

ONTOGENY OF HUMAN LATERALIZATION

Our understanding of the ontogenesis of cerebral lateralization in humans has changed no less radically in the past few years than our understanding of its phylogenesis. Beginning when nineteenth-century neurologists (including Sigmund Freud, 1891/1953) noted a relatively high incidence of aphasia following right hemisphere damage in children, some assumed that the left and right sides of the brain were functionally equivalent in infancy and that lateralization of language to the left hemisphere was not complete until the time of puberty. These two concepts—equipotentiality and progressive lateralization—formed the basis for Lenneberg's (1967) influential account of the biological basis of language development. Ironically, these basic assumptions about the development of hemispheric specialization, having persisted in neurology for a century, were discredited only a few years after Lenneberg popularized them (Kinsbourne, 1975; Segalowitz and Gruber, 1977; Woods and Teuber, 1978).

Criticism of the equipotentiality and progressive lateralization doctrines stems from two general sources: findings from children with unilateral brain damage and studies of behavioral and electrophysiologic asymmetry in children.

Clinical Evidence

Childhood Aphasia   The equipotentiality and progressive lateralization hypotheses are largely based on reports of language disturbance (aphasia) occurring in children that have suffered right hemisphere damage. A series reviewed by Basser (1962), in which 35% of children with acquired speech disturbance had sustained right-sided lesions, particularly influenced Lenneberg's (1967) thinking. Yet this evidence cannot withstand scrutiny. In the first place, Krashen (1973) pointed out that only Basser's data for children below the age of 5 years suggest any significant incidence of aphasia following right hemisphere damage. The data for older children are similar to data for adults with aphasia, i.e., aphasia is rarely associated with lesions restricted to the right hemisphere (e.g., Russell and Espir, 1961).

Krashen's (1973) observation reduced to about 5 years the time frame within which progressive lateralization supposedly occurs, but it did not necessitate abandoning the concept. Kinsbourne (1975) and Kinsbourne and Hiscock (1977) took the more radical position that even the aphasia data for children younger than 5 years do not constitute satisfactory evidence of incomplete language lateralization. Kinsbourne and Hiscock (1977) cautioned that the childhood aphasia data are vulnerable to distortion from several sources, among which is the selective reporting of cases. Insofar as unusual cases are more noteworthy than ordinary ones, exceptional cases will be overrepresented in published case material. Consequently, the incidence of aphasia in association with right hemisphere lesions almost certainly will be inflated if cases are culled from the medical literature. Kinsbourne and Hiscock also pointed out that many children who become aphasic suffer from medical conditions that put them at risk for recurrent damage to the brain. If the right hemisphere lesion associated with aphasia had been preceded by other brain damage, then the previous damage may have caused a transfer of language representation to the right hemisphere. The results of such cases cannot be considered representative of what one would find in brains without preexisting disease.

Kinsbourne and Hiscock (1977) also argued that in many of the published reports of childhood aphasia, lax criteria were used, not only for diagnosing aphasia but also for ascertaining the unilaterality of the cerebral lesion. They undertook a survey of records at their own institution, a large pediatric hospital, and found that, out of 30 children aged 5 years and under who were reported to have acquired aphasia as a consequence of unilateral cerebral damage, only 4 (13%) had right-sided lesions. When strict criteria for the presence of aphasia were applied, the number of cases was reduced to eight, none of which had a right hemisphere lesion.

The argument against equipotentiality and progressive lateralization was reinforced by Woods and Teuber (1978), who found few cases of aphasia among children who had sustained right hemisphere damage after they had begun to acquire speech. Although 25 of 34 (74%) children with left hemisphere damage showed some disturbance of language, only 4 of 31 (13%) children with right hemisphere damage had any language disruption (and 2 of those 4 children were known to have been left-handed prior to the lesion). Of the 15 known right-handers who became aphasic as a result of their lesion, 14 had left-sided lesions and only 1 had a right-sided lesion. After reviewing the literature on aphasia acquired in childhood, Woods and Teuber (1978) concluded that only studies conducted prior to the 1930s yielded a relatively high incidence of aphasia following right hemisphere damage. Excluding known left-handers, most recent studies find only about 5% of childhood aphasias to be associated with right-sided damage. Woods and Teuber (1978) attributed this dramatic shift in outcome to the introduction of antibiotics and mass immunization in the 1930s and 1940s. Before then, aphasias and hemiplegias often occurred as complications of systemic bacterial infections. Such infections might also produce a diffuse encephalopathy involving the opposite hemisphere as well, which would account for the aphasia. Woods and Teuber note that many of Basser's cases were accumulated in the 1930s and 1940s and thus may have been contaminated by the same artifacts that presumably distort the earlier findings.

The childhood aphasia data were reanalyzed by Satz and his colleagues (Carter, Hohenegger, and Satz, 1982; Satz and Bullard-Bates, 1981), using a statistical method previously applied to infer the incidence of left-sided, right-sided, and bilateral language representation in adults (Carter, Hohenegger, and Satz, 1980; Satz, 1979). Their results are generally consistent with early language lateralization, the "developmental invariance" position (Kinsbourne, 1975). Considering only post-1940 cases and excluding data from Basser's study, Carter et al. (1982) estimated that 84% of right-handed children below the age of 5 years have left hemisphere speech and the other 16% have bilateral speech. However, the 16% estimate for bilateral speech did not differ significantly from zero; the null hypothesis that no children have bilateral speech could not be rejected. These analyses illustrate the importance of inclusion and exclusion criteria such as age, premorbid handedness, evidence for speech development prior to the lesion, unilaterality of the lesion, and criteria for aphasia. For example, even though Carter et al. began by considering a sample of 171 children, their "purest" subsample of young children with right hemisphere lesions consisted of only four children, none of whom had become aphasic.

Another argument for incomplete left lateralization in young children relies on the alleged lack of differentiation of distinct aphasic syndromes after early left focal cerebral damage (Lenneberg, 1967). But an increasing literature refutes this claim, documenting adultlike syndromes at least down to age 3 years (Van Hout, 1992).

Hemispherectomy   Also in defense of equipotentiality and progressive lateralization in the immature brain, Lenneberg (1967) cited Basser's (1962) summary of 113 cases of hemispherectomy (surgical removal of a cerebral hemisphere) to support his argument that children's speech functions may be served satisfactorily by either hemisphere. He reasoned that unilateral left hemisphere lesions acquired during childhood have no deleterious effect on language capacity because language may be subserved by the healthy right hemisphere. When the diseased left hemisphere is subsequently removed, speech is seldom affected. In contrast, when left hemisphere malignancy appears during adulthood, removal of the left hemisphere produces aphasic symptoms (Burklund and Smith, 1977), though long-term outcome cannot be ascertained on account of tumor recurrence.

This traditional distinction between the results of hemispherectomy in children and hemispherectomy in adults has been challenged in two ways. Reports that following hemispherectomy during adolescence (Ogden, 1988) or adulthood (Crockett and Estridge, 1951; Smith, 1966; Zollinger, 1935) the nondominant right hemisphere of adults may support the recovery of substantial language capacity argue against a critical period limiting the right hemisphere's potential for language compensation. That compensation is complete in the immature right hemisphere has also been contested. Dennis and her colleagues (Dennis, 1980; Dennis and Kohn, 1975; Dennis, Lovett, and Wiegel-Crump, 1981; Dennis and Whitaker, 1976) have argued that the isolated right hemisphere in children cannot support as complete a development of language as can the isolated left hemisphere. More recent studies, in which the unilaterality of the cerebral lesions was well controlled (see Aram, 1988, for a review), support this point. Children with early left hemisphere damage are particularly impaired on syntactic production (Aram, Ekelman, and Whitaker, 1986). Children with right-sided lesions have spatial impairments (Vargha-Khadem, O'Gorman, and Watters, 1985). However, Bishop (1983, 1988) has pointed out that the language-related studies are all inconclusive on account of flawed methodology, including inappropriate statistical analysis and lack of control data. Therefore Lenneberg's notion of early complete hemispheric equipotentiality for language has not been disconfirmed.

Both the presence of right hemisphere language in adults and possible subtle limitations of right hemisphere language in children mitigate the sharp distinction drawn by Basser (1962) and Lenneberg (1967) between the consequences of late and early lesions. This distinction was further challenged by St. James-Roberts (1981), who argued that recovery of function following hemispherectomy is variable among individuals for reasons other than the age at which the brain damage occurred; these reasons include lesion etiology, length of recovery time, and experience following the damage.

Recovery of Function   Lenneberg's (1967) argument for equipotentiality and progressive lateralization was also based on his conclusion from meta-analysis that recovery from aphasia is much more complete in children than in adolescents and adults. Lenneberg inferred that children's brains have greater capacity for functional reorganization of language following injury than more mature brains. This he attributed to the as yet incomplete hemispheric specialization in children and the consequent ability of the not yet spatially dedicated right hemisphere to assume language functions following their loss in the left hemisphere.

This argument raises the issue of neuroplasticity, the ability of the damaged brain to recover functions that are disrupted by the damage. Of special relevance to equipotentiality and progressive lateralization are these questions: (1) Does plasticity decrease with age?, and, (2) if so, is the greater plasticity of the younger brain a result of the incomplete lateralization of language? The first question is controversial (cf. Isaacson, 1975; Satz and Fletcher, 1981; Smith, 1983; St. James-Roberts, 1981). Perhaps, as Rudel (1978) has suggested, the degree to which the young brain is plastic differs according to the function being observed. Whereas recovery of speech and sensory processes after early hemisphere injury is impressive, and most of these children learn to read in the normal way (Aram, Gillespie, and Yamashita, 1990), other functions, especially complex functions, tend not to develop normally following early brain damage, either in humans (Hebb, 1942) or animals (Schneider, 1979).

Even if neuroplasticity for speech does decrease with increasing age, it does not follow that hemispheric specialization is absent from the young brain. The damaged left hemisphere sometimes retains control of the speech function. If the right hemisphere does "take over" speech control following damage to the left hemisphere, speech may nonetheless have been under exclusive left hemisphere control prior to the lesion. In the words of Rudel (1978):

With left hemispherectomy or with a lesion encroaching directly upon the speech area, language in the child is taken over by other areas (Milner, 1974). This need not be ascribed to a shift of language function to the other side, but rather as a release of a latent potential for language in the right hemisphere, a potential inhibited in the course of normal speech development in the left hemisphere. (p. 292)

The same compensatory mechanism, which leads to right hemisphere control of speech, has been shown by intracarotid amobarbital sodium (Amytal Sodium) studies to account for residual speech in a large proportion of aphasic adults (Czopf, 1972; Kinsbourne, 1971). If that recovery is less complete in adults than in children, that may be due to decreasing plasticity rather than the absence of hemispheric specialization in the children.

Evidence about nonverbal functioning following hemispherectomy is sparse. Early left lateralized lesions result in more mathematical difficulties than do right-sided lesions (Ashcraft, Yamashita, and Aram, 1992). The report by Nass and Koch (1987) of more temperamental problems, involving mood and rhythmicity, after right than after left hemispherectomy, also points to an early origin of hemispheric specialization.

Neuroanatomic Asymmetry According to Dennis and Whitaker (1977), the apparently identical shape of the infant's cerebral hemispheres was one of the main arguments for functional identity, or equipotentiality. It is now clear, however, that the anatomic differences between the left and right hemispheres of adults (Geschwind and Levitsky, 1968; LeMay and Culebras, 1972; Wada, Clarke, and Hamm, 1975) are also present in the infant brain (Chi, Dooling, and Gilles, 1977; Teszner et al., 1972; Wada et al., 1975; Weinberger et al., 1982; Witelson and Pallie, 1973). The evidence that anatomic asymmetries in either the infant or adult brain are related to functional asymmetries is sparse (Yeo et al., 1987). But the structural asymmetries known to exist in the mature brain are neither absent nor less prominent in the immature brain.

Asymmetries in the Normal Infant

The clinical evidence concerning the ontogeny of hemispheric specialization is complemented by evidence of early asymmetry in normal children, and this evidence is even more conclusive.

Orientation   Asymmetric postures and orienting suggest that the left side of the brain is prepotent in infancy. More specifically, the fact that infants preponderantly orient or turn toward the right side suggests an activation imbalance between the left and right sides of the brain such that the left side is more highly activated (Kinsbourne, 1972, 1974a,b). The asymmetric tonic neck reflex (ATNR) attitude, in which the head is turned sideward with ipsilateral limbs extended and contralateral limbs flexed, can be observed during the first 4 weeks of life. Most infants turn to the right most of the time (Gesell, 1938; Gesell and Ames, 1950). This rightward bias predisposes the infant to coordinate his or her gaze with pointing or reaching by the right hand when these behaviors emerge and, more generally, to orient toward the right side of space. Both spontaneously or in response to external stimuli, infants favor rightward turning over leftward turning (Coryell and Michel, 1978; Harris and Fitzgerald, 1983; Liederman and Kinsbourne, 1980; Michel, 1981; Siqueland and Lipsitt, 1966; Turkewitz, Gordon, and Birch, 1965; Turkewitz et al., 1967). When these infants turn to the right they turn farther than when they turn to the left (Liederman, 1987). These turning tendencies reflect parental handedness (Liederman and Kinsbourne, 1980) and predict the child's subsequent hand preference (Coryell, 1985; Coryell and Michel, 1978; Goodwin and Michel, 1981; Michel, 1981; Viviani, Turkewitz, and Karp, 1978).

A study by MacKain et al. (1983) links infants' orienting behavior to speech perception (see Lempert and Kinsbourne, 1985) and implicates the left hemisphere in both processes. MacKain et al. showed that 6-month-old infants could detect the correspondence between the acoustic and visual components of an adult's speech articulation, but only when looking to the right side. This finding suggests that, in addition to the general, tonic prepotency of the left hemisphere that tends to bias orientation toward the right side in various situations, there is also a speech-specific, phasic activation of the left hemisphere that potentiates rightward turning within a linguistic context.

Manual Activity   No infant asymmetry is more difficult to characterize than asymmetry of manual activity (see Provins, 1992; Young et al., 1983a). As Liederman (1983a) noted, "... during early infancy, lateral preferences often fluctuate, the proportion of right-sidedness is lower than in adulthood, and there may even be periods when left-sidedness is predominant" (p. 71). She concluded: "Most behavior will be dominated by the left hemisphere—right hand—but this is due to the conjoint influence of many factors that themselves can operate relatively independently, rather than a single mechanism that reveals itself over time" (p. 89).

Despite this variability, certain manual asymmetries can be demonstrated at a very early age. Infants as young as 17 days on average grasp objects for a longer time with the right hand than with the left (Caplan and Kinsbourne, 1976; Hawn and Harris, 1983; Petrie and Peters, 1980), and the right arm tends to be more active than the left during the first 3 months of life (Coryell and Michel, 1978; Liederman, 1983b; von Hofsten, 1982). Although there has been confusion regarding early asymmetries in precision grasping, object manipulation, and reaching, the right hand is generally preferred throughout the first 4 months of life for "directed, target-related" acts (Young et al., 1983b). The confusion may have arisen from a tendency by infants to engage in more nondirected activity (e.g., passive holding, reflexive movements, hand and finger movements in the absence of arm movements) with the left hand than with the right during this period (Young et al., 1983b). Furthermore, if there is more left- than right-hand activity in response to stimulation, this asymmetry may very well reflect a decrease in right-hand activity rather than an increase in left-hand activity (Liederman, 1983b). Liederman (1983b) has argued that the left-sided bias reported in some studies of infant arm movements (e.g., McDonnell, Anderson, and Abraham, 1983) represents a "generalized disinhibition of movement" with the left arm, which is "a lag, rather than a lead, in development" (p. 329).

As noted previously, Liederman (1983b) proposed that infant asymmetries are multiply determined. One potential determinant of early manual asymmetry is the activity's meaning, or functional significance, to the infant (Peters, 1983a,b). Early asymmetry in an activity, its subsequent disappearance, and its ultimate reemergence, may reflect structural and functional changes in the neural substrate of that activity. A superficial constancy in the topography of a movement may mask a shift in underlying processes. Peters's view is supported by evidence of a temporal linkage between hand preference and language milestones; discontinuities in the developmental course of manual asymmetry coincide with transitions between stages of language development (Ramsay, 1985). "Cycles" in the development of handedness have been attributed to fluctuations in the degree to which speech interferes with use of the dominant hand (Bates et al., 1986). Such interference is thought to be due to the proximity of these two control processes in "functional cerebral space" (Kinsbourne and Hicks, 1978) within the same hemisphere. From the correlation of language competence and right-hand bias in children between the ages of 13 and 28 months, Bates et al. concluded that speech interferes maximally with right-hand activity while children are mastering a new problem in language development. When the problem is mastered, interference abates and the right-hand bias reverts to its usual level, at which it remains until the next problem in language development is encountered.

Perception Perceptual asymmetries can be found in infants. Entus (1977) showed that infants between 22 and 140 days of age could detect transitions from one CV nonsense word to another more readily at the right ear than at the left ear. In this paradigm, the presentation of CV stimuli is made contingent on the infant's non-nutritive sucking, which causes the sucking rate to rise above the baseline level. After the same pair of stimuli is presented repeatedly, the rate of sucking declines, indicating habituation. Then the signal arriving at one ear is changed while the signal at the other ear remains unchanged. If the infant detects the change in the stimulus, this will produce another increase in sucking rate (dishabituation). According to Entus (1977), not only were consonant shifts more likely to be detected when they occurred at the right ear but shifts from one musical sound to another (e.g., cello to bassoon) were more likely to be detected at the left ear. Entus concluded that hemispheric asymmetry is manifest by 3 weeks of age.

Vargha-Khadem and Corballis (1979), applying the non-nutritive sucking paradigm to somewhat younger children, failed to replicate Entus's (1977) results. Nonetheless, subsequent studies using a measure of cardiac habituation in lieu of sucking did yield asymmetries comparable to those described by Entus (Best, Hoffman, and Glanville, 1982; Glanville, Best, and Levenson, 1977). Both Hammer (1977) and Young and Gagnon (1990) found that newborns turn more often to the right than the left when they hear speech sounds. Perceptual asymmetries may even antedate full fetal development. Using accelerometers to measure limb tremor, Segalowitz and Chapman (1980) compared premature infants (average gestational age, 36 weeks) who had been repeatedly exposed to speech with ones exposed repeatedly to music and with a control group. The neonates exposed to speech showed a disproportionate reduction ("stilling") of right-sided movement, whereas those exposed to music showed the opposite asymmetry.

Electroencephalographic and Evoked Potentials Electrophysiologic studies that provide additional evidence that the left and right sides of the brain are functionally differentiated early in life are discussed by Segalowitz and Berge in chapter 19.

Interpretation Inconsistencies notwithstanding, the numerous findings of asymmetry in infants strongly suggest that the human brain is functionally asymmetric long before language and other higher cognitive skills have developed. What underlying processes do these early asymmetries represent? We suggest that these asymmetries do not indicate that the lateralized neural processors that will manifest themselves later in development are already present, but indicate precursors of these lateralized processors. Given the relative immaturity of the newborn's cerebrum (Dobbing and Sands, 1973), these precursors are likely to be represented not cerebrally but rather at the level of basal ganglia and thalamus, structures now known to share in the complementary specialization that is familiar in the case of the cerebral hemispheres. The concept of precursors, which is an important explanatory construct for much of early behavior (Kinsbourne and Hiscock, 1977), allows us to appreciate that lateralization of a behavior (or, to be more precise, lateralization of certain early developing components of a behavior) may precede the expression of the behavior itself.

Childhood Asymmetries

Insofar as equipotentiality is functional equivalence of the left and right sides of the neonatal brain, the early appearance of asymmetries—especially asymmetries that may be regarded as precursors of a more mature form of hemispheric specialization for perceptual, motor, and cognitive functions (Kinsbourne and Hiscock, 1977)—is inconsistent with equipotentiality. The infant data, nonetheless, are not necessarily inconsistent with a weak form of progressive lateralization. As the lateralized precursors evolve into increasingly mature behaviors, the degree of asymmetry may increase (Moscovitch, 1977). It has been suggested, for example, that developmental changes in the lateralization of linguistic processing depend on the level of the processing required (Porter and Berlin, 1975). Lower-level acoustic and phonological processes are hypothesized to be fully lateralized early in development, whereas the lateralization of semantic processes would come later. The question of increasing lateralization cannot be answered using the infant data alone: Data from older children are also needed. However, tasks that can be used with infants are usually inappropriate for older children. Investigators consequently have had to rely on studies of normal children above age 2 years as the primary means of determining whether asymmetries increase in magnitude during development. Dichotic listening studies have been a major source of evidence.

Dichotic Listening Hiscock and Decter (1988) contrasted two approaches to studying listening asymmetry in preschool children. One approach entails applying stimulus material and tasks designed for adults and older children to young children. The other approach involves modifying the material or the task, or both, to optimize the performance of even the youngest children tested. Whereas the results of studies employing the first approach have been mixed, studies employing the second approach consistently have yielded REAs in children as young as 2 and 3 years old (e.g., Bever, 1971; Gilbert and Climan, 1974; Ingram, 1975; Lokker and Morais, 1985; Piazza, 1977; Yeni-Komshian and Paul-Brown, 1982).

Replacing the free report method with signal detection or selective listening procedures has yielded some very large REAs in preschool children, REAs larger than those typically obtained with older children or adults (Hiscock and Kinsbourne, 1977; Kinsbourne and Hiscock, 1977). When signal detection and selective listening methods are applied to children across a wider age range, there is no suggestion of a developmental increase in the magnitude of the REA (e.g., Anderson and Hugdahl, 1987; Eling, Marshall, and van Galen, 1981; Geffen, 1978; Hiscock and Kinsbourne, 1980). Thus, as Morris et al. (1984) suggested, some of the ambiguous or anomalous outcomes in the childhood dichotic listening literature may be attributable to use of the problematic free report technique instead of a method that allows better control over the child's strategies and biases.

A multitude of free report dichotic listening studies nonetheless contains only a small minority in which the REA for verbal material either increases in magnitude or becomes more frequent with increasing age (Bryden, 1970, and Bryden and Allard, 1978; not replicated by Bryden and Allard, 1981, and Satz et al., 1975). A few additional studies had ambiguous outcomes, including a large longitudinal study by Morris et al. (1984), but in the large majority the REA remains constant across the childhood years (see recent reviews by Hahn, 1987; Hiscock, 1988; Hiscock and Decter, 1988). The typical developmental study yields a significant REA and an age-related increase in overall performance, but no significant age-related change in the magnitude of the REA (e.g., Berlin et al., 1973; Goodglass, 1973; Hiscock and Kinsbourne, 1980; Hynd and Obrzut, 1977; Kinsbourne and Hiscock, 1977; Schulman-Galambos, 1977). Nonverbal dichotic studies also have failed to show a developmental change in direction or degree of listening asymmetry (e.g., Knox and Kimura, 1970; Sidtis, Sadler, and Nass, 1987).

Other Manifestations of Laterality   There are numerous studies of other kinds of asymmetry in normal children, e.g., asymmetries of visual perception, of tactile (haptic) perception, and of interference between two tasks performed concurrently. Each of these laterality methods differs from the others not only with respect to the modality being tested and the associated experimental details but also in the rationale for asymmetric performance. Some of the methods are limited in their usefulness for addressing developmental questions. Visual half-field studies, for example, cannot be used to obtain information about asymmetric verbal processing in children who have not yet learned to read. In spite of this diversity, the various studies converge on the same conclusion, viz., the absence of developmental changes in the direction or degree of asymmetry. Age-related laterality changes have been reported often in children of one gender but not the other (e.g., Witelson, 1976), but none of the methods has yielded a consistent pattern of age-related change in degree or direction of asymmetry (see reviews by Beaumont, 1982; Hahn, 1987; Hiscock, 1988; Witelson, 1977; Young, 1982). As for the possibility that some asymmetries increase in degree very early in life, this has to be evaluated against the alternative possibility that the function under consideration was not even represented prior to the emergence of the asymmetry. A "blank slate" prior to the beginnings of hemispheric specialization is not the same as functional equivalence of the hemispheres.

Anatomic Studies   Whereas the relative size of various cerebral territories remains rather constant across development, increases in absolute brain weight occur almost entirely before birth and in the first 2 years of life. Over 90% of human brain growth is completed by the age of 6 years (Blinkov and

Glezer, 1968; Coppoletta and Wolbach, 1933). In contrast, head circumference continues to increase well beyond that age. Thus, in school-age children, growth in head circumference does not directly reflect brain growth (contrary to claims by Epstein, 1980).

Morphologic brain asymmetries at the population level have already been referred to. Of these, at least the planum temporale asymmetry is already present in the fetal brain (Chi et al., 1977; Wada et al., 1975). Petalia (right anterior–left posterior preponderance of volume) is also observable in the fetus (LeMay, 1984). While these anatomic laterality findings conform to the principle of invariant lateralization in that precursors of adult asymmetries are present very early in development, evidence of a direct relationship between morphologic mass and functional capability at the level of the individual is still lacking. Certainly, language is in some people lateralized to the smaller of paired brain structures (Piedniadz et al., 1983; Ratcliffe et al., 1980).

NEUROLOGIC MECHANISMS OF CEREBRAL LATERALIZATION

We have summarized evidence that bears on the phylogeny and ontogeny of cerebral lateralization. We now ask whether this evidence provides any clues as to the nature of hemispheric specialization per se. What is hemispheric specialization? What is lateralized? Do animal asymmetries implicate a particular mechanism that is responsible for lateralization of the brain? Do infant asymmetries suggest a mechanism? Is there one general principle of asymmetric neural organization that applies across functions, species, and maturational stages? Or does brain lateralization describe dozens of independent asymmetries misconstrued as indicators of some covert basic asymmetry of the nervous system?

We begin by drawing conclusions from the evidence concerning animal asymmetries and early asymmetries in the human. These conclusions do not pertain directly to the specific question of neural mechanisms, but contribute indirectly. In particular, our understanding of hemispheric specialization depends on whether there is some common basis for the diverse asymmetries that have been observed in different species.

Phylogenetic Trends

The animal evidence is not consistent with the hypothesis that degree of hemispheric specialization covaries across species with degree of behavioral complexity. Even rank-ordering species on the basis of behavioral complexity is itself problematic. Different species adapt in qualitatively different ways to different environments. This often precludes meaningful comparison with respect to any hypothesized general domain of behavioral complexity (Hodos and Campbell, 1969). Nevertheless, if we make intuitive judgments about major differences in behavioral complexity, as in judging primates to be behaviorally more complex than rodents, we still find no obvious relationship between behavioral complexity and degree of asymmetry. For example, the asymmetry of song control in passerine birds is more striking than the asymmetry of circling in rats, which, in turn, is more pronounced than the asymmetry of hand use in nonhuman primates. If behavioral complexity increases from passerine birds to rats and then to primates, one could even argue for an inverse relationship between behavioral complexity and the degree to which the selected species-specific behavior is lateralized.

Perhaps the relationship between behavioral complexity and degree of laterality could be addressed by quantifying the degree to which a target behavior is lateralized in a small number of species forming a "quasi-evolutionary sequence" (Hodos and Campbell, 1969; Kolb and Whishaw, 1990; Masterton and Skeen, 1972). Reaching asymmetry, for example, might be compared under comparable conditions in the bush baby, rhesus monkey, chimpanzee, and human. In the absence of such information, there is no basis for concluding that asymmetries in relatively complex species are more frequent or more marked than asymmetries in relatively rudimentary organisms. There is no reason to dispute Corballis's (1983) conclusion that the asymmetries observed in different species "have evolved in relatively isolated and independent contexts, and do not represent some common evolutionary thread" (p. 121).

Adaptive Significance

Given that the structures and functions known (or thought) to be lateralized vary from one species to another, do these characteristics have particular adaptive significance for the respective species? This important question is difficult to answer. It is no easy matter to determine the adaptive significance of specified characteristics. Whereas manual dexterity has obvious survival value for primates, the significance of turning tendencies in rodents is less clear. Also, bilateral symmetry, i.e., the absence of lateralization, is often adaptive in many instances, and specifically for orienting and moving toward either side of space. Corballis (1983) emphasizes that "bilateral symmetry is itself an evolutionary adaptation" (p. 121) and "for bilateral symmetry to have emerged in so precise and comprehensive a fashion, there must have been adaptive advantages associated with symmetry sufficiently strong to overcome a natural organic predisposition to asymmetry" (p. 122).

One such advantage may have arisen from the neural network characteristic of the forebrain and from the hemispheric representations of contralateral turning. Activation of each vertebrate half-brain occasions contralateral turning (see Kinsbourne, 1974b, for a review). The processing of information relative to a target is best accomplished in the hemisphere opposite its location because there the processing and orienting operations are congruent. Processing ipsilateral to the target would incur cross-talk interference between the hemispheres (Kinsbourne, 1970).

Mental operations not targeted to specific points in ambient space (e.g., emotions, language, problem solving) need not be bilaterally represented, and the relaxation of the need for bisymmetry may be a sufficient condition for lateralization to evolve (Kinsbourne, 1978). Whether beyond this, lateralization in humans confers an adaptive advantage remains questionable, given the persisting failure of investigators to demonstrate any substantial cognitive deficiencies in non-right-handers (Hardyck, Petrinovitch, and Goldman, 1976), although some 70% of them appear to be bilateralized for both language and spatial functions (Satz, 1979).

We now draw upon the broad database on animal asymmetries summarized above to address the perennially interesting issue of how human language evolved.

Language Origins

Behavioral   While extreme claims for the uniqueness of human language (Chomsky, 1966) must be regarded as dogma rather than knowledge (e.g., Beer, 1976; Steklis and Raleigh, 1979), there is indeed little to be observed in nonhuman primates in nature that might represent a language precursor or analog (Andrew, 1976). As for human ancestors, the lack of useful evidence leaves us unable either to support or to refute the currently fashionable view that tool use was a language antecedent (Hewes, 1973). We therefore turn to a less direct source of evidence about language phylogeny: the ontogeny of speech in the human infant.

Haeckel's (1879) law, that ontogeny recapitulates phylogeny, is overstated if it is construed to claim that infants transiently display functional mechanisms characteristic of mature individuals from phylogenetically earlier species. Certainly, the human infant exhibits no elaborated communication system before language emerges. But more properly construed as recapitulating antecedent stages in immature form (von Baer, 1828, cited in Lamendella, 1976), the principle retains heuristic value (Lamendella, 1976), and its applicability has often been demonstrated (DeBeer, 1951). It offers the opportunity for explaining transient behaviors in immature humans that in themselves seem devoid of adaptive rationale. We focus on two such behaviors: babbling and pointing ("deixis").

Babbling is promising as a speech antecedent in that it is known to encompass a wide range of speech sounds. These include sounds not represented in the infant's own prospective language. Therefore babbling cannot be regarded as imitative, a point that can also be inferred from the occurrence of initially normal babbling in deaf infants. At first babbling neither conveys external reference nor expresses the emotional state. Emotional vocalizations of limbic origin, which humans have in common with nonhuman primates (and which remain intact even in global aphasia), are quite distinct, and not related to ongoing speech (Myers, 1976). Why would such a conspicuous stage in behavioral development, i.e., babbling, unfold if it has no adaptive utility? Perhaps because it represents, in immature form, what was an earlier form of communication, now superseded by later emerging speech.

Just as babbling represents an immature communication system (not yet ripe for communicative use), so does pointing, with which babbling is often coordinated. Whereas infants do not otherwise gesture, they frequently and freely point. Pointing is usually classified among gestures. But if gestures are defined as communicative, early pointing is not a gesture and gives no grounds for a gestural theory of language origins. This is because early emerging pointing is devoid of communicative intent (Lempert and Kinsbourne, 1985). For the 9- to 12-month-old infant, pointing is not indicating, at least not to another, and occurs regardless of whether another is even present. Early pointing is a component of a selective orienting response to a salient (bright, moving, novel) stimulus. Early naming is similarly communicatively neutral. It too refers to salient stimuli and is coordinated with the pointing movement. If another person is present, he or she may derive signaling value from these actions, but this is not their purpose. Only after the age of 13 months do infants point things out to others, by gesture and name. This is now incipient speech-as-communication (Lancaster, 1975).

Apes do not speak, point, or babble. Thus the tight relationship between hand use and speech (e.g., Kimura and Archibald, 1974) does not compel belief in speech origin through tool use or gesture. In fact, when infants use their hands instrumentally, speech is suppressed (Nelson and Bonvillian, 1973). Through pointing, the hand participates in a perceptual function: reference. If ontogeny reveals phylogeny, we would conclude that speech emerged from reference enriched by differential vocalization, the signaling value of which only later became a means for modifying the behavior of others, i.e., communicating (Kinsbourne and Lempert, 1980).

Neurologic Phylogenetically, bilateral reference probably is antecedent to human verbal reference. Left hemisphere specialization in humans transcends the language function to include diverse forms of nonlinguistic reference. Analogous cognitive operations in nonhuman primates, such as visual object identification, are bilaterally represented, in posterior temporo-occipital cortex (Mishkin, Ungerleider, and Macko, 1983). This bilateral representation is not diffuse, however, but is itself part of a complementarity comparable to that between hemispheres in humans: the ventral vs. dorsal stream of visual information, two cortical systems subserving object and spatial vision respectively (Desimone and Ungerleider, 1989). A comparable dichotomy, between space- and object-centered decision, extends to the prefrontal lobe (Fuster, 1989). Therefore specialization and lateralization must be distinguished. Dichotomous specialization can occur other than along the lateral plane. We envisage a phylogenetic shift from dorsal-ventral to right-left complementarity in a hominid ancestor (Kinsbourne and Duffy, 1990). If so, investigators may have been looking in the wrong place when pitting the animal hemispheres against each other in their search for an analog to the overriding lateral specializations of the human brain.

Premack (1976) has pointed out that categorical perception of auditory stimuli is fairly widespread among species—e.g., chinchilla (Kuhl and Miller, 1975) and rhesus monkey (Morse and Snowdon, 1975)—and therefore presumably is not dependent on brain lateralization. Categorical perception in human verbal communication apparently takes advantage of a phylogenetically ancient perceptual phenomenon. Marin (1976) remarks that lateralization characterizes speech output more than perception, and he postulates that the midline organ for speech production, being bilaterally innervated, might otherwise be at risk of conflicting instructions. But the bilateralized parrot and the often bilateralized normal left-handed human are cases in point that weaken this argument.

Corballis (1989) suggested that although left hemisphere language may have been present in hominids who lived more than 2 million years ago, the flexible, rapid speech of modern humans (*Homo sapiens sapiens*) did not evolve until 150,000 to 200,000 years ago. According to Corballis, modern human language and the construction of complex tools mark the emergence of "generativity," the ability to combine elements according to rules so as to form "novel assemblages, be they words, sentences, or multipart tools" (p. 499). Corballis argues that generativity depends largely on the left hemisphere. This account of left hemisphere specialization is vulnerable to the criticism that deviation from the norm of left hemisphere speech representation apparently does not impair cognitive skill or generativity. Corballis (1991) specifically repudiates the implication that individuals who lack laterality are "throwbacks" to a more rudimentary form. Instead, he asserts that "There are probably advantages to a more symmetrical representation that must be weighed against the advantages of lateralization, and the optimum may be a balance between the two ..." (Corballis, 1991, p. 195).

The following facts must be accommodated by any theory of the brain basis of emerging language:

1. In the great majority of humans, language is left-lateralized.

2. In a substantial minority, language is bilateralized, without any substantial detriment to its efficiency.

3. In the presence of an intact left hemisphere, speech production (but not comprehension) remains limited to the left side, even if the hemispheres are callosally disconnected.

4. When the left hemisphere has been excised or is substantially lesioned, the right hemisphere proves quite capable of programming speech.

It follows that both hemispheres have neuronal substrate for generating speech. The left hemisphere usually suppresses the right hemisphere's speech potential by inhibitory interaction at the brainstem level (Kinsbourne, 1974c).

Left brain damage may release the right hemisphere's speech capability from inhibition. But the absence of this hypothesized asymmetric inhibition does not impair speech development.

SUMMARY

Structural and functional brain asymmetries exist in nonhuman vertebrates. It is no longer tenable to view brain lateralization as an exclusively, or even primarily, human attribute. Yet the animal data fail to suggest a general principle relating brain lateralization to behavior.

Insofar as some of the more striking animal asymmetries are observed in species with relatively primitive behavioral repertoires, the data disconfirm the traditional assumption that brain lateralization covaries across species with degree of behavioral refinement. Natural selection favors bisymmetric organization in motile organisms. Only when selection pressure for bisymmetry is relaxed do asymmetries appear in a species.

Human brain asymmetries arise much earlier in ontogeny than previously believed. Both structural and functional differences between the left and right sides of the brain are present at birth, if not earlier. The early emergence of behavioral asymmetries, and the character of the asymmetries themselves, imply that a subcortical mechanism underlies infantile lateralization. The better-known cortical asymmetries may be extrapolations from the corresponding subcortical asymmetries. Although it is difficult to quantify change in asymmetry against a background of a rapidly maturing brain and rapidly emerging behavioral capabilities, evidence from various sources converges on the conclusion that the asymmetries of infancy do not become more pronounced as children grow older.

We cannot subsume the diverse asymmetries observed in different species under a single organizing principle. The mechanism and functional significance of each manifestation of hemispheric specialization must be clarified individually. With respect to human language, we suggest that hemispheric specialization (as well as hemispheric specialization for other cognitive and emotional processes) reflects a relaxation of selection pressure favoring bisymmetry. The keys to understanding the ontogenesis of language lateralization consist of two language precursors—babbling and pointing—both of which represent primitive communication systems that the human infant initially uses for non-communicative purposes, but ultimately uses for signaling to others (Kinsbourne and Lempert, 1980).

Specifying the neural basis of human language lateralization necessitates accounting for the fact that right hemisphere language performance varies dramatically according to the state of the left hemisphere. The human "language acquisition device" is not referable to a uniquely dedicated language module. Instead, the left and right hemispheres are both equipped to perform linguistic functions, but the right hemisphere's role in language is normally suppressed by the left hemisphere.

REFERENCES

Adams, C. L., Molfese, C., and Betz, J. C. (1987). Electrophysiological correlates of categorical speech perception for voicing contrasts in dogs. *Developmental Neuropsychology, 3,* 175–189.

Anderson, B., and Hugdahl, K. (1987). Effects of sex, age and forced attention on dichotic listening in children: A longitudinal study. *Developmental Neuropsychology, 3,* 191–208.

Andrew, R. J. (1976). Use of formants in the grunts of baboons and other nonhuman primates. *Annals of the New York Academy of Sciences, 280,* 673–693.

Andrew, R. J., Mench, J., and Rainey, C. (1982). Right-left asymmetry of response to visual stimuli in the domestic check. In D. J. Ingle, M. A. Goodale, and R. J. W. Mansfield (Eds.), *Analysis of visual behavior* (pp. 197–209). Cambridge, MA: MIT Press.

Aram, D. M. (1988). Cognitive sequelae of unilateral lesions acquired in early childhood. In D. L. Molfese and S. J. Segalowitz (Eds.), *Brain lateralization in children* (pp. 617–636). New York: Guilford Press.

Aram, D. M., Ekelman, B. L., and Whitaker, H. A. (1986). Spoken syntax in children with acquired hemisphere lesions. *Brain and Language, 27,* 75–100.

Aram, D. M., Gillespie, L. L., and Yamashita, T. S. (1990). Reading among children with left and right brain lesions. *Developmental Neuropsychology, 6,* 301–318.

Arbuthnott, G. W., and Crow, T. J. (1971). Relation of contraversive turning to unilateral release of dopamine from the nigrostriatal pathway in rats. *Experimental Neurology, 30,* 484–491.

Arnold, A. P., and Bottjer, S. W. (1985). Cerebral lateralization in birds. In S. D. Glick (Ed.), *Cerebral lateralization in nonhuman species* (pp. 11–39). Orlando, FL: Academic Press.

Ashcraft, M. H., Yamashita, T. S., and Aram, D. M. (1992). Mathematics performance in left and right brain lesioned children and adults. *Brain and Cognition, 19,* 208–252.

Basser, S. (1962). Hemiplegia of early onset and the faculty of speech with special reference to the effects of hemispherectomy. *Brain, 85,* 427–460.

Bates, E., O'Connell, B., Vaid, J., Sledge, P., and Oakes, L. (1986). Language and hand preference in early development. *Developmental Neuropsychology, 2,* 1–15.

Beaumont, J. G. (1982). Developmental aspects. In J. G. Beaumont (Ed.), *Divided visual field studies of cerebral organisation* (pp. 113–128). London: Academic Press.

Beecher, M. D., Peterson, M. R., Zoloth, S. R., Moody, D. B., and Stebbins, W. C. (1979). Perception of conspecific vocalizations by Japanese macaques: Evidence for selective attention and neural lateralization. *Brain and Behavioral Evolution, 16,* 443–460.

Beer, C. (1976). Some complexities in the communication behavior of gulls. *Annals of the New York Academy of Sciences, 280,* 413–432.

Benton, A. L., Varney, N. R., and Hamsher, K. deS. (1978). Visuospatial judgment: A clinical test. *Archives of Neurology, 35,* 364–367.

Berlin, C. I., Hughes, L. F., Lowe-Bell, S. S., and Berlin, H. L. (1973). Dichotic right ear advantage in children 5 to 13. *Cortex, 9,* 394–402.

Best, C. T. (1988). The emergence of cerebral asymmetries in early human development: A literature review and a neuroembryological model. In D. L. Molfese and S. J. Segalowitz (Eds.), *Brain lateralization in children* (pp. 5–34). New York: Guilford Press.

Best, C. T., Hoffman, H., and Glanville, B. B. (1982). Development of infant ear asymmetries for speech and music. *Perception and Psychophysics, 35,* 75–85.

Bever, T. G. (1971). The nature of cerebral dominance in speech behavior of the child and adult. In R. Huxley and E. Ingram (Eds.), *Language acquisition: Models and methods* (pp. 231–261). London: Academic Press.

Bishop, D. V. M. (1983). Linguistic impairment after left hemidecortication for infantile hemiplegia? A reappraisal. *Quarterly Journal of Experimental Psychology, 35A*, 199–207.

Bishop, D. V. M. (1988). Can the right hemisphere mediate language as well as the left? A critical review of recent research. *Cognitive Neuropsychology, 3*, 353–367.

Blinkov, S. M., and Glezer, I. I. (1968). *The human brain in figures and tables*. New York: Basic Books.

Bowers, D., and Heilman, K. M. (1980). Material-specific hemispheric activation. *Neuropsychologia, 18*, 309–320.

Bradley, P., Horn, G., and Bateson, P. (1981). Imprinting: An electron microscopic study of chick hyperstriatum ventrale. *Experimental Brain Research, 41*, 115–120.

Braitenberg, V., and Kemali, M. (1970). Exceptions to bilateral symmetry in the epithalamus of lower vertebrate. *Journal of Comparative Neurology, 38*, 137–146.

Bruner, J. S. (1968). *Processes of cognitive growth: Infancy* (Heinz Werner Memorial Lecture Series, Vol. 3). Worcester, MA: Clark University Press.

Bryden, M. P. (1970). Laterality effects in dichotic listening: Relations with handedness and reading ability in children. *Neuropsychologia, 8*, 443–450.

Bryden, M. P. (1982). *Laterality: Functional asymmetry in the intact brain*. New York: Academic Press.

Bryden, M. P., and Allard, F. A. (1978). Dichotic listening and the development of linguistic processes. In M. Kinsbourne (Ed.), *Asymmetrical function of the brain* (pp. 392–404). New York: Cambridge University Press.

Bryden, M. P., and Allard, F. A. (1981). Do auditory perceptual asymmetries develop? *Cortex, 17*, 313–318.

Bryden, M. P., Hécaen, H., and DeAgostini, M. (1983). Patterns of cerebral organization. *Brain and Language, 20*, 249–262.

Buckenham, K. E., and Yeomans, J. S. (1993). An uncrossed tectopontine pathway mediates ipsiversive circling. *Experimental Brain Research, 54*, 11–22.

Burklund, C. W., and Smith, A. (1977). Language and the cerebral hemispheres: Observations of verbal and non-verbal responses during eighteen months following left ("dominant") hemispherectomy. *Neurology, 27*, 627–633.

Butler, C. R. (1968). A memory-record for visual discrimination habits produced in both cerebral hemispheres of a monkey when only one hemisphere has received direct visual information. *Brain Research, 10*, 152–167.

Camp, D. M., Robinson, T. E., and Becker, J. B. (1984). Sex differences in the effects of early experience on the development of behavioral and brain asymmetries in rats. *Physiology and Behavior, 33*, 433–439.

Caplan, P. J., and Kinsbourne, M. (1976). Baby drops the rattle: Asymmetry of duration of grasp by infants. *Child Development, 47*, 532–534.

Carlson, J. N., and Glick, S. D. (1989). Cerebral lateralization as a source of interindividual differences in behavior. *Experientia, 45*, 788–798.

Carter, R. L., Hohenegger, M. K., and Satz, P. (1980). Handedness and aphasia: An inferential method for determining the mode of cerebral speech specialization. *Neuropsychologia, 18,* 569–574.

Carter, R. L., Hohenegger, M. K., and Satz, P. (1982). Aphasia and speech organization in children. *Science, 218,* 797–799.

Castellano, M. A., Diaz-Palarea, M. D., Barroso, J., and Rodriguez, M. (1989). Behavioral lateralization in rats and dopaminergic system: Individual and population laterality. *Behavioral Neuroscience, 103,* 46–53.

Chi, J. G., Dooling, E. C., and Gilles, F. H. (1977). Gyral development of the human brain. *Annals of Neurology, 1,* 86–93.

Chomsky, N. (1966). *Cartesian linguistics.* New York: Harper & Row.

Cipolla-Neto, J., Horn, G., and McCabe, B. J. (1982). Hemispheric asymmetry and imprinting: The effect of sequential lesions to the hyperstriatum ventrale. *Experimental Brain Research, 48,* 22–27.

Cobb, S. (1964). A comparison of the size of an auditory nucleus (n. mesencephalicus lateralis, pars dorsalis) with the size of the optic lobe in twenty-seven species of birds. *Journal of Comparative Neurology, 122,* 271–280.

Coppoletta, J. M., and Wolbach, M. D. (1933). Body length and organ weights of infants and children. *American Journal of Pathology, 9,* 55–70.

Corballis, M. C. (1983). *Human laterality.* New York: Academic Press.

Corballis, M. C. (1989). Laterality and human evolution. *Psychological Review, 96,* 492–505.

Corballis, M. C. (1991). *The lopsided ape: Evolution of the generative mind.* New York: Oxford University Press.

Corballis, M. C., and Beale, I. L. (1976). *The psychology of left and right.* Hillsdale, NJ: Lawrence Erlbaum Associates.

Coryell, J. (1985). Infant rightward asymmetries predict right-handedness in childhood. *Neuropsychologia, 23,* 269–271.

Coryell, J., and Michel, G. F. (1978). How supine postural preferences of infants can contribute toward the development of handedness. *Infant Behavior and Development, 1,* 245–257.

Crockett, H. G., and Estridge, N. M. (1951). Cerebral hemispherectomy. *Bulletin of the Los Angeles Neurological Society, 16,* 71–87.

Czopf, J. (1972). Über die Rolle der nicht dominanten Hemisphäre in der Restitution der Sprache der Aphasischen. *Archiv für Psychiatrie und Nervenkrankheiten, 216,* 162–171.

DeBeer, G. R. (1951). *Embryos and ancestors.* Oxford: Clarendon Press.

Denenberg, V. H., Gall, J. S., Berrebi, A. S., and Yutzey, D. A. (1986). Callosal mediation of cortical inhibition in the lateralized rat brain. *Brain Research, 397,* 327–332.

Denenberg, V. H., Garbanati, J., Sherman, G., Yutzey, D. A., and Kaplan, R. (1978). Infantile stimulation induced brain lateralization in rats. *Science, 201,* 1150–1152.

Denenberg, V. H., Hofmann, M., Garbanati, J. A., Sherman, G. F., Rosen, G. D., and Yutzey, D. A. (1980). Handling in infancy, taste aversion, and brain laterality in rats. *Brain Research, 200,* 123–133.

Denenberg, V. H., and Yutzey, D. A. (1985). Hemispheric laterality, behavioral asymmetry, and the effects of early experience in rats. In S. D. Glick (Ed.), *Cerebral lateralization in nonhuman species* (pp. 109–133). Orlando, FL: Academic Press.

Ontogeny and Developmental Disabilities

Dennis, M. (1980). Capacity and strategy for syntactic comprehension after left or right hemidecortication. *Brain and Language, 10,* 287–317.

Dennis, M., and Kohn, B. (1975). Comprehension of syntax in infantile hemiplegics after cerebral hemidecortication: Left-hemisphere superiority. *Brain and Language, 2,* 475–486.

Dennis, M., Lovett, M., and Wiegel-Crump, C. A. (1981). Written language acquisition after left or right hemidecortication in infancy. *Brain and Language, 12,* 54–91.

Dennis, M., and Whitaker, H. A. (1976). Language acquisition following hemidecortication: Linguistic superiority of the left over the right hemisphere. *Brain and Language, 3,* 404–433.

Dennis, M., and Whitaker, H. A. (1977). Hemispheric equipotentiality and language acquisition. In S. J. Segalowitz and F. A. Gruber (Eds.), *Language development and neurological theory* (pp. 93–106). New York: Academic Press.

Desimone, R., and Ungerleider, L. G. (1989). Neural mechanisms of visual processing in monkeys. In F. Boller and J. Grafman (Eds.), *Handbook of neuropsychology,* Vol. 2 (pp. 267–299). Amsterdam: Elsevier.

Dewson, J. H. (1977). Preliminary evidence of hemispheric asymmetry of auditory function in monkeys. In S. Harnad, R. W. Doty, L. Goldstein, J. Jaynes, and G. Krauthamer (Eds.), *Lateralization in the nervous system* (pp. 63–71). New York: Academic Press.

Dobbing, J., and Sands, J. (1973). Quantitative growth and development of human brain. *Archives of Disease in Childhood, 48,* 757–767.

Downer, J. L. de C. (1962). Interhemispheric integration in the visual system. In V. B. Mountcastle (Ed.), *Interhemispheric relations and cerebral dominance* (pp. 87–100). Baltimore: Johns Hopkins Press.

Ebner, F. F., and Myers, R. E. (1962a). Corpus callosum and interhemispheric transmision of tactual learning. *Journal of Neurophysiology, 25,* 380–391.

Ebner, F. F., and Myers, R. E. (1962b). Direct and transcallosal induction of touch memories in the monkey. *Science, 138,* 51–52.

Ehret, G. (1987). Left hemisphere advantage in the mouse brain for recognizing ultrasonic communication calls. *Nature, 325,* 249–251.

Eling, P., Marshall, J. C., and van Galen, G. (1981). The development of language lateralization as measured by dichotic listening. *Neuropsychologia, 19,* 767–773.

Entus, A. K. (1977). Hemispheric asymmetry in processing of dichotically presented speech and nonspeech stimuli by infants. In S. J. Segalowitz and F. A. Gruber (Eds.), *Language development and neurological theory* (pp. 63–73). New York: Academic Press.

Epstein, H. T. (1980). Phrenoblysis: Special brain and mind growth periods. 1. Human brain and skull development. *Developmental Psychobiology, 13,* 629–631.

Ettlinger, G. (1987). Primate handedness: How nice if it were really so. *Behavioral and Brain Sciences, 10,* 271–273.

Fagot, J., and Vauclair, J. (1991). Manual laterality in nonhuman primates: A distinction between handedness and manual specialization. *Psychological Bulletin, 109,* 76–89.

Freud, S. (1953). *On aphasia* (E. Stengel, Trans.). New York: International Universities Press. (Original work published 1891)

Fuster, J. M. (1989). *The prefrontal cortex,* ed 2. New York: Raven Press.

Galaburda, A., Sherman, G., and Geschwind, N. (1985). Cerebral lateralization: Historical note on animal studies. In S. D. Glick (Ed.), *Cerebral lateralization in nonhuman species.* (pp. 1–10). Orlando, FL: Academic Press.

Garbanati, J. A., Sherman, G. F., Rosen, G. D., Hofmann, M., Yutzey, D. A., and Denenberg, V. H. (1983). Handling in infancy, brain laterality and muricide in rats. *Behavioural Brain Research, 7*, 351–359.

Geffen, G. (1978). The development of the right ear advantage in dichotic listening with focused attention. *Cortex, 14*, 169–177.

Geschwind, N., and Levitsky, W. (1968). Human brain: Left-right asymmetries in temporal speech regions. *Science, 161*, 181–187.

Gesell, A. (1938). The tonic neck reflex in the human infant. *Journal of Pediatrics, 13*, 455–464.

Gesell, A., and Ames, L. B. (1950). Tonic neck reflex and symmetrotonic behavior. *Journal of Pediatrics, 35*, 165–178.

Gilbert, J. H. V., and Climan, I. (1974). Dichotic studies in 2–3 year olds: A preliminary report. In *Speech communication seminar Stockholm*, Vol. 2. Uppsala, Sweden: Almqvist & Wiksell.

Glanville, B. B., Best, C. T., and Levenson, R. A. (1977). Cardiac measure of cerebral asymmetries in infant auditory perception. *Developmental Psychology, 13*, 55–59.

Glick, S. D., and Cox, R. D. (1978). Nocturnal rotation in normal rats: Correlation with amphetamine-induced rotation and effects of nigro-striatal lesions. *Brain Research, 150*, 149–161.

Glick, S. D., Hinds, P. A., and Baird, J. L. (1988). Two kinds of nigrostriatal asymmetry: Relationship to dopaminergic drug sensitivity and 6-hydroxydopamine lesion effects in Long-Evans rats. *Brain Research, 450*, 334–341.

Glick, S. D., Jerussi, T. P., Waters, D. H., and Green, J. P. (1974). Amphetamine-induced changes in striatal dopamine and acetylcholine levels and relationship to rotation (circling behavior) in rats. *Biochemical Pharmacology, 23*, 3223–3225.

Glick, S. D., Jerussi, T. P., and Zimmerberg, B. (1977). Behavioral and neuropharmacological correlates of nigrostriatal asymmetry in rats. In S. Harnad, R. W. Doty, L. Goldstein, J. Jaynes, and G. Krauthamer (Eds.), *Lateralization in the nervous system* (pp. 213–249). New York: Academic Press.

Glick, S. D., and Ross, D. A. (1981). Right-sided population bias and lateralization of activity in normal rats. *Brain Research, 205*, 222–225.

Glick, S. D., and Shapiro, R. M. (1984). Functional and neurochemical asymmetries. In N. Geschwind and A. M. Galaburda (Eds.), *Cerebral dominance: The biological foundations* (pp. 147–166). Cambridge, MA: Harvard University Press.

Glick, S. D., and Shapiro, R. M. (1985). Functional and neurochemical mechanisms of cerebral lateralization in rats. In S. D. Glick (Ed.), *Cerebral lateralization in nonhuman species* (pp. 157–183). Orlando, FL: Academic Press.

Goldberg, E., and Costa, L. D. (1981). Hemispheric differences in the acquisition and use of descriptive systems. *Brain and Language, 14*, 144–173.

Goodglass, H. (1973). Developmental comparisons of vowels and consonants in dichotic listening. *Journal of Speech and Hearing Research, 16*, 744–756.

Goodwin, R. S., and Michel, G. F. (1981). Head orientation position during birth and in infant neonatal period, and hand preference at nineteen weeks. *Child Development, 52*, 819–826.

Greenewalt, C. H. (1968). *Bird song, acoustics and Physiology*. Washington, DC: Smithsonian Institution Press.

Haeckel, E. (1879). *The evolution of man*. New York: D. Appleton & Co.

Hahn, W. K. (1987). Cerebral lateralization of function: From infancy through childhood. *Psychological Bulletin, 101*, 376–392.

Hamilton, C. R. (1977a). An assessment of hemispheric specialization in monkeys. *Annals of the New York Academy of Sciences, 299,* 222–232.

Hamilton, C. R. (1977b). Investigations of perceptual and mnemonic lateralization in monkeys. In S. Harnad, R. W. Doty, J. Jaynes, L. Goldstein, and G. Krauthamer (Eds.), *Lateralization in the nervous system* (pp. 45–62). New York: Academic Press.

Hamilton, C. R. (1983). Lateralization for orientation in split-brain monkeys. *Behavioural Brain Research, 10,* 399–403.

Hamilton, C. R., and Gazzaniga, M. S. (1964). Lateralization of learning of colour and brightness discriminations following brain bisection. *Nature, 201,* 220.

Hamilton, C. R., and Lund, J. S. (1970). Visual discrimination of movement: Midbrain or forebrain? *Science, 170,* 1428–1430.

Hamilton, C. R., Tieman, S. B., and Farrell, W. S., Jr. (1974). Cerebral dominance in monkeys? *Neuropsychologia, 12,* 193–198.

Hamilton, C. R., and Vermeire, B. A. (1982). Hemispheric differences in split-brain monkeys learning sequential comparisons. *Neuropsychologia, 20,* 691–698.

Hamilton, C. R., and Vermeire, B. A. (1983). Discrimination of monkey faces by split-brain monkeys. *Behavioural Brain Research, 9,* 263–275.

Hamilton, C. R., and Vermeire, B. A. (1988). Complementary hemispheric specialization in monkeys. *Science, 242,* 1691–1694.

Hamilton, C. R., and Vermeire, B. A. (1991). Functional lateralization in monkeys. In F. L. Kitterle (Ed.), *Cerebral laterality: Theory and research* (pp. 19–34). Hillsdale, NJ: Lawrence Erlbaum Associates.

Hammer, M. (1977). Lateral differences in the newborn infant's response to speech and noise stimuli. *Dissertation Abstracts International, 38,* 1493B.

Hardyck, C., Petrinovitch, L. F., and Goldman, R. D. (1976). Left-handedness and cognitive deficit. *Cortex, 12,* 266–279.

Harris, L. J., and Fitzgerald, H. E. (1983). Postural orientation in human infants: Changes from birth to three months. In G. Young, S. J. Segalowitz, C. M. Corter, and S. E. Trehub (Eds.), *Manual specialization and the developing brain* (pp. 285–305). New York: Academic Press.

Hatta, T., and Koike, M. (1991). Left-hand preference in frightened mother monkeys in taking up their babies. *Neuropsychologia, 29,* 207–209.

Hawn, P. R., and Harris, L. J. (1983). Hand differences in grasp duration and reaching in two- and five-month-old human infants. In G. Young, S. J. Segalowitz, C. M. Corter, and S. E. Trehub (Eds.), *Manual specialization and the developing brain* (pp. 71–92). New York: Academic Press.

Hebb, D. O. (1942). The effect of early and late brain injury upon test scores and the nature of normal adult intelligence. *Proceedings of the American Philosophy Society, 85,* 265–292.

Heffner, H. E., and Heffner, R. S. (1984). Temporal lobe lesions and perception of species-specific vocalizations by macaques. *Science, 226,* 75–76.

Hewes, G. W. (1973). Primate communication and the gestural origin of language. *Current Anthropology, 14,* 5–24.

Hiscock, M. (1988). Behavioral asymmetries in normal children. In D. L. Molfese and S. J. Segalowitz (Eds.), *Brain lateralization in children: Developmental implications* (pp. 85–169). New York: Guilford Press.

Hiscock, M., and Decter, M. H. (1988). Dichotic listening in children. In K. Hugdahl (Ed.), *Handbook of dichotic listening: Theory, methods and research* (pp. 431–473). Chichester, England: John Wiley & Sons.

Hiscock, M., and Kinsbourne, M. (1977). Selective listening asymmetry in preschool children. *Developmental Psychology, 13,* 217–224.

Hiscock, M., and Kinsbourne, M. (1980). Asymmetries of selective listening and attention switching in children. *Developmental Psychology, 16,* 70–82.

Hodos, W., and Campbell, C. B. G. (1969). Scala naturae: Why there is no theory in comparative psychology. *Psychological Review, 76,* 337–350.

Hopkins, W. D., Fagot, J., and Vauclair, J. (1993). Mirror-image matching and mental rotation problem solved by baboons (*Papio papio*): Unilateral input enhances performance. *Journal of Experimental Psychology: General, 122,* 61–72.

Hopkins, W. D., Morris, R. D., and Savage-Rumbaugh, E. S. (1991). Evidence for asymmetrical hemispheric priming using known and unknown warning stimuli in two language-trained chimpanzees. *Journal of Experimental Psychology: General, 104,* 46–56.

Hopkins, W. D., Morris, R. D., Savage-Rumbaugh, E. S., and Rumbaugh, D. M. (1992). Hemispheric priming by meaningful and nonmeaningful symbols in language-trained chimpanzees (*Pan troglodytes*): Further evidence of a left hemisphere advantage. *Behavioral Neuroscience, 106,* 575–582.

Hopkins, W. D., Washburn, D. A., and Rumbaugh, D. M. (1989). Note on hand use in the manipulation of joysticks by rhesus monkeys (*Macaca mulatta*) and chimpanzees (*Pan troglodytes*). *Journal of Comparative Psychology, 103,* 91–94.

Hörster, W., and Ettlinger, G. (1985). An association between hand preference and tactile discrimination performance in the rhesus monkey. *Neuropsychologia, 23,* 411–413.

Howard, K. J., Rogers, L. J., and Boura, A. L. A. (1980). Functional lateralization of the chicken forebrain revealed by use of intracranial glutamate. *Brain Research, 188,* 369–382.

Hynd, G. W., and Obrzut, J. E. (1977). Effects of grade level and sex on the magnitude of the dichotic ear advantage. *Neuropsychologia, 15,* 689–692.

Ingram, D. (1975). Cerebral speech lateralization in young children. *Neuropsychologia, 13,* 103–105.

Isaacson, R. L. (1975). The myth of recovery from early brain damage. In N. R. Ellis (Ed.), *Aberrant development in infancy: Human and animal studies* (pp. 1–25). Hillsdale, NJ: Lawrence Erlbaum Associates.

Jason, G. W., Cowey, A., and Weiskrantz, L. (1984). Hemispheric asymmetry for a visuospatial task in monkeys. *Neuropsychologia, 22,* 777–784.

Jerussi, T. P., and Glick, S. D. (1974). Amphetamine-induced rotation in rats without lesions. *Neuropharmacology, 13,* 283–286.

Jerussi, T. P., and Glick, S. D. (1976). Drug-induced rotation in rats without lesions: Behavioral and neurochemical indices of a normal asymmetry in nigro-striatal function. *Psychopharmacology, 47,* 249–260.

Kimura, D. (1961). Cerebral dominance and the perception of verbal stimuli. *Canadian Journal of Psychology, 15,* 166–171.

Kimura, D., and Archibald, Y. (1974). Motor functions of the left hemisphere. *Brain, 97,* 337–350.

Kinsbourne, M. (1970). The cerebral basis of lateral asymmetries in attention. *Acta Psychologica, 33*, 193–201.

Kinsbourne, M. (1971). The minor cerebral hemisphere as a source of aphasic speech. *Archives of Neurology, 25*, 302–306.

Kinsbourne, M. (1972). Eye and head turning indicates cerebral lateralization. *Science, 176*, 539–541.

Kinsbourne, M. (1973). The control of attention by interaction between the two hemispheres. In S. Kornblum (Ed.), *Attention and performance*, Vol. 4 (pp. 239–256). New York: Academic Press.

Kinsbourne, M. (1974a). Direction of gaze and distribution of cerebral thought processes. *Neuropsychologia, 12*, 279–281.

Kinsbourne, M. (1974b). Lateral interactions in the brain. In M. Kinsbourne and W. L. Smith (Eds.), *Hemispheric disconnection and cerebral function* (pp. 239–259). Springfield, IL: Charles C Thomas.

Kinsbourne, M. (1974c). Mechanisms of language in relation to lateral action. In M. Kinsbourne and W. L. Smith (Eds.), *Hemispheric disconnection and cerebral function* (pp. 260–285). Springfield, IL: Charles C Thomas.

Kinsbourne, M. (1975). The ontogeny of cerebral dominance. *Annals of the New York Academy of Sciences, 263*, 244–250.

Kinsbourne, M. (1978). Evolution of language in relation to lateral action. In M. Kinsbourne (Ed.), *Asymmetrical function of the brain* (pp. 553–566). Cambridge: Cambridge University Press.

Kinsbourne, M., and Bruce, R. (1987). Shift in visual laterality within blocks of trials. *Acta Psychologica, 66*, 139–156.

Kinsbourne, M., and Duffy, C. J. (1990). The role of dorsal/ventral processing dissociation in the economy of the primate brain. *Behavioral and Brain Sciences, 13*, 553–554.

Kinsbourne, M., and Hicks, R. E. (1978). Functional cerebral space: A model for overflow, transfer and interference effects in human performance. In J. Requin (Ed.), *Attention and performance*, Vol. 7 (pp. 345–362). Hillsdale, NJ: Lawrence Erlbaum Associates.

Kinsbourne, M., and Hiscock, M. (1977). Does cerebral dominance develop? In S. J. Segalowitz and F. A. Gruber (Eds.), *Language development and neurological theory* (pp. 171–191). New York: Academic Press.

Kinsbourne, M., and Lempert, H. (1980). Does left brain lateralization of speech arise from right-biased orienting to salient precepts? *Human Development, 22*, 270–276.

Knox, C., and Kimura, D. (1970). Cerebral processing of nonverbal sounds in boys and girls. *Neuropsychologia, 8*, 227–237.

Kokkinidis, L. (1987). Amphetamine-elicited perseverative and rotational behavior: Evaluation of directional preference. *Pharmacology, Biochemistry, and Behavior, 26*, 527–532.

Kokkinidis, L., and Anisman, H. (1977). Perseveration and rotational behavior elicited by d-amphetamine in a Y-maze exploratory task: Differential effects of intraperitoneal and unilateral intraventricular administration. *Psychopharmacology (Berlin), 52*, 123–128.

Kolb, B., and Whishaw, I. Q. (1990). *Fundamentals of human neuropsychology* (3rd ed.). San Francisco: WH Freeman & Co.

Krashen, S. (1973). Lateralization, language learning and the critical period: Some new evidence. *Language Learning, 23*, 63–74.

Kubos, K. L., Pearlson, G. D., and Robinson, R. G. (1982). Intracortical kainic acid induces an asymmetrical behavioral response in the rat. *Brain Research, 239*, 303–309.

Kubos, K. L., and Robinson, R. G. (1984). Cortical undercuts in the rat produce asymmetrical behavioral response without altering catecholamine concentrations. *Experimental Neurology, 83*, 646–653.

Kuhl, P., and Miller, J. (1975). Speech perception by the chinchilla: Voiced-voiceless distinction in alveolar plosive consonants. *Science, 190*, 69–72.

Lamendella, J. T. (1976). Relations between the ontogeny and phylogeny of language: A neorecapitulationist view. *Annals of the New York Academy of Sciences, 280*, 396–412.

Lancaster, J. B. (1975). *Primate behavior and the emergence of human culture.* New York: Holt.

Leehey, S. C., Carey, S., Diamond, R., and Cahn, A. (1978). Upright and inverted faces: The right hemisphere knows the difference. *Cortex, 14*, 411–419.

LeMay, M. (1984). Radiological, developmental, and fossil asymmetries. In N. Geschwind and A. M. Galaburda (Eds.), *Cerebral dominance: The biological foundations* (pp. 26–42). Cambridge, MA: Harvard University Press.

LeMay, M., and Culebras, A. (1972). Human brain—Morphologic differences in the hemispheres demonstrable by carotid arteriography. *New England Journal of Medicine, 287*, 168–170.

Lempert, H., and Kinsbourne, M. (1985). Possible origin of speech in selective orienting. *Psychological Bulletin, 97*, 62–73.

Lenneberg, E. H. (1967). *Biological foundations of language.* New York: John Wiley & Sons.

Liederman, J. (1983a). Mechanisms underlying instability in the development of hand preference. In G. Young, S. J. Segalowitz, C. M. Corter, and S. E. Trehub (Eds.), *Manual specialization and the developing brain* (pp. 71–92). New York: Academic Press.

Liederman, J. (1983b). Is there a stage of left-sided precocity during early manual specialization? In G. Young, S. J. Segalowitz, C. M. Corter, and S. E. Trehub (Eds.), *Manual specialization and the developing brain* (pp. 321–330). New York: Academic Press.

Liederman, J. (1987). Neonates show an asymmetric degree of head rotation but lack an asymmetric tonic neck reflex asymmetry: Neuropsychological implications. *Developmental Neuropsychology, 3*, 101–112.

Liederman, J., and Kinsbourne, M. (1980). The mechanism of neonatal rightward turning bias: A sensory or motor asymmetry? *Infant Behavior and Development, 3*, 223–238.

Lokker, R., and Morais, J. (1985). Ear differences in children at two years of age. *Neuropsychologia, 23*, 127–129.

Lovejoy, O. C. (1981). The origin of man. *Science, 221*, 341–350.

Luria, A. R. (1973). *The working brain.* London: Penguin.

MacKain, K., Studdert-Kennedy, M., Spieker, S., and Stern, D. (1983). Infant intermodal speech perception is a left hemisphere function. *Science, 214*, 1347–1349.

MacNeilage, P. F., Studdert-Kennedy, M. G., and Lindblom, B. (1987). Primate handedness reconsidered. *Behavioral and Brain Sciences, 10*, 247–303.

MacNeilage, P. F., Studdert-Kennedy, M. G., and Lindblom, B. (1988). Primate handedness: A foot in the door. *Behavioral and Brain Sciences, 11*, 737–746.

Marin, O. S. M. (1976). Neurobiology of language: An overview. *Annals of the New York Academy of Sciences, 280*, 868–884.

Masterton, B., and Skeen, L. C. (1972). Origins of anthropoid intelligence: Prefrontal system and delayed alternation in hedgehog, tree shrew and bushbaby. *Journal of Comparative and Physiological Psychology, 81,* 423–433.

Mayberg, H., Moran, T. H., and Robinson, R. G. (1990). Remote lateralized changes in cortical ^{3}H spiperone binding following focal frontal cortex lesions in the rat. *Brain Research, 516,* 127–131.

McDonnell, P. M., Anderson, V. E. S., and Abraham, W. C. (1983). Asymmetry and orientation of arm movements in three- to eight-week-old infants. *Infant Behavior and Development, 6,* 287–298.

Michel, G. F. (1981). Right handedness: A consequence of infant supine head-orientation preference? *Science, 212,* 685–687.

Milner, B. (1974). Sparing of language after unilateral brain damage. *Neuroscience Research Program Bulletin, 12,* 213–217.

Mishkin, M., Ungerleider, L. G., and Macko, K. A. (1983). Object vision and spatial vision: Two cortical pathways. *Trends in the Neurosciences, 6,* 414–417.

Moran, T. H., Sanberg, P. R., Kubos, K. L., Goldrich, M., and Robinson, R. G. (1984). Asymmetrical effects of unilateral cortical suction lesions: Behavioral characterization. *Behavioral Neuroscience, 98,* 747–752.

Morgan, M. J. (1977). Embryology and inheritance of asymmetry. In S. Harnad, R. W. Doty, L. Goldstein, J. Jaynes, and G. Krauthamer (Eds.), *Lateralization in the nervous system* (pp. 173–194). New York: Academic Press.

Morris, R., Bakker, D., Satz, P., and Van der Vlugt, H. (1984). Dichotic listening ear asymmetry: Patterns of longitudinal development. *Brain and Language, 22,* 49–66.

Morris, R. D., and Hopkins, W. D. (1993). Perception of human chimeric faces by chimpanzees? Evidence for a right hemisphere advantage. *Brain and Cognition, 21,* 111–222.

Morris, R. D., Hopkins, W. D., and Bolser-Gilmore, L. (1993). Assessment of hand preference in two language-trained chimpanzees (*Pan troglodytes*): A multimethod analysis. *Journal of Clinical and Experimental Neuropsychology, 15,* 487–502.

Morse, P. A., and Snowdon, C. (1975). An investigation of categorical speech discrimination by rhesus monkeys. *Perception and Psychophysics, 17,* 9–16.

Moscovitch, M. (1977). The development of lateralization of language functions and its relation to cognitive and linguistic development: A review and some theoretical speculations. In S. J. Segalowitz and F. A. Gruber (Eds.), *Language development and neurological theory* (pp. 193–211). New York: Academic Press.

Myers, R. E. (1976). Comparative neurology of vocalization and speech: Proof of a dichotomy. *Annals of the New York Academy of Sciences, 280,* 745–757.

Nass, R., and Koch, D. (1987). Temperamental differences in toddlers with early unilateral right- and left-brain damage. *Developmental Neuropsychology, 3,* 93–99.

Nelson, K. E., and Bonvillian, J. D. (1973). Concepts and words in the 18-month old: Acquiring concept names under controlled conditions. *Cognition, 2,* 435–440.

Nottebohm, F. (1971). Neural lateralization of vocal control in a passerine bird. I. Song. *Journal of Experimental Zoology, 177,* 229–261.

Nottebohm, F. (1976). Phonation in the orange-winged Amazon parrot, *Amazona amazonica. Journal of Comparative Physiology, 108,* 157–170.

Nottebohm, F. (1977). Asymmetries in neural control of vocalization in the canary. In S. Harnad, R. W. Doty, L. Goldstein, J. Jaynes, and G. Krauthamer (Eds.), *Lateralization in the nervous system* (pp. 23–44). New York: Academic Press. Nottebohm, F., Manning, E., and Nottebohm, M. E. (1979). Reversal of hypoglossal dominance in canaries following syringeal denervation. *Journal of Comparative Physiology, 134,* 227–240.

Nottebohm, F., Stokes, T. M., and Leonard, C. M. (1976). Central control of song in the canary, *Serinus canarius. Journal of Comparative Neurology, 165,* 457–486.

Ogden, J. A. (1988). Language and memory functions after long recovery periods in left-hemispherectomized subject. *Neuropsychologia, 26,* 645–659.

Overman, W. H., Jr., and Doty, R. W. (1982). Hemispheric specialization displayed by man but not macaques for analysis of faces. *Neuropsychologia, 20,* 113–128.

Pazo, J. H., Murer, G. M., and Segal, E. (1993). D_1 and D_2 receptors and circling behavior in rats with unilateral lesion of the entopeduncular nucleus. *Brain Research Bulletin, 30,* 635–639.

Pearlson, G. D., Kubos, K. L., and Robinson, R. G. (1984). Effect of anterior-posterior lesion location on the asymmetrical behavioral and biochemical response to cortical suction ablations in the rat. *Brain Research, 293,* 241–250.

Pearlson, G. D., and Robinson, R. G. (1981). Suction lesions of the frontal cerebral cortex in the rat induce asymmetrical behavioral and catecholaminergic responses. *Brain Research, 218,* 233–242.

Perrett, D. I., Rolls, E. T., and Caan, W. (1982). Visual neurons responsive to faces in the monkey temporal cortex. *Experimental Brain Research, 47,* 329–342.

Peters, M. (1983a). Differentiation and lateral specialization in motor development. In G. Young, S. J. Segalowitz, C. M. Corter, and S. E. Trehub (Eds.), *Manual specialization and the developing brain* (pp. 141–159). New York: Academic Press.

Peters, M. (1983b). Lateral bias in reaching and holding at six and twelve months. In G. Young, S. J. Segalowitz, C. M. Corter, and S. E. Trehub (Eds.), *Manual specialization and the developing brain* (pp. 367–374). New York: Academic Press.

Peterson, M. R., Beecher, M. D., Zoloth, S. R., Green, S., Marler, P. R., Moody, D. B., and Stebbins, W. C. (1984). Neural lateralization of vocalization by Japanese macaques: Communicative significance is more important than acoustic structure. *Behavioral Neuroscience, 98,* 779–790.

Petrie, B. N., and Peters, M. (1980). Handedness: Left/right differences in intensity of grasp response and duration of rattle holding in infants. *Infant Behavior and Development, 3,* 215–221.

Piazza, D. M. (1977). Cerebral lateralization in young children as measured by dichotic listening and finger tapping tasks. *Neuropsychologia, 15,* 417–425.

Piedniadz, J. M., Naeser, M. A., Koff, E., and Levine, H. L. (1983). CT scan cerebral hemispheric asymmetry measurements in stroke cases with global aphasia: Atypical asymmetries associated with improved recovery. *Cortex, 19,* 371–391.

Pohl, P. (1983). Central auditory processing V: Ear advantages for acoustic stimuli in baboons. *Brain and Language, 20,* 44–53.

Pohl, P. (1984). Ear advantages for temporal resolution in baboons. *Brain and Cognition, 3,* 438–444.

Porter, R. J., Jr., and Berlin, C. I. (1975). On interpreting developmental changes in the dichotic right-ear advantage. *Brain and Language, 2,* 186–200.

Premack, D. (1976). Mechanisms of intelligence: Preconditions for language. *Annals of the New York Academy of Sciences, 280,* 544–561.

Provins, K. A. (1992). Early infant motor asymmetries and handedness: A critical evaluation of the evidence. *Developmental Neuropsychology, 8,* 325–365.

Ramsay, D. S. (1985). Fluctuations in unimanual hand preference in infants following the onset of duplicated syllable babbling. *Developmental Psychology, 21,* 318–324.

Ratcliffe, G., Dila, C., Taylor, L., and Milner, B. (1980). The morphological asymmetry of the hemispheres and cerebral dominance: A possible relationship. *Brain and Language, 11,* 87–98.

Robinson, R. G. (1979). Differential behavior and biochemical effects of right and left hemispheric cerebral infarction in the rat. *Science, 205,* 707–710.

Robinson, R. G. (1985). Lateralized behavioral and neurochemical consequences of unilateral brain injury in rats. In S. D. Glick (Ed.), *Cerebral lateralization in nonhuman species* (pp. 135–156). Orlando, FL: Academic Press.

Robinson, R. G., and Bloom, F. E. (1977). Pharmacological treatment following experimental cerebral infarction: Implications for understanding psychological symptoms of human stroke. *Biological Psychiatry, 12,* 669–680.

Robinson, R. G., Shoemaker, W. J., and Schlumpf, M. (1980). Time course of changes in catecholamines following right hemispheric cerebral infarction in the rat. *Brain Research, 181,* 202–208.

Robinson, R. G., Shoemaker, W. J., Schlumpf, M., Valk, T., and Bloom, F. E. (1975). Effect of experimental cerebral infarction in rat brain on catecholamines and behaviour. *Nature, 255,* 332–334.

Robinson, R. G., and Stitt, T. G. (1981). Intracortical 6-hydroxydopamine induces an asymmetrical behavioral response in the rat. *Brain Research, 213,* 387–395.

Rogers, L. J. (1980a). Functional lateralisation in the chicken fore-brain revealed by cycloheximide treatment. In R. Nohring (Ed.), *Acta XVII Congressus Internationalis Ornithologici* (pp. 653–659). Berlin: Verlag der deutschen Ornithologen-Gesellschaft.

Rogers, L. J. (1980b). Lateralization in the avian brain. *Bird Behaviour, 2,* 1–12.

Rogers, L. J. (1982). Light experience and asymmetry of brain function in chickens. *Nature, 297,* 223–225.

Rudel, R. G. (1978). Neuroplasticity: Implications for development and education. In J. S. Chall and A. F. Mirsky (Eds.), *Education and the brain. Seventy-seventh yearbook of the National Society for the Study of Education* (pp. 269–307). Chicago: University of Chicago Press.

Russell, W. R., and Espir, M. L. (1961) . *Traumatic aphasia: A study of aphasia in war wounds of the brain.* New York: Oxford University Press.

St. James-Roberts, I. (1981). A reinterpretation of hemispherectomy data without functional plasticity of the brain. *Brain and Language, 13,* 31–53.

Satz, P. (1979). A test of some models of hemispheric speech organization in the left- and right-handed. *Science, 203,* 1131–1133.

Satz, P., Bakker, D. J., Teunissen, J., Goebel, R., and Van der Vlugt, H. (1975). Developmental parameters of the ear asymmetry: A multivariate approach. *Brain and Language, 2,* 171–185.

Satz, P., and Bullard-Bates, C. (1981). Acquired aphasia in children. In M. T. Sarno (Ed.), *Acquired aphasia* (pp. 399–426). New York: Academic Press.

Satz, P., and Fletcher, J. M. (1981). Emergent trends in neuropsychology: An overview. *Journal of Consulting and Clinical Psychology, 49,* 851–865.

Schneider, G. E. (1979). Is it really better to have your brain lesion early? A revision of the "Kennard principle." *Neuropsychologia, 17,* 557–583.

Schulman-Galambos, C. (1977). Dichotic listening performance in elementary and college students. *Neuropsychologia, 15,* 577–584.

Segalowitz, S. J., and Chapman, J. S. (1980). Cerebral asymmetry for speech in neonates: A behavioral measure. *Brain and Language, 9,* 281–288.

Segalowitz, S. J., and Gruber, F. A. (Eds.). (1977). *Language development and neurological theory.* New York: Academic Press.

Shapiro, R. M., Camarota, N. A., and Glick, S. D. (1987). Nocturnal rotational behavior in rats: Further neurochemical support for a two-population model. *Brain Research Bulletin, 19,* 421–427.

Shapiro, R. M., Glick, S. D., and Camarota, N. A. (1987). A two-population model of rat rotational behavior: Effects of unilateral nigrostriatal 6-hydroxydopamine on striatal neurochemistry and amphetamine-induced rotation. *Brain Research, 426,* 323–331.

Shapiro, R. M., Glick, S. D., and Hough, L. B. (1986). Striatal dopamine uptake asymmetries and rotational behavior in unlesioned rats: Revising the model? *Psychopharmacology, 89,* 25–30.

Sherman, G. F., Garbanati, J. A., Rosen, G. D., Hofmann, M., Yutzey, D. A., and Denenberg, V. H. (1983). Lateralization of spatial preference in the female rat. *Life Sciences, 33,* 189–193.

Sherman, G. F., Garbanati, J. A., Rosen, G. D., Yutzey, D. A., and Denenberg, V. H. (1980). Brain and behavioral asymmetries for spatial preference in rats. *Brain Research, 192,* 61–67.

Sidtis, J. J., Sadler, A. E, and Nass, R. D. (1987). Dichotic complex pitch and speech discrimination in 7 to 12 year old children. *Developmental Neuropsychology, 3,* 227–238.

Siqueland, E. R., and Lipsitt, L. P. (1966) . Conditioned head turning in human newborns. *Journal of Experimental Child Psychology, 4,* 356–357.

Smith, A. (1966). Speech and other functions after left (dominant) hemispherectomy. *Journal of Neurology, Neurosurgery and Psychiatry, 29,* 467–471.

Smith, A. (1983). Overview or "underview": A comment on Satz and Fletcher's "Emergent trends in neuropsychology: An overview." *Journal of Consulting and Clinical Psychology, 51,* 768–775.

Spellacy, F., and Blumstein, S. (1970) . The influence of language set on ear preference in phoneme recognition. *Cortex, 6,* 430–439.

Spemann, H., and Falkenberg, H. (1919). Über asymmetrische Entwicklung und Situs inversus bei Zwillingen und Doppelbildungen. *Wilhelm Roux Archiv für Entwicklungsmechanik, 45,* 371–422.

Steklis, H. D., and Raleigh, M. J. (Eds.). (1979). *Neurobiology of social communication in primates: An evolutionary perspective.* New York: Academic Press.

Teszner, D., Tzavaras, A., Gruner, J., and Hécaen, H. (1972). Étude anatomique de l'asymétrie droite-gauche du planum temporale. *Revue Neurologie (Paris), 126,* 444–462.

Turkewitz, G., Gordon, E. W., and Birch, H. G. (1965). Head turning in the human neonate: Spontaneous patterns. *Journal of Genetic Psychology, 107,* 143–148.

Turkewitz, G., Moreau, T., Gordon, E. W., Birch, H. G., and Crystal, D. (1967). Relationships between prior head positions and lateral differences in responsiveness to somesthetic stimulation in the human neonate. *Journal of Experimental Child Psychology, 5,* 548–561.

Ungerstedt, U. (1971). Striatal dopamine release after amphetamine or nerve degeneration revealed by rotational behaviour. *Acta Physiologica Scandinavica Supplement 367*, 49–68.

Ungerstedt, U., and Arbuthnott, G. W. (1970). Quantitative recording of rotational behavior in rats after 6-hydroxy-dopamine lesions of the nigrostriatal dopamine system. *Brain Research, 24*, 485–493.

Van Hout, A. (1992). Acquired aphasias in children. In S. J. Segalowitz and I. Rapin (Eds.), *Handbook of neuropsychology*, Vol. 7, Section 10, Part 2: *Child neuropsychology* (pp. 139–161). R. Boller and J. Grafman (section Eds.). Amsterdam: Elsevier.

Van Lancker, D., and Fromkin, V. A. (1977). Hemispheric specialization for pitch and "tone." Evidence from Thai. *Journal of Phonetics, 1*, 101–109.

Vargha-Khadem, F., and Corballis, M. C. (1979). Cerebral asymmetry in infants. *Brain and Language, 8*, 1–9.

Vargha-Khadem, F, O'Gorman, A. M., and Watters, G. V. (1985). Aphasia and handedness in relation to hemispheric side, age at injury and severity of cerebral lesions during childhood. *Brain, 108*, 677–696.

Vauclair, J., Fagot, J., and Hopkins, W. D. (1993). Rotation of mental images in baboons when the visual input is directed to the left cerebral hemisphere. *Psychological Science, 4*, 99–103.

Vermeire, B. A., and Hamilton, C. R. (1988). Laterality in monkeys discriminating inverted faces. *Neuroscience Abstracts, 14*, 1139.

Viviani, J., Turkewitz, G., and Karp. E. (1978) . A relationship between laterality of functioning at 2 days and at 7 years of age. *Bulletin of the Psychonomic Society, 12*, 189–192.

von Hofsten, C. (1982). Eye-hand coordination in the newborn. *Developmental Psychology, 18*, 450–461.

Wada, J. A., Clarke, R., and Hamm, A. (1975). Cerebral hemispheric asymmetry in humans. *Archives of Neurology, 32*, 239–246.

Ward, J. P. (1991). Prosimians as animal models in the study of neural lateralization. In F. L. Kitterle (Ed.), *Cerebral laterality: Theory and research* (pp. 1–17). Hillsdale, NJ: Lawrence Erlbaum Associates.

Warren, J. M. (1980). Handedness and laterality in humans and other animals. *Physiological Psychology, 8*, 351–359.

Warren, J. M., Abplanalp, J. M., and Warren, H. B. (1967). The development of handedness in cats and rhesus monkeys. In H. W. Stevenson, E. H. Hess, and H. L. Rheingold (Eds.), *Early behavior: Comparative developmental approaches* (pp. 73–101). New York: John Wiley & Sons.

Webster, W. G. (1972). Functional asymmetry between the cerebral hemispheres of the cat. *Neuropsychologia, 10*, 75–87.

Webster, W. G. (1981). Morphological asymmetries of the cat brain. *Brain, Behavior and Evolution, 18*, 72–79.

Webster, W. G., and Webster, I. H. (1975). Anatomical asymmetries of the cerebral hemispheres of the cat brain. *Physiology and Behavior, 14*, 867–869.

Weinberger, D. R., Luchins, D. J., Morihisa, J., and Wyatt, R. J. (1982). Asymmetrical volumes of the right and left frontal and occipital regions of the human brain. *Annals of Neurology, 11*, 97–99.

Wise, R. A., and Holmes, L. J. (1986). Circling from unilateral VIA morphine: Direction is controlled by environmental stimuli. *Brain Research Bulletin, 16*, 267–269.

Witelson, S. F. (1976). Sex and the single hemisphere: Right hemisphere specialization for spatial processing. *Science, 193,* 425–427.

Witelson, S. F. (1977). Early hemisphere specialization and interhemisphere plasticity: An empirical and theoretical review. In S. J. Segalowitz and F. A. Gruber (Eds.), *Language development and neurological theory* (pp. 213–287). New York: Academic Press.

Witelson, S. F., and Pallie, W. (1973). Left hemisphere specialization for language in the newborn: Neuroanatomical evidence of brain asymmetry. *Brain, 96,* 641–646.

Woods, B. T., and Teuber, H.-L. (1978). Changing patterns of childhood aphasia. *Annals of Neurology, 32,* 239–246.

Yeni-Komshian, G. H., and Paul-Brown, D. (1982). Perception of temporally competing speech stimuli in preschool children. *Brain and Language, 17,* 166–179.

Yeo, R. A., Turkheimer, E., Raz, N., and Bigler, E. D. (1987). Volumetric asymmetries of the human brain: Intellectual correlates. *Brain and Cognition, 6*(1), 15–23.

Young, A. W. (1982). Asymmetry of cerebral hemispheric function during development. In J. W. T. Dickerson and H. McGurk (Eds.), *Brain and behavioural development* (pp. 168–202). Glasgow: Blackie.

Young, G., and Gagnon, M. (1990). Neonatal laterality, birth stress, familial sinistrality, and left-brain inhibition. *Developmental Neuropsychology, 6,* 127–150.

Young, G., Segalowitz, S. J., Corter, C. M., and Trehub, S. E. (Eds.). (1983a). *Manual specialization and the developing brain.* New York: Academic Press.

Young, G., Segalowitz, S. J., Misek, P., Alp, I. E., and Boulet, R. (1983b). Is early reaching left-handed? Review of manual specialization research. In G. Young, S. J. Segalowitz, C. M. Corter, and S. E. Trehub (Eds.), *Manual specialization and the developing brain* (pp. 13–32). New York: Academic Press.

Zappia, J. V., and Rogers, L. J. (1983). Light experience during development affects asymmetry of forebrain function in chickens. *Developmental Brain Research, 11,* 93–106.

Zimmerberg, B., Glick, S. D., and Jerussi, T. P. (1974). Neurochemical correlate of a spatial preference in rats. *Science, 185,* 623–625.

Zollinger, R. (1935). Removal of left cerebral hemisphere. Report of a case. *Archives of Neurology and Psychiatry, 34,* 1055–1064.

19 Functional Asymmetries in Infancy and Early Childhood: A Review of Electrophysiologic Studies and Their Implications

Sidney J. Segalowitz and Brenda E. Berge

WHY HEMISPHERIC ASYMMETRIES IN INFANCY AND CHILDHOOD?

It has been obvious for a long time from clinical cases that the adult cerebral hemispheres harbor major functional asymmetries, and despite empirical challenges in demonstrating such asymmetries, there are not many philosophical difficulties with this fact. The philosophical problems which do remain center primarily on questions surrounding the notion of consciousness and whether or not it is unitary, but this sort of problem is basic to all reductionist neuroscience and not just models of lateralization (e.g., Churchland, 1986; Dennett and Kinsbourne, 1992).

When we extrapolate the notion to infants, however, new issues arise concerning what we might mean by functional asymmetries of the hemispheres. For example, for a long time it was supposed that the brains of infants, by their very nature, could not be functionally asymmetric for language processes simply because infants do not yet have language. Coupling this with the then-current clinical suggestions that both right and left unilateral damage could lead to aphasic symptoms, the conclusion that infants and young children do not have functionally asymmetric brains (for language, at least) seemed well supported (Lenneberg, 1967).

This situation has, of course, changed dramatically in the last 25 years and functional asymmetries in infants and children are now well documented (e.g., Kinsbourne and Hiscock, 1983; Molfese and Segalowitz, 1988; Segalowitz and Gruber, 1977). What may have been seen as a logjam was broken with two developments: First, Eimas and his co-workers (1971) reported that very young infants are indeed sensitive to phonological elements of language. This and many other studies with infants led to the now not-so-startling notion that very young babies are adept at processing and structuring the information around them and that these structurings are pivotal in the development of the higher cognitive functions we associate with cerebral asymmetries.

The second change reflects a movement away from Luria's formulation that the more abstract the cognitive function, the more likely it is to be functionally asymmetric in the brain (Luria, 1973; Moscovitch, 1979). As he suggested, some "high level" functions are considered to be highly lateralized, such as syntactic and morphologic knowledge, but others are less so, such as some semantic information and perhaps even symbolic procedures. By the same token, some "low level" functions may exhibit little asymmetry, such as some aspects of sensory detection (e.g., Lederman, Jones, and Segalowitz, 1984), and others may be the basis for some asymmetries in visual perception, such as Sergent's (1987) controversial claims about spatial-frequency analysis. Once we begin to abandon generalizations about brain lateralization based on a straightforward reductionist principle, several difficulties with developmental hypotheses disappear.

First of all, it becomes unnecessary to specify a priori what is a higher- or lower-level function, or to link this notion together with cerebral asymmetries. In fact, it becomes unclear what is indeed "high level" and what is "low level," especially from a developmental perspective. For example, consider the case of speech sound processing involving fewer computations for adults than for infants, with infants showing less lateralization. Would this be because more automatized processing of speech sounds by adults is more focalized in the left hemisphere, or because speech sounds are more linguistic to adults, or because the processing of novel stimuli in the infants also involves the right hemisphere? In contrast, consider a higher-level function such as word processing. If meaningful words give evidence of different functional asymmetry in adults compared to children, and words are processed further in adults (have greater spreading activation) than in children, we cannot make any statement about children being more or less lateralized since the processes are not comparable. The general problem here is that what is "high" level for adults may be "low" level for children or vice versa. The developmental pathway of infant asymmetry to adult asymmetry may be a linear one, but the relationship between such a reductionist principle (high vs. low level of function) and hemispheric organization may differ from function to function.

Considering these limitations to theorizing about development, in this chapter we focus primarily on demonstrated hemispheric asymmetries in infancy and early childhood. We also limit our review to electrophysiologic studies. There are several reasons for doing this. First, assessment of asymmetries in infants by behavioral means almost inevitably requires response paradigms that are not appropriate either for slightly older children or adults (e.g., Bertoncini et al., 1989; Entus, 1977; Segalowitz and Chapman, 1980). With electrophysiologic responses, we can present a variety of stimuli in more normal contexts since we are not restricted to visual half-field or dichotic presentation. Another benefit is that we do not require the same kind of behavioral cooperation since the "responses" in electrophysiologic studies are not based on response conditioning or reinforcement. This allows us, in theory at least, to freely examine many different aspects of information processing in various contexts.

A second reason for focusing on electrophysiologic studies in this review is that the use of this paradigm for information on lateralization in infants and children is quickly growing, with new applications appearing at a rapid pace.

LIMITATIONS OF THIS REVIEW

There are many sources for more general reviews of hemispheric asymmetries in childhood and infancy (e.g., Hahn, 1991; Hiscock, 1988; Kinsbourne and Hiscock, 1983; Segalowitz, 1983; Witelson, 1977, 1985). The major thrust of these reviews is that there are indeed cerebral asymmetries in children and infants for language functions and several nonlinguistic functions. What brain processes these asymmetries reflect is usually not an issue that can be directly assessed with the behavioral techniques.

In this chapter, we do not assume a background in electrophysiologic methods on the part of the reader, nor do we dwell on methodologic issues except as we see them pertaining to developmental issues in laterality. There are many excellent sources for general and specific reviews of electrophysiologic techniques (Cacioppo and Tassinary, 1990; Martin and Venables, 1980; Picton, 1988; Rohrbaugh, Parasuraman, and Johnson, 1990; Regan, 1989; Steinschneider, Kurtzberg, and Vaughan, 1992). We do, however, outline briefly the three primary approaches to utilizing electrophysiologic information for questions of brain localization of cognitive functions.

ELECTROPHYSIOLOGIC APPROACHES: ACTIVATION VS. PROCESSING

Studies of functional specialization ask two primary questions that are different enough to demand very different research paradigms. The first concerns specialization as reflected in generalized activation. For example, if language processing is primarily mediated by tissue in the central area of the left hemisphere, then we would expect that this area would generate more electrical activity of the sort that represents information processing. This approach addresses the question of localized tissue specialization without specifying the details of the information processing involved. Examples of this approach are common in electrophysiologic studies of laterality with adults, and three paradigms have been used with babies.

1. The first paradigm involves measuring the general peak-to-trough or baseline-to-peak amplitude of the event-related potentials (ERPs), which, in this chapter, refer to electrical potential fluctuations recorded at the scalp and, unless indicated otherwise, are averaged over many trials. ERPs are taken to the stimuli of interest (such as speech sounds vs. musical sounds), and from these we get a measure of overall sensitivity of the tissue that contributes to the electrical signal at the various sites on the scalp. Although a stable, general sort of response is obtained, this analysis does not divide ERP responses into components sensitive to the particular attributes of the stimulus. Peak analyses

often center around the standard ERP responses to auditory and visual stimuli, that is, the amplitude of the first major negative or positive peak that reflects the signal arriving at the primary sensory area of the cortex and the later major peaks (such as the N2 and P3 at approximately 200 and 300–500 ms) that reflect attentional and memory processing associated with the processing of the stimuli. The traditional peak analysis approach has its strength in summarizing major cognitive processes during stimulus evaluation (e.g., detection vs. recognition vs. semantic evaluation) that are mostly independent of subtle aspects of the stimulus.

2. A second approach has involved the use of tone probes that are presented incidental to the stimulation of interest. Such probes evoke standard responses and can be compared over different conditions (Papanicoloau and Johnstone, 1984). Presumably, any differences between conditions reflect differences in generalized activity level due to the stimulation. For example, ongoing verbal stimulation that promotes more activation of the left temporal lobe would also affect the incidental tone probes at left hemisphere sites more than ongoing musical stimulation. From such an asymmetric effect on tone probes, we can infer asymmetric activation patterns due to the stimulation.

3. The third approach to be outlined here utilizes frequency analysis of the electroencephalographic (EEG) signal. General arousal level of cortical tissue is reflected in the EEG spectrum, which can be analyzed in many different ways. A relatively simple and standard method is to compare the extent of slow-wave activity (such as alpha) across conditions. This is predicated on the notion that when slow-wave activity is prominent, the tissue generating it cannot simultaneously actively process information. Although rather insensitive to the characteristics of specific stimuli except as they promote activation of one region vs. another, the advantage of this method is that mood states that are not elicited by discrete stimuli can be measured. Another advantage is that this method also allows continuous stimulation.

The second primary question involves much more focused aspects of the processing of specific information. This approach is a continuation of the research that demonstrated different hemispheric responses to speech and music. After this asymmetry was amply demonstrated, the next step was to zero in on specific processes in the information flow in the brain. We can illustrate these two steps with an example from speech processing. A traditional question in lateralization research would pit verbal against nonverbal processing and a traditional ERP strategy would involve comparing the amplitude of some component such as the N1 (at around 100 ms) or the P3 that resulted from presentations of some verbal stimuli with those associated with some musical or noise stimuli (e.g., Molfese, Freeman, and Palermo, 1975). By focusing on these well-studied components, we are able to rest on the massive research associated with them, such as that relating the N1 complex to detection of the stimulus and the P3 to its recognition (Parasuraman, Richer, and Beatty, 1982). However, using this paradigm presupposes that the stimuli are processed in such a way as to take advantage of the perceptual and cognitive attributes of these components. For example, consider the ERPs that result from hearing consonant-vowel (CV) syllables such as /ba/ vs. /ga/. With infants or neonates as subjects, can we be sure that the detection and recognition of such stimuli are processes that resemble those in adults?

One strategy to get around this problem is to use a statistical method that captures the subtle variations in the ERP that reflect the differences in stimuli as they are being processed throughout the brain. Let us take the cell assembly model of how the cortex processes information literally (Hebb, 1949) and assume that whenever a stimulus reaches the cortex, it reverberates within a network of activity throughout many regions of the cortex. Presumably on the way to parsing a speech sound, subcomponents of this process influence the shape of the wave throughout the brain in electrical activity that reflects those processes. These subtle fluctuations would not likely be picked up by examining only the major N1 and P3 peaks and ignoring the rest of the ERP wave.

The statistics in this approach involve first doing a principal components analysis (PCA) on the ERPs with time points as variables. The factor scores are then entered into an analysis of variance (ANOVA) that checks to see if they are affected by the experimental conditions, such as stimulus type and electrode site. This approach, which is described in more detail below, makes several assumptions about the data which may or may not be justified in any particular situation, although it probably is the case that any complex and highly sensitive statistical procedure based on the general linear model will have such assumptions.

One assumption is, as suggested above, that any part of the entire wave may be relevant to speech perception. This assumption is safe because if most of the wave is irrelevant to the processing of the particular stimulus, then the factor scores will not be related to the stimulus variables. Thus, this approach does not a priori insist that the relevant parts of the wave occur at specific times, such as around 100 and 350 ms after the stimulus presentation as for N1 and P3, but is sensitive to their occurrence at any time.

Another assumption of the PCA-ANOVA approach is that speech processing is a common mechanical procedure so that there is minimal latency jitter, i.e., the part of the wave reflecting the critical distinction between two sounds does not vary widely from one person to another. There is some concern that serious amounts of latency jitter can force the PCA to produce misleading factors (Möcks, 1986; Wastell, 1981; see Wood and McCarthy, 1984, and Möcks and Verleger, 1986, for discussions of the orthogonality assumption).

As is usual with any statistical procedure used in empirical psychology, the assumptions are contravened regularly and proof of whether or not this matters is empirical: Does the effect replicate, and is it robust? We return to an examination of these issues later.

The PCA-ANOVA technique can be summarized as follows. First, gather averaged ERPs to the stimuli of interest from various sites on the scalp. The sections of the waves that capture the variability across sites and stimuli can be captured by a PCA. The PCA treats the EEG samples making up the ERP as variables and each averaged ERPs as cases. Doing the PCA reduces the ERP waveform from, say, 100 time samplings (e.g., every 5 ms of EEG) that are somewhat contingent on one another, to a manageable set of orthogonal factors, each representing a cluster of time points. For example, consider a time segment of an ERP that acts functionally as a unit. We can predict the rest of the segment fairly well from knowing the amplitude of a part. Often it is the case that the period of time points from 300 to 400 ms after the stimulus acts as a unit, either moving together to produce a large P3 peak or a small one. This particular cluster might, however, be quite independent of a cluster of time points at 80 to 160 ms or 450 to 550 ms. Once the wave is divided into such factors, then the PCA assigns factor scores (weights) relating these factors to each ERP collected. But each ERP came from a particular electrode site and particular stimulus, so we can enter the factor scores into a standard ANOVA to see if they are systematically related to some stimulus or site variable of the study. We may find that a particular segment of ERP (say, 150–200 ms) is sensitive to a particular acoustic feature of the stimuli (say, second formant structure) that is manipulated in the study (i.e., present in some stimuli and absent or different in others), and this sensitivity may be present at some electrode sites and not others (say, T3 and not T4). When this happens, it is fair to conclude that the EEG at the time segment of the ERP represented by that factor differentiates the stimuli at a particular site, e.g., something may happen to generate a second formant transition discrimination at T3 and not T4, presumably representing a lateralized function.

Although the PCA-ANOVA technique sounds like a complicated procedure to initiate, once it is set up it is quite straightforward since the statistical work is mechanical and no judgment calls are needed. The strength of the technique is that it can, in theory, capture all the signal in the averaged ERP. When we have no a priori reason to presuppose or even expect that particular peaks will be important in the processing of the stimuli, this technique guides us in exploring the ERP in its full complexity (as we will see below).

DETERMINING LATERALITY WITH ELECTROPHYSIOLOGIC METHODS

Simple, Exclusive, and Complementary Dominance: Three Meanings of Laterality

An evaluation of the electrophysiologic methods and their usefulness for developmental neuropsychology rests on the type of research question one has. The notion that the brain's functional asymmetries can be reflected in electrophysiologic data is entirely dependent on our notion of functional asymmetry, three of which are outlined here.

Simple Dominance   In one model of asymmetric organization, a particular hemisphere dominates in decision making of a certain sort, but this does not mean that the other is incapable of making such decisions. For example, the right hemisphere is dominant when it comes to making decisions about facial expression (Levy et al., 1983). Let us call this situation "simple dominance," where one side may inhibit and dominate the other while it can. Surgery or incapacity of the dominant side may immediately release the other's hidden competence.

Exclusive Dominance   In another view of functional asymmetry, one hemisphere may not have the programs to perform certain tasks (e.g., the right hemisphere lacking phonological manipulation). In contrast to the first meaning, we could call this "exclusive dominance." We often think of certain basic speech and language skills as falling into this category. After brain damage, it may be the case that the right hemisphere is capable of subserving those processes, but this usually takes time to develop and therefore falls more within the realm of neural plasticity. One could make the argument that such recovery of function cannot reflect a true regeneration of the information processing that was lost, but rather that the previously nondominant hemisphere develops its own way of dealing with the information. This Sinatra-esque ("I'll do it my way") principle is simply another way of indicating that the function in question must be developed at the appropriate time in the organism's history. By the time recovery of function occurs, the brain has passed too many crossroads to allow for a repeat of its developmental history (Isaacson, 1975).

Complementary Dominance   A third notion of functional asymmetry, complementary dominance, has both hemispheres playing critical but highly differentiated roles in some task. Our usual behavioral techniques for determining laterality have focused, for idiosyncratic reasons, on only certain aspects of the task, producing a laterality that is more apparent than real. For example, consider the classic right hemisphere superiority in facial recognition. Ross and Turkewitz (1981) demonstrated that the tachistoscopic superiority of the left visual field is dependent on the cognitive approach to the task that subjects bring with them. Those subjects who use more global cues demonstrate a left visual field advantage while those who use a more analytic approach demonstrate a right visual field advantage. If our tasks require or favor a global approach, then we should expect a left visual field advantage. Similarly, with dichotic listening for speech, one might argue that making the distinctions between stimuli based on contrasts between stop consonants, one will facilitate finding left hemisphere dominance for speech. One could conclude from much of Molfese's work cited below, however, that this would not be the case if dichotic listening stimuli were based on phonological distinctions other than place of articulation. (Along these lines, it is intriguing to consider Previc's [1991] suggestion that dichotic listening and language lateralization effects are due to the right ear's greater sensitivity to the 1000- to 4000-Hz band, which is where most of speech formant transition information appears.)

These three notions of dominance do not represent clear-cut divisions. For any one process that is made up of multiple subprocesses, one sense of dominance shades into another. However, we would be naive if we expect that all studies of laterality utilizing different techniques should produce the same results. Each technique emphasizes certain aspects of the information to be processed, and it should not surprise us that laterality results from different techniques do not agree with one another (Segalowitz, 1986).

Electrophysiologic Techniques and Their Laterality

We might not expect each of the electrophysiologic techniques described in this chapter to be influenced identically by each of these processes, and they certainly may not agree with behavioral techniques for the same reason. For example, dichotic listening and visual half-field viewing are situations where one side is pitted against the other in such a way as to maximize interference or inhibition from one to the other. In such a situation, lateralized performance is highly influenced by dominance factors, blurring the distinction between simple and exclusive dominance. Complementary dominance is completely ignored in these paradigms since there is no way for different aspects of the task to demonstrate their dominance separately.

Traditional electrophysiologic techniques, on the other hand, do not differentiate well between simple and complementary dominance, where both hemispheres are actively monitoring the task situation. In the case of simple dominance, only one hemisphere will determine in the end the behavioral response, while in complementary dominance both will participate. In both cases, however, there may be electrical potential changes over both hemispheres that reflect the decision making. There also may be cases, on the other hand, where simple dominance is reflected in greater activation by one hemisphere during the specialized task, just as we would expect to be the case with exclusive dominance. In such situations one hemisphere would show greater electrophysiologic sensitivity, and we would not expect such measures to be able to tell the difference between simple and exclusive dominance. Since simple and exclusive dominance easily shade into each other, this should not bother us. However, the distinction between these two and complementary dominance should produce marked differences in ERP response.

ELECTROPHYSIOLOGIC ASYMMETRIES FOUND IN INFANCY AND CHILDHOOD

We have tried to include in this brief review all research with infants or young children (less than 5 years old) using electrophysiologic techniques that test for and report results concerning functional hemispheric asymmetries. There are, of course, many other studies that focus on general electrical responses, without reporting on lateralization effects.

As mentioned earlier, there have been many behavioral studies of functional asymmetries in very young children and even infants (e.g., Gilbert and Climan, 1974; Bertoncini et al., 1989; Prescott and DeCasper, 1991) and these almost always focus on left hemisphere dominance for speech processing. Electrophysiologic techniques allow us to examine aspects of speech and nonspeech processing in an intensive way not available with behavioral methods. In this section, we focus first on some demonstrations of simple left-right dichotomies; these indicate that the asymmetries we expect to find in adults and older children are also detectable in very young children and babies. Many of these demonstrations can be interpreted as indicating that asymmetries can be couched in terms of modality-specific processing, e.g., the left hemisphere for auditory stimuli and the right for visual. The next section deals with intensive examination of which speech factors may underlie speech lateralization. The last section deals with the growing evidence of asymmetries associated with experiencing certain emotions of differing valence.

Throughout these summaries, we should keep in mind two issues concerning lateralization. First, a wealth of evidence indicates that it is no longer possible to dismiss examples of functional asymmetries in infants as exceptions; localization of function in the brain in general (of which lateralization is only one aspect) is the rule for very young brains as well as mature ones. In fact, young brains may have more functional asymmetries than older ones. Second, there need not be (and probably is not) any simple single dichotomy or even continuum that will define a left vs. right specialization principle. The global picture is one of complex brain modules interacting dynamically.

General Modality-based Asymmetries

It has been popular for a long time to consider the hemispheres as having different growth rates, whether it be a left advantage (Corballis and Morgan, 1978; Bever, 1975), a right advantage (deSchonen and Mathivet, 1989), or some more complex gradient (Best, 1988). Fundamental to this argument is that certain cognitive functions associated with one hemisphere become dominant because that hemisphere is more "ready" than the other to be the substrate of that function when the infant is developing it. For example, perhaps the left hemisphere becomes dominant for speech and praxis because it has a developmental advantage, while the right hemisphere gets the leftover functions of visual and spatial skills (Bever, 1975). On the other hand, perhaps the right hemisphere is more advanced developmentally at first and so is more likely to take on the information-processing functions that are most critical for infants, i.e., face processing, visual and spatial memory, and emotional processing and expression. This would leave language and perhaps some analytic functions to the later-developing left hemisphere (Carmon et al., 1972; deSchonen and Mathivet, 1989). Of course, this argument is of the sort that cannot be settled. We have too many variables to manipulate (left vs. right; early vs. late maturity; what is really necessary as a first function) and not enough empirical constraints. For example, we cannot tell whether language develops with left dominance and later than some other cognitive skills because the left hemisphere is programmed to take it on but only matures later, or whether the left hemisphere matures later at just the right time when children are ready to start integrating the learned speech code into semantic and grammatical sequences (cf. Scheibel, 1990).

The empirical work should, by this time, have warned us off trying to gauge the merits of maturational maps of the cortex (and such models almost always restrict themselves to cortical areas), no matter how enticing such models are. While Crowell and colleagues (1973) in fact used their finding of an early right hemisphere advantage in photic driving to bolster a maturational model, Molfese, Freeman, and Palermo (1975), Barnet, Vicentini, and Campos (1974), Gardiner and Walter (1977), and Davis and Wada (1977) shortly afterward demonstrated that dissociable interactions can be shown, where each hemisphere has its specialization, as early as electrophysiologic responses can be measured (see tables 19.1 and 19.3 for a summary).

As mentioned earlier, such early modality-based asymmetries naturally lead to speculation that some single or at least simple factor can account for the hemispheric specializations that are apparent in adults. For example, in theory it is possible that a predisposition of the right hemisphere to preferentially process visual stimuli could promote a right lateralization for visual and spatial memory, while a predisposition for the left hemisphere to deal with auditory stimulation could evolve into a language preference (e.g., Segalowitz, 1977). While finding such a "snowball" model attractive because of its simplicity, we should note that this model is counter to the data linking sign language aphasia in deaf adults to the left hemisphere in much the same way as spoken languages (Poizner, Klima, and Bellugi, 1987).

Maturational models are increasingly strained, especially in light of the complex maturational data being reported. For example, Thatcher and his colleagues (Thatcher, Walker, and Giudice, 1987; Thatcher, 1991, 1992) have found electrophysiologic growth patterns that belie any simple lateralized growth gradient. There are left hemisphere advantages at certain ages for certain regions and right hemisphere advantages for other regions at the same time (Thatcher et al., 1987). Similarly, the pattern of hemispheric differences is highly dependent on the particular measure used. There is a relatively simple

Table 19.1 Studies of general electrophysiologic asymmetries in infants or children

Study	Age of subjects	Sites	Stimuli	Results and inferences
Thatcher et al. (1987)	2 mo to adulthood	Full 19 sites of the international 10–20 system	Coherence and phase during resting EEG	Right frontal coherence is greater than left during childhood. There was greater left frontotemporal EEG phase increment (growth spurt) during 4–6 yr and greater right-sided increment during 8–10 yr. There is no simple left-to-right gradient (or vice versa) since specific regions of the left (LH) and right (RH) hemispheres may be leading at any time with intra-hemispheric coherence changes. Mean absolute phase gradually grows in RH, asymptoting at 10 yr, while the LH spurts at 2–4 yr, continues to rise to a plateau by 6 yr, only slowly increases until 11–12 yr, then overshoots adult levels by 14 yr, and gradually returns by late teens.
Crowell et al. (1973)	2 days	O2-A2, O1-A2	Bilateral photic stimulation	Measured photic driving of a 3-Hz flash, producing spectral coherence around 3 Hz. Of the 18 babies that showed unilateral photic driving, 16 were of the RH and 2 of the LH. Eighteen others showed bilateral driving. Since adults respond bilaterally, results are considered to reflect maturational factors, with the unilateral driving interpreted as evidence of a lack of interhemispheric integration. Also, they suggest photic driving may be an early index of cerebral dominance.
Davis and Wada (1977)	5 wk avg (2–10 wk range)	T3, T4, O1, O2 referenced to linked ears	Flash stimuli by photostimulator; click stimuli: 65 dB 8000-Hz tone, 100-ms duration	Clicks produced greater coherence over LH sites, with no asymmetry for flashes. Clicks produced greater temporal than occipital responses (6–12 Hz power), with flashes doing the opposite. In addition, this pattern was significant on the left side for clicks and on the right side for flashes.
Gardiner and Walter (1977)	6 mo	P3, P4, and over left and right Wernicke's area	Conversational speech, unspecified ratio or tape music	Greater activation (lower 3–5 Hz power) in LH during speech and greater activation in RH during music.
Barnet et al. (1974)	5–12 mo (avg 8 mo)	C3, C4	Clicks, name of child	Significant Hemisphere × Stimulus interaction: greater P2-N2 amplitude for names in LH and for clicks in RH.

and intriguing story to tell if one examines mean absolute EEG phase. With this measure, the right hemisphere appears to mature steadily and evenly until adult patterns are reached by late teens, while the left hemisphere spurts at 2 to 6 years, slows down its growth rate until 13 to 14 years, and then shoots past adults levels by 16 years, only to retreat by the late teens. One could, no doubt, construct a cognitive growth model based on this accounting for early childhood spurts in language and adolescent spurts in formal operational thinking. However, without longitudinal data mapping EEG phase onto growth in cognitive functions, it is all too easy to be misled by cohort effects. There are just too many interesting developmental changes occurring at any one time to be able to conclude, without direct comparison data, that EEG changes necessarily relate to the cognitive construct that fascinate psychologists at the moment. Besides, when one examines more intrahemispherically based patterns of coherence, there appear to be regular cycles that vary across hemisphere and region (Thatcher et al., 1987). It is clear that any grand model will involve many maturational variables simultaneously. However, there is no doubt that the hemispheres are not identical in structure and function from the youngest ages.

Another complicating factor in any developmental model is that boys and girls may not have identical maturational patterns. For example, Shucard and colleagues (1981) and Shucard and Shucard (1990), using a probe technique that employed verbal vs. musical passages, suggest there are consistent sex differences in hemispheric maturation. They find that for boys at 3 months of age, the right hemisphere produces larger ERP responses to the tone probes, while for girls the left hemisphere does, whether the main task is listening to verbal or to musical stimuli. At 6 months, the boys are still showing the same pattern while the girls are producing the verbal/musical split across hemispheres that we would expect with adults (table 19.2). Although Molfese and Radtke (1982) dispute the Shucard et al. (1981) conclusions on statistical grounds, similar sex differences in speech laterality have since been reported by Shucard and Shucard (1990), Molfese (1990), and Molfese, Burger-Judisch, and Hans (1991).

Speech and Language Processing

Despite several decades' work on the question, we still do not know what it is about language that leads it to be the most clearly lateralized cognitive function. A good place to start asking the question is in the presumably simpler nervous system found in infants who, while not verbal in the usual sense, still process speech. This question has been painstakingly analysed by Molfese and his colleagues (tables 19.3a and 19.3b; see Molfese and Betz, 1988, for a review). By examining the ERP responses to highly controlled speech stimuli, they have narrowed down the possibilities and reshaped the question from one of laterality to a highly dynamic mechanism involving many brain areas in both hemispheres and multifaceted speech variables. For

Table 19.2 Studies using probe event-related potentials (ERPs) with infants

Study	Age of subjects	Sites	Stimuli	Results and inferences
Shucard et al. (1981)	10–13 wk: 8 male, 8 female	T3 and T4 referenced to Cz	Probe tone pips during presentation of Verbal, Musical, and baseline passages	Males had greater N2 and P3 amplitudes in the RH and females greater in the LH in the Verbal and Music conditions collapsed together. This sex difference was not present in a baseline condition (no stimulation). There was no condition by hemisphere interaction, suggesting that asymmetries are not found using this technique at this age.
Shucard and Shucard (1990)	6 mo: 10 male, 10 female	T3 and T4 referenced to Cz	Probe tone pips during presentation of Verbal, Musical, and baseline (noise) passages	Girls had greater N1-P2 and P2-N2 peak-to-peak amplitudes in the LH during the Verbal condition and in the RH during the Music condition, entirely due to a change in the LH amplitudes. Boys showed a main effect of greater amplitudes during the Verbal condition and a main effect of greater RH amplitudes for both conditions. For boys, there was no hemisphere-by-condition interaction. ERP amplitude differences were consistently positively related to girls' handedness, while for boys the relation was positive only for the Music condition and was negative for the Verbal condition. Taken together with Shucard et al. (1981), these results suggest that girls' LH may mature faster than their RH, while the opposite holds for boys, and by 6 mo, girls' hemispheric functional pattern has matured while the boys' is still immature.

Table 19.3a Studies of speech with neonates

Study	Age of subjects	Sites	Stimuli	Results and inferences
Molfese and Molfese (1980)	36 wk (C.A.)	T3, T4 referenced to linked ears	/bae/ and /gae/ with formant widths of 60, 90, and 120 Hz, simulated CVs with 1-Hz-wide formants, and analog speech and nonspeech using formants not possible from the human vocal tract	LH differentiated between the phonetic and nonphonetic transitions for the consonants /b/ and /g/ and between nonphonetic /b/ and /g/, and LH differentiated phonetic from nonphonetic transition stimuli with speech formant structure. Some of the mechanisms that may be lateralized early in development change after birth.
Molfese (1977)	Exp. 3: 24 hr	T3, T4 referenced to linked ears	/ba/-/pa/ CVs with 0-, 20-, 40-, and 60-ms VOT, and /da/ with 0-ms VOT	LH and RH show amplitude dishabituation for VOT change across the voicing boundary (20–40 ms). No dishabituation for change to /da/ or within voicing categories.
Molfese and Molfese (1979)	21 hr	T3, T4 referenced to linked ears	Four CV syllables; normal (NF) and sine wave (SF) formant, and initial F2 consonant transitions (/b/, /g/); all stimuli had three formants	One AER factor differentiated between NF /b/ and /g/ in both hemispheres while another earlier component showed only the LH doing this. Conclusion: hemisphere differences at birth appear to be due to asymmetric distribution of a specialized perceptual system sensitive to changes in specific acoustic cues.
Molfese et al. (1976)	48 hr	T3, T4 referenced to linked ears	/gae/, /ae/, pure tones at same formant frequencies, and a 500-Hz tone	One ERP component differentiating hemispheres. No hemisphere interaction with formant transitions or bandwidths.
Molfese et al. (1991)	19 boys and 19 girls, <48 hr old	T3, T4, FL, FR, PL, PR	/bi/ and /gi/ with formant widths of 60, 90, and 120 Hz, and simulated CVs with 1-Hz-wide formants	Girls showed FL and PL differentiation of consonants (80–330 ms) and of speech/nonspeech at LH sites (520–700 ms) while boys did not. Many bilateral effects. FR and PL also differentiated speech and nonspeech (520–700 ms) for boys and girls.
Molfese and Molfese (1985)	36 hr (mean gestational age = 38.6 wk)	T3, T4	6 stimuli (/bi/, /bae/, /bo/, /gi/, /gae/, /gɔ/) generated with 3 formants of bandwidth 60, 90, and 120 Hz, and 6 with bandwidths of 1 Hz	Children with high language function at 3-yr follow-up showed at birth an AER component differentiating speech /b/ from /g/ over the LH site only and nonspeech /b/ from /g/ over the RH. No similar effects for low-language children. Vowels were discriminated over the LH around 400 ms.

CV, consonant-vowel; VOT, voice onset time; AER, auditory evoked response.

Table 19.3b Studies of speech with infants and children

Study	Age of subjects	Sites	Stimuli	Results and inferences
Molfese and Molfese (1978)	Exp. 1: 3–mo Exp. 2: 24 hr	T3, T4	/pa/-/ba/ CVs with 0-, 20-, 40-, and 60-ms VOT	Exp. 1: Factor 2 (920 ms) differentiated VOT over RH only. Factor 3 showed that girls differentiated VOT categories more than boys. Other main effects of hemisphere and VOT. Exp. 2: Main effects of hemisphere only.
Molfese et al. (1975)	1 wk–10 mo vs. 6 yr and adult controls	T3, T4	/ba/, /dae/ "Boy," "dog," C-major paino chord, noise burst @ 250–4000 Hz	N1-P2 RH amplitudes were greater for the music and noise stimuli; words and syllables produced greater LH amplitudes. Asymmetry for noise and music in the infants was greater than in child or adult controls, and greater asymmetry for the verbal stimuli in infants and children than in adults.
Molfese and Searcock (1986)	ERPs at 12 mo and language at 3 yr	T3, T4 referenced to linked ears	Three synthesized vowels (/i/, /ae/, /ɔ/), each with 60-, 90-, 120-Hz formants, and three similar nonspeech sounds with formant bandwidth of 1 Hz	Several RH components differentiated nonspeech formants in the high-language group. As well, some bilateral components differentiated nonspeech stimuli, while other RH and LH components were variously sensitive to vowel contrasts.
Molfese and Molfese (1988)	3 yr	T3, T4 referenced to linked ears	0-, 20-, 40-, and 60-ms VOT speechlike stimuli with three formants (identified as /ga/ and /ka/), and four nonspeech two-tone stimuli with similar onsets (0-, 20-, 40-, 60-ms TOT)	RH activity at 180 and 400 ms discriminated 0- and 20-ms from 40- and 60-ms stimuli. The 180-ms component also differentiated 0- from 20-ms stimuli over the RH and 40- from 60-ms stimuli over the LH. A 320-ms component discriminated VOT and TOT stimuli over the RH of girls and over the LH and RH of the boys (plus other sex differences). These results replicate VOT and TOT results from adults.
Molfese and Hess (1978)	4.4 yr	T3, T4	Four computer-generated CV speech syllables with 0-, 20-, 40-, and 60-ms VOT	A factor linking activity at 120, 312-, and 444-ms differentiated stimuli along the expected categorical lines (0- and 20- vs. 40- and 60-ms VOT), but only over the RH. No component differentiated VOT over the LH.

TOT, tone onset stimuli. For other abbreviations, see footnote, table 19.3a.

example, let us consider the acoustic factors involved defining stop consonants, place of articulation (POA), voice onset time (VOT), and formant band-
width. POA (where the tongue touches the upper surface of the mouth to stop
the airflow) is defined acoustically by formant patterns that, for example,
distinguish between bilabial, dental, and alveolar restrictions of air (/b/ and
/p/ vs. /d/ and /t/ vs. /g/ and /k/). Molfese and Molfese (1985) found that
neonates 36 hours after birth demonstrate an ERP segment that is sensitive
only over the left hemisphere to the /b/ vs. /g/ distinction in three different
vowel contexts. This association between place of articulation and some
unique left hemisphere mechanism was also found in two earlier studies with
neonates (Molfese and Molfese, 1979, 1980). Molfese and Molfese (1985) also
found a segment that made the same differentiation over the right hemisphere
only when the stimuli were nonspeech analogs. (A nonspeech analog is a
computer-generated simulation where the formant bandwidths are reduced
to 1 Hz.)

In contrast to the POA issue, the VOT distinction differentiates /b/ from
/p/, /d/ from /t/, and /g/ from /k/ where the second of each pair has the
voicing (vocal fold vibration) commence approximately 30 ms after the air
release while the first has it commence sooner than 30 ms. VOT is perceived
categorically in that VOT values less than 30 ms are perceived by adults as
similar to one another but different from those after the boundary, which are
perceived as belonging to a different category. That is, a 20-ms VOT difference that crosses the boundary is perceived as a change in stimulus category,
while a 20-ms VOT difference that does not cross the boundary is not perceived as a change in stimulus. VOT is interesting because not only are young
babies able to discriminate the boundary in a way similar to adults (Eimas et
al., 1971) but so are some other mammals, such as chinchillas and monkeys
(Kuhl and Miller, 1975; Kuhl and Padden, 1983). The ERP testing method
involves recording auditory ERPs to computer-generated stimuli with VOT
values of 0, 20, 40, and 60 ms and examining the PCA-ANOVA results to see
which factors differentiate the stimuli on a categorical basis. Surprisingly,
Molfese (1978) had found that this distinction was represented at right and
not left hemisphere sites in adults, and found the same results when the stimuli
were nonspeech analogs (Molfese, 1980). Asymmetry effects are the same in
children, with categorical VOT being differentiated by right hemisphere electrode sites (Molfese and Hess, 1978; Molfese and Molfese, 1978, 1988). Similar results were found in young monkeys (Molfese et al., 1986; Morse et al.,
1987) and in dogs (Adams, Molfese, and Betz, 1987) (table 19.4). These asymmetries were in addition to bilateral effects, which are difficult to interpret in
this paradigm (see below, Types of bilateral effects).

Vowels have always been less likely to produce a right ear advantage in
dichotic listening, and therefore vowel processing has not been considered a
highly lateralized function (Spellacy and Blumstein, 1970; Studdert-Kennedy
and Shankweiler, 1970). The same ambiguity is the case with infants: Molfese
and Molfese (1985) found in neonates that a late left hemisphere component

Table 19.4 Event-related potential (ERP) studies of speech laterality in nonhumans

Study	Age of subjects	Sites	Stimuli	Results and inferences
Molfese et al. (1986)	1-yr-old control monkeys and two lead-treated groups	T3, T4, P3, P4	Two versions of /dae/ and /gae/	The RH of control monkeys differentiated /dae/ and /gae/ syllables, while the LH of the pernatally lead-treated monkeys did so in a later portion. Postnatal lead-treated group did not differentiate stimuli in this matter.
Morse et al. (1987)	Same as above	T3, T4, P3, P4	0-, 20-, 40-, and 60-ms VOT CV syllables (/ba/, /pa/)	T4 discriminated /ba/ from /pa/ stimuli (0-, 20- vs. 40-, 60-ms VOT) with a late AER component for all groups. This parallels results on VOT with humans. Other within-category differentiations were made at various sites.
Adams et al. (1987)	15-wk-old Border collies	TL, TR, PL, PR	0-, 20-, 40-, and 60-ms VOT CV syllables (/ga/, /ka/)	All sites differentiated within and between VOT categories, but only the RH sites (50–180 ms) differentiated between /ga/ and /ka/ and not also within the phoneme categories.

For abbreviations, see table 19.3a.

differentiated three vowel sounds, while Molfese and Searock (1986), in a study with 1-year-olds, found both left and right hemisphere components that were sensitive to vowel contrasts.

Molfese and his colleagues have also looked at word processing in infants and children, both by examining the ERP deflections upon hearing real words and by introducing new words to infants. Molfese (1990) recorded ERPs from 16-month-olds' left and right sides at frontal, temporal, and parietal locations while playing to them a word that their parents were sure they knew and a word that they did not know (different words for each child). A PCA factor at 180 to 340 ms differentiated known from unknown words in both girls and boys at the left temporal site, while it did so in the boys also at both left and right frontal sites. A late negativity (570–700 ms) also marked the unknown words, with a positivity for known words, at all left hemisphere sites in the girls and over both hemispheres in the boys. As was found with the Shucards' studies described above, such sex differences do not answer the question of whether there are simply maturational differences between boys and girls or differences in brain organization.

In a different paradigm, Molfese, Morse, and Peters (1990) presented 15-month-olds with two CVCV syllables, "gibu" and "bidu," which they paired with specific objects over a training period. They then examined the ERPs taken to matched and mismatched word-object pairings. They found two components that were sensitive to the word-object match: an early (30–120 ms) frontally based, bilateral one and a later (520–600 ms) one confined to the left hemisphere. This may reflect some immediate frontal response to the match, perhaps reflecting some memory component, and a later cognitive or linguistic aspect to the processing, although there is considerable debate as to whether one can draw localization conclusions from the recording paradigm used (Steinschneider et al., 1992).

Considering that for a child to know the meaning of a word also requires that the sound of the word be familiar, Molfese (1989) compared the effects of familiarity with knowing the meaning (table 19.5). Experiment 1 was similar to Molfese (1990); 14-month-olds heard a word they knew and a word they did not know. ERP activity between 30 and 220 ms for all sites, except for that over the right parietal area, discriminated the known word from the unknown word; i.e., the asymmetry for word knowledge appeared only at parietal sites. A later region between 270 and 380 ms varied across all sites, across both left and right hemispheres, and discriminated known from unknown words. Finally, between 380 and 500 ms, both parietal sites differentiate the known from the unknown word. In Experiment 2, Molfese examined familiarity instead of meaning by familiarizing the infant with one of two CVCV syllables. ERP activity discriminated between familiar and unfamiliar CVCVs only at frontal sites around 360 ms. Molfese argues that at least in early stages of processing, both hemispheres are involved in the process of learning to relate word sounds to word meanings, and that different brain regions respond differently over time in the two hemispheres. The hemi-

Table 19.5 Studies of word recognition and familiarity within infants

Study	Age of subjects	Sites	Stimuli	Results and inferences
Molfese (1989)	14 mo	T3, T4, FL, FR, PL, PR linked-ears reference	Exp. 1: A known vs. unknown word (different for each infant) Exp. 2: Two CVCV bisyllabic nonsense stimuli	Exp. 1: AER activity at 30–220 ms for T3, T4, FL, FR, and PL discriminated known (K) from unknown (U) word, showing an asymmetry only at parietal sites, while at 270–380 ms all sites produced larger peak-to-peak amplitudes for K. At 380–500 ms, both parietal sites differentiate K from U. Exp. 2 examined familiarity instead of meaning. AER activity discriminated between familiar and unfamiliar CVCVs only at frontal sites around 360 ms.
Molfese and Wetzel (1992)	14 mo	T3, T4, FL, FR, PL, PR linked-ears reference	/gigi/ and /toto/ nonsense CVCVs; subjects were familiarized with one only	After a 2-day "training" period, infants were presented with the familiar and unfamiliar CVCV. FL and FR discriminated familiar from unfamiliar stimuli (280–470 ms). A later component (410–560 ms) differentiated stimuli at all sites.
Molfese (1990)	16 mo	T3, T4, FL, FR, PL, PR	A known word and an unknown word, rated by the parents from a list of ten words	Activity at 180–340 ms differed for the K and U at T3 in females, and at FL, FR, and T3 in males. A late negativity (570–700 ms) over the LH (all sites) in females marked, with a positivity for K. Males showed same effect over the LH and RH.
Molfese et al. (1990)	15 mo	T3, T4, FL, FR, PL, PR linked-ears reference	Infants were trained to pair two CVCV stimuli ("gibu" and "bidu") with two objects; ERPs were then taken to match and mismatch word-object pairings	An early frontally based, bilateral AER component was sensitive to the word-object matching as was a later LH-only component, suggesting an immediate frontal response to the word-object match and some later cognitive or linguistic effect. A split-half reanalysis of the data produced the same results.

For abbreviations, see footnote, table 19.3a.

spheres initially differentiate known from unknown words over almost all sites, followed by a restriction of this differentiation to parietal regions of both the left and right hemispheres, while both frontal sites seem to be sensitive to familiarity. This frontal sensitivity to familiarity was replicated by Molfese and Wetzel (1992).

One might conclude from these results that whatever promotes left hemisphere dominance for speech processing is not something inherent in all vocal tract sounds and is not necessarily going to come into play with full word comprehension. As discussed earlier, this has serious implications for what we might mean by the notion of "language dominance." Molfese and his colleagues stress the dynamic nature of information processing in the brain, and in fact discourage us from focusing solely on issues of left vs. right hemisphere processing in the brain.

Social and Emotional Functioning

The expansion of issues of brain lateralization to developmental questions in social and emotional behavior represent the most exciting development in brain laterality research in the last decade. Bridging the gap between cognitive information processing and social and emotional behavior has always been difficult for psychology, and for neuropsychology to manage this through examination of brain activity is a real breakthrough. In this section, we review the work of primarily two research groups: that of Davidson and Fox, and that of Dawson and her colleagues. Both come from a clinical perspective. That is, both expect that there should be individual differences in the balance of hemispheric processes (among others) and not just individual differences in brain organization among, say, left- vs. right-handers or males vs. females. This approach has been conspicuously lacking from the research reviewed so far, and in fact is counter to some of the statistical assumptions in the research designs used. Of course, one could argue that assuming a lack of such individual differences is absolutely necessary in order to map out the basic pattern from which to build models. We must, however, keep in mind that the assumption of uniformity is only an assumption of convenience.

The social and emotional laterality issue has taken a form rather different from the traditional laterality issue of the right hemisphere dominance for face perception (Borod et al., 1986) and for emotional tone in verbal material (Saxby and Bryden, 1984, 1985). Tucker et al. (1981) and Davidson et al. (1979) have shown with adults that brain localization for experiencing emotions rests on important issues of valence. Experiencing certain positive emotions and certain negative emotions appears to be related to activation processes that are associated with left vs. right frontal regions. When adults experience negative, depressive feelings, there is a relative electrophysiologic activation of the right frontal region compared to the left, and vice versa for happy or elative feelings. These differences are not apparent at parietal electrode sites. The developmental questions thus involve two primary issues: Are

these patterns of activation apparent in babies, and if so, are they trait correlates of temperament or socialization styles, or both, that will come to characterize much of their lives? The first has clearly been answered in the positive
while the second question on traits is now the topic of intensive study.

In a primary study with 10-month-old infants, Davidson and Fox (1982)
found asymmetric slow-wave power output from frontal sites when babies
were watching a video of an actress showing great mirth compared with the
same actress expressing great sadness (table 19.6). To an adult, the film clips
seem to induce in the viewer the positive and negative moods portrayed and
possibly the film had similar effects on the babies. The theoretical importance
of this effect has led to a number of associated studies leading to questions of
the nature of infant temperament and factors controlling socialization processes. In a later study, Davidson and Fox (1989) found that babies that cried
when their mothers left the room were more likely to have greater right than
left frontal activation during a baseline period before the mother-leaving episode when there was no emotional negativity shown. One possible conclusion from this is that infants have temperament differences, some being more
easily upset by such things as unwanted or unpredicted changes in the environment, as when mother leaves the room, and these differences are traits
reflected in frontal lobe activation asymmetries. If this is the case, then it could
be the basis of the individual differences in temperament that play so great a
role in the socialization and attachment of the young child (see Davidson and
Fox, 1988, for a review; see Fox, Bell, and Jones, 1992, for preliminary support
for a trait characterization of frontal asymmetry). For example, temperamental
inhibition—the tendency to withdraw from novel experiences more than
peers—is seen in this light as a response to any stimulus, not just social
stimuli. Similarly, the opposite temperament is seen as a tendency to approach
novel objects and new experiences. Fox and Davidson (1986) found that while
sucrose (presumably a positive stimulus) elicits greater left-sided frontal activation in neonates, plain water elicited greater right-sided activation.

Further evidence in support of the valence association with hemisphere
activation come from Fox and Davidson (1988; see also Fox and Davidson,
1987). In this study, EEGs were taken while 10-month-olds were approached
by their mothers and by a stranger. Their reactions were noted, especially
when their smiles were accompanied by obicularis muscle activity, which is
present when the smile is a genuine reflection of spontaneous joy ("felt"
smiles) as opposed to a tense ("unfelt") smile. Crying activity was associated
with greater right activation; felt smiles were associated with left frontal
activation and unfelt smiles with right frontal activation.

Dawson and her colleagues (table 19.7) have further support for the relevance of frontal asymmetries to positive vs. negative emotions. Dawson et al.
(1992a) coded 21-month-old babies' expressions while the mother left the
room, was outside, and returned. During angry and neutral expressions, there
was greater left frontal activation, while during sad expressions there was
greater right frontal activation. Parietal sites were not sensitive to mood

Table 19.6 EEG asymmetry studies related to affective state of the infant

Study	Age of subjects	Sites	Stimuli	Results and inferences
Fox and Davidson (1986)	2–3-day-old neonates	F3, F4, P3, P4 referred to Cz	Water vs. sucrose vs. referred to citric acid tastes	Water stimulation elicited greater right activation at both frontal and parietal sites (less 3–6 Hz and less 6–12 Hz power) than left, while sucrose elicited greater left-sided activation. Citric acid produced no asymmetries.
Davidson and Fox (1982)	10 mo	F3, F4, P3, P4 referred to Cz	Videotape of female actress generating happy and sad faces	Study 1: Infants showed greater left than right frontal activation (less 1–12 Hz power) in response to happy faces, but no asymmetry at parietal sites. Study 2: Replicated results of study 1, with closer monitoring of infants' attention to stimuli.
Davidson and Fox (1989)	10 mo	F3, F4, P3, P4 referred to Cz	Maternal approach and maternal separation	Babies who cried upon MS demonstrated more right frontal activation, (less 6–8 Hz power) during a pretest baseline period, while noncriers show more left frontal activation, although there were no behavioral differences between criers and noncriers during baseline. Parietal regions showed no asymmetry.
Fox and Davidson (1987)	10 mo	F3, F4, P3, P4 referred to Cz	Mother-enter (ME), mother-reach (MR), and mother-separation (MS) conditions	Left frontal activation (less 6–8 Hz power) is higher during ME compared with MR episodes with no difference at parietal sites. Left frontal activation was correlated with infant's vocalization during both episodes. Those who cried during MS showed greater left frontal activation (lower 3–5 Hz power) during MR than MS, while noncriers showed the opposite. During separation, criers show more right frontal activation than noncriers.
Fox and Davidson (1988)	10 mo	F3, F4, P3, P4 referred to Cz	Maternal and stranger approach and separation	"Felt" smiles (to mother approach) showed increased left frontal activation compared to "unfelt" smiles (in response to stranger approach) which displayed more right frontal activation. Crying was associated with greater right frontal activation vs. noncrying and angry or sad conditions.
Fox et al. (1992)	I. 14 and 24 mo	F3, F4, P3, P4 referred to Cz	I. Strange Situation: EEG while watching *Sesame Street* and bubble blowing	I. 6–9 Hz power asymmetries in Strange Situation with 60-sec artifact-free data in both situations. Criers (n = 3) vs. noncriers (n = 9) had less left frontal activation (asymmetry: P = .05). (Note: EEG was measured 4–8 wk after Strange Situation.) No parietal effects.
	II. 7–12 mo		II. MS vs. EEG as above	II. Thirteen 7–12 mo-olds tested monthly on latency to crying upon maternal separation and EEG asymmetries. Frontal sites: noncriers (n = 8) have greater left activation.

Table 19.7 EEG asymmetry studies related to social/attachment challenges

Study	Age of subjects	Sites	Stimuli	Results and inferences
Dawson et al. (1992c)	14 mo (11–17 mo)	F3, F4, P3, P4 referred to Cz	1. Baseline EEG 2. Peekaboo 3 and 4. Maternal and stranger approach and separation	During baseline and peekaboo conditions, insecurely attached infants of depressed mothers (DM) showed increased left frontal activity (lower 6–9 Hz power) compared to insecurely attached infants of nondepressed mothers (NDM), while securely attached infants showed the opposite trend. When mother left the room, infants of NDM show an increase in right frontal activity, while those of DM show greater left frontal activity. This is especially so for insecurely attached infants. There were no asymmetries at parietal sites.
Dawson et al. (1992b)	14 mo (11–17 mo)	F3, F4, P3, P4 referred to Cz	1. Baseline EEG; *Sesame Street* with (happy, sad, neutral faces inserted); "Peekaboo"; Stranger Enter, Stranger Looming and Stranger Out; Mother Leaving; Mother Out; Mother returning	All asymmetries occurred at frontal sites only. Neither infants of DM nor infants of NDM showed asymmetries during baseline. During peekaboo, infants of NDM showed greater left activation, while infants of DM showed no asymmetries. During Mother Leaving, infants of DM showed left activation, while those of NDM had no asymmetry. There were no asymmetries during Mother Out. Stranger Enter produced no asymmetry differences between groups (both mildly greater left activation), while Stranger Looming raised left activation of infants of DM and lowered it for infants of NDM. Stranger Out reversed this pattern. Conclusion: maternal depression reverses the frontal asymmetries of infants during emotional settings.
Dawson et al. (1992a)	21 mo	F3, F4, T3, T4 referenced to Cz	Babies' facial expression coded for Angry, Neutral, Sad when mother leaves room, stays out, and returns	During Angry and Neutral expressions, there was greater left frontal activation (lower 6–9 Hz power) while during Sad periods there was greater right frontal activation. There was no mood by hemispheric interaction at parietal sites.

changes. These data again support asymmetry in activation associated with sad vs. non-sad feelings.

Dawson et al. (1992b) then went on to examine the asymmetries in 14-month-old infants of mothers who were clinically depressed. These results relate to the question of how such infants' attachment process may differ, assuming that the asymmetries noted by Davidson and Fox really do reflect approach vs. withdrawal processes. They generally found that infants of depressed mothers displayed frontal asymmetries opposite to those of infants whose mothers were not clinically depressed. For example, when a stranger loomed overhead, the infants of nondepressed mothers had lowered left frontal activation while those of depressed mothers had raised left frontal activation. During a peekaboo game, infants of nondepressed mothers showed greater left frontal activation, while infants of depressed mothers showed no change. The reverse was found while mother left the room. Similarly, Dawson et al. (1992c) report that infants of nondepressed mothers show an increase in right frontal activation when mother leaves the room, but infants of depressed mothers show an increase in left frontal activation. This was especially so for insecurely attached infants. As well, baseline and peekaboo conditions produced greater left hemisphere activation in securely attached infants of nondepressed mothers compared to securely attached infants of depressed mothers. Clearly, the clinical position of the mother has considerable effect on the infant and may potentially put the child at risk for attachment and socialization processes. If left hemisphere activation can generally be taken to indicate greater positive, approach-related, or at least non-sad mood, infants of depressed mothers are happier when they are insecurely attached to their mothers and the mother leaves the room. The critical issue here is the quality of the relationship between infant and mother, since it may be that infants that are insecurely attached to depressed mothers are in fact apprehensive when mother is around. They may, of course, be securely attached to someone else.

A primary issue not completely resolved here is whether the tendency for a frontal asymmetry of one sort or another is a trait that infants have and maintain through childhood. Presumably the baseline data from the studies of Dawson and colleagues imply that general traits can be changed: infants of depressed mothers come to view standard settings in a way that is different from the infants of nondepressed mothers. However, we do not know whether these baseline conditions truly reflect the long-term prospects for the child or are the results of temperament status at a particularly critical time in the development of the attachment process. It will take longitudinal studies to sort out these issues.

PROBLEMS OF INTERPRETATION

Does the Tripartite Distinction Matter?

Recall our previous distinction among single, exclusive, and complementary dominance. If there is hemispheric specialization of function, why should we worry about the exact dynamics of the information processing involved in these distinctions? For many functions, this division would be close to hair-splitting, as in the case of speech vs. musical processing or the case of grammatical vs. emotional processing, where the relative difference in asymmetry is so great that distinctions among the three types of dominance probably would not account for much variance.

However, as we begin to examine specific modes of processing in a detailed way, such distinctions become important. We saw this with speech processing where there appears to be a highly dynamic interplay across many brain regions when speech is being processed. Of the electrophysiologic techniques available, only PCA-ANOVA is sensitive to the multivariate aspects of complementary dominance and, therefore, is in a position to reflect them (although with caveats that we discuss below).

One way of viewing this division among dominances is in terms of the classic holist-localizationist debate, now rephrased as hemispheric dominance vs. network integration. There is a current trend in the field to give more than lip service to the notion that the brain is an integrated network of systems. In such a network view, information processing comprises distinctive computations, and a differentiation of ERP activity could capture this. Unfortunately, at the moment we have no way of distinguishing whether such an ERP sensitivity reflects a tissue's contribution to the computational network. It could be that some ERP sensitivity indicates some "negative" appreciation. For example, suppose the right hemisphere receives inhibitory signals from the left concerning speech processing. These would show up as an ERP differentiation, although the right hemisphere is not really contributing to the process that leads to understanding or control of that speech episode. Similarly, the right hemisphere might receive excitation through callosal transfer of information, making it a "passive" appreciator of the stimulus. "Negative" and "passive" appreciation certainly suggest that such differentiation is part of a network (the whole brain works together), but does not address the same localization issue (exclusive dominance) in the way that traditional clinical studies do.

TYPES OF BILATERAL EFFECTS

This inability to differentiate "negative" and "passive" activation from the contrasting "active" ERP sensitivity produces a problem of interpretation for two types of ERP results: bilateral effects and crossover interactions.

In a bilateral stimulus effect, the two hemispheres show similar sensitivity to the stimulus factor (such as VOT). If we conclude from this that the stimulus is processed equally by the two hemispheres, we are implying that a bilateral effect proves the null hypothesis. Given that in many PCA-ANOVA studies, bilateral and asymmetric effects are found simultaneously, it seems reasonable to doubt the bilaterality of the stimulus processing. The bilateral effect could be reflecting a "passive" activation that masks or is in addition to an asymmetric ERP response.

PCA-ANOVA studies also often produce crossover interactions, where one hemisphere shows a stimulus effect in one direction and the other hemisphere shows an effect in the opposite direction. This does suggest that different things are going on in each hemisphere, although interpreting this difference can be difficult from the statistical analysis. For example, if one hemisphere induces an inhibitory response in the other hemisphere, both sides will appear active but for very different reasons. The PCA-ANOVA cannot indicate which pattern is an inhibitory process and which is excitatory. The only interaction that demonstrates an asymmetry unambiguously is the type where an ERP at sites in one hemisphere shows a differentiation not apparent at sites in the other.

Implications of Infancy Studies for Developmental Models of Laterality

Does laterality develop? First of all, we should differentiate between the laterality issues of information processing and the laterality issues of state (and trait). The latter are reflected in studies of EEG, the former in ERP studies. They may not coincide because the factors leading to a state (e.g., mood, arousal) are not necessarily involved in lateralized information processing (e.g., speech).

Rather than view laterality as a "normal" developmental phenomenon where infants have less of it, children have more, and adults have most, the infancy studies of laterality suggest a rather different model: the infant's brain is highly differentiated in the functions that it has. The traditional notion of laterality that we have adopted for the infant and child comes essentially from clinical and experimental work with adults, where we see many cases of exclusive and simple dominance and we tend to ignore the issue of complementary dominance. This is especially so with clinical studies on aphasias and agnosias. Partly because of the need to use nonbehavioral measures with infants, such as ERPs, we are in more of a position to think about complementary processes in the brain. The complementary pattern of hemispheric processes in infants may change as they grow, so that it may be the case that speech processing involves more of a mixture of right and left hemisphere subsystems in infants than in adults. Or, of course, the opposite may be true. We really do not have enough applications of the same paradigm with many age groups in order to tell, although Molfese and his colleagues are building such a database for speech processing.

This fundamental question—Does laterality develop?—turns out to be not quite so simple, although we can be sure that the simple model of the young brain being unlateralized is wrong. Many asymmetries of cerebral function can be demonstrated in neonates, infants, and children. However, these asymmetries may not be comparable to those traditionally found in adults, and therefore laterality may very well change over time. In fact, it seems sensible to expect that laterality is not going to remain constant when the brain, the functional repertoire, and the mental needs of the child do not.

WHERE DO WE GO FROM HERE?

Despite the very large number of methodologic studies done on electrophysiologic techniques, there are still a number of remaining questions that relate directly to studies of laterality in children. In this section, we outline what we see as some critical issues to be resolved for the electrophysiology of laterality in infants. Some of these issues are empirical and can only be resolved by performing the necessary experiments. Others may be worked out through discussion within the scientific community.

Reliability

Experimental psychologists tend not to doubt the psychometric worth of their measures. No one normally doubts the usefulness of an EEG spectrum if, after all the effort that goes into conducting such a study, they find that a relationship between EEG and processing is indeed apparent. However, it is important to be able to document the statistical reliability of these measures, a task that is rarely undertaken. Unfortunately, when it is in fact undertaken, we cannot assume that the reliability found will generalize to a new age group, especially from adults to children and infants. It may be that under certain controlled (or uncontrolled) conditions, EEG power or ERP waveshape are not particularly reliable, while they may be robust under others. It turns out that with adolescents and presumably adults, the standard ERP peak values are highly reliable even over a 2-year time spread (Segalowitz and Barnes, 1993). These results suggest that within certain given controlled task paradigms (in this case, auditory oddball), the ERP peaks may be taken as traits of the individual. Whether or not this is the case with more stimuli that require more complex processing is unknown at the moment (Fabiani et al., 1987). Whether these optimistic results can be generalized to infants and very young children is not known.

Similar arguments can be made concerning the reliability of EEG power analyses that are so important for studying laterality of mood in infants. Recently, Tomarken and colleagues (1992) demonstrated high stability of alpha asymmetry in a large group of adults. We have no reason to expect that they or their equivalents are not also stable in infants (see Fox et al., 1992, for some longitudinal data from infants).

The issue of PCA factor structures being reliable in laterality paradigms has never really been addressed, but there are some relevant data in other contexts. Molfese's research suggests that a systematic examination is possible to isolate those aspects that are consistent across studies, although, at present, no such summary has been offered. There are several ways that reliability can be viewed within the PCA-ANOVA framework. We can ask whether the factor structure itself is replicable, whether the individual differences captured by the PCA are reliable, and whether the experimental effects are replicable independent of specific factor structure. As indicated earlier, the PCA-ANOVA technique assumes that the latency and waveshape for specific components are fixed (Fabiani et al., 1987). Variance due to shifts in the latency of underlying wave components will be reflected in the PCA structure, which of course means that the factor structure under such conditions will not replicate. This will be the case especially when the number of trials per ERP average is small (Möcks, 1986; Wood and McCarthy, 1984). However, despite the potential misallocation of variance, the PCA is the only method available to extract subcomponents from a given set of ERPs. What is needed is some sense of the stability of the PCA structure given certain types of stimuli in the subject population of interest, e.g., speech perceived by infants. In the classic oddball P300 paradigm using adult subjects with simple stimuli, visual inspection suggested that the first two components (of four) were rather reliable while factors 3 and 4 were not (Fabiani et al., 1987). Since the authors were concerned with whatever component reflected the P300, this was adequate. However, since it is often the later factors that have been of interest in the PCA-ANOVA paradigm with infants, such unreliability may be problematic.

Individual differences in factor scores were not found to be reliable in the study of Fabiani et al. (1987) of the P300 as reflected by PCA components. We do not know whether this same instability is the case with infants. In addition, we must keep in mind that PCA structures give us information about the latency of components only through latency-amplitude interactions. In fact, as mentioned earlier, the analysis assumes that there are not latency differences in the underlying components across conditions or sites.

Perhaps the reliability function of most interest, however, is the one relating to experimental replication: Is the study replicable despite whatever variations in factor structure appear due to idiosyncratic latency shift variance? Such a question must be highly dependent on the hypothesis of concern and the strength of the effects. Molfese has shown that certain effects are replicable in different samples and with different stimuli (e.g., the VOT × Hemisphere and POA × Hemisphere effects), while Segalowitz and Cohen (1989) replicated the Molfese (1978) right hemisphere VOT effect using different stimuli, different vowel contexts, and slightly different electrode placements. They also presented a Monte Carlo simulation with the data to check for inflated Type I error probabilities. That the factor structure they found did not match Molfese's is not surprising since the stimuli and task parameters were not the same. However, the experimental hypothesis concerning a VOT by hemisphere interaction was supported.

One advantage of the PCA-ANOVA approach is that the experimenter need not decide on a scoring system since the PCA essentially takes care of that. Such is not the case with EEG power and with ERP peak analysis. While standards for ERP analysis have been addressed many times and some consensus has been reached (Fabiani et al., 1987; Regan, 1989), it is still unclear exactly which EEG power metric is appropriate or most robust (although Tomarken et al., 1992, and Pivik et al., 1993, do address some of these issues). For example, the studies reviewed here sometimes use 1 to 12 Hz, 6 to 8 Hz, 3 to 5 Hz, 6 to 12 Hz, etc. Generally speaking, difference scores are used in the ANOVAs. However, there are well-known statistical problems with using difference scores (Chapman and Chapman, 1988; Cronbach and Furby, 1970; Woody and Constanzo, 1990). The extent to which these difficulties apply to the EEG power asymmetry paradigms is a matter for discussion.

Interpreting ERPs

As with any dependent measure in psychology, we can try to interpret ERP analyses either in an explanatory way or in a descriptive way. For an explanatory analysis, one needs to have a way of verifying that the measures (the ERP peaks or factors) have useful construct validity, i.e., some relationship to processes that would interest us. For many of the traditional peaks, there is a long history of linking them to specific aspects of the information-processing requirements of the task, as well as intuitive meaning: the larger the peak amplitude, the greater the response; when the stimulus is not processed, the response diminishes (Polich, 1986).

For descriptive uses, however, peaks and PCA "factors" do not need interpretation, only documented asymmetries. Such analyses can imply some processing differences between data from two sites. But factors derived from the PCA-ANOVA technique cannot be interpreted cognitively as they are not independently motivated (they are defined by the data set itself) and may be highly dependent on the particular variance space in the particular ERP set. For example, not only does the VARIMAX rotation make the factors partly dependent on variance due to latency jitter (Möcks and Verleger, 1986) but it seems to us that they must be also depend on one another. The extraction of the first orthogonal factor depends to some extent on the clustering for the second factor (in order to keep the factors orthogonal), and so on. This in turn must influence the allocation of factor scores, which of course determines the outcome of the ANOVA. In other words, how the factors turn out will depend on the particular data set and, as discussed above, may not be replicable (although the ANOVA results may replicate). Thus, interpreting the factors from a particular data set without external validation is problematic at best. This does not, of course, compromise their utility in descriptive analysis.

These caveats have special force in the context of laterality studies since ERPs are sensitive to all electrical activity, including that due to nonexclusive forms of dominance of functioning (simple and complementary dominance). Given the potential complications in such interacting systems, it would be extremely difficult to predict ahead of time the nature of the variance space.

Generator Sources

The primary localization question of course concerns the generator source of the EEG and the ERP components that we find differentiate hemispheres according to stimuli. While Kinsbourne and Hiscock (1983) have suggested that the electrophysiologic asymmetries found in infancy may be driven by activation differences in the brainstem, the general consensus is that EEG sources are primarily cortical, especially those reflecting time-locked ERP components (Desmedt, 1989). Far-field effects primarily influence low-amplitude, high-frequency signals that are not relevant to EEG and ERP recordings, while near-field transmission falls off as the cube of the distance from the generator (Regan, 1989, p. 16). This does not prevent us from attempting to measure high-frequency, distant ERP generators by averaging over a very large number of trials (as in brainstem auditory ERPs), but it does suggest that what we measure in the paradigms discussed in this paper are cortical phenomena (Regan, 1989). An interesting demonstration of this is Freeman and Thibos' (1973) report of corrected astigmatism in adults still producing deficient ERPs that could only be mediated at the cortical level.

SOME RESEARCH QUESTIONS FOR THE FUTURE

Longitudinal Studies

The finding of very early asymmetries for linguistic and social development suggest that both of these processes have an early start, and that there are early biological structures that may influence later development. However, this does not preclude important subsequent environmental influences on these biological substrates (Gottlieb, 1983). With this in mind, we need to ask whether the asymmetries related to social behaviors are traits or temporary reactions (states) those individuals bring to the test conditions. Dawson's work and Davidson and Fox's work are compatible with either a trait or a state view of the asymmetries. Hopefully, the question of whether early individual differences in temperament can be related to asymmetries of frontal activation will soon be settled empirically.

N = 1 Studies

The work of Molfese and his colleagues suggests that electrophysiologic techniques may be able to capture the flow of speech as it is being perceived through the brain. One difficulty with interpretation of PCA-ANOVA results is, as we discussed, that the technique does not deal well with individual differences. However, it may prove itself to be more stable in an N = 1 paradigm, where individual difference variance is not confounded with other sources. It is reasonable, after all, to consider that all babies' processing of phonetic features is not identically organized in the brain or identically timed.

Nor should we expect the exuberant projections to be identically patterned (Diamond, 1990, xvi–xix). If it is the case that the PCA-ANOVA catches all the perturbations that the stimulation induces in the brain, surely it will also catch variations among subjects, adding variance that the PCA might misallocate to the factor structure. In a study of a single subject (or a series of them), the factor structure may be more stable. A case study that was longitudinal would provide evidence of the stability of the models involving dynamic phonetic feature by brain region by time interactions that Molfese's work clearly point to at the moment.

The Use of Electrophysiologic Data for Laterality

Can electrophysiology be used to detect specific hemispheric specialization of function? The picture we have drawn so far suggests that when we consider studies of the processing of specific information, the interactions in the brain are too dynamic for a simple left-right dichotomy. The normal processing of stimuli is complex and may not be decipherable in left-right terms from ERPs. This sensitivity in normal functioning is quite different from the notion of laterality taken from cases of unilateral brain damage, since electrophysiologic measures may not be sensitive to a construct of exclusive hemispheric dominance either in infancy or adulthood.

To some extent, electrophysiologic research on localization speaks to two audiences, one concerned with finding early evidence for specific mental functions of interest, the other in how the brain organizes such functions. In other words, the issue of laterality of function is an addendum to the purely developmental issues. In order to derive laterality results from the electrophysiologic paradigms discussed in this chapter, we must admit two constraining features. The first involves constraining the notion of laterality used, as we saw in the tripartite division suggested here. The second involves constraining the analysis of the data to specifically find functional asymmetries. The complexity of each reflects the complexity of information processing in even the infant's brain.

ACKNOWLEDGMENTS

We thank Dennis Molfese, Jane Dywan, and Doug Cross for comments on the original manuscript.

REFERENCES

Adams, C. L., Molfese, D. L., and Betz, J. C. (1987). Electrophysiological correlates of categorical speech perception for voicing contrasts in dogs. *Developmental Neuropsychology, 3*, 175–189.

Barnet, A. B., Vincentini, M., and Campos, S. M. (1974). EEG sensory evoked responses (ERs) in early infancy malnutrition. Presented to Society for Neuroscience, St. Louis, MO.

Bertoncini, J., Morais, J., Bijeljac-Babic, R., McAdams, S., Peretz, I., and Mehler, J. (1989). Dichotic perception and laterality in neonates. *Brain and Language, 37,* 591–605.

Best, C. T. (1988). The emergence of cerebral asymmetries in early human development: A literature review and a neuroembryological model. In D. L. Molfese and S. J. Segalowitz (Eds.), *Brain lateralization in children* (pp 5–34). New York, NY: Guilford Press.

Bever, T. (1975). Cerebral asymmetries in humans are due to the differentiation of two incompatible processes: Holistic and analytic. In D. Aronson and R. W. Reiber (Eds.), *Developmental psycholinguistics and communication disorders.* New York, NY: New York Academy of Sciences.

Borod, J. C., Koff, E., Lorch, M. P., and Nicholas, M. (1986). The expression and perception of facial emotion in brain-damaged patients. *Neuropsychologia, 24,* 169–180.

Cacioppo, J. T., and Tassinary, L. G. (1990). *Principles of psychophysiology.* Cambridge, England: Cambridge University Press.

Carmon, A., Harishanu, E., Lowinger, E., and Lavy, S. (1972). Asymmetries in hemispheric blood volume and cerebral dominance. *Behavioural Biology, 7,* 853–859.

Chapman, L. J., and Chapman, J. P. (1988). Artifactual and genuine relationships of lateral difference scores to overall accuracy in studies of laterality. *Psychological Bulletin, 104,* 127–136.

Churchland, P. S. (1986). *Neurophilosophy.* Cambridge, MA: MIT Press.

Corballis, M. C., and Morgan, M. J. (1978). On the biological basis of human laterality: I. Evidence for a maturational left-right gradient. *Behavioral and Brain Sciences, 2,* 261–336.

Cronbach, L. J., and Furby, L. (1970). How we should measure "change"—or should we? *Psychological Bulletin, 74,* 68–80.

Crowell, D. H., Jones, R. H., Kapuniai, L. E., and Nakagawa, J. K. (1973). Unilateral cortical activity in newborn humans: An early index of cerebral dominance? *Science, 180,* 205–208.

Davidson, R. J., and Fox, N. A. (1982). Asymmetrical brain activity discriminates between positive and negative affective stimuli in human infants. *Science, 218,* 1235–1236.

Davidson, R. J., and Fox, N. A. (1988). Cerebral asymmetry and emotion: Developmental and individual differences. In D. L. Molfese and S. J. Segalowitz (Eds.), *Brain lateralization in children: Developmental implications* (pp 191–206). New York, NY: Guilford Press.

Davidson, R. J., and Fox, N. A. (1989). Frontal brain asymmetry predicts infants' response to maternal separation. *Journal of Abnormal Psychology, 98,* 127–131.

Davidson, R. J., Schwartz, G. E., Saron, C., Bennett, J., and Goleman, D. J. (1979). Frontal versus parietal EEG asymmetry during positive and negative affect. *Psychophysiology, 16,* 202–203.

Davis, A. E., and Wada, J. A. (1977). Hemispheric asymmetries in human infants: Spectral analysis of flash and click evoked potentials. *Brain and Language, 4,* 22–31.

deSchonen, S., and Mathivet, E. (1989). First come, first served: A scenario about the development of hemispheric specialization in face recognition during infancy. *European Bulletin of Cognitive Psychology, 9,* 3–44.

Dawson, G., Panagiotides, H., Klinger, L., and Hill, D. (1992a). The role of frontal lobe functioning in the development of infant self-regulatory behavior. *Brain and Cognition, 20,* 152–175.

Dawson, G., Klinger, G. L., Panagiotides, H., Hill, D., and Spieker, S. (1992b). Frontal lobe activity and affective behaviour of infants of mothers with depressive symptoms. *Child Development, 63,* 725–737.

Dawson, G., Klinger, G. L., Panagiotides, H., Spieker, S., and Frey, K. (1992c). Infants of mothers with depressive symptoms: Electroencephalographic and behavioural findings related to attachment status. *Development and Psychopathology, 4,* 67–80.

Dennett, D., and Kinsbourne, M. (1992). Time and the observer: The where and when of consciousness in the brain. *Behavioural and Brain Sciences, 15*, 183−201.

Desmedt, J. E. (1989). Topographic mapping of generators of somatosensory evoked potentials. In K. Maurer (Ed.), *Topographic brain mapping of EEG and evoked potentials* (pp 76−89). Berlin: Springer-Verlag.

Diamond, A. (1990). The development and neural bases of memory functions as indexed by the AB and delayed response tasks in human infants and infant monkeys. *Annals of the New York Academy of Sciences, 608*, 267−317.

Eimas, P. D., Siqueland, E., Jusczyk, P., and Vigorito, J. (1971). Speech perception in infants. *Science, 171*, 303−306.

Entus, A. K. (1977). Hemispheric asymmetry in processing of dichotically presented speech and nonspeech stimuli by infants. In S. J. Segalowitz and F. A. Gruber (Eds.), *Language development and neurological theory* (pp 63−73). New York, NY: Academic Press.

Fabiani, M., Gratton, G., Karis, D., and Donchin, E. (1987). Definition, identification, and reliability of measurement of the P300 component of the event-related brain potential. In P. K. Ackles, J. R. Jenning, and M. G. H. Coles (Eds.), *Advances in psychophysiology*, Vol 2 (pp 1−78). London: JAI Press Ltd.

Fox, N. A., Bell, M. A., and Jones, N. A. (1992). Individual differences in response to stress and cerebral asymmetry. *Developmental Neuropsychology, 8*, 161−184.

Fox, N. A., and Davidson, R. J. (1986). Taste-elicited changes in facial signs of emotion and the asymmetry of brain electrical activity in human newborns. *Neuropsychologia, 24*, 417−422.

Fox, N. A., and Davidson, R. J. (1987). Electroencephalogram asymmetry in response to the approach of a stranger and maternal separation in 10-month-old infants. *Developmental Psychology, 23*, 233−240.

Fox, N. A., and Davidson, R. J. (1988). Patterns of brain electrical activity during facial signs of emotion in 10-month-old infants. *Developmental Psychology, 24*, 230−236.

Freeman, R. D., and Thibos, L. N. (1973). Electrophysiological evidence that abnormal early visual experience can modify the human brain. *Science, 180*, 876−878.

Gardiner, M. F., and Walter, D. O. (1977). Evidence of hemispheric specialization from infant EEG. In S. Harnad, R. W. Doty, L. Goldstein, J. Jaynes, and G. Krauthamer (Eds.), *Lateralization in the nervous system*. New York, NY: Academic Press.

Gilbert, J. H., and Climan, I. (1974). Dichotic studies in 2−3 year olds: A preliminary report. Speech Communication Seminar, Stockholm, Aug 1−3, 1974.

Gottlieb, G. (1983). The psychobiological approach to developmental issues. In M. M. Haith and J. J. Campos (Eds.), *Infancy and developmental psychobiology* (pp 1−26), Vol 2 of the *Handbook of child psychology*, P. H. Mussen (Series Ed.).

Hahn, W. K. (1991). Cerebral lateralization of function: From infancy through childhood. *Psychological Bulletin, 101*, 376−392.

Hebb, D. O. (1949). *The organization of behavior*. New York, NY: John Wiley & Sons.

Hiscock, M. (1988). Behavioural asymmetries in normal children. In D. L. Molfese and S. J. Segalowitz (Eds.), *Brain lateralization in children: Developmental implications* (pp 85−170). New York, NY: Guilford Press.

Isaacson, R. L. (1975). The myth of recovery from early brain damage. In N. E. Ellis (Ed.), *Aberrant development in infancy*. London: John Wiley & Sons.

Kinsbourne, M., and Hiscock, M. (1983). The normal and deviant development of functional lateralization of the brain. In M. M. Haith and J. J. Campos (Eds.), *Infancy and developmental psychobiology* (pp 157–280), Vol 2 of the *Handbook of child psychology*, P. H. Mussen (Series Ed.). New York: Wiley.

Kuhl, P., and Miller, J. (1975). Speech perception by the chinchilla: Voiced-voiceless distinction in alveolar plosive consonants. *Science, 190,* 69–72.

Kuhl, P., and Padden, D. (1983). Enhanced discriminability at the phonetic boundaries for the voicing feature in macaques. *Perception and Psychophysics, 32,* 542–550.

Lederman, S. J., Jones, B., and Segalowitz, S. J. (1984). Lateral symmetry in the tactual perception of roughness. *Canadian Journal of Psychology, 38,* 599–609.

Lenneberg, E. H. (1967). *Biological foundations of language.* New York, NY: John Wiley & Sons.

Levy, J., Heller, W., Banich, M. T., and Burton, L. A. (1983). Asymmetry of perception in free viewing of chimeric faces. *Brain and Cognition, 2,* 404–419.

Luria, A. R. (1973). *The working brain: An introduction to neuropsychology.* London: Penguin.

Martin, I., and Venables, P. (1980). Techniques of psychophysiology. New York, NY: John Wiley & Sons.

Möcks, J. (1986). The influence of latency jitter in principal component analysis of event-related potentials. *Psychophysiology, 23,* 480–484.

Möcks, J., and Verleger, R. (1986). Principal component analysis of event-related potentials: A note on misallocation of variance. *Electroencephalography and Clinical Neurophysiology, 65,* 393–398.

Molfese, D. L. (1977). Infant cerebral asymmetry. In S. J. Segalowitz and F. A. Gruber (Eds.), *Language development and neurological theory* (pp 21–35). New York, NY: Academic Press.

Molfese, D. L. (1978). Neuroelectrical correlates of categorical speech perception in adults. *Brain and Language, 5,* 25–35.

Molfese, D. L. (1980). Hemispheric specialization for temporal information: Implications for the perception of voicing cues during speech perception. *Brain and Language, 11,* 285–299.

Molfese, D. L. (1989). Electrophysiological correlates of word meanings in 14-month-old human infants. *Developmental Neuropsychology, 5,* 79–103.

Molfese, D. L. (1990). Auditory evoked responses recorded from 16-month-old human infants to words they did and did not know. *Brain and Language, 38,* 345–363.

Molfese, D. L., and Betz, J. C. (1988). Electrophysiological indices of the early development of lateralization for language and cognition, and their implications for predicting later development. In D. L. Molfese and S. J. Segalowitz (Eds.), *Brain lateralization in children: Developmental implications* (pp 171–190). New York, NY: Guilford Press.

Molfese, D. L., Burger-Judisch, L. M., and Hans, L. L. (1991). Consonant discrimination by newborn infants: Electrophysiological differences. *Developmental Neuropsychology, 7,* 177–195.

Molfese, D. L., Freeman, R. B., and Palermo, D. S. (1975). The ontongeny of brain lateralization for speech and nonspeech stimuli. *Brain and Language, 2,* 356–368.

Molfese, D. L., and Hess, T. M. (1978). Hemispheric specialization for VOT perception in the preschool child. *Journal of Experimental Child Psychology, 26,* 71–84.

Molfese, D. L., Laughlin, N. K., Morse, P. A., Linnville, S. E., Wetzel, W. F., and Erwin, R. J. (1986). Neuroelectrical correlates of categorical perception for place of articulation in normal and lead-treated rhesus monkeys. *Journal of Clinical and Experimental Neuropyschology, 8,* 860–696.

Molfese, D. L., and Molfese, V. J. (1978). VOT distinctions in infants: Learned or innate? In H. Whitaker and H. A. Whitaker (Eds.), *Studies in neurolinguistics*, Vol 4. New York, NY: Academic Press.

Molfese, D. L., and Molfese, V. J. (1979). Hemisphere and stimulus differences as reflected in the cortical responses of newborn infants to speech stimuli. *Developmental Psychology, 15,* 505–511.

Molfese, D. L., and Molfese, V. J. (1980). Cortical responses of preterm infants to phonetic and nonphonetic speech stimuli. *Developmental Psychology, 16,* 574–581.

Molfese, D. L., and Molfese, V. J. (1985). Electrophysiological indices of auditory discrimination in newborn infants: The bases for predicting later language development? *Infant Behavior and Development, 8,* 197–211.

Molfese, D. L., and Molfese, V. J. (1988). Right-hemisphere responses from preschool children to temporal cues to speech and nonspeech materials: Electrophysiological correlates. *Brain and Language, 33,* 245–259.

Molfese, D. L., Morse, P. A., and Peters, C. J. (1990). Auditory evoked responses to names for different objects: Cross-modal processing as a basis for infant language acquisition. *Developmental Psychology, 26,* 780–795.

Molfese, D. L., Nunez, V., Siebert, S. M., and Ramanaiah, N. V. (1976). Cerebral asymmetry: Changes in factors affecting its development. *Annals of the New York Academy of Sciences, 280,* 821–833.

Molfese, D. L., and Radtke, R. C. (1982). Statistical and methodological issues in "Auditory evoked potentials and sex-related differences in brain development." *Brain and Language, 16,* 338–341.

Molfese, D. L., and Searock, K. J. (1986). The use of auditory evoked responses at one-year-of-age to predict language skills at 3-years. *Australian Journal of Human Communication Disorders, 14,* 35–46.

Molfese, D. M., and Segalowitz, S. J. (Eds.) (1988). *Brain lateralization in children: Developmental implications.* New York, NY: Guilford Press.

Molfese, D. L., and Wetzel, W. F. (1992). Short- and long-term auditory recognition memory in 14-month-old human infants: Electrophysiological correlates. *Developmental Neuropsychology, 8,* 135–160.

Morse, P. A., Molfese, D. L., Laughlin, N. K., Linnville, S., and Wetzel, F. (1987). Categorical perception for voicing contrasts in normal and lead-treated rhesus monkeys: Electrophysiological indices. *Brain and Language, 30,* 63–80.

Moscovitch, M. (1979). Information processing and the cerebral hemispheres. In M. S. Gazzaniga (Ed.), *Handbook of behavioral neurobiology*, Vol 2: *Neuropsychology* (pp 379–446). New York, NY: Plenum Press.

Papanicoloau, A. C., and Johnstone, J. (1984). Probe evoked potentials: Theory, method and applications. *International Journal of Neuroscience, 24,* 107–131.

Parasuraman, R., Richer, F., and Beatty, J. (1982) Detection and recognition: Concurrent processes in perception. *Perception and Psychophysics, 31,* 1–12.

Picton, T. (1988). *Human event-related potentials.* Amsterdam: Elsevier.

Pivik, R. T., Broughton, R. G., Croppolla, R., Davidson, R. T., Fox, N., and Newer, M. R. (1993). Guidelines for recording and quantitative analysis of the electroencephalographic activity in research contexts. *Psychophysiology, 6,* 547–558.

Poizner, H., Klima, E., and Bellugi, U. (1987). *What the hands reveal about the brain*. Cambridge, MA: MIT Press.

Polich, J. (1986). Attention, probability, and task demands as determinants of P300 latency from auditory stimuli. *Electroencephalography and Clinical Neurophysiology, 63*, 251–259.

Prescott, P. A., and DeCasper, A. J. (1991). Human perception of speech and nonspeech is functionally lateralized at birth. Unpublished manuscript, University of North Carolina at Greensboro.

Previc, F. H. (1991). A general theory concerning the prenatal origins of cerebral lateralization. *Psychological Review, 98*, 299–334.

Regan, M. D. (1989). *Human brain electrophysiology: Evoked potentials and evoked magnetic fields in science and medicine*. Amsterdam: Elsevier.

Rohrbaugh, J. W., Parasuraman, R., and Johnson, R., Jr. (1990). *Event-related brain potentials*. New York, NY: Oxford University Press.

Ross, P., and Turkewitz, G. (1981). Individual differences in cerebral asymmetries for facial recognition. *Cortex, 17*, 199–214.

Saxby, L., and Bryden, M. P. (1984). Left-ear superiority in children for processing auditory emotional material. *Developmental Psychology, 20*, 99–103.

Saxby, L., and Bryden, M. P. (1985). Left visual-field advantage in children for processing visual emotion stimuli. *Developmental Psychology, 21*, 253–261.

Segalowitz, S. J. (1977) Why is language lateralized to the left? In S. J. Segalowitz and F. A. Gruber (Eds.), *Language development and neurological theory* (pp 165–169). New York, NY: Academic Press.

Segalowitz, S. J. (1983). Cerebral asymmetries for speech in infancy. In S. J. Segalowitz (Ed.), *Language functions and brain organization* (pp 221–229). New York, NY: Academic Press.

Segalowitz, S. J. (1986). Validity and reliability of noninvasive measures of brain lateralization. In J. Obrzut and D. Hines (Eds.), *Child neuropsychology: Empirical issues* (pp 191–208). New York, NY: Academic Press.

Segalowitz, S. J., and Barnes, K. L. (1993). The reliability of ERP components in the auditory oddball paradigm. *Psychophysiology, 30*, 451–459.

Segalowitz, S. J., and Chapman, J. S. (1980). Cerebral asymmetry for speech in neonates: A behavioral measure. *Brain and Language, 9*, 281–288.

Segalowitz, S. J., and Cohen, H. (1989). Right hemisphere EEG sensitivity to speech. *Brain and Language, 37*, 220–231.

Segalowitz, S. J., and Gruber, F. A. (Eds.) (1977). *Language development and neurological theory*. New York, NY: Academic Press.

Sergent, J. (1987). Failures to confirm the spatial-frequency hypothesis: Fatal blow or healthy complication? *Canadian Journal of Psychology, 41*, 412–428.

Scheibel, A. B. (1990). Dendritic correlates of higher cognitive function. In A. B. Scheibel and A. F. Wechsler (Eds.), *Neurobiology of higher cognitive function* (pp 239–270). New York, NY: Guilford Press.

Spellacy, F., and Blumstein, S. (1970). The influence of language set on ear preference in phoneme recognition. *Cortex, 6*, 430–439.

Shucard, J. L., and Shucard, D. W. (1990). Auditory evoked potentials and hand preference in 6-month-old infants: Possible gender-related differences in cerebral organization. *Developmental Psychology, 26*, 923–930.

Shucard, J. L, Shucard, D. W., Cummins, K. R., and Campos, J. J. (1981). Auditory evoked potentials and sex-related differences in brain development. *Brain and Language, 13*, 91–102.

Steinschneider, M., Kurtzberg, D., and Vaughan, H. (1992). Event-related potentials in developmental neuropsychology. In I. Rapin and S. J. Segalowitz (Eds.), *Child neuropsychology* (pp 238–300), Vol 6 of *Handbook of neuropsychology*. F. Boller and J. Grafman (Series Eds). Amsterdam: Elsevier.

Studdert-Kennedy, M., and Shankweiler, D. (1970). Hemispheric specialization for speech perception. *Journal of the Acoustical Society of America, 48*, 579–594.

Thatcher, R. W. (1991). Maturation of the human frontal lobes: Physiological evidence for staging. *Developmental Neuropsychology, 7*, 397–419.

Thatcher, R. W. (1992). Cyclic cortical reorganization during early childhood. *Brain and Cognition, 20*.

Thatcher, R. W., Walker, R. A., and Guidice, S. (1987). Human cerebral hemispheres develop at different rates and ages. *Science, 236*, 1110–1113.

Tomarken, A. J., Davidson, R. J., Wheeler, R. E., and Kenney, L. (1992). Psychometric properties of resting anterior EEG asymmetry: Temporal stability and internal consistency. *Psychophysiology, 29*, 576–592.

Tucker, D. M., Stenslie, C. E., Roth, R. S., and Shearer, S. L. (1981). Right frontal lobe activation and right hemisphere performance decrement during a depressed mood. *Archives of General Psychiatry, 38*, 169–174.

Wastell, D. G. (1981). On the correlated nature of evoked brain activity: Biophysical and statistical considerations. *Biological Psychology, 13*, 51–69.

Witelson, S. F. (1977). Early hemispheric specialization and interhemispheric plasticity: An empirical and theoretical review. In S. J. Segalowitz and F. A. Gruber (Eds.), *Language development and neurological theory* (pp 213–289). New York, NY: Academic Press.

Witelson, S. F. (1985). On hemispheric specialization and cerebral plasticity from birth: Mark II. In C. T. Best (Ed.), *Hemispheric function and collaboration in the child* (pp 33–85). New York, NY: Academic Press.

Wood, C. C., and McCarthy, G. (1984). Principal component analysis of event-related potentials: Simulation studies demonstrate misallocation of variance across components. *Electroencephalography and Clinical Neurophysiology, 59*, 249–260.

Woody, E. Z., and Costanzo, P. R. (1990). Does marital agony precede marital ecstasy? A comment on Gottman and Krokoff's "Marital interaction and satisfaction: A longitudinal view." *Journal of Consulting and Clinical Psychology, 58*, 499–501.

20 Learning Disabilities: Neuroanatomic Asymmetries

George W. Hynd, Richard Marshall, Josh Hall, and Jane E. Edmonds

More than 100 years have passed since the first reports of children with learning disabilities appeared in the literature (Bastian, 1898; Hinshelwood, 1900; Kussmaul, 1877; Morgan, 1896). Many of the reports attempted to explain why an estimated 3% to 6% of the school-age population could not learn consistent with what would be expected considering their intellectual ability and repeated attempts at instruction (Gaddes, 1985; Yule and Rutter, 1976). These early reports were often quite rich in clinical detail and provided insights that are remarkably consistent with present research findings.

In fact, in reviewing the early literature, Hynd and Willis (1988) concluded that by 1905 the number of observations that had emerged from the evolving literature was such that a number of tentative conclusions could be offered. Overall, the literature by 1905 supported the following: (1) reading disability (congenital word blindness) could manifest in children with normal ability, (2) males seemed to be more often affected than females, (3) children presented with varied symptoms, but all suffered a core deficit in reading acquisition, (4) normal or even extended classroom instruction did not significantly improve reading ability, (5) some reading problems seemed to be transmitted genetically, and (6) the core symptoms seemed similar to those seen in adults with left temporoparietal lesions.

While no one would contest the idea that learning disabilities may differentially manifest in many areas of learning, including arithmetic, writing, spelling, and so on, there is little doubt that it is with reading disabilities, or dyslexia, where most researchers have concentrated their efforts. For this reason and because so many researchers from neuropsychology, neurology, and neurolinguistics have focused their efforts on reading disabilities, we will examine this literature in an attempt to draw some meaning from the volumes of research that have investigated brain-behavior relationships in this most common of learning disabilities. In fact, an understanding of this literature and the theoretical ideas concerning the meaning of lateralized function and potentially associated deviations in brain morphology may well assist future scholars in their investigation of the neurobiological basis of other forms of learning disabilities.

As the early case studies suggested, learning disabilities have always been thought to have a neurologic origin and present definitions of learning disability reflect this perspective (Wyngaarden, 1987). However, the literature supporting this perspective has generated a great deal of controversy. As Golden (1982) and Taylor and Fletcher (1983) have pointed out, much if not most of the literature through the early part of the 1980s was correlational in nature.

For example, some research indicates that reading-disabled children have an increased incidence of electrophysiologic abnormalities (Duffy et al., 1980) and perhaps differentially so in subtypes of reading disabilities (e.g., Fried et al., 1981). Soft signs are also more frequently found in reading-disabled children (Peters, Romine, and Dykman, 1975) and few would argue that reading-disabled children have a higher incidence of left- or mixed handedness (Bryden and Steenhuis, 1991). Further, reading-disabled children are often inferred to have weak or incomplete laterality, as evidenced on perceptual measures such as dichotic listening (Obrzut, 1991). In fact, volumes summarizing the research in this area have been written (Bakker and van der Vlugt, 1989; Gaddes, 1985; Kershner and Chyczij, 1992; Obrzut and Hynd, 1991), but we are still to a significant degree left with inferential or correlative evidence supporting the presumption of a neurologic etiology for learning disabilities. Typical of such inferential evidence were studies that found that children with learning disabilities performed more poorly than normal children on any given task (cognitive or perceptual) but did better than children with documented brain damage (e.g., Reitan and Boll, 1973). Needless to say, the inference was often made that the learning-disabled children suffered "minimal brain dysfunction" because their level of performance was somewhere between normality and known brain damage. This was clearly an inference and while not without merit theoretically, it did not directly correlate a known neurologic deviation of any kind (e.g., developmental, traumatic) with observed behavioral or cognitive deficits, as we might find in learning-disabled children.

This absence of confirming evidence is certainly not due to a shortage of theories or research, however. Historically relevant is the theory of Orton (1928) who proposed that as children become more linguistically competent, the left cerebral hemisphere becomes progressively more dominant for speech and language. He believed that motor dominance and its evolution in the developing child reflected this process of progressive lateralization. Consequently, according to Orton, children who had mixed cerebral dominance, as might be reflected in poor language skills, reading words or letters backward and inconsistent handedness, were most likely delayed in cerebral lateralization and therefore neither cerebral hemisphere, particularly the left, was dominant for linguistic processes. While decades of research documented that learning-disabled children were indeed deficient in language processes, especially phonological coding, the model of progressive lateralization has not been supported by the research (Benton, 1975; Kinsbourne and Hiscock, 1981; Satz 1991).

Actually, there is a growing body of evidence that indicates that very young children, including infants, are lateralized for language processing (Molfese and Molfese, 1986). Thus, none would refute the notion that in the majority of cases language is lateralized to the left cerebral hemisphere. However, while language abilities clearly develop over the course of human ontogeny, language remains lateralized as it was early in infant development. What may devolve is the capacity for plasticity of function; i.e., the capacity for the other cerebral hemisphere to assume language functions when the dominant hemisphere is severely damaged may decrease significantly with the course of development (Piacentini and Hynd, 1988).

What neurologic structures or deficient neuropsychological systems underlie the behavioral and cognitive symptoms we associate with learning disabilities, particularly reading disabilities? While there are likely many different ways in which one could begin to address this question, we will approach this question from a neurolinguistic-neuroanatomic perspective. We first present a discussion of the lateralized system of language and associated reading processes and then examine its impact and relation to research that employs brain-imaging procedures to investigate morphologic differences in the brains of reading-disabled children and adolescents. In this fashion we hope to directly tie deviations in lateralized brain processes (e.g., language, reading) to potentially associated deviations in brain structure.

NEUROLINGUISTIC-NEUROANATOMIC MODEL

For over a century, those concerned with reading and language disorders have attempted to correlate observed functional deficits with the location of known brain lesions (Bastian, 1898; Dejerine, 1892; Dejerine and Vialet, 1893; Dejerine and Dejerine-Klumpke, 1901; Geschwind, 1974; Head, 1926; Kussmaul, 1877; Wernicke, 1910). These scholars and others interested in the lateralization and localization of language and reading processes contributed to a literature that resulted in a neurolinguistic model of language and reading referred to by some as the Wernicke-Geschwind model (Mayeux and Kandel, 1985). While Wernicke and Dejerine deserve the most credit for the development of this model, it is clear that Geschwind (1974) did much to revive interest in the perspective first proposed in part by Bastian (1898), Liepmann (1915), Marie (1906), and others, whose ideas were controversial even when they were first proposed. As Head (1926) suggested over 60 years ago, "localization of speech became a political question; the older conservative school, haunted by the bogey of phrenology, clung to the conception that the 'brain acted as a whole,' whilst the younger liberals and Republicans passionately favored the view that different functions were exercised by the various portions of the cerebral hemispheres" (p. 25).

Even among the "diagram makers" (Head, 1926) controversy existed. For example, Bastian (1898) argued strongly against the popular perspective

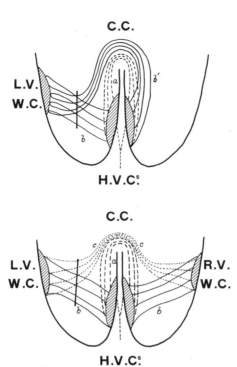

Figure 20.1 A comparison of Dejerine's and Bastain's views on the neuroanatomic basis of "pure word blindness" as presented by Bastian (1898). (*Above*) A simplified diagram representing Dejerine's views as to the mode of production of pure word blindness. The *dark line* indicates the site of a lesion which would cut off the left visual word center (L.V.W.C.) from the half-vision center (H.V.C.) of each side. (*Below*) A diagram representing Bastian's views as to the mode of production of pure word blindness. C.C., corpus callosum.

advocated by Dejerine whose views so influenced Geschwind in his thinking. Bastian proposed that bilateral visual word centers existed in the brain, each of which was involved in visual perception, low-level feature analysis, and cross-modal integration with the central language centers. Dejerine's views prevailed, however, as the accumulation of case studies supported the notion that there was indeed a left-lateralized "word center," most notably, it seemed, in the region of the angular gyrus. Figure 20.1 graphically contrasts Dejerine and Bastian's views on the posterior cortex involved in reading.

Based on the contributions of Broca, Wernicke, and the others noted above, a more complete neurolinguistic model of language and reading evolved. This model presupposes that visual stimuli such as words are registered in the bilateral primary occipital cortex, meaningful low-level perceptual associations occur in the secondary visual cortex, and this input is shared with further input from other sensory modalities in the region of the angular gyrus in the left cerebral hemisphere. This sequential neurocognitive process presumably then associates linguistic-semantic comprehension with input from the region of the angular gyrus; a process which involves the cortical region of the left

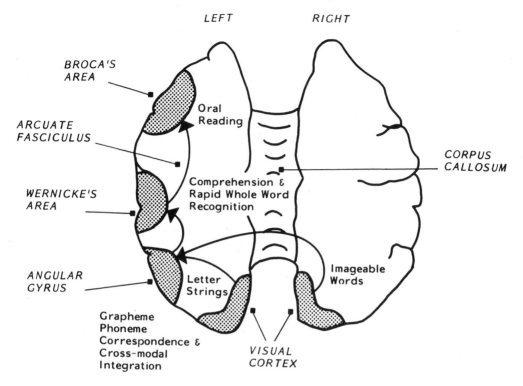

LEFT　　　　RIGHT

BROCA'S
AREA

ARCUATE
FASCICULUS

WERNICKE'S
AREA

ANGULAR
GYRUS

CORPUS
CALLOSUM

Oral
Reading

Comprehension &
Rapid Whole Word
Recognition

Letter
Strings

Imageable
Words

Grapheme
Phoneme
Correspondence &
Cross-modal
Integration

VISUAL
CORTEX

Figure 20.2 The brain as viewed in horizontal section. The major pathways and cortical regions thought to be involved in reading are depicted. Neurolinguistic processes important in reading are also noted.

posterior superior temporal region, including the region of the planum temporale. Then the process is completed when interhemispheric fibers connect these regions with Broca's area in the left inferior frontal region. Figure 20.2 presents this model, and the prevailing view of Dejerine's theory regarding the left lateralized "word center" can be seen in the posterior aspect of the figure.

It was Geschwind (1974), of course, who revived interest in this neurolinguistic-neuroanatomic model. He contributed significantly, however, by focusing attention on the natural left-sided asymmetry of the region of the planum temporale. Reports by early investigators (Flechsig, 1908; von Economo and Horn, 1930) encouraged Geschwind and Levitsky (1968) to investigate asymmetries associated with the region of the planum temporale. They examined 100 normal adult brains and found that the region of the planum temporale (the most posterior aspect of the superior temporal lobe) is larger on the left in 65% of brains, whereas it is larger on the right in only 11% of brains. These findings were taken as evidence of a specialized and asymmetric neuroanatomic region in support of language functions. Studies by other investigators documented the finding of plana asymmetry in both adult and infant brains (Kopp et al., 1977; Rubens, Mahuwald, and Hutton, 1976; Wada,

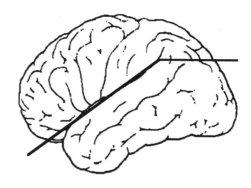

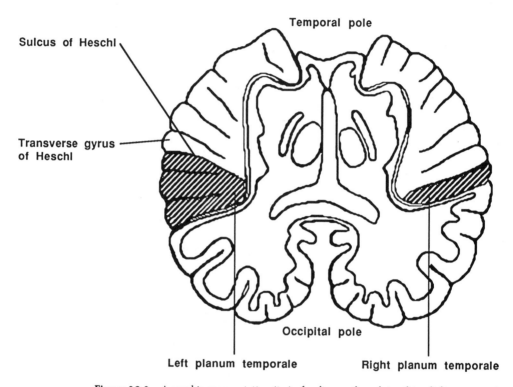

Figure 20.3 A graphic representation (*top*) of a slice up the sylvian (lateral) fissure exposing the posterior portion of the superior temporal region. The planum temporale is shaded bilaterally (*bottom*) and it can be seen that it is generally larger on the left.

Clarke, and Hamm, 1975; Witelson and Pallie, 1973). Figure 20.3 shows the left-sided asymmetry typically found in normal brains that is thought to subserve the evolution of higher-order neurolinguistic processes.

The research that was encouraged by the findings of Geschwind and Levitsky (1968) was significant in that other morphologic asymmetries in the human brain were soon reported. For example, Weinberger and colleagues (1982) found evidence that in approximately 75% of normal brains the right frontal volume (R) exceeds that of the left frontal cortex (L). Also this pattern of L < R asymmetry seems evident in fetal development as early as 20 weeks. Other documented asymmetries include the left anterior speech region (pars opercularis and pars triangularis of the third frontal convolution) favoring the left side (Falzi, Perrone, and Vignolo, 1982) and cytoarchitectonic asymmetries favoring the left inferior parietal lobe (Eidelberg and Galaburda, 1984), the left auditory cortex (Galaburda and Sanides, 1980), and the posterior thalamus (Eidelberg and Galaburda, 1982).

Based on these as well as other research findings, Geschwind (1974, 1984) and especially Geschwind and Galaburda (1985a–c) argued that these natural asymmetries may be associated in a meaningful manner with language processes and, in cases of reversed asymmetry or symmetry, they may underlie the deficits we observe in severe reading disabilities. While the theory outlined by Geschwind and Galaburda (1985a–c) addresses the possible relations between male gender differentiation, the effects of testosterone on neuronal assemblies, and correlated asymmetries in brain morphology, immune function, and left-handedness, we are especially interested in our research with the idea that deviations in natural brain asymmetries may be related to the deficient linguistic and reading processes we observe in reading-disabled children. Thus, in this context, the remainder of this chapter will address the brain-imaging literature and examine the findings in relation to whether or not evidence exists in support of the notion that deviations in natural asymmetries in the language-reading system in the brain are indeed related in some fashion to the cognitive or behavioral deficits we observe in these children.

BRAIN IMAGING

Many different methodologies have been employed to investigate laterality and asymmetries in human performance. Certainly, visual half-field and dichotic listening experiments have assisted us greatly in better understanding perceptual asymmetries that underly linguistic and visuospatial perception. Dual-task paradigms have helped develop a better understanding of the lateralization of hemispheric attentional mechanisms and handedness—manual preference inventories have likewise helped in documenting variability in human laterality. All of these methodologies rely on the recording of a behavioral response which in turn leads to a measure of laterality.

The documentation of morphologic asymmetries in the human brain that seemed to favor the left hemisphere central language zones encouraged speculation that variability in these patterns of asymmetry might be related to the behavioral deficits we see in such conditions as severe reading disability. Geschwind and his colleagues deserve much of the credit for encouraging this perspective. In this context then, measures of manual preference or perceptual asymmetries might still be of interest but they could not provide a window from which to actually view the brain and its associated morphology.

Table 20.1 Brain imaging studies of subjects with developmental dyslexia

Study	Type	No. of subjects	Mean age (yr)	Diagnostic criteria	Conclusions
Hier et al. (1978)	CT	24	25	Less than 5th-grade reading level on Gray Oral Reading Test or > 2-yr delay in reading while in school	Dyslexic subjects with reversed posterior asymmetry had lower verbal IQ 33% had normal L > R posterior asymmetry; 67% had symmetry or reversed (L < R) posterior asymmetry
LeMay (1978)	CT	27 dyslexic subjects[a] 317 controls	NR	NR	33% of dyslexic subjects had normal (L > R) posterior asymmetry compared to 70% of right-handed controls Left-handed controls evidenced more symmetry and reversed (L < R) asymmetry of posterior region
Leisman and Ashkenazi (1980)	CT	8 dyslexic subjects 2 controls	8.2—dyslexic subjects 7.6—normals	NR	100% of dyslexic subjects had symmetry or received asymmetry (L < R) of posterior region
Rosenberger and Hier (1980)	CT	53	6–45 (range)	Two grade levels below actual grade; large verbal-performance IQ discrepancy	42% of dyslexic subjects had reversed asymmetry (L < R) of posterior region Asymmetry index correlated with verbal-performance IQ discrepancy ($r = .38$, $P < .02$)
Haslam et al. (1981)	CT	26 dyslexic subjects 8 controls	11.7—dyslexic subjects 9.8—controls	Reading performance at least 2 yr below expected level based on IQ	46% of dyslexic subjects showed normal (L > R) posterior asymmetry while 87% controls did No relationship between IQ and posterior symmetry or asymmetry
Rumsey et al. (1986)	MRI	10	22.6	Childhood history of reading disability; median Gray Oral Reading Test was 3.7 grade equivalent	90% of dyslexic subjects showed symmetry of posterior regions
Parkins et al. (1987)	CT	44 dyslexic subjects 254 controls	57	Childhood history of reading and spelling disability; psychometrc evidence of dyslexia	Concluded that reversed posterior asymmetries are not characteristic of right-handed dyslexic subjects, but left-handed dyslexic subjects may evidence more symmetry

Table 20.1 (cont.)

Study	Type	No. of subjects	Mean age (yr)	Diagnostic criteria	Conclusions
Larsen et al. (1990)	MRI	19 dyslexic subjects 19 normals	15.1—dyslexic subjects 15.4—controls	Highly significant difference between normals and dyslexic subjects in word recognition; selected prior to study by schools as dyslexic	Measured the patterns of asymmetry in the region of the planum temporale: 70% of dyslexic subjects evidenced symmetry, while only 30% of nondyslexic subjects did All dyslexic subjects with plana asymmetry demonstrated significant phonological coding deficits
Hynd et al. (1990)[b]	MRI	10 dyslexic subjects 10 ADDH children 10 normals	9.9—dyslexic subjects 10.0—ADDH children 11.8—normals	IQ ≥ 85, positive family history, reading achievement ≥ 20 standard score points below full-scale IQ on tests of word recognition and passage comprehension	Both dyslexic subjects ADDH children had smaller right frontal widths (more frontal symmetry than normals) 70% of normal and ADDH children demonstrated L > R plana asymmetry, while only 10% of dyslexic subjects did; plana symmetry or reversed asymmetry seems characteristic of dyslexia
Semrud-Clikeman et al. (1991)	MRI	Same as Hynd et al. (1990)	Same as Hynd et al. (1990)	NR	Frontal width symmetry/reversed asymmetry (L ≥ R) associated with very significant delay in word attack skills Symmetry/reversed asymmetry of plana associated with poor confrontational naming, rapid naming, and passage comprehension
Leonard et al. (1993)	MRI	9 dyslexic subjects 10 relatives 11 controls	15–65 6–63 14–52	Primarily by clinical report and history	Dyslexic subjects had exaggerated left plana asymmetry for the temporal band and right asymmetry for the parietal bank Higher incidence of cerebral anomalies bilaterally

Modified from Hynd and Semrud-Clikeman (1989)

Key: ADDH, attention-deficit hyperactivity disorder; NR, not reported.

[a] LeMay (1981) used all subjects of Hier et al. (1978) adding three of her own in addition to the controls.

[b] Semrud-Clikeman et al. (1991) employed these subjects to examine the relationship between deviations in patterns of brain morphology and neurolinguistic ability in developmental dyslexics.

Computed tomography (CT) and magnetic resonance imaging (MRI) were obviously technologic advances that could help researchers examine directly structure-function relations in living humans. CT, of course, is considered an invasive procedure as there is some limited exposure to radiation, whereas with MRI scans there are no known risk factors. Until MRI became more readily available, CT was the method employed to examine deviations in normal patters of asymmetry in the brains of reading-disabled children and adults. CT studies typically employed a scan between 0 and 25 degrees above the acanthomedial line to examine for posterior asymmetries. With the increased sophistication of MRI scanning procedures it became possible to obtain thinner slices and extreme lateral sagittal scans were used to examine sulcul topography as well. Most scanning facilities now have the capability to obtain three-dimensional volumetric scan data so that later reconstructions can be made on any plane desired. These technological advances have been accompanied by very significant methodologic challenges with regard to head positioning, using a standardized grid system to normalize data acquisition across scans, and other difficulties in defining morphologic boundaries that may have functional significance. Nonetheless, these studies have been revealing and have encouraged increasing interest in using brain-imaging procedures to investigate many issues important to the study of lateralized functioning.

As can be seen in table 20.1, 11 studies using either CT or MRI have been conducted to examine whether or not deviations in normal patterns of asymmetry in brain morphology are associated with the manifestation of reading disabilities. The first such study was reported by Hier and colleagues (1978) who employed CT to investigate posterior asymmetries in 24 dyslexic subjects. They found that only 33% of the dyslexic group had a wider left posterior region while 67% had either symmetry or reversed asymmetry of the posterior region. Since fully 66% of the normal population is expected to show the expected L > R asymmetry, this lower incidence among the dyslexic group was taken as support for Geschwind's (1974) idea that patterns of asymmetry were meaningfully associated with linguistic functioning.

In a further study, Rosenberger and Hier (1980) found that a brain asymmetry index correlated with verbal performance intelligence quotient (IQ) discrepancies, whereas lower verbal IQ was correlated with symmetry or reversed asymmetry in the posterior region in the dyslexic subjects. This study actually was the first to examine whether there was any psychometric or behavioral relationship between asymmetry patterns and performance. In this respect this study was unique and an entire decade elapsed before several new studies also examined behavioral relationships to brain morphology data. Thus, most of the early literature was characterized by examining the rather straightforward issue as to whether there was any deviation from normal patterns of brain asymmetry in subjects with severe reading disability.

In 1981, Haslam et al. found in their sample of dyslexic subjects that 46% had L > R asymmetry similar to the normals, but in contrast to Rosenberger and Hier (1980), no relationship was found with regard to verbal ability. As Hynd and Semrud-Clikeman (1989) have pointed out, however, the criteria employed by Haslam et al. for defining language delay were less strict than in the Rosenberger and Hier study. Nonetheless, Haslam et al. (1981) did note that fewer dyslexic subjects had the normal L > R posterior asymmetry.

The mid-1980s marked a time of transition in that fewer CT studies were reported with increasingly more studies employing MRI procedures as MRI scanners became more available to the research community. In fact, the last CT study reported was by Parkins et al. (1987) who found that there existed some relationship of handedness to deviations from normal patterns of asymmetry by dyslexic subjects. They found in their older adult sample (mean age, 57 years) that symmetry of the posterior region was characteristic only in the left-handed dyslexic subjects. The results of this study are unusual because previously and in the studies to follow, handedness may have differentiated the normal from the severely reading-disabled sample, but no relationship was ever reported with handedness. The mean age of this sample is also unusual as these were reading-disabled adults who may represent an unusual part of the reading disability spectrum in that their reading disability persisted to such a severe degree well into advanced adulthood. Most other studies typically employed subjects in early adolescence through young adulthood.

The first reported MRI study was reported in 1986 by Rumsey et al. who found in their brief report that 90% of the dyslexic subjects showed evidence of posterior asymmetry. In a sense, this study was typical of the rather unsophisticated methodology that characterized the studies at that time in that determination of asymmetry, symmetry, and reversed asymmetry of the posterior region most often relied on the clinical judgment of a radiologist or other expert in reading scans. Rarely were data presented as to the morphometric measurements that were obtained, if any, and for this reason it was difficult to compare results across studies. About the only conclusion that could reasonably be advanced was that deviations in normal patterns of posterior asymmetry may be found more frequently in the brains of severe reading-disabled persons. Based entirely on the Rosenberger and Hier (1980) study, there was limited but tantalizing evidence that symmetry or reversed asymmetry may somehow be associated with poor verbal-linguistic ability as is often found in dyslexic children.

To this point most studies had focused on posterior asymmetries, but theory had continued to emphasize the region of the planum temporale as being vitally important in verbal-linguistic processes, particularly phonological coding. In fact, Galaburda et al. (1985) summarized their four consecutive autopsy cases and reported that the focal dysplasias clustered preferentially in the left superior posterior temporal region by a ratio of 11 : 1. Thus, there was good reason to shift the attention of researchers away from simple posterior asymmetries toward attempts at measuring asymmetry of the region of the planum temporale. The focal dysplasias, Galaburda and colleagues reported, certainly could not be visualized on MRI scans, but different method could be employed in attempting to measure either the area or length of this region bilaterally in the brains of persons with dyslexia.

Two studies employed different methodologies aimed at investigating asymmetries in the region of the planum temporale in dyslexic persons. Using MRI to examine the size and patterns of asymmetry in this region in adolescents with dyslexia, Larsen, and colleagues (1990) found that 70% of their dyslexic group had symmetry in the region of the plana in contrast to 30% of the normals. In addition to the importance of this finding, Larsen et al. also found that when symmetry of the plana was present in dyslexia, the subjects demonstrated phonological deficits. They concluded that some relationship may exist between brain morphology patterns and neurolinguistic process, consistent with Rosenberger and Hier's (1980) conclusions.

That same year, Hynd et al. (1990) also reported a study employing MRI in which the relative specificity of patterns of plana morphology were investigated in relation to a population of normal controls and clinic control children. In this case the clinic control group comprised children with attention-deficit hyperactivity disorder (ADDH). For this reason, the study was unique in that of all studies reported previously, none had included a clinic contrast group but rather compared dyslexic subjects only with normal controls. While such an approach has value in determining whether a line of investigation might be productive, the results only suggested differences from normals. There was no way to address the specificity of deviations in brain morphology in relation to the behavioral deficits seen in any one clinical syndrome such as reading. Based on the previous literature, it was hypothesized that if differences existed in the brains of the dyslexic children in the region of the plana, similar differences would not be evident in the brains of the ADDH children who were carefully diagnosed so that this group did not include children with reading or learning disabilities.

Similar to Larsen et al. (1990), Hynd, et al. (1990) found that the dyslexic group was characterized by either symmetry or reversed asymmetry ($L < R$) of the plana. Underscoring the importance of this region scientifically, they found that in 70% of the normals *and* ADDH children, $L > R$ plana asymmetry existed. This is what would be expected according to the normative data provided originally by Geschwind and Levitsky (1968). Fully 90% of the dyslexic children demonstrated symmetry or reversed asymmetry of the plana. In a follow-up study, Semrud-Clikeman and colleagues (1991) reported that symmetry and reversed asymmetry of the planum temporale was associated with significant deficits in confrontational naming, rapid naming, and neurolinguistic processes in general.

If one compares the Larsen et al. (1990) and Hynd et al. (1990) studies, differences seem evident in the way in which the plana were measured. Hynd et al. (1990) measured the length of the plana on extreme lateral sagittal MRI scans. Larsen et al. (1990), however, took measurements from sequential scans so that a measurement of area could be derived. Both studies found that significant indices of symmetry or reversed asymmetry characterized the brains of dyslexic children even though different methodologies were employed. A point to derive from this discussion is that there are no agreed-upon standardized methodologies, although the method employed by Larsen et al. (1990) most likely provides more reliable data. Further, in examining the literature regarding the neuroanatomic morphology of the plana, one quickly realizes that there may be different sulcul patterns associated with whether or not a parietal bank of the planum temporale exists.

In the most recent study, reported by Leonard et al. (1993), the morphology of the posterior superior temporal region was examined bilaterally including the relative contribution of the temporal and parietal banks to an asymmetry index. The results of this study are particularly revealing in several ways. First, it turns out that nearly all dyslexic subjects and normals demonstrated a natural leftward asymmetry in the temporal bank and a rightward asymmetry in the parietal bank. When they examined intrahemispheric asymmetry, some dyslexic subjects had an anomalous intrahemispheric asymmetry between the temporal and planar banks in the right hemisphere because of an increased proportion of the plana being in the parietal bank. What this suggests is that consideration in future studies must be given to measuring both the temporal and parietal banks of the planum temporale and the relative contribution of both banks bilaterally in deriving asymmetry indexes. To quickly illustrate this issue the reader may wish to refer to figure 20.3 which illustrates the typical fashion in which the plana were described in the literature. By looking at the figure at the top where the slice location is noted, one can see at the end of the sylvian fissure where the slice line cuts horizontally that there is a small ascending ramus that is actually part of the planum. By not including this parietal aspect in lateral measures of asymmetry, the Larsen et al. (1990) and Hynd et al. (1990) studies were incomplete, although at the time they were published they were excellent studies. Finally, the Leonard et al. (1993) study documented that the dyslexic persons were more likely to evidence anomalies such as missing or duplicated gyri bilaterally in the region of the posterior end of the lateral fissure. These cerebral anomalies most likely evolve somewhere between the 24 and 30th week of fetal gestation when gyration occurs and represent a neurodevelopmental anomaly possibly related to a genetic etiology. Figure 20.4 presents sample MRI scans from the Leonard et al. (1993) study showing the anomalous cortex in the dyslexic subjects.

What does this evolving literature suggest about cerebral morphology and lateralized function in reading-disabled or dyslexic children? First, it suggests that asymmetry may indeed be characteristic of most normal brains. Second, in the region of the planum temporale there may be an increased incidence of symmetry or reversed asymmetry if one only measures the temporal bank. If one measures the bilateral temporal and parietal banks in the dyslexic group one may actually end up with these persons having more leftward asymmetry because of intrahemispheric variation in the right hemisphere, at least according to Leonard et al. (1993). As the Leonard et al. (1993) study clearly indicates,

CONTROLS

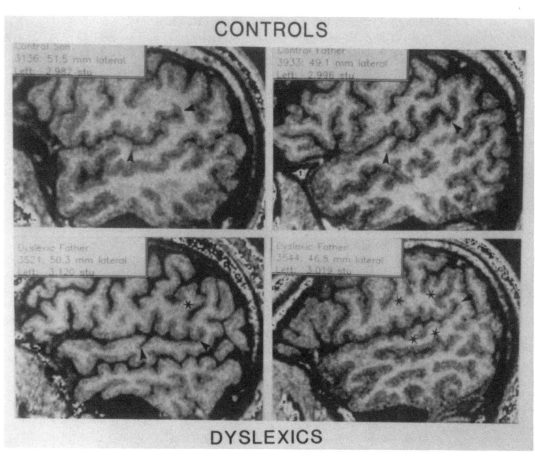

DYSLEXICS

Figure 20.4 Magnetic resonance image of two controls and two dyslexic subjects from the Leonard, et al. (1993) study. The controls have either the typical bifurcation (*left*) or an ascending parietal bank (*right*) that enters a clearly demarcated supramarginal gyrus. Arrowheads mark the borders of the temporal bank of the planum. The two dyslexic subjects have multiple primary sulci and extra gyri in the parietal operculum (stars) and/or multiple Heschl's gyri (stars in lower right), or all of these anomalies.

measuring highly variable brain regions in different subject groups is fraught with complications, and decisions that must be made in terms of what to measure can dramatically influence outcomes. Finally, as Rosenberger and Hier (1980) first suggested, there may indeed be relationships between deviations in brain morphology and neurolinguistic processes. The Larsen et al. (1990) and Semrud-Clikeman et al. (1991) studies provide further support for this important aspect of the theory advanced by Geschwind (1974, 1984).

UNANSWERED QUESTIONS AND FUTURE RESEARCH AGENDA

There should be little doubt that brain-imaging procedures offer much promise in investigating issues related to possible relationships between brain structure morphology and behavioral observations, whether these observations be clinical or experimental. What needs to be kept in mind, however, is that across all of these studies in which over 200 subjects have been scanned, not one brain of a reading-disabled subject was judged to be abnormal in structure (other than asymmetry patterns). In other words, no evidence of brain damage was found. This should underscore the important findings of Galaburda and colleagues (1985) who find developmental anomalies in the brains of dyslexic persons. The anomalous cortex identified by Leonard et al. (1993) provides further data implicating neurodevelopmental processes as underlying the behavioral symptomatology we see in dyslexia. It appears that reasonable evidence exists implicating unusual developmental processes sometime during the fifth to seventh month of fetal gestation in dyslexia. Clearly, the exact cause of these neurodevelopmental anomalies is one of the most important unanswered questions.

However, with regard to measures of brain asymmetry, it must be pointed out that if 65% of the normal population has L > R asymmetry in the region of the plana, then some 35% have some other pattern (L ≤ R) that does not seem to put them at risk for exclusion from the normal control population. That is, symmetry or reversed asymmetry is not sufficient to cause or predict deficient linguistic processes or dyslexia since some 35% of normals may likewise have brains with symmetry or reversed asymmetry of the plana.

There are two points to make in this regard. First, as Rosenberger and Hier (1980) suggested, symmetry or reversed asymmetry may not be a sufficient cause of reading or language problems but rather, in the context of a predisposition for language or reading difficulty (e.g., genetically at risk), symmetry or reversed asymmetry may act as an additional risk or potentiating factor. Second, to date no one has examined variability in brain morphology either with regard to asymmetry or sulcul patterns in normal persons for whom extensive neuropsychological, experimental, or behavioral data exist. It may well be that symmetry or less common sulcul topography is related to the significant variability we observe in the normal range of what would be considered individual differences. Investigating this issue should be a clear priority in future studies, especially since by using three-dimensional whole-brain acquisitions, reconstructions can be made in any plane and, if desired, volumetric data can be generated for any region. However, the value of volumetric data at present is questionable since functional, cytoarchitectural, and sulcul-lobe boundaries do not necessarily correlate well. Therefore, dividing the brain up into sections based on qualitative judgments may lead to unreliable and theoretically questionable results. One hopes, however, that future investigators will be able to address this issue in some fashion. For example, it is possible to obtain brain metabolic scans (e.g., positron emission tomography or single photon emission CT) and overlay MRI scans to identify more clearly areas or regions of increased metabolic activity in response to some cognitive task demands. One could then define the functional boundaries in the brain for certain tasks and use this topographically derived area as a starting point for examining how deviations in morphology (perhaps sulcul patterns) relate to levels and perhaps topographic distribution of functional activation. Integrating multiple sources of brain-imaging data with behavioral data should be a priority, especially in regard to answering some questions about hemispheric laterality.

While research aimed at better understanding the neurobiological basis of learning disabilities has shown significant progress over the past several decades, it is still not known with any certainty why focal deviations in the cellular architecture occur or how they relate to the deficient learning abilities in dyslexic children. Equally, those engaged in MRI work with dyslexic children still do not have a good idea as to how exactly deviations in patterns of expected brain morphology cause or relate to the linguistic deficits we observe in these children. In a rather discouraging sense we are left in the same position as those who inferred brain damage or dysfunction on the basis of psychometric tests; we infer that there is some meaningful relationship between deviations in asymmetry or morphology and learning disabilities. We seem to overlook the fact that these anomalies also occur, perhaps at a lower incidence for some anomalies, in the presumably normal population. This needs to be kept in mind as our enthusiasm grows, in hopes of eventually uncovering the invariably complex interactions that must exist between the morphology of the brain, its many neurotransmitter systems, and the behaviors we deem important enough to study.

REFERENCES

Bakker, D. J., and van der Vlugt, H. (Eds.) (1989). *Learning disabilities*, Vol 1. *Neuropsychological correlates and treatment.* Amsterdam: Swets & Zeitlinger.

Bastian, H. C. (1898). *A treatise on aphasia and other speech defects.* London: H. K. Lewis.

Benton, A. L. (1975). Developmental dyslexia: Neurological aspects. In W. J. Friedlander (Ed.), *Advances in neurology.* New York, NY: Raven Press.

Bryden, M. P., and Steenhuis, R. (1991). The assessment of handedness in children. In J. E. Obrzut and G. W. Hynd (Eds.), *Neuropsychological foundations of learning disabilities: A handbook of issues, methods, and practice* (pp 411–436). New York, NY: Academic Press.

Dejerine, J. (1892). Contribution à l'étude anatomopathologique et clinique des differentes variétés de cécité verbale. *Mémoires de la Societé de Biologie, 4,* 61–90.

Dejerine, J., and Dejerine-Klumpke, A. (1901). *Anatomie des centres nerveux,* Vol 2 (pp 109–114). Paris: Rueff et Cie.

Dejerine, J., and Vialet, P. (1893). Contribution à l'étude de la localisation anatomique de la cécité verbale pure. *Comptes rendus des Seánces de la Societé de Biologie, 45,* 790–793.

Duffy, F. H., Denckla, M. B., Bartels, P. H., Sandini, G., and Kiessling, L. S. (1980). Dyslexia: Automated diagnosis by computerized classification of brain electrical activity. *Annals of Neurology, 7,* 421–428.

Eidelberg, D., and Galaburda, A. M. (1982). Symmetry and asymmetry in the human posterior thalamus: I. Cytoarchitectonic analysis in normal persons. *Archives of Neurology, 39,* 325–332.

Eidelberg, D., and Galaburda, A. M. (1984). Inferior parietal lobule: Divergent architectonic asymmetries in the human brain. *Archives of Neurology, 41,* 843–852.

Falzi, G., Perrone, P., and Vignolo, L. A. (1982). Right-left asymmetry in anterior speech region. *Archives of Neurology, 39,* 239–240.

Flechsig, P. (1908). Bemerkungen über die Hemisphären des menschlichen Gehirns. *Neurologisches Zentralblatt, 27,* 50–57.

Fried, I., Tanguay, P. E., Boder, E., Doubleday, C., and Greensite, M. (1981). Developmental dyslexia: Electrophysiological evidence of clinical subgroups. *Brain and Language, 12,* 14–22.

Gaddes, W. H. (1985). *Learning disabilities and brain function: A neuropsychological approach,* ed 2. New York, NY: Springer-Verlag.

Galaburda, A. M., and Sanides, F. (1980). Cytoarchitectonic organization in the human auditory cortex. *Journal of Comparative Neurology, 190,* 597–610.

Galaburda, A. M., Sherman, G. F., Rosen, G. D., Aboitiz, F., and Geschwind, N. (1985). Developmental dyslexia: Four consecutive cases with cortical anomalies. *Annals of Neurology, 18,* 222–233.

Geschwind, N. (1974). The development of the brain and the evolution of language. In N. Geschwind (Ed.), *Selected papers on language and the brain* (pp 122–146). Dordrecht, Netherlands: D. Reidel.

Geschwind, N. (1984). Cerebral dominance in biological perspective. *Neuropsychologia, 22,* 675–683.

Geschwind, N., and Galaburda, A. M. (1985a). Cerebral lateralization: Biological mechanisms, associations, and pathology, I. A hypothesis and program for research. *Archives of Neurology, 42,* 428–459.

Geschwind, N., and Galaburda, A. M. (1985b). Cerebral lateralization: Biological mechanisms, associations, and pathology, II. A hypothesis and program for research. *Archives of Neurology, 42,* 521–552.

Geschwind, N., and Galaburda, A. M. (1985c). Cerebral lateralization: Biological mechanisms, associations, and pathology. III. A hypothesis and program for research. *Archives of Neurology, 42,* 634–654.

Geschwind, N., and Levitsky, W. (1968). Human brain: Left-right asymmetries in temporal speech region. *Science, 161,* 186–187.

Golden, G. S. (1982). Neurobiological correlates of learning disabilities. *Annals of Neurology, 12,* 409–418.

Haslam, R. H., Dalby, J. T., Johns, R. D., and Rademaker, A. W. (1981). Cerebral asymmetry in developmental dyslexia. *Archives of Neurology, 38,* 679–682.

Head, H. (1926). *Aphasia and kindred disorders of speech.* Cambridge, England: Cambridge University Press.

Hier, D. B., LeMay, M., Rosenberger, P. B., and Perlo, V. P. (1978). Developmental dyslexia: Evidence for a subgroup with a reversal of cerebral asymmetry. *Archives of Neurology, 35,* 90–92.

Hinshelwood, J. (1900). Word-blindness and visual memory. *Lancet, 2,* 1564–1570.

Hynd, G. W., and Semrud-Clikeman, M. (1989). Dyslexia and brain morphology. *Psychological Bulletin, 106,* 447–482.

Hynd, G. W., Semrud-Clikeman, M., Lorys, A. R., Novey, E., and Eliopulos, D. (1990). Brain morphology in developmental dyslexia and attention deficit disorder/hyperactivity. *Archives of Neurology, 47,* 919–926.

Hynd, G. W., and Willis, W. G. (1988). *Pediatric neuropsychology.* Needham Heights, MA: Allyn & Bacon.

Kershner, J., and Chyczij, M. (1992). Lateral preference in six to nine year old children: Relationships to language lateralization and cognitive ability. *Learning and Individual Differences, 4,* 347–367.

Kinsbourne, M., and Hiscock, M. (1981). Cerebral lateralization and cognitive development: Conceptual and methodological issues. In G. W. Hynd and J. E. Obrzut (Eds.), *Neuropsychological assessment and the school-age child* (pp 125–166). New York, NY: Grune & Stratton, Inc.

Kopp, N., Michel, F., Carrier, H., Biron, A., and Duvillard, P. (1977). Étude de certaines asymétries hémisphériques de cerveau humain. *Journal of the Neurological Sciences, 34,* 349–363.

Kussmaul, A. (1877). A disturbance of speech. *Cylopedia of Practical Medicine, 14,* 581–875.

Larsen, J. P., Hoien, T., Lundberg, I., and Odegaard, H. (1990). MRI evaluation of the size and symmetry of the planum temporal in adolescents with developmental dyslexia. *Brain and Language, 39,* 289–301.

Leisman, G., and Ashkenazi, M. (1980). Aetiological factors in dyslexia: IV. Cerebral hemispheres are functionally equivalent. *Neuroscience, 11,* 157–164.

LeMay, M. (1981). Are there radiological changes in the brains of individuals with dyslexia? *Bulletin of the Orton Society, 31,* 135–141.

Leonard, C. M., Voeller, K. K. S., Lombardino, L. J., Morris, M., Hynd, G. W., Alexander, A. W., Anderson, H. G., Garofalakis, M., Honeyman, J. C., Mao, J., Agee, O. F., and Staab, E. V. (1993). Anomalous cerebral morphology in dyslexia revealed with MR imaging. *Archives of Neurology, 50,* 461–469.

Liepmann, H. (1915). Diseases of the brain: Normal and pathological physiology of the brain. In C. W. Burr (Ed.), *Text-book on nervous disease* (pp 445–552). Philadelphia, PA: Blakiston.

Marie, P. (1906). Revision de la question de l'aphasie: La 3 circonvolution frontale gauche ne joue aucun rôle spécial dans la fonction du langage. *Semaine Médicale, 21* (May 23), 241–247.

Mayeux, R., and Kandel, E. R. (1985). Natural language, disorders of language, and other localizable disorders of cognitive functioning. In E. R. Kandel and J. H. Schwartz (Eds.), *Principles of neural science,* (ed. 2) (pp 688–703). New York, NY: Elsevier.

Molfese, D. L., and Molfese, V. J. (1986). Psychophysiological indices of early cognitive processes and their relationship to language. In J. E. Obrzut and G. W. Hynd (Eds.), *Child neuropsychology: Theory and practice.* Vol 1 (pp 95–115). New York, NY: Academic Press.

Morgan, W. P. (1896). A case of congenital word-blindness. *British Medical Journal, 2,* 1978.

Obrzut, J. E. (1991). Hemispheric activation and arousal asymmetry in learning disabled children. In J. E. Obrzut and G. W. Hynd (Eds.). *Neuropsychological foundations of learning disabilities: A handbook of issues, methods, and practice* (pp 179–198). New York, NY: Academic Press.

Obrzut, J. E., and Hynd, G. W. (Eds.) (1991). *Neuropsychological foundations of learning disabilities: A handbook of issues, methods, and practice.* New York, NY: Academic Press.

Orton, S. T. (1928). Specific reading disability—strephosymbolia. *Journal of the American Medical Association, 90,* 1095–1099.

Parkins, R., Roberts, R. J., Reinarz, S. J., and Varney, N. R. (1987). *Asymmetries in adult developmental dyslexics*. Paper presented at the annual convention of the International Neuropsychological Society, Washington, DC, January 1987.

Peters, J. E., Romine, J. S., and Dykman, R. A. (1975). A special neurological examination of children with learning disabilities. *Developmental Medicine and Child Neurology, 17*, 63–78.

Piacentini, J. C., and Hynd, G. W. (1988). Language after dominant hemispherectomy: Are plasticity of function and equipotentiality viable concepts? *Clinical Psychology Review, 8*, 595–609.

Reitan, R. M., and Boll, T. J. (1973). Neuropsychological correlates of minimal brain dysfunction. *Annals of the New York Academy of Sciences, 205*, 65–68.

Rosenberger, P. B., and Hier, D. B. (1980). Cerebral asymmetry and verbal intellectual deficits. *Annals of Neurology, 8*, 300–304.

Rubens, A. B., Mahuwold, M. W., and Hutton, J. T. (1976). Asymmetry of the lateral (sylvian) fissures in man. *Neurology, 26*, 620–624.

Rumsey, J. M., Dorwart, R., Vermess, M., Denckla, M. B., Kruest, M. J. P., and Rapoport, J. L. (1986). Magnetic resonance imaging of brain anatomy in severe developmental dyslexia. *Archives of Neurology, 43*, 1045–1046.

Satz, P. (1991). The Dejerine hypothesis: Implications for an etiological reformulation of developmental dyslexia. In J. E. Obrzut and G. W. Hynd (Eds.), *Neuropsychological foundations of learning disabilities: A handbook of issues, methods, and practice* (pp 99–112). New York, NY: Academic Press.

Semrud-Clikeman, M., Hynd, G. W., Novey, E., and Eliopulos, D. (1991). Dyslexia and brain morphology: Relationships between neuroanatomical variation and neurolinguistic performance. *Learning and Individual Differences, 3*, 225–242.

Taylor, H. G., and Fletcher, J. M. (1983). Biological foundations of "specific developmental disorders": Methods, findings, and future directions. *Journal of Clinical Child Psychology, 12*, 46–65.

Von Economo, C. and Horn, L. (1930). *Zeitschrift für die gesamte Neurologie und Psychiatrie, 130*, 678.

Wada, J. A., Clarke, R., and Hamm, A. (1975). Cerebral hemispheric asymmetry in humans. *Archives of Neurology, 32*, 239–246.

Weinberger, D. R., Luchins, D. J., Morihisa, J., and Wyatt, R. J. (1982). Asymmetrical volumes of the right and left frontal and occipital regions of the human brain. *Neurology, 11*, 97–100.

Wernicke, C. (1910). The symptom-complex of aphasia. In A. Church (Ed.), *Modern clinical medicine: Diseases of the nervous system* (pp 265–324). New York, NY: D. Appleton & Co.

Witelson, S. F., and Pallie, W. (1973). Left hemisphere specialization for language in the newborn. *Brain, 96*, 641–646.

Wyngaarden, J. E. (1987). *Learning disabilities: A report to the Congress*. Washington, DC: National Institutes of Health, Interagency Committee on Learning Disabilities.

Yule, W., and Rutter, M. (1976). Epidemiology and social implications of specific reading retardation. In R. M. Knights and D. J. Bakker (Eds.), *The neuropsychology of learning disorders: Theoretical approaches*. Baltimore, MD: University Park Press.

21 Perceptual Laterality in Developmental Learning Disabilities

Carol A. Boliek and John E. Obrzut

There exists a group of children who exhibit significant deficiencies performing tasks that require semantic-linguistic or visuospatial skills, or both. Characteristics of children with developmental learning disabilities have been well documented over the past several decades and have often been compared to adult patients with known brain lesions. General observations of these children have been summarized by Hynd and Willis (1988) to include a congenital form of learning difficulty which has been demonstrated to affect more males than females. Also, whereas manifestations of this disability vary in terms of patterns and severity of deficits, habilitation by regular classroom educational methods has not proved effective. Finally, it has been hypothesized that the disorder may be related to a neurodevelopmental process primarily affecting the left hemisphere.

Over the years, researchers have studied various factors thought to be related to developmental learning disabilities and have done so from diverse theoretical orientations, levels of measurement, and with specific subpopulations of children suffering from this disorder. Our investigations have been designed to observe laterality performance in children who exhibit primarily auditory-linguistic impairment. This chapter is intended to integrate our observations and current working hypotheses into the broader neurobiological theory of developmental learning disabilities. We present some current data as well as outline a future research agenda which we think will advance our understanding of brain-behavior relationships in the auditory-linguistic subtype of learning disabilities.

ONTOGENY OF HEMISPHERIC SPECIALIZATION

In a recent paper by Satz, Strauss, and Whitaker (1990), the ontogeny of hemispheric specialization was reexamined. These authors presented compelling arguments encouraging laterality researchers to take a renewed look at two hypotheses that attempt to explain the ontogeny of hemispheric specialization. Specifically, *equipotentiality* and *progressive lateralization* hypotheses were reconceptualized within the context of Hughlings Jackson's three Cartesian coordinates used to explain the human nervous system. As interpreted by

Kinsbourne and Hiscock (1983), the vertical coordinate (y-axis) delineates a progression from the spinal cord to the neocortex, the lateral dimension (x-axis) is representative of left-right hemisphere differences in the cerebral cortex, and the z-axis represents an anteroposterior cerebral progression. Satz et al. (1990) and Satz (1991) argue that the term *equipotentiality* should not refer to bisymmetry of function but rather connote not only "the capacity of structures in the intact right hemisphere, but also the left hemisphere, to subserve speech and language functions after perturbations to the left hemisphere" (p. 600). The argument for conceptualizing equipotentiality in this manner comes from studies of aphasia which showed that lesions occurring prior to the age of 2 years result in speech reorganization in the contralateral hemisphere, whereas later-occurring lesions (after the age of 6 years) resulted in more instances of aphasia and speech arrest (Penfield and Roberts, 1959; Rassmussen and Milner, 1977; Satz et al., 1988). Satz et al. (1990) also suggest that the equipotentiality hypothesis addresses both interhemispheric and intrahemispheric reorganization.

Progressive lateralization has been traditionally defined as a function that is bilaterally represented initially but becomes localized to a specific hemisphere as the brain matures. Satz et al. (1990), however, support an alternative definition of progressive lateralization derived from Lurian theory (Luria, 1973) which states that lateralization of functions progress from primary cortical areas to secondary and tertiary areas as the child matures. According to Luria's theory, the brain consists of highly specialized cortical regions that are interconnected with other cortical and subcortical areas producing complex functional systems. Luria postulated that the brain was divided into three functional units: (1) the arousal unit, (2) the sensory receptive and integrative unit, and (3) the planning and organizational unit. The second and third units are organized into three hierarchic zones. The *primary zone* is responsible for sorting and recording incoming sensory information. The *secondary zone* organizes and codes information from the primary zone. The *tertiary zone* is where data are merged from multiple sources of input and collated as the basis for organizing complex behavioral responses. Luria's dynamic progression of lateralized function parallels Jackson's Cartesian coordinates with respect to progression of function from the brainstem to cortical regions (vertical), laterally (left hemisphere specialization for language functions), and implies anteroposterior progression (Satz et al., 1990). Based on anatomic (postmortem) and clinical aphasia studies, these authors suggested that whereas the left hemisphere is structurally preprogrammed for speech and language, the time when structures within the left hemisphere reach functional maturity is variable. The functional maturity concept therefore explains *sparing* and *recovery* of speech and other functions following early brain injury as a result of structures within the left and right hemispheres not reaching full maturity at the same time (Campbell and Whitaker, 1986; Satz, 1991; Satz et al., 1990).

Many researchers have traditionally accepted the *developmental invariance hypothesis* which describes hemispheric specialization as being preprogrammed early (perhaps prenatally) with functions of the left and right hemispheres remaining invariant throughout development (e.g., Kinsbourne and Hiscock, 1983; Witelson, 1977; Molfese and Molfese, 1979). Satz et al. (1990) have suggested that perhaps developmental invariance describes the lateral (x-axis) dimension of asymmetry, whereas their current formulation of equipotentiality and progressive lateralization hypotheses better describe vertical (subcortical-cortical) and horizontal (anteroposterior) progression during infancy and early childhood. Ironically, most laterality research has been conducted using paradigms that observe only left-right hemisphere differences as described by Jackson's lateral (x-axis) Cartesian coordinate. Most research designed to address laterality issues in developmental disabilities (i.e., learning disabilities) has not dealt systematically with subcortical-cortical development or anteroposterior progressions.

Models of Laterality in Relationship to Learning-disabled Children

Laterality hypotheses have been advanced primarily with data obtained from infants, children, and adults with known lesion sites. Developmental dysfunction of the same brain areas as described in acquired disorders (i.e., acquired aphasia) may be the basis of developmental learning disabilities (Dawson, 1988; Obrzut, 1991). However, as Isaacson (1975) cautions, when making comparisons between symptoms of an acquired neuropsychological syndrome and similar symptoms from an atypically developing brain, the underlying source may be very different.

As originally proposed by Orton (1937), it is now generally assumed that persons with learning disabilities have abnormal cerebral organization including atypical or weak patterns of hemispheric specialization (see reviews by Bryden, 1988; Corballis, 1983; Obrzut, 1988). Two competing hypotheses have been advanced to account for deficient hemispheric lateralization in learning-disabled populations. First, the *developmental lag hypothesis*, as proposed by Lenneberg (1967), suggests that learning-disabled persons are slower to develop language-based skills and demonstrate weak hemispheric specialization for language tasks. This hypothesis would predict that eventually, these developmental delays would be resolved. There is little empirical evidence, however, demonstrating that laterality changes with increasing age (Bryden, 1982; Bryden and Saxby, 1986; Obrzut et al., 1981). However, if one tested the Satz et al. (1990) reformulation of the progressive lateralization hypotheses, it may be found that subcortical-cortical and anteroposterior progressions have a differential developmental course with populations of learning-disabled children and adults compared to control subjects or those with acquired syndromes.

Since learning-disabled children exhibit deficient performance on a variety of tests presumed to measure perceptual laterality, and evidence of weak laterality has been found across various modalities (auditory, visual, tactile) as well as when two modalities are combined (i.e., verbal-manual tasks), it is likely these children experience *abnormal cerebral organization*, as suggested by Corballis (1983) and Obrzut (1988). The basic premise is that dysfunction in the structure of the central nervous system, either prenatally or during early postnatal development, results in atypical cerebral organization and associated functional specialization required for lateralized processing of both language and nonlanguage information. It is thought that cortical and subcortical dysfunction which results from aberrant patterns of activation or arousal (Obrzut, 1991), inter- and intrahemispheric transmission deficits, or inadequate resource allocation (Kershner, 1988), or any combination of these, may further compromise hemispheric specialization in learning-disabled populations. However, the abnormal cerebral organization hypothesis and related models of activation, transmission, and resource allocation must be viewed within a larger theoretical context. Doing so, will clarify further the precise nature of the presumed abnormality in cerebral organization and perhaps lead to a better understanding of developmental learning disabilities.

LEARNING DISABILITIES AND NEUROBIOLOGICAL THEORY

If there is focal insult to the left hemisphere prior to the age of 6 to 8 years, and effective sparing or recovery processes have occurred, there will be little or no evidence of speech, language, or reading deficit. However, if focal damage to the left hemisphere occurs after this period the result will likely be a speech-language type of neuropsychological syndrome (see review by Satz, 1991). Based on findings from acquired lesion studies of infants and young children, Satz (1990) postulated that developmental learning disabilities were the result of prenatal or early postnatal damage to both the left and right cerebral hemispheres. Bilateral damage during this time of morphogenesis would result in the prevention of hemispheric reorganization and sparing, leading to permanent forms of learning disabilities (Dennis and Whitaker, 1976; Kinsbourne and Hiscock, 1977, 1983; Satz, 1991).

Evidence of bilateral involvement has come from various in vivo studies that examine anatomic, physiologic, and neurochemical parameters of learning disabilities as well as in vitro studies such as the postmortem cytoarchtectonic studies conducted by Galaburda, Geschwind, and their colleagues (Galaburda, 1986; Galaburda and Eidelberg, 1982; Galaburda et al., 1985) and previously by Drake (1968). The results of these studies have indicated that neurodevelopmental abnormalities exist in the brains of developmentally dyslexic adults, perhaps due to deviations in the developing brain between the fifth and seventh gestational month. These postmortem studies indicated that not only were certain structures symmetric (e.g., the temporal plana) but abnormal cell migration and organization were found in both left and right regions of the anterior cortex and the left temporal cortex (Galaburda et al., 1985) as well as regions of the right temporal lobe (Drake, 1968). Hynd and Semrud-Clickman, in their 1989 review, began to link the postmortem findings described above with specifically impaired behaviors often observed in learning-disabled persons. For example, language-related impairments pertaining to issues of prosody and emotional aspects may be part of the functional-linguistic system featured by the right frontal and central perisylvian cortex.

Further neurobiological evidence of atypical cerebral organization in learning-disabled populations comes from in vivo studies including neuroimaging methods and electrophysiology measures (see reviews by Hynd and Semrud-Clikeman, 1989; Hynd, Semrud-Clikeman, and Lyytinen, 1991). Recent work using magnetic resonance imaging (MRI) by Plante and her colleagues (Plante, 1991; Plante, Swisher, and Vance, 1989; Plante et al., 1991) found symmetry and reversed asymmetry of the left-right parasylvian regions in a small sample of language-disabled children as well as in several of their siblings and biological parents. Another MRI study conducted by Hynd et al. (1990) examined three groups of children (dyslexic, attention-deficit hyperactivity disorder (ADDH), normal control children) and found the dyslexic group to have symmetric or reversed asymmetry of the plana length. Whereas 90% of the dyslexic group exhibited this pattern, only 30% of the ADDH group and normals showed this same pattern. These authors found that reversed or symmetric frontal regions were correlated with behavioral deficits in word attack skills but not passage comprehension. Further, Larsen et al. (1989) reported that 70% of their sample of adolescents with dyslexia compared to 30% of normals exhibited symmetric left-right plana temporale.

Other neuroimaging approaches have been used to examine brain organization in learning-disabled populations, including positron emission tomography (PET) and regional cerebral blood flow (rCBF). One such study using PET and a radioactive glucose tracer (rCMRGLu), found that during reading tasks, dyslexic subjects showed active bilateral participation of the insular cortex (Gross-Glenn et al., 1986). Recent rCBF studies also have indicated that recruitment of both left and right central and posterior cortical regions were observed in dyslexic subjects during the reading of a narrative text (Hynd et al., 1987; Huettner, Rosenthal, and Hynd, 1989).

Electrophysiologic studies have been conducted more extensively on various subgroups of learning-disabled populations and show promise as an approach to advancing our understanding of functional laterality in learning-disabled populations. For example, bilateral temporal indices in spontaneous electroencephalography (EEG) were indicated for a group of learning-disabled children (Morris, Obrzut, and Coulthard-Morris, 1989). Studies have been conducted on subgroups of learning-disabled persons using brain electrical activity mapping (BEAM), which is a form of a multivariate procedure used by Duffy and colleagues (Duffy et al., 1980, 1988). The findings from these studies provide support that learning-disabled children have dysfunction in cortical language zones, and patterns of disturbances may be related to specific subgroups of disabled readers. However, whereas these data provide insight into the neuroanatomic differences in learning-disabled persons, further replication of these investigations is warranted.

Harter (1991) reported differential visual evoked potentials to language stimuli by two groups of reading-disabled children. The results from his study suggested one subgroup with enhanced occipitoparietal involvement and the other with enhanced occipitotemporal involvement. In another study, Segalowitz, Wagner, and Menna (1992) used event-related potentials (ERPs) to examine hemispheric asymmetry for language, signal processing efficiency, hemisphericity, and frontally based attentional control in good vs. poor adolescent readers. The results of their study indicated that hemisphericity differences accounted for reading skill level only among good readers but that frontally generated attentional ERP (contingent negative variation) accounted for reading skill among poor readers. Whereas good readers demonstrated the expected ERP asymmetries, the poor readers did not. The authors suggested, however, that below some "crucial" reading threshold, frontal attentional skill may be a better predictor of reading disability, whereas above this threshold good reading is predicted by hemisphericity.

From the review above, studies using neuroimaging and electrophysiologic paradigms with learning-disabled populations have provided results that are in support of a neurobiological basis of developmental learning disorders. As these approaches become more refined, and researchers employ carefully diagnosed and clearly defined subgroups of learning-disabled persons, more meaningful comparisons across studies will be forthcoming. Innovative use of neuroimaging techniques will advance our knowledge of brain-behavior relationships as they specifically relate to learning disabilities.

Evidence derived from neurobiological studies, as well as data derived from our current investigations using behavioral paradigms, have led to the conclusion that for a large subset of learning-disabled children, atypical cerebral organization and unusual patterns of laterality, attention, and arousal may underlie deficits in auditory and visual, language, and nonlanguage information-processing abilities. In the following section we discuss preferred experimental approaches, the strengths and weaknesses of these methods, some current findings, and a future research agenda.

FUNCTIONAL LATERALITY AND LEARNING-DISABLED CHILDREN

Dichotic Listening Methods

We have found the most commonly used and valid behavioral technique for assessing auditory laterality is dichotic listening. The dichotic listening paradigm presumably measures how the brain processes linguistic and nonlinguistic auditory information (Obrzut, 1991). The premise in using performance patterns derived from dichotic listening paradigms with learning-disabled children is that inferences can be made regarding functional laterality and its relationship to deviant academic performance. Based on extensive reviews of behavioral measures of functional lateralization including handedness, dichotic listening, visual half-field, and dichhaptic techniques, Bryden (1988) and

Obrzut (1988) suggested that the most valid laterality measures for observing auditory receptive language and nonlanguage lateralization in learning-disabled children are *directed attention–dichotic listening* paradigms. Although free recall paradigms are most commonly used in this endeavor, directed attention dichotic studies control for the attentional bias on perceptual asymmetries.

The original theory is based on the notion that if linguistic stimuli are employed in a free recall dichotic listening paradigm, then one would expect a right ear advantage (REA) reflective of left hemisphere specialization for language processing in normally developing right-handed children. It was hypothesized by Kimura (1961, 1967) that this phenomenon is due to the following: (1) the prepotency of the contralateral pathways over ipsilateral pathways in the auditory system; (2) that when differentially activated, the left hemisphere is preprogrammed to selectively attend to the right side of space (i.e., the right ear); (3) ipsilateral perception is suppressed by contralateral input; and (4) input from the nondominant hemisphere must traverse the corpus callosum in order to be processed by the dominant cerebral hemisphere (Bradshaw and Nettleton, 1988). This conceptualization has primary relevance for examining cerebral organization in learning-disabled populations. However, other factors such as memory requirements, task difficulty, order of report, stimuli, and statistical manipulation can potentially have confounding effects on the magnitude and direction of ear advantage (see Hugdahl, 1988; Obrzut, 1991). We concern ourselves here with the issues of attention and arousal because they are perhaps the most intriguing factors known to interact with dichotic asymmetries in both normal and learning-disabled populations.

Issues of Selective Attention on Dichotic Listening Performance

The manipulation of attention and arousal in experimental dichotic listening paradigms has advanced our understanding of functional laterality and cerebral organization in learning disabled children (see Obrzut, 1991). In a free report paradigm, a subject may invoke various attending and memory strategies that could influence overall performance patterns. There have been several recent attempts to manipulate attention and levels of arousal in dichotic listening paradigms with normal children and adults. The signal detection procedure outlined by Hiscock and Decter (1988) requires the subject to listen for a single target that occurs randomly at either ear. Response patterns yield information that differentiates asymmetric sensitivity and asymmetric response bias. Earlier, Bryden, Munhall, and Allard (1983) employed an attentional paradigm where subjects were required to report from one ear over a block of trials in an effort to eliminate any natural attentional bias. However, the results indicated a persistent REA for both right- and left-directed conditions and more intrusions from the unattended right ear (RE) were noted. In contrast, Hugdahl and Andersson (1986) found that directing attention did have an effect on intrusions differentially for females and males and for adults and children.

Verbal cuing has been the most commonly used technique for manipulating attention in dichotic listening paradigms (see Obrzut, 1988). Data from these studies have found that verbal cuing prior to each trial will have a greater impact on ear report than cuing prior to a block of trials (Murray, Allard, and Bryden, 1988). These observations have led Mondor and Bryden (1991) to conclude that the timing between the prestimulus cue and stimulus presentation, as well as the type of cue used, may also have an effect on the ability to orient attention during dichotic listening tasks. Based on the visuo-spatial attention studies of Yantis and Jonides (1990) and Muller and Rabbit (1989), Mondor and Bryden (1991) designed a study to advance the notion that a *pull cue* (one which is automatically processed) may be better at capturing attention than a *push cue* (one which requires a voluntary action by the subject such as verbal cuing). In one study they used a right and left visual field letter identification task and a lexical decision task, and employed a pull cue (a cue presented in a location approximate to where the proceeding stimuli will appear) to orient attention. In addition, the onset of the cue and the onset of the stimulus (stimulus onset asynchrony, SOA) were also manipulated. The results indicated that a right visual field (RVF) advantage for both tasks was apparent at short SOAs, but was eliminated at longer SOAs. The authors concluded that given sufficient opportunity to focus attention, stimuli presented to the "nondominant" side of space can be processed as well as when presented to the "dominant" side of space.

Based on the results of their visual half-field study, Mondor and Bryden (1991) designed a parallel study using a pull cue within a dichotic listening consonant-vowel (CV) paradigm. The idea was that when one is verbally directed to attend to the right or left ear, this direction must be voluntarily acted upon (push cue), whereas if a cue were presented in the same ear just prior to the stimulus event, then attention is automatically captured in that direction. A tone cue was used and as with the visual field experiment, SOAs were varied. The results indicated that sizeable REAs were apparent at the shortest SOA (150 ms) but were significantly attenuated at longer SOA intervals (450 and 750 ms). The SOAs were also found to have a much larger effect of left ear (LE) compared to RE reporting. The authors concluded that a pull cue was effective in orienting attention and perhaps provided a better estimation of attentional effects on the dichotic asymmetries. The overall findings of this study also suggested that there is an attentional bias to the RE for language processing.

The above studies have shown that directed attention conditions have been employed successfully to control for the effects of individual attention strategies. Directed attention paradigms have also been widely employed with learning-disabled children and have demonstrated lateralized performance differences between these children and control children (e.g., Boliek, Obrzut, and Shaw, 1988; Hugdahl and Andersson, 1987; Kershner and Micallef, 1992; Obrzut, Hynd, and Obrzut, 1983). In addition, directed attention performances have been shown to differ among other anomalous groups such as left-handed and bilingual children (Obrzut, Conrad, and Boliek, 1989; Obrzut et al., 1988).

There is now a reasonably large number of studies that have examined patterns of laterality in learning-disabled children and adults using some form of behavioral task such as dichotic listening, visual half-field, and tactual dich-haptic paradigms. Bryden (1988) reviewed 51 such studies and found that 30 of those studies indicated that learning-disabled children (poor readers) were less lateralized than normal readers. There is also now a sufficient number of studies that have employed some specific form of controlled attention in dichotic listening paradigms with learning-disabled children to systematically examine performance patterns from various laboratories. The following is a summary of the general trends found in a meta-analysis related to selective attention, handedness, and functional laterality in learning-disabled children.

Selective Attention and Laterality Issues in Handedness and Reading Ability: A Meta-Analysis

A meta-analysis was used to synthesize data regarding the influence of selective attention, handedness, and reading ability on the REA in dichotic listening (Obrzut, Bryden, and Boliek, 1992). One of the most frequent reasons for failure to replicate handedness and reading ability effects on dichotic outcome has been inadequate statistical power, due mainly to small sample sizes or to a limited amount of dichotic trials. As a result, each data set is certain to have low reliability and any difference in asymmetry would tend to be lost in random noise. The specific research question asked was: What is the influence of selective attention on dichotic listening relative to the variables of age, reading ability, and handedness?

Based on meta-analysis formulation (Glass, 1976; Kavale, 1988) our research domain was defined as follows: (1) subjects ranged in age from 6.0 to 12.11 years; (2) intelligence levels had to be above 85 on a standardized test of intelligence; (3) stimuli were male-voiced, synthesized CV syllables; (4) reading achievement rated as good or poor based on standard reading achievement measures or reading error analyses; (5) handedness rated as left- or right-handed based on a handedness index; and (6) dichotic conditions that had a free report condition or directed left and directed right conditions. As can be seen in table 21.1, a total of 15 studies met the above research criteria (14 published and 1 submitted for publication).

Coding of the data involved converting all means and standard deviations to percent correct report for LE and RE scores across groups and conditions. Individual studies ranged from 12 to 96 subjects with a total of 953 children across reading group, age, handedness, and dichotic condition. Effect sizes (ES) were computed on RE-LE for dichotic conditions (free recall, directed left, directed right), by Reader Group (good, poor), Age (younger, older), and Handedness (left, right). The statistical aggregation of results involved taking the mean ES with calculated standard deviations for RE-LE for each variable

Table 21.1 Studies included in the meta-analysis and their respective criteria characteristics

Study	n	Subject groupings	Age (yr)	Gender	Stimulus conditions	Handedness
Boliek et al. (1988)	50	25 average readers 25 poor readers	6–13 7–13	M & F	Free recall, Directed left and right	Right
Hugdahl and Andersson (1986)	36	Average readers	8–9	M & F	Free recall, Directed left and right	Right
Hugdahl and Andersson (1987)	60	20 good readers 20 average readers 20 poor readers	8–9	M & F	Free recall, Directed left and right	Right
Hugdahl et al. (1990)	48	Average readers	7	M & F	Free recall, Directed left and right	Right and left
Hynd and Obrzut (1977)	40	Average readers	6–12	M & F	Free recall	Right
Hynd et al. (1979)	96	48 good readers 48 poor readers	7–11	M & F	Free recall	Right
Kershner and Micallef (1992)	90	60 average readers 30 poor readers	7–12	Males	Free recall Directed left and right	Right
Morton and Siegel (1991)	80	40 average readers 40 poor readers	8–10	Males	Directed left and right	Right
Obrzut et al. (in press)	96	48 average readers 48 poor readers	6–12	M & F	Free recall	Right
Obrzut et al. (1986)	12	Average readers	9–12	M & F	Free recall, Directed left and right	Right
Obrzut et al. (1989)	60	30 average readers 30 poor readers	7–12	M & F	Free recall, Directed left and right	Right and left

Table 21.1 (cont.)

Study	n	Subject groupings	Age (yr)	Gender	Stimulus conditions	Handedness
Obrzut et al. (1988)	45	30 average readers 15 poor readers	6–13	M & F	Free recall, Directed left and right	Right and left
Obrzut et al. (1980)	96	48 average readers 48 poor readers	7–12	M & F	Free recall	Right
Obrzut et al. (1981)	64	32 average readers 32 poor readers	7–13	M & F	Free recall, Directed left and right	Right
Obrzut et al. (1985)	32	16 average readers 16 poor readers	7–12	M & F	Free recall, Directed left and right	Right

and conducting follow-up one-sample *t*-tests (significance from zero) on the mean ES for each variable.

In the *free recall* condition, Age × Reader Group comparisons revealed that all groups of children demonstrated an REA except the younger poor readers. With age collapsed for the Handedness × Reader Group comparisons, right-handed good and poor readers demonstrated an REA, whereas left-handed good readers had no ear advantage (NEA). Left-handed poor readers demonstrated an LEA in the free recall condition. In the *directed left* condition, Age × Reader Group comparisons indicated that both reader groups and age groups exhibited NEA. However, when age was collapsed for the Handedness × Reader Group comparisons, right-handed good readers demonstrated an REA, left-handed good readers and right-handed poor readers demonstrated NEA, whereas left-handed poor readers exhibited an LEA. In the *directed right* condition, both younger and older good and poor reading groups demonstrated an REA. When collapsed by age, it was found that right-handed good and poor readers had an REA whereas left-handed good and poor readers had NEA.

Based on this meta-analysis it is clear that there is an interaction among handedness, age, and reading ability on auditory verbal dichotic tasks. Further, it is apparent that attentional manipulation differentially affects ear report among these groups. Younger and older good readers and older poor readers shift attention in the directed left condition, whereas younger poor readers shift attention in the directed right condition. When age is combined, left- and right-handed *good readers* do not shift attention in either directed condition. In contrast, when age is combined, left- and right-handed *poor readers* shift attention in the directed conditions but in a reversed direction from one another. The lack of attentional shifting for left- and right-handed good readers supports a structural theory of lateralization, whereas the degree and direction of attentional shifting for left- and right-handed poor readers is suggestive of interhemispheric transfer difficulties and atypical cerebral organization.

Current Research

In an effort to further understand the construct of selective attention as it relates to perceptual asymmetries in learning-disabled children, Obrzut, Mondor, and Uecker (1992) designed a study using the paradigm developed by Mondor and Bryden (1991). The basic premise was that the tone (pull) cue may more effectively capture attention than the verbal instructions used in prior directed attention dichotic tasks. The authors predicted that for normal control children, the magnitude of the REA would be reduced as the time available to orient attention increased. Learning-disabled children were also expected to show a change in the magnitude of the REA with varying SOAs, but that the rate of that change would be deviant from controls. A total of 51 (34 control, 17 learning-disabled) children (6–12 years of age) participated in the study. All subjects were right handed and had average to above-average intelligence quotients (IQs). The learning-disabled children all demonstrated a significant disability in the area of reading and related language skills. Identical to the procedures used by Mondor and Bryden (1991), a tone was presented to either one ear or the other prior to every dichotic CV trial. SOAs were presented at 150, 450, and 750 ms.

For the control children, the results confirmed that the REA for verbal discriminations obtained in standard dichotic listening experiments is quite dependent on attentional processes. There was a tendency by both groups to more often report the item from the unattended RE than from the unattended LE, which indicated an attentional bias toward the RE. In addition, a subgroup of mixed learning-disabled and control children had difficulty performing the dichotic task at above-chance levels because they were unable to effectively orient attention to the cue. Perhaps their inability to effectively orient attention is related either to an underlying atypically organized functional (or structural) system or to a lack of motivation. Interestingly, the learning-disabled subjects who could perform the task identified the "to-be-attended" and "to-be-unattended" items equally often, which may be indicative of children who experience selective attention deficits but whose performance tends to fluctuate depending on task involvement.

Although the authors concluded that the data from this study support the hypothesis that auditory perceptual asymmetries in children are the result of the interaction of hemispheric capability and attentional factors, it was not decisively shown that the tone cue was more effective than verbal cuing for orienting attention in children with learning disabilities. Additional studies need to be designed and conducted to further define the role of attention on dichotic performance in control and learning-disabled children. It remains unclear whether inadequate attentional systems are a symptom of atypical cerebral organization, perhaps involving dysfunctional frontal regions as indicated by electrophysiologic and neuroimaging studies, or a function of weak hemispheric specialization in developmental learning-disabled children.

Studies such as those discussed above have led others to formulate more specific models of maladaptive lateralization. For example, Kershner and Morton (1990) have described four models of maladaptive laterality and predicted related dichotic listening response patterns. These models include: (1) poor structural lateralization (PSL), (2) right hemisphere excessive activation (RHA), (3) left hemisphere excessive activation (LHA), and (4) bidirectional excessive hemisphere activation (BHA). In his review of these four models, Obrzut (1991) pointed out that:

Regardless of the particular model one subscribes to, the results [data from studies with learning-disabled populations] support the view that, in contrast to a fixed laterality deficit, learning-disabled children experience an attentional dysfunction which interferes with left-hemisphere language processing by overengaging either hemisphere. In addition, pronounced asymmetry in the relative magnitude of the ear effects at each channel also suggests greater interference in learning-disabled children between the systems controlling auditory-linguistic attention and lateral orienting. (p. 191)

There is no doubt, many more questions about attention and perceptual asymmetries exist for both normally developing and learning-disabled children. Further, we know less about listening asymmetries in relation to right hemisphere functioning in learning-disabled children. For example, Witelson (1977) reported that there were learning-disabled–normal differences in right hemisphere function as assessed by dichhaptic tests, and suggested that the difficulty for learning-disabled children lay not in the representation of language in the left hemisphere but in the crowding of left hemisphere functions by spatial functions that would normally be executed by the right hemisphere. It has been further postulated that associations among learning disorders, immune disorders, and non-right-handedness may be due to prenatal testosterone acting independently of the developing thymus and brain and this prenatal exposure to excess testosterone results in delayed growth in the left hemisphere with likely concomitant right hemisphere deficiency (Geshwind and Galaburda, 1985a,b).

To assess the relationship between left- and right-hemisphere processing, left- and right-handed good readers and poor readers were given both CVs and nonverbal (tonal) dichotic listening tasks (Obrzut et al.,1989). These data suggested that right hemisphere processing was generally unaffected by left hemisphere dysfunction and neither handedness nor attentional manipulation was found to affect such processing for any of the groups. The authors hypothesized that the source of the reading-disabled child's difficulties may be primarily due to the inability of either the left or right hemisphere to assume a dominant role in the processing of verbal information.

A more recent study (Obrzut et al., 1994), has further examined left and right hemisphere tasks among control and learning-disabled males and females at three different age levels. It was hypothesized that learning-disabled children may be less lateralized for both linguistic and nonlinguistic tasks. A total of 82 (44 control, 38 learning-disabled) male and female children (ages 6–12 years) participated in the study. These children were further subdivided into younger, intermediate, and older age groups. All subjects were right-handed and demonstrated average to above-average performance on IQ measures from standardized tests. The learning-disabled children demonstrated a significant disability in the auditory-linguistic domain resulting in significantly deviant reading and related language skills. The traditional dichotic listening CVs were presented to each child. In addition, each child was administered a tone task originally developed by Sidtis (1981). For each type of tone stimulus (simple tone, complex tone) a dichotic probe stimulus technique was employed where half the probes were the same as one member of the dichotic pair (distributed randomly and equally to each channel), and half were different. The data indicated that control children demonstrated the expected hemisphere shift in laterality which appears to be related to stimulus characteristics (REA for CVs and LEA for tones). However, learning-disabled children exhibited a general processing bias to the same hemisphere (left hemisphere for some subjects, right hemisphere for others) regardless of stimulus characteristics. Consequently, it could be implied that doing both verbal and nonverbal processing with the same hemisphere is deleterious, and that persons who do so are likely to show deficits in cognitive processing and are apt to be labeled as learning-disabled.

To summarize, the nature of learning disabilities presents us with a heterogeneous population. As a consequence, subject selection and clear subject description has made cross-study comparisons difficult (see reviews by Obrzut, 1988, 1991). Perhaps some clear universals for learning-disabled subtypes could be formally proposed and outlined by those working with this population. Moreover, there exists a persistent disadvantage with regard to linking listening asymmetries with theoretical models. For example, data from dichotic listening studies have clearly demonstrated differences between learning-disabled and nondisabled children, essentially in the lateral (left-right hemisphere) plane as proposed by Jackson and described in the beginning of this chapter. However, it is difficult, if not impossible, to test whether observed differences in laterality and attention are due to anomalies in subcortical-cortical or anteroposterior progressions as described by Satz et al. (1990). With the rapid technological advances in neuroimaging, we may soon have the capability to superimpose neurometabolic (PET) images on structural (MRI) images which may begin to show us how deviations in structure relate to functional disturbances. Neuroanatomic data can then be correlated with behavioral paradigms such as dichotic listening to reveal in-depth analyses of atypically functioning information-processing systems.

FUTURE LATERALITY STUDIES AND LEARNING-DISABLED CHILDREN

Probably the direction of study with the highest priority will involve the continued advancement of neurobiological correlates of developmental learning disabilities. As progress is made in neuroimaging technologies like MRI, PET, single positron emission computed tomography (SPECT), and BEAM, more precise measurements of brain-behavior phenomena can be conducted. However, as Hynd, et al. (1991) point out, neuroimaging data that differentiate learning-disabled from other anomalous groups are only relevant if they can advance theory and promote our understanding of etiologic factors in this population.

The advancement of genetic theories holds promise in uncovering etiologic information in children with learning disabilities. Several such genetic studies are currently underway including the Colorado Reading Project (DeFries, 1985; DeFries, Fulker, and LaBuda, 1987) and molecular genetic studies (e.g., Smith et al., 1983). DeFries and Gillis (1991) have provided evidence through twin studies conducted as a part of the Colorado Reading Project, that individual differences in reading attainment are highly heritable. Data derived from molecular genetics indicate clear evidence of genetic linkage to various manifestations of learning disabilities (see review by Lubs et al., 1991).

In addition to scientific advances in neuroimaging and genetic endeavors, innovative developments will continue to occur using behavioral measures with learning-disabled children. The studies presented below represent examples of the types of innovations in research designs that are expected to contribute to our knowledge of brain-behavior relationships in children with developmental learning disabilities.

Existing studies have contrasted laterality performance patterns in anomalous groups of children such as males and females, developmental cross sections, left- and right-handed subjects, good and poor readers, monolingual and bilingual populations (Obrzut et al., 1988, 1989, 1992). However, in order to further understand similarities and differences between developmental disorders and acquired neuropsychological disorders, studies need to be conducted that contrast developmental learning disorders to disorders related to specific acquired lesions. For example, one such study conducted by Cohen, Hynd, and Hugdahl (1992) contrasted three subtypes of children with reading disabilities to a clinical group of children with left temporal lobe brain tumors. Dichotic listening performances yielded observable laterality differences among dyslexic subgroups and between children with acquired left temporal lesions. Future studies such as these should include contrasts between learning-disabled children and other types of acquired cortical and subcortical injuries.

In order to further our understanding of cerebral organization in children with learning disabilities, it will be beneficial to continue to pursue the various factors affecting dichotic listening performance. For example, Tallal and Stark (1981), and Cohen and colleagues (1991) have designed studies to examine the relationship between temporal and spectral characterisics of speech and nonspeech material and dichotic listening performance.

Finally, we have become increasingly aware of the relationship between learning disabilities and social skill development. It is likely that children with concomitant learning and social deficits constitute a group of children with "nonverbal" learning disabilities (Semrud-Clikeman and Hynd, 1990). Johnson and Myklebust (1971) first described this disorder as the inability to process environmental cues including those used in communication (gestures, facial expressions, vocal intonation). These children often have difficulties in processing other (noncommunicative) information such as visuospatial skills and certain types of arithmetic problems. Whereas children with these types of deficits have been identified in the subtype literature (e.g., Rourke and Fisk, 1981; Voeller, 1986), little is known about their patterns of performance on laterality measures. Hynd and Semrud-Clikeman (1989) have implicated thalamic dysfunction as it relates to attention resources which is consistent with others who implicate the role of the thalamic nuclei in visuospatial input and emotional expression (Kelly, 1985). Obviously, this subtype of nonverbal learning-disabled children warrants further study not only for heuristic value but for advancing more effective differential intervention strategies. Studies such as these should provide some insight into perceptual and cognitive processes of learning-disabled children throughout the next decade and beyond.

REFERENCES

Boliek, C. A., Obrzut, J. E., and Shaw, D. (1988). The effects of hemispatial and asymmetrically focused attention on dichotic listening with normal and learning-disabled children. *Neuropsychologia, 26*, 417–423.

Bradshaw, J. L., and Nettleton, N. C. (1988). Monaural asymmetries. In K. Hugdahl (Ed.), *Handbook of dichotic listening* (pp 45–69). New York, NY: John Wiley & Sons.

Bryden, M. P. (1982). *Laterality*. New York, NY: Academic Press.

Bryden, M. P. (1988). Does laterality make any difference? Thoughts on the relation between cerebral asymmetry and reading. In D. L. Molfese and S. J. Segalowitz (Eds.), *Brain lateralization in children: Developmental implications* (pp 509–525). New York, NY: Guilford Press.

Bryden, M. P., Munhall, K., and Allard, F. (1983). Attentional biases and the right-ear effect in dichotic listening. *Brain and Language, 18*, 236–248.

Bryden, M. P., and Saxby, L. (1986). Developmental aspects of cerebral organization. In J. E. Obrzut and G. W. Hynd (Eds.), *Child neuropsychology*, Vol. I: *Theory and research* (pp 73–94). Orlando, FL: Academic Press.

Campbell, S., and Whitaker, H. A. (1986). Cortical maturation and developmental neurolinguistics. In J. E. Obrzut and G. W. Hynd (Eds.), *Child neuropsychology* (pp 55–72). New York, NY: Academic Press.

Cohen, H., Gelinas, C., Lassonde, M., and Geoffroy, G. (1991). Audiotory lateralizaiton for speech in language-impaired children. *Brain and Language, 41*, 395–401.

Cohen, M., Hynd, G., and Hugdahl, K. (1992). Dichotic listening performance in subtypes of developmental dyslexia and a left temporal lobe brain tumor contrast group. *Brain and Language, 42*, 187–202.

Corballis, M. C. (1983). *Human laterality*. New York, NY: Academic Press.

Dawson, G. (1988). Cerebral lateralization in autism: Clues to its role in language and affective development. In D. L. Molfese and S. J. Segalowitz (Eds.), *Brain lateralization in children: Developmental implications* (pp 437–461). New York, NY: Guilford Press.

DeFries, J. C. (1985). Colorado reading project. In D. B. Gray and J. F. Kavanagh (Eds.), *Biobehavioral measures of dyslexia* (pp 107–122). Parkton, MD: York Press.

DeFries, J. C., Fulker, D. W., and LaBuda, M. C. (1987). Evidence for a genetic aetiology in reading disability of twins. *Nature, 329*, 537–539.

DeFries, J. C., and Gillis, J. J. (1991). Etiology of reading deficits in learning disabilities: Quantitative genetic analysis. In J. E. Obrzut and G. W. Hynd (Eds.), *Neuropsychological foundations of learning disabilities: A handbook of issues, methods, and practice* (pp 29–47). San Diego, CA: Academic Press.

Dennis, M., and Whitaker, H. A. (1976). Language acquisition following hemidecortication: Linguistic superiority of the left over the right hemisphere. *Brain and Language, 3*, 404–433.

Drake, W. E. (1968). Clinical and pathological findings in a child with a developmental learning disability. *Journal of Learning Disabilities, 1*, 486–502.

Duffy, F. H., Denckla, M. B., Bartels, P. H., and Sandini, G. (1980). Dyslexia: Regional differences in brain electrical activity by topographic mapping. *Annals of Neurology, 7*, 412–420.

Duffy, F. H., Denckla, M. B., McAnulty, G. B., and Holmes, J. A. (1988). Neurophysiological studies in dyslexia. In F. Plum (Ed.), *Language, communication and the brain* (pp 149–170). New York, NY: Raven Press.

Galaburda, A. M. (1986). *Human studies on the anatomy of dyslexia.* Paper presented at the annual conference of the Orton Dyslexia Society, Philadelphia, PA, November, 1986.

Galaburda, A. M., and Eidelberg, P. (1982). Symmetry and asymmetry in the human posterior thalamus. II. Thalamic lesions in a cae of developmental dyslexia. *Archives of Neurology, 39,* 333–336.

Galaburda, A. M., Sherman, G. F., Rosen, G. D., Aboitiz, F., and Geschwind, N. (1985). Developmental dyslexia: Four consecutive patients with cortical anomalies. *Annals of Neurology, 18,* 222–233.

Geschwind, N., and Galaburda, A. M. (1985a). Cerebral lateralization: Biological mechanisms, associations, and pathology: I. A hypothesis and a program for research. *Archives of Neurology, 42,* 428–459.

Geschwind, N., and Galaburda, A. M. (1985b). Cerebral lateralization: Biological mechanisms, associations, and pathology: II. A hypothesis and a program for research. *Archives of Neurology, 42,* 428–459.

Glass, G. V. (1976). Primary, secondary and meta-analysis of research. *Educational Researcher, 5,* 3–8.

Gross-Glenn, K., Duara, R., Yoshii, F., Barker, W., Chang, J., Apicella, A., Boothe, T., and Lubs, H. (1990). PET-scan reading studies: Familial dyslexics. In G. T. Pavlidis (Ed.), *Dyslexia: A neuropsychological and learning perspective,* vol. 1 (pp 109–118). New York, NY: John Wiley & Sons.

Harter, M. R. (1991). Event-related potential indicies: Learning disabilities and visual processing. In J. E. Obrzut and G. W. Hynd (Eds.), *Neuropsychological foundations of learning disabilities: A handbook of issues, methods, and practice* (pp 437–473). San Diego, CA: Academic Press.

Hiscock , M., and Decter, M. H. (1988). Dichotic listening in children. In K. Hughdahl (Ed.), *Handbook of dichotic listening: Theory, methods, and research.* New York, NY: John Wiley & Sons.

Huettner, M. I. S., Rosenthal, B. L., and Hynd, G. W. (1989). Regional cerebral blood flow (rCBF) in normal readers: Bilateral activation with narrative speech. *Archives of Clinical Neuropsychology, 4,* 71–78.

Hugdahl, K. (Ed.) (1988). *Handbook of dichotic listening: Theory, methods, and research.* New York, NY: John Wiley & Sons.

Hugdahl, K., and Andersson, L. (1986). The forced-attention paradigm in dichotic listening to CV syllables: A comparison between adults and children. *Cortex, 22,* 417–432.

Hugdahl, K., and Andersson, L. (1987). Dichotic listening and reading acquisition in children: A one-year follow-up. *Journal of Clinical and Experimental Neurophychology, 9,* 631–649.

Hugdahl K., Andersson, L., Asbjornsen, A., and Dalen, K. (1990). Dichotic listening, forced attention, and brain asymmetry in right-handed and left-handed children. *Journal of Clinical and Experimental Neuropsychology, 12,* 539–548.

Hynd, G. W., Hynd, C. R., Sullivan, H. G., and Kingsbury, T., Jr. (1987). Regional cerebral blood flow (rCBF) in developmental dyslexia: Activation during reading in a surface and deep dyslexic. *Journal of Learning Disabilities, 20,* 294–300.

Hynd, G. W., and Obrzut, J. E. (1977). Effects of grade level and sex on the magnitude of the dichotic ear advantage. *Neuropsychologia, 15,* 689–692.

Hynd, G. W., Obrzut, J. E., Weed, W., and Hynd, C. R. (1979). Development of cerebral dominance: Dichotic listening asymmetry in normal and learning-disabled children. *Journal of Experimental Child Psychology, 28*, 445–454.

Hynd, G. W., and Semrud-Clickman, M. (1989). Dyslexia and brain morphology. *Psychological Bulletin, 106*, 447–482.

Hynd, G. W., Semrud-Clickman, M., Lorys, A. R., Novey, E. S., and Eliopolos, D. (1990). Brain morphology in developmental dyslexia, attention deficit disorder/hyperactivity. *Archives of Neurology, 47*, 919–926.

Hynd, G. W., Semrud-Clickman, M., and Lyytinen, H. (1991). Brain imaging in learning disabilities. In J. E. Obrzut and G. W. Hynd (Eds.), *Neuropsychological foundations of learning disabilities: A handbook of issues, methods, and practice* (pp 475–511). San Diego, CA: Academic Press.

Hynd, G. W., and Willis, W. G. (1988). *Pediatric neuropsychology.* Orlando, FL: Grune & Stratton, Inc.

Isaacson, R. L. (1975). The myth of recovery after early brain damage. In J. E. Ellis (Ed.), *Aberrant development in infancy.* London: John Wiley & Sons.

Johnson, D. J., and Myklebust, H. R. (1971). *Learning disabilities.* New York, NY: Grune & Stratton, Inc.

Kavele, K. A. (1988). Using meta-analysis to answer the question: What are the important, manipulable influences on school learning? *School Psychology Review, 17*, 644–650.

Kelly, J. P. (1985). Anatomical basis of sensory perception and motor coordination. In E. R. Kandel and J. H. Schwartz (Eds.), *Principles of neural science*, ed 2, (pp 222–243). New York, NY: Elsevier.

Kershner, J., and Micallef, J. (1992). Consonant-vowel lateralization in dyslexic children: Deficit or compensatory development? *Brain and Language, 43*, 66–82.

Kershner, J., and Morton, L. (1990). Directed attention dichotic listening in reading disabled children: A test of four models of maladaptive lateralization. *Neuropsychologia, 28*, 181–198.

Kershner, J. R. (1988). Dual processing models of learning disability. In D. L. Molfese and S. J. Segalowitz (Eds.), *Brain lateralization in children: Developmental implications* (pp 527–546). New York, NY: Guilford Press.

Kimura, D. (1961). Cerebral dominance and the perception of verbal stimuli. *Canadian Journal of Psychology, 15*, 166–171.

Kimura, D. (1967). Functional asymmetry of the brain in dichotic listening. *Cortex, 3*, 163–178.

Kinsbourne, M., and Hiscock, M. (1977). Does cerebral dominance develop? In S. Segalowitz and F. Gruber (Eds.), *Language development and neurological theory* (pp 171–191). New York, NY: Academic Press.

Kinsbourne, M., and Hiscock, M. (1983). The normal and deviant development of functional lateralization of the brain. In P. Mussen, M. Haith, and J. Campos (Eds.), *Handbook of child psychology*, (ed 4.). New York, NY: John Wiley & Sons.

Larsen, J., Hoien, T., Lundberg, I., and Odegaard, H. (1989). MRI evaluation of the size and symmetry of the planum temporale in adolescents with developmental dyslexia. Stavenger, Norway: Center for Reading Research.

Lenneberg, E. (1967). *Biological foundations of language.* New York, NY: John Wiley & Sons.

Lubs, H. A., Rabin, M., Carland-Saucier, K., Wen, X. L., Gross-Glenn, K., Duara, R., Levin, B., and Lubs, M. L. (1991). Genetic bases of developmental dyslexia: Molecular studies. In J. E. Obrzut and G. W. Hynd (Eds.), *Neuropsychological foundations of learning disabilities: A handbook of issues, methods, and practice* (pp 49–77). San Diego, CA: Academic Press.

Luria, A. R. (1973). *The working brain.* New York, NY: Basic Books.

Molfese, D. L., and Molfese, V. J. (1979). Hemisphere and stimulus differences as reflected in the cortical responses of newborn infants to speech stimuli. *Developmental Psychology, 15,* 505–511.

Mondor, T. A., and Bryden, M. P. (1991). The influence of attention on the dichotic REA. *Neuropsychologia, 29,* 1179–1190.

Morris, G. L., Obrzut, J. E., and Coulthard-Morris, L. (1989). Electroencephalographic and brain stem evoked responses from learning-disabled and control children. *Developmental Neuropsychology, 5,* 187–206.

Morton, L. L., and Siegel, L. S. (1991). Left ear dichotic listening performance on consonant-vowel combinations and digits in subtypes of reading-disabled children. *Brain and Language, 40,* 162–180.

Muller, H., and Rabbit, P. (1989). Refexive and voluntary orienting of visual attention: Time course of activation and resistance to interruption. *Journal of Experimental Psychology: Human Perception and Performance, 15,* 315–330.

Murray, J., Allard, F., and Bryden M. P. (1988). Expectancy effects: Cost-benefit analysis of monaurally and dichotically presented speech. *Brain and Language, 35,* 105–118.

Obrzut, J. E. (1988). Deficient lateralization in learning-disabled children: Developmental lag or abnormal cerebral organization? In D. L. Molfese and S. J. Segalowitz (Eds.), *Brain lateralization in children: Developmental implications* (pp 567–589). New York, NY: Guilford Press.

Obrzut, J. E. (1991). Hemispheric activation and arousal asymmetry in learning-disabled children. In J. E. Obrzut and G. W. Hynd (Eds.), *Neuropsychological foundations of learning disabilities: A handbook of issues, methods, and practice* (pp 179–198). San Diego, CA: Academic Press.

Obrzut, J. E., Boliek, C. A., Bryden, M. P., and Nicholson, J. A. (1994). Age and sex-related differences in left and right hemisphere processing by learning disabled children. *Neuropsychology, 8,* 75–82.

Obrzut, J. E., Boliek, C. A., and Obrzut, A. (1986). The effect of stimulus type and directed attenton on dichotic listening with children. *Journal of Experimental Child Psychology, 41,* 198–209.

Obrzut, J. E., Bryden, M. P., and Boliek, C. A. (1992). *Dichotic listening, handedness, and reading ability: A meta-analysis.* Paper presented at the Twentieth Annual Meeting of the International Neuropsychological Society, San Diego, CA, February 1992.

Obrzut, J. E., Conrad, P. F., and Boliek, C. A. (1989). Verbal and nonverbal auditory processing among left- and right-handed good readers and reading-disabled children. *Neuropsychologia, 27,* 1357–1371.

Obrzut, J. E., Conrad, P. F., Bryden, M. P., and Boliek, C. A. (1988). Cued dichotic listening with right-handed, left-handed, bilingual and learning-disabled children. *Neuropsychologia, 26,* 119–131.

Obrzut, J. E., Hynd, G. W., and Obrzut, A. (1983). Neuropsychological assessment of learning disabilities: A discriminant analysis. *Journal of Experimental Child Psychology, 35,* 46–55.

Obrzut, J. E., Hynd, G. W., Obrzut, A., and Leitgeb, J. L. (1980). Time sharing and dichotic listening asymmetry in normal and learning-disabled children. *Brain and Language, 11,* 181–194.

Obrzut, J. E., Hynd, G. W., Obrzut, A., and Pirozzolo, F. J. (1981). Effect of directed attention on cerebral asymmetries in normal and learning-disabled children. *Developmental Psychology, 17,* 188–125.

Obrzut, J. E., Mondor, T. A., Uecker, A. (1993). The influence of attention on the dichotic REA in normal and learning-disabled children. *Neuropsychologia, 3,* 1411–1416.

Obrzut, J. E., Obrzut, A., Bryden, M. P., and Bartels, S. G. (1985). Information processing and speech lateralization in learning disabled children. *Brain and Language, 25,* 87–101.

Orton, S. T. (1937). *Reading, writing and speech problems in children.* New York, NY: W. W. Norton & Co., Inc.

Penfield, W., and Roberts, L. (1959). *Speech and brain mechanisms.* Princeton, NJ: Princeton University Press.

Plante, E. (1991). MRI findings in the parents and siblings of specifically language-impaired boys. *Brain and Language, 41,* 67–80.

Plante, E., Swisher, L., and Vance, R. (1989). Anatomical correlates of normal and impaired language in a set of dizygotic twins. *Brain and Language, 37,* 643–655.

Plante, E., Swisher, L., Vance, R., and Rapcsak, S. (1991). MRI findings in boys with specific language impairment. *Brain and Language, 41,* 52–66.

Rasmussen, T., and Milner, B. (1977). The role of early left-brain injury in determining lateralization of cerebral speech functions. *Annals of the New York Academy of Sciences, 299,* 355–369.

Rourke, B. P., and Fisk, J. L. (1981). Socio-emotional disturbances of learning disabled children: The role of central processing deficits. *Bulletin of the Orton Society, 31,* 77–88.

Satz, P. (1990). Developmental dyslexia: An etiological reformulation. In G. Pavlidis (Ed.), *Perspectives on dyslexia.* Vol. 1. *Neurology, neuropsychology and genetics* (pp 3–26). New York, NY: John Wiley & Sons.

Satz, P. (1991). The Dejerine hypotheses: Implications for an etiological reformulation of developmental dyslexia. In J. E. Obrzut and G. W. Hynd (Eds.), *Neuropsychological foundations of learning disabilities: A handbook of issues, methods, and practice* (pp 99–112). San Diego, CA: Academic Press.

Satz, P., Strauss, E., Wada, J., and Orsini, D. L. (1988). Some correlates of intra- and interhemispheric speech organization after left focal brain injury. *Neuropsychologia, 26,* 345–350.

Satz, P., Strauss, E., and Whitaker, H. (1990). The ontogeny of hemispheric specialization: Some old hypotheses revisited. *Brain and Language, 38,* 596–614.

Segalowitz, S. J., Wagner, W. J., and Menna, R. (1992). Lateral versus frontal ERP predictors of reading skill. *Brain and Cognition, 20,* 85–103.

Semrud-Clikeman, M., and Hynd, G. W. (1990). Right hemispheric dysfunction in nonverbal learning disabilities: Social, academic, and adaptive functioning in adults and children. *Psychological Bulletin, 107,* 196–207.

Sidtis, J. J. (1981). The complex tone test: Implications for assessment of auditory laterality effects. *Neuropsychologia, 19,* 102–112.

Smith, S. D., Kimberling, W. J., Pennington, B. F., and Lubs, H. A. (1983). Specific reading disability: Identification of an inherited form through linkage analysis. *Science, 219,* 1345.

Tallal, P., and Stark, R. E. (1981). Developing and language-impaired children. *Journal of the Acoustical Society of America, 69,* 568–573.

Voeller, K. S. (1986). Right hemisphere deficit syndrome in children. *American Journal of Psychiatry, 143,* 1004–1011.

Witelson, S. F. (1977). Early hemisphere specialization and interhemispheric plasticity: An empirical and theoretical reveiw. In S. Segalowitz and F. Gruber (Eds.), *Language development and neurological theory* (pp 33–84). New York, NY: Academic Press.

Yantis, S., and Jonides, J. (1990). Abrupt visual onsets and selective attention: Voluntary versus automatic allocation. *Journal of Experimental Psychology: Human Perception and Performance, 16,* 121–134.

IX   Psychopathology

Cerebral Laterality and Psychopathology: Perceptual and Event-Related Potential Asymmetries in Affective and Schizophrenic Disorders

Gerard E. Bruder

Considerable research on the relation of psychopathology and cerebral laterality has been undertaken since the original report by Flor-Henry (1969) that among psychotic patients with temporal lobe epilepsy left foci were associated with schizophrenia and right foci were associated with manic-depressive illness. This chapter focuses on recent studies of cerebral laterality in psychiatric disorders that have used behavioral measures of perceptual asymmetry and event-related brain potential (ERP) measures of hemispheric activity. A convergence of findings across these behavioral and electrophysiologic domains provides new evidence of abnormalities of lateralized hemispheric processing in affective and schizophrenic disorders. Although the neurophysiologic basis for these abnormalities is not well understood, several theoretical formulations are discussed that can serve to direct future research in this area.

METHODOLOGY

Clinical Issues

A number of methodologic concerns that arise when doing laterality research in psychiatric patients, e.g., diagnosis, clinical state of patients, or medication control, have been discussed elsewhere and are not dealt with here (see Bruder, 1988, 1991). One additional issue that has proved to be of importance in this area is the heterogeneity of affective and schizophrenic disorders. For instance, we have found differences in perceptual asymmetry among diagnostic subtypes of depression, i.e., between unipolar vs. bipolar depression or between melancholic vs. atypical depression. It is therefore important to specify the diagnostic subtypes of patients and, where possible, to compare findings across subtypes so as to determine those that do or do not display a given abnormality of laterality. The relationship of laterality effects to specific symptoms of schizophrenia, e.g., positive symptoms of hallucinations or thought disorder, has also provided some insight into specific clinical characteristics associated with abnormalities of laterality. Another approach for dealing with diagnostic heterogeneity is to compare findings in patients that respond to a standard medication and in those that do not. Yet another strategy is to divide patients into subgroups on the basis of their laterality scores and to compare them for differences on clinical or biological measures (e.g., Wexler et al., 1989). This strategy recognizes the possibility that individual differences in laterality among patients might ultimately be of some value in identifying pathologically distinct subtypes.

Perceptual Asymmetry Measures

A variety of dichotic listening and visual half-field tests have been used to assess perceptual asymmetry for verbal and nonverbal material. Dichotic listening tests consist of presenting a different syllable, word, or tone simultaneously to the two ears. One of the most frequently used verbal dichotic tests involves the simultaneous presentation of a different consonant-vowel (CV) syllable /ba/, /da/, /ga/, /pa/, /ta/, or /ka/ to each ear; the subject reports the two syllables using a multiple-choice answer sheet (Berlin et al., 1973). This test has consistently yielded a mean right ear (left hemisphere) advantage of 10% to 15% in normal adults (for reviews, see Speaks, Niccum, and Carney, 1982; Bruder, 1988). Other dichotic nonsense syllable or word tests use synthesized and natural speech to yield dichotic pairs that fuse to form a single percept and the subject thereby reports only one syllable or word (Wexler and Heninger, 1979; Wexler and Halwes, 1983, 1985). These "fused" dichotic tests have the advantage of reducing extraneous variance due to factors such as memory load, report order, or attentional bias. The fused rhymed words test introduced by Wexler and Halwes (1983) is particularly attractive for use with severely disturbed psychiatric patients because of the simplicity of the task. It also has excellent test-retest reliability ($r = .85-.90$) and there is evidence for the validity of this test in measuring hemispheric dominance for language (Zatorre, 1989; Wexler and King, 1990).

Other dichotic listening tests have been designed to measure hemispheric dominance for nonverbal processing of melodies, musical chords, or tones. The Complex Tone Test (Sidtis, 1981) is one of the most reliable and well validated of these nonverbal tests (Sidtis and Volpe, 1988; Bruder, 1988; Tenke et al., 1993). A different complex tone is presented simultaneously to the two ears followed by a binaurally presented probe tone. Subjects use a nonverbal response to indicate whether or not the probe tone matches one of the dichotic stimuli. The Complex Tone Test yields a mean left ear (right hemisphere) advantage of 5% to 10% in normal adults.

Visual half-field tests have traditionally been used to provide measures of visual-field advantage for perceiving verbal or nonverbal stimuli (Bryden, 1982). In these tests, the subject fixates on a central point, and stimuli, such as syllables, words, or dots, are briefly flashed (usually for less than 200 ms) to either the left or right visual field. Use of adequate procedures for maintaining subject fixation is of critical importance in these tests. Levy and Reid (1976) introduced a consonant-vowel-consonant (CVC) nonsense syllable task with a built-in control for subject fixation. At trial onset, a central fixation point is replaced by a central digit (1–9) and by a syllable in either the left or right field. Subjects are required to first report the central digit and then pronounce the syllable. Normal adults show a mean right field (left hemisphere) advantage of about 10% on this task (Gur, 1978; Bruder et al., 1989).

We have developed a nonverbal visual half-field test that is an adaptation of the dot enumeration task of Kimura (1966). At trial onset, the subject views a moderately dense visual mask with a central fixation point. The mask and fixation point are replaced by a digit at central fixation and by two to six dots in either the left or right visual field. Subjects use a nonverbal response to indicate whether or not the number of dots in the lateral field matched the central digit. Both the original version of the dot enumeration task (Kimura, 1966; McGlone and Davidson, 1973) and our modified version (Bruder et al., 1992a) yield a mean left visual field (right hemisphere) advantage of 5% to 10% in normal adults. Our nonverbal dot enumeration task has the advantage of providing control over central fixation and has improved test-retest reliability ($r = .61$).

Individual Differences in Perceptual Asymmetry

Although the above tests typically yield a right ear/field advantage for verbal tasks and a left ear/field advantage for nonverbal tasks, considerable individual differences are found in the magnitude and direction of perceptual asymmetry. For instance, only about 75% of normal right-handed adults show the expected direction of ear advantages for dichotic listening tests. Researchers are now beginning to realize the theoretical and clinical significance of differences in laterality. There is evidence that differences among right handers in dichotic ear advantages (Hellige and Wong, 1983; Bruder, 1991; Kim and Levine, 1992) and visual field advantages (Levy et al., 1983; Kim, Levine, and Kertesz, 1990; Luh, Rueckert, and Levy, 1991; Kim and Levine, 1992) are reliable and reflect real individual differences in relative activation or utilization of the right and left hemisphere. Levy et al. (1983) hypothesized that between-subject variations in perceptual asymmetry among right-handed adults are due more to task-independent differences in characteristic arousal asymmetry than to hemispheric specialization. They developed a free-field chimeric faces test to measure characteristic perceptual asymmetry. Using a principal components factor analysis, it was shown that about half of the variation of asymmetry scores on this free-field test and on a series of other visual laterality tests could be accounted for by a common factor that they refer to as characteristic perceptual asymmetry (Kim et al., 1990; Luh et al., 1991). Kim and Levine (1992) similarly found that about 50% of between-subject variation in dichotic listening asymmetry could be attributed to characteristic perceptual asymmetry and that both modality-specific and modality-general components contribute to asymmetries. Also, individual differences among normal adults in ear advantages for dichotic pitch discrimination were found to be closely related to differences in hemispheric asymmetry, as measured by regional cerebral blood flow (Coffey et al., 1989) and brain ERPs (Tenke et al., 1993).

ERP Measures of Hemispheric Activity

Although perceptual asymmetry measures can provide reliable and valid data concerning cerebral laterality, they do not in themselves provide sufficient information concerning the neurophysiologic basis of abnormal laterality in psychiatric disorders. For instance, decreased left ear advantage for nonverbal dichotic testing could stem from right hemisphere dysfunction, left hemisphere overactivation, or some combination of both. While the use of *both* verbal and nonverbal laterality tests and absolute accuracy scores can aid in interpreting perceptual asymmetry findings (e.g., Bruder, 1991), converging evidence from more direct measures of brain function or morphology is needed to draw more definitive conclusions. The use of brain imaging techniques such as positron emission tomography (PET) or magnetic resonance imaging (MRI) scans has obvious value in this regard, but the costs and complications of these techniques often limit sample sizes, which in turn can limit their value for examining issues related to the heterogeneity of psychiatric disorders or to the generalizability of findings.

Brain ERPs provide a noninvasive and cost-effective means for measuring physiologic correlates of cognitive processing during laterality tasks. ERPs have the major advantage of being time-locked to test stimuli and therefore provide measures of brain potentials occurring at the very time that subjects are actively perceiving stimuli and formulating a cognitive decision. Measures of ERPs during dichotic or visual half-field tasks can yield information about the stage of information processing in which perceptual asymmetries arise. For instance, measurement of ERPs during a dichotic pitch discrimination task revealed that hemispheric asymmetries related to perceptual asymmetries peaked at about 350 to 550 ms after stimulus onset and are thus more likely to reflect later cognitive processes, such as perceptual evaluation, memory, or decision processes, rather than early sensory or attentional processes (Tenke et al., 1993). This same approach should be of value in determining the stages of information processing underlying abnormalities of cerebral laterality in psychiatric disorders. Thus, comparison among patient groups and normal controls can be made for early ERP components such as N1, a negative peak associated with sensory and attentional processes (Näätänen and Picton, 1987), and for later ERP components such as P3, a positive peak associated with stimulus evaluation (Donchin and Coles, 1988).

One disadvantage of ERPs is that their scalp distribution does not clearly indicate what regions of the brain are active. New techniques are, however, beginning to provide more fine-grained topographic mapping of ERPs and may give information on putative sources underlying ERP components (Perrin et al., 1989; Giard et al., 1990). Moreover, the measurement of ERPs over left and right hemiscalp to stimuli in dichotic or visual half-field tasks provides two converging lines of evidence concerning cerebral laterality: (1) ERPs can be related to the side on which the stimuli were presented, e.g., contralateral or ipsilateral to the recording site; and (2) hemispheric asymmetries of ERPs can be related to behavioral measures of perceptual asymmetry for the same subjects. Findings from our recent studies in depressed patients illustrate the strategy of using combined ERP and behavioral measures to study cerebral laterality in psychiatric disorders.

STUDIES IN AFFECTIVE DISORDERS

Theoretical Formulations

Initial research on cerebral laterality in affective disorders focused on evaluating the hypothesis of right hemisphere dysfunction in these disorders (Gruzelier and Venables, 1974; Flor-Henry, 1976; Kronfol et al., 1978; Yozawitz et al., 1979). Although these and more recent studies have found some support for this hypothesis, it has also become clear that more elaborate theories that take into account not only right-left but also anteroposterior and cortical-subcortical dimensions will be needed to account for the full range of laterality findings in depressed patients.

More recent attempts to account for abnormal behavioral or electrophysiologic asymmetries in depression have implicated frontal and posterior regions (Tucker et al., 1981; Tucker, 1981; Levy et al., 1983; Kinsbourne and Bemporad, 1984; Davidson and Tomarken, 1989). Tucker et al. (1981) hypothesized that right frontal activation during depressed mood, as indicated by electroencephalographic (EEG) alpha asymmetry, represents an inhibitory function that acts to suppress the information-processing capacity of more posterior regions of the right hemisphere. This model has the advantage of being readily testable by examining relationships between EEG measures of right frontal activation and performance measures of right hemisphere function. It could account for the state-dependent reductions of visuospatial processing in depression (Kronfol et al., 1978; Tucker et al., 1981; Davidson, Chapman, and Chapman, 1987). Other theories have been advanced to account for more "trait-like" alterations of laterality in depression. Levy et al. (1983) suggested that depression and negative self-evaluation are associated with characteristically low right hemisphere arousal. This is supported by electrophysiologic evidence of reduced right posterior activation in normothymic depressive patients (Henriques and Davidson, 1990) and by lack of a right hemisphere advantage for dichotic complex tones in depressed patients before and after successful treatment (Bruder et al., 1990). Henriques and Davidson (1990, 1991) have also reported evidence of left frontal inactivation in subjects having a unipolar major depression and in subjects who had a previous episode of depression. This is in accord with findings that major depression following stroke is associated with left frontal lesions (Robinson and Szetela, 1981; Robinson and Starkstein, 1991).

Given the clinical heterogeneity of depressive disorders, e.g., as reflected in distinctions between unipolar and bipolar or melancholic and nonmelancholic depression, it is unlikely that any one of these theoretical formulations could account for the laterality alterations that exist in depressive disorders. A possible "integrative theory" was suggested by Kinsbourne and Bemporad (1984), which postulates that two types of depression may exist. They review evidence from studies of focally brain-damaged patients indicating that depression is most likely to result from either left anterior or right posterior lesions. This integrative theory is also consistent with EEG findings of both left frontal and right posterior inactivation in depression (Davidson and Tomarken, 1989; Henriques and Davidson, 1990). Furthermore, the perceptual asymmetry and ERP findings reviewed below indicate that different subtypes of depression are associated with different abnormalities of lateralized hemispheric function.

Dichotic Listening in Depressed Patients

Studies of dichotic listening in affective disorders have generally found reduced or absent left ear (right hemisphere) advantages for nonverbal tasks (Bruder, 1988; Overby et al., 1989). The reduction of right hemisphere advantage has been found to be related to important clinical features of depressive disorders. In examining its relation to diagnostic subtype, we compared the perceptual asymmetry of melancholic vs. nonmelancholic and bipolar vs. unipolar subtypes (Bruder et al., 1989). Melancholia is a severe form of depression characterized by pervasive anhedonia, nonreactivity of mood, and endogenous features such as worse in morning, insomnia, anorexia, and weight loss (American Psychiatric Association, 1987). Our nonmelancholic contrast group had an atypical depression, which is characterized by having symptoms that are in some respects the opposite of those of melancholia (Liebowitz et al., 1988). The symptoms of atypical depression include reactivity of mood with preserved pleasure capacity and associated features such as hypersomnia and overeating. The melancholic patients had an abnormally large right ear (left hemisphere) advantage for a dichotic syllables test, but had *no* left ear (right hemisphere) advantage for a complex tone test. In contrast, patients having an atypical depression did not differ significantly from normal controls on either test. These results are consistent with other evidence that "endogenomorphic depression" with pervasive anhedonia and nonreactivity of mood is associated with a neurophysiologic central nervous system (CNS) disorder (Klein et al., 1980). Our finding that the abnormally large right ear advantage for syllables in melancholic patients was due to significantly poorer left ear accuracy when compared to normal controls was taken as evidence supporting the hypothesis of right hemisphere dysfunction. While the distinc-

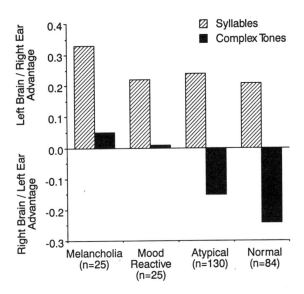

Figure 22.1 Mean ear advantages (*e* scores) for dichotic syllable and complex tone tests.

tion between melancholic and atypical depression was of importance, bipolar and unipolar subtypes did not differ on these dichotic tests.

We have continued to test unmedicated depressed patients on the dichotic syllable and complex tone tests so as to confirm, in larger samples, the above differences in perceptual asymmetry between diagnostic subtypes and normal controls. The larger sample of depressed patients made it possible to compare the findings not only for melancholic and atypical depression but also an additional subgroup of patients having a simple mood reactive depression. This subgroup is characterized by the presence of reactive mood but no other symptoms of atypical depression (Quitkin et al., 1989). Figure 22.1 shows the perceptual asymmetry findings for these subgroups and normal controls on the dichotic syllable and complex tone tests. A positive asymmetry score (*e* score) indicates a relative right ear (left hemisphere) advantage, while a negative score indicates a relative left ear (right hemisphere) advantage. Melancholic patients differed from normal controls in showing both a marked right ear advantage for syllables and *no* left ear advantage for complex tones. Accuracy scores for these tests indicated that this was due primarily to the poor left ear accuracy in melancholic patients. Moreover, patients having a simple mood reactive depression resembled melancholic patients in failing to show a left ear (right hemisphere) advantage for complex tones. Patients having an atypical depression were intermediate, showing a somewhat smaller left ear advantage than normal controls.

The absence of a right hemisphere advantage in melancholia and simple mood reactive depression is also of interest because these subgroups share an important clinical feature, i.e., they both respond equally well to treatment with either a tricyclic or monoamine oxidase inhibitor (MAOI) antidepressant.

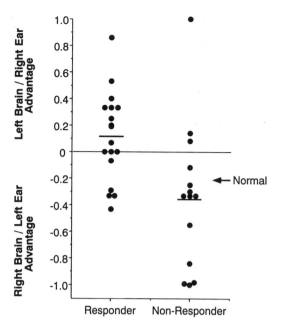

Figure 22.2 Ear advantages (*e* scores) for complex tone test in tricyclic antidepressant responders and nonresponders.

In contrast, atypical depression responds better to treatment with an MAOI than a tricyclic antidepressant (Stewart et al., 1980, 1989; McGrath et al., 1986; Quitkin et al., 1989).

We have examined the relationship between perceptual asymmetry and outcome of treatment with antidepressants by comparing dichotic listening and visual half-field asymmetry scores for subgroups formed on the basis of response to treatment with a tricyclic or MAOI antidepressant (Bruder et al., 1990). The most striking finding was the failure of tricyclic responders to show a right hemisphere advantage for complex tones. Figure 22.2 shows the asymmetry scores for patients who were judged to be treatment responders or nonresponders on the basis of a research psychiatrist's ratings on the Clinical Global Impression Scale. Treatment responders were rated to be much improved or better at the end of 6 weeks of treatment with a tricyclic antidepressant. Nonresponders showed the normal mean left ear (right hemisphere) advantage, whereas treatment responders did not. No comparable differences were found in perceptual asymmetry for MAOI responders and nonresponders.

The above differences in perceptual asymmetry between diagnostic or treatment-responsive subgroups do not appear to be state-dependent because there were no changes following treatment with antidepressants. A comparison was made of the dichotic listening asymmetry scores of depressed patients who were retested after 6 weeks of treatment with an antidepressant (imipramine or phenelzine in most cases). An ANOVA (analysis of variance) of the initial and retest asymmetry scores for 19 melancholic patients, 12 mood reactive patients, 63 atypical patients, and 62 normal controls who were retested on the syllable and complex tone tests showed no changes in asymmetry across the pre- and posttreatment sessions. Similarly, we found no pre- vs. posttreatment changes in dichotic listening asymmetry for tricyclic responders who showed marked clinical improvement (Bruder et al., 1990; Bruder, 1991). Thus, these findings suggest that abnormalities of perceptual asymmetry for nonverbal dichotic tasks in diagnostic or treatment-responsive subgroups of depression are state-independent (trait) characteristics.

Findings for depressed patients on verbal dichotic listening tests have been less consistent (see Bruder, 1988 for a review). Although some studies have found reduced right ear advantages in depressed patients, this finding appears to be related to the patient's clinical state (Moscovitch, Strauss, and Olds, 1981; Johnson and Crockett, 1982). There are also two reports relating individual differences in perceptual asymmetry on dichotic fused words or syllables tests to biological measures in depressed patients. Wexler et al. (1989) divided patients having affective disorders into two subgroups on the basis of a difference in ear advantages for dichotic fused words and syllables. These laterality-defined subgroups differed in their serum testosterone level and in the relationship between testosterone level and symptom severity. Similarly, Otto et al. (1991) found that right ear advantages for depressed patients on a fused words task were correlated with plasma cortisol levels and outcome of treatment. Wexler et al. suggest that dichotic listening tests might be able to define pathologically distinct subtypes and that testosterone-related alterations in left hemisphere function may play a role in a subtype of affective illness. Evidence for the effects of testosterone on the development of cerebral laterality has been reviewed by Geschwind and Galaburda (1985), and testosterone has also been related to mood status and affective disorders (Wexler et al., 1989).

Visual Field Asymmetry in Depression

Studies measuring visual field asymmetries for *nonverbal* stimuli have found evidence of right hemisphere involvement in depression. Jaeger, Borod, and Peselow (1987) tested unipolar depressed patients and normal controls on the free-field chimeric faces test developed by Levy et al. (1983). The depressed patients failed to show the left hemispatial bias for perceiving emotion in faces that is seen in normal adults. Liotti et al. (1991) tested depressed outpatients on a visual reaction time task. In addition to a group of patients who met DSM-III-R criteria for dysthymic disorder or depressive neurosis (American Psychiatric Association, 1987), the authors also tested patients having a generalized anxiety disorder. Depressed patients had longer reaction times for detecting a light square in the left field than in the right field, while patients having an anxiety disorder showed a nonsignificant trend for the opposite direction of visual field asymmetry. They interpret their findings as consistent

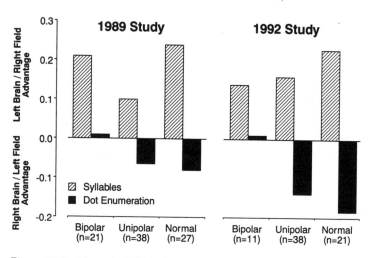

Figure 22.3 Mean visual field advantages (*e* scores) for syllable and dot enumeration tests.

with other evidence for right hemisphere involvement in depression and left hemisphere involvement in anxiety disorders.

The depressed patients in our 1989 study were tested on verbal and nonverbal visual half-field tests (Bruder et al., 1989). We found a difference between bipolar and unipolar subtypes of depression in visual field asymmetry on the nonverbal test. Depressed patients who met research diagnostic criteria (RDC) (Spitzer, Endicott, and Robins, 1978) for bipolar disorder (all but one had a bipolar 2 disorder with a history of hypomania) differed from unipolar depressed patients and normal controls in failing to show a left visual field (right hemisphere) advantage for a visuospatial dot enumeration test. We have recently replicated this finding in new samples (Bruder et al., 1992a). Figure 22.3 shows visual field asymmetry (*e* scores) on the syllable identification and dot enumeration tasks for the bipolar, unipolar, and normal control groups in our 1989 and 1992 studies. All groups showed the expected right field (left hemisphere) advantage for syllables, whereas bipolar patients did not show the left field (right hemisphere) advantage for dot enumeration seen in both unipolar patients and normal controls. The difference in visual field asymmetry among groups was statistically significant for the dot enumeration test, but not for the syllable test. The lack of a left visual field advantage in bipolar patients was clearly due to their poor left field accuracy. There was a significant difference among groups in left field accuracy, but not in right field accuracy. Bipolar depressed patients in both our 1989 and 1992 studies had poorer left field accuracy when compared to either unipolar patients or normal controls. The dot enumeration performance for bipolar patients resembles the findings for brain-damaged patients with right temporal lesions, who likewise performed poorer than controls only for dots in the contralateral *left* field (Warrington and James, 1967).

In our 1989 study, we noted a nonsignificant trend for unipolar depressed patients to have a smaller right field advantage for the syllables when compared to normal controls. This trend was also evident in the 1992 study (see figure 22.3), but again did not achieve statistical significance. A prior study did find reduced right visual field advantage for a verbal task in women having a major depressive disorder (Silberman et al., 1983), and we found evidence of this abnormality in depressed patients who respond to a tricyclic antidepressant (Bruder et al., 1990). There may therefore be a subgroup of unipolar depressed patients who exhibit reduced left hemisphere advantage for verbal material in visual half-field tests. Evidence from ERP findings, discussed below, suggests that this abnormality may be related to a slowing of cognitive processing of stimuli in the right hemifield.

Accuracy for identifying syllables in the half-field task increased following treatment in tricyclic antidepressant responders but not in nonresponders (Bruder et al., 1990). Despite this improvement in perceptual accuracy following successful antidepressant treatment, there was no change in visual field asymmetry. We also compared the pre- vs. posttreatment performance of bipolar and unipolar patients that were retested on the visual half-field tests following about 6 weeks of antidepressant treatment. An analysis of the test and retest data for 18 bipolar patients, 50 unipolar patients, and 44 normal controls showed no changes in visual field advantages. There were, however, changes in *accuracy* across sessions, with bipolar patients improving more on the dot enumeration task than the syllables task, and unipolar patients improving more on the syllables task than on the dot enumeration task. Further study would seem warranted on the differential effects of antidepressant treatment on visual perception in bipolar and unipolar subtypes.

ERP Findings in Depressed Patients

Most of the early ERP studies in depressed patients used an "oddball" task (Roth et al., 1986). Detection of target tones in an oddball task may be too simple a task to reveal the lateralized cognitive dysfunctions that have been hypothesized to exist in affective disorders. In our initial study, we measured ERPs during cognitively challenging audiospatial and temporal discrimination tasks. In the spatial task, subjects discriminated a difference in the apparent location of standard and test stimuli, and in the temporal task, they discriminated a small difference in duration of standard and test stimuli. These tests were selected because of the association of audiospatial processing with right hemisphere dominance (Ruff, Hersh, and Pribram, 1981) and fine temporal processing with left hemisphere dominance (Hammond, 1982). The hypothesis of right hemisphere dysfunction in affective disorders led us to predict that depressed patients would be more likely to show abnormal ERPs during the audiospatial task. The auditory stimuli in this study were presented in either the right or left hemifield, which enabled us to examine whether ERP differences between depressed patients and controls were related to hemifield of stimulation. Moreover, dichotic listening and visual half-field data available for the patients in this study made it possible to relate abnormalities of perceptual asymmetry to ERP laterality effects.

When we compared the ERP data for patients having a typical major depression (melancholia or simple mood reactive depression), patients having an atypical depression, and normal controls, there were two main findings (Bruder et al., 1991). First, these groups showed a task-related difference in latency of the cognitive P3 component. Patients having a typical depressive disorder had considerably longer P3 latency than atypical depressives or normal controls in the audiospatial task but not in the temporal task. This abnormality was equally present in patients having a melancholic or simple mood reactive depression, and was highly correlated with ratings of insomnia on the Hamilton Depression Scale. Second, in both the audiospatial and temporal discrimination tasks, patients having a typical depressive disorder also had longer P3 latency for stimuli in the right than left hemifield, whereas patients having an atypical depression and normal controls did not. Importantly, this abnormal asymmetry of P3 latency was correlated with perceptual asymmetry scores on the visual syllable identification test. Longer P3 latency for right than for left hemifield stimuli was associated with less right visual field advantage for syllables. Thus, while the first finding for typical depression is suggestive of a deficit in audiospatial processing for which the right hemisphere is dominant, the second finding is more indicative of a disturbance in left hemisphere function. These data are therefore consistent with the hypothesis that aspects of *both* left frontal and right posterior inactivation are involved in depressive disorders (Kinsbourne and Bemporad, 1984).

In the same study, we also found that patients having a bipolar depression were particularly likely to show an asymmetry of N1 for test stimuli in the audiospatial and temporal discrimination tasks, and this was related to their abnormal visual-field asymmetry for dot enumeration (Bruder et al., 1992a). Bipolar patients showed less N1 amplitude for stimuli in the left than right hemifield, while unipolar patients and normal controls did not. This N1 asymmetry was significantly correlated with visual field asymmetry (*e* scores) on the dot enumeration test. The bipolar patients' failure to show a left visual field (right hemisphere) advantage was associated with smaller amplitude of N1 for test stimuli in the left than right hemifield. This relationship is important for two reasons. First, it indicates that an abnormal asymmetry in bipolar depression is present at a relatively early stage in processing, roughly 100 ms after stimulus onset. It is therefore more likely to involve sensory or attentional processes than later cognitive processes associated with P3. Second, there is evidence that N1 is generated in temporoparietal regions and is modulated by an "attention-related process" in the frontal lobes (Knight et al., 1980; Näätänen and Picton, 1987). Knight et al. noted the tendency for unilateral frontal lesions to *increase* N1 to stimuli contralateral to the lesion. On this basis they concluded that frontal cortex has an inhibitory influence on N1

Table 22.1 Principal component analysis (PCA) of asymmetry scores for patients and normal controls*

Task	Factor 1	Factor 2	Factor 3
Dichotic syllables	.042	**.739**	.179
Dichotic complex tones	.004	**.717**	−.189
Visual syllables	.185	−.454	**−.665**
Visual dot enumeration	**.873**	−.003	−.150
N1 amplitude asymmetry	**−.769**	−.033	−.288
P3 latency asymmetry	.196	−.188	**.762**
Eigenvalue	1.469	1.303	1.196
Proportion of variance	.254	.236	.172

* This PCA was performed using a standard VARIMAX rotation. Unrotated factor loadings were essentially the same for factor 1.

to contralateral stimuli. Conversely, increased right frontal activation could, through an inhibitory mechanism similar to that proposed by Knight et al., result in reduced N1 and accuracy for stimuli in the left hemifield in bipolar depression. This would be consistent with the model proposed by Tucker et al. (1981) to explain the effects of depression on right hemisphere function. Alternatively, the abnormal asymmetries in bipolar depression could result directly from decreased activation of right temporoparietal regions that are known to be involved in mediating hemispheric arousal and visuospatial attention (Heilman and Watson, 1977; Posner et al., 1984).

A principal components analysis (PCA) of our ERP and perceptual asymmetry scores was also conducted to evaluate whether one overall factor, such as characteristic perceptual asymmetry (Levy et al., 1983; Kim et al., 1990), could account for the individual differences in asymmetry among depressed patients and normal controls. The PCA was performed on six asymmetry measures obtained from 51 depressed patients and 23 normal controls who were tested on both the behavioral and ERP measures in our 1989 and 1992 studies. The four perceptual asymmetry measures were *e* scores on the verbal and nonverbal dichotic listening and visual half-field tests. The two ERP asymmetry measures were the N1 amplitude and P3 latency asymmetry scores for our audiospatial and temporal tasks. VARIMAX rotated principal components were extracted from the correlation matrix for these asymmetry scores (BMDP-4M). The results in table 22.1 show that three factors that had eigenvalues greater than 1 combined to account for 66% of the total variance of asymmetry scores. The first factor had high loadings on the dot enumeration and N1 amplitude asymmetry scores, i.e., the measures that differentiated bipolar and unipolar subtypes, and may correspond to an asymmetric arousal or attentional asymmetry. The second factor had high loadings on the two dichotic listening tests and may therefore represent individual differences related to auditory perceptual asymmetry. The third factor had high loadings on the visual field advantages for syllables and P3 latency asymmetry. This appears to correspond to individual differences

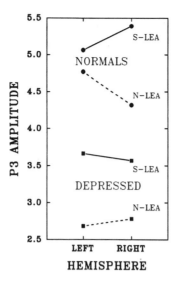

Figure 22.4 Mean P3 amplitude over left and right hemispheres for depressed and normal subjects with a strong left ear advantage (S-LEA) or no left ear advantage (N-LEA).

in speed or efficiency of processing stimuli in the right as compared to the left hemifield. The results of this PCA suggest that there are *multiple* factors that contribute to the differences in ERP and behavioral asymmetry among depressed patients and normal controls.

One weakness of the audiospatial and temporal tasks used in our initial ERP study is that neither task yielded significant behavioral asymmetries. To remedy this, we began to measure ERPs during the dichotic Complex Tone Test (Sidtis, 1981). ERPs of 20 normal adults were recorded from homologous sites over the left and right hemisphere (Tenke et al., 1993). The subjects showed the expected mean left ear advantage for complex tones, and, most important, they showed hemispheric asymmetries of late positive ERPs, which were related to their behavioral asymmetries. The relationship between individual differences in perceptual asymmetry and P3 asymmetry was examined by splitting the subjects at the median behavioral asymmetry. Subjects with a strong left ear advantage (S-LEA) greater than the median had larger P3 amplitudes over the right than the left hemisphere, whereas subjects with little or no left ear advantage (N-LEA) tended to show the opposite hemispheric asymmetry of P3 (figure 22.4).

We have also measured the ERPs of 46 unmedicated depressed patients during the Complex Tone Test. The depressed patients did not differ from the normal adults in sex, age, or handedness (all but one subject in each group was right-handed). Unlike normal adults, the depressed patients showed no significant left ear advantage for complex tones and they did not show behavior-related hemispheric asymmetries of P3. In the same manner as normal adults, depressed patients were divided into two subgroups—one with an S-LEA greater than the median for normal adults (n = 16) and one with N-LEA (n = 30). As can be seen in figure 22.4, depressed patients had considerably smaller P3 amplitudes when compared to normal adults. This finding was not a reflection of poorer performance in depressed patients, in that there was no difference in overall accuracy between groups. The different hemispheric asymmetries of P3 seen for normal adults with an S-LEA vs. N-LEA were not found for depressed patients. Even patients with an S-LEA failed to show any evidence of greater P3 over the right hemisphere. These findings suggest that the abnormal perceptual asymmetry for dichotic complex tones in depressed patients involves a relatively late stage of cognitive processing, which is reflected in abnormalities of P3.

Summary of Findings for Affective Disorders: Toward a Multifactorial Theory

The findings reviewed for dichotic listening, visual half-field, and ERP measures indicate that abnormalities of cerebral laterality in depression are related to the patient's clinical features, e.g., diagnostic subtype and outcome of treatment. An analysis of individual differences in laterality among depressed patients suggested that three factors could contribute to these abnormalities.

One factor, perhaps involving asymmetric arousal or attention, may account for differences in perceptual asymmetry on a visuospatial test and in N1 asymmetry. This factor appears to be most abnormal in depressed patients having a bipolar disorder. It may involve early processing in subcortical sites in the temporal lobe. The neural system that is thought to mediate hemispheric arousal and attention includes extensive connections to limbic and midbrain structures in this region (Heilman and Watson, 1977; Mesulam, 1981; Posner et al., 1984). The possibility that bipolar depression may involve right subcortical areas is also suggested by mood disorders in patients with brain lesions (Starkstein et al., 1991; Robinson and Starkstein, 1991). Patients having secondary bipolar disorders had subcortical lesions mainly involving the right head of the caudate and right thalamus.

The second factor is associated with abnormal dichotic listening asymmetry, which was most evident among depressed patients having a melancholic or simple mood reactive depression. This could represent an abnormality of a modality-specific component of characteristic perceptual asymmetry (Levy et al., 1983; Kim and Levine, 1992). The lack of a left ear advantage for complex tones could involve cortical inactivation of right posterior temporal lobe regions that have been implicated in pitch discrimination (Zattore, 1988; Coffey et al., 1989). The relationship of perceptual asymmetry for complex tones to P3, but not N1, argues that the abnormal dichotic listening asymmetry in depressed patients is related to later cognitive processes, such as stimulus evaluation or memory (Donchin and Coles, 1988). The temporoparietal junction appears to be important for modulating the P3 component (Knight et al., 1989), and cortical inactivation in this region could therefore account for abnormal P3 findings in depressed patients for pitch discrimination and audiospatial tasks (Roth et al., 1986; Blackwood et al., 1987; Bruder et al., 1991).

A third factor is associated with reduced right visual-field advantage for syllables and longer P3 latency for auditory stimuli in the right than left hemifield. This could reflect a slowing of cognitive processing for stimuli in the right hemifield and may stem from left frontal inactivation, which has been found to occur in patients having a unipolar depression (Davidson and Tomarken, 1989; Henriques and Davidson, 1990). Davidson and Tomarken suggested that this frontal asymmetry in depression may reflect a state-independent deficit in neural structures that regulate approach motivation, which could be clinically manifested in features such as psychomotor retardation, low energy, and absence of motivation toward positive hedonic stimuli. In mood disorders following stroke, major depression was similarly associated with lesions of the left frontal region (Robinson and Szetela, 1981), and severity of depression correlated with the proximity of the lesion to the frontal pole (Robinson et al., 1984). Also, Robinson and Starkstein (1991) found that patients having a major depression who also met criteria for a generalized anxiety disorder were more likely to have a left cortical lesion than patients with major depression without prominent anxiety symptoms, who were likely to have a left subcortical lesion. Further research should therefore examine whether or not there are differences in left frontal activation between depressed patients with and without an anxiety disorder.

The above findings are supportive of an "integrative theory" that postulates the existence of *both* left frontal and right posterior dysfunctions in depressive disorders (Kinsbourne and Bemporad, 1984). Moreover, the clinical heterogeneity of depressive disorders may be related, in part, to variations in hemispheric dysfunctions along not only a right-left dimension but also anteroposterior and cortical-subcortical dimensions.

STUDIES IN SCHIZOPHRENIA

Theoretical Formulations

Early theories concerning abnormal cerebral laterality in schizophrenia focused on the role of the left hemisphere. The association of left-sided foci in patients with temporal lobe epilepsy with schizophrenic-like symptoms and neuropsychological test results led Flor-Henry (1969, 1976) to hypothesize the existence of left hemisphere dysfunction in schizophrenia. Other findings, however, have led to an hypothesis of left hemisphere overactivation in schizophrenia (Nachshon, 1980) and evidence has also been presented to support a formulation of both left hemisphere dysfunction and overactivaton in schizophrenia (Gur, 1978; Walker and McGuire, 1982). There were also some attempts to deal with the heterogeneity of schizophrenia. Differences in laterality findings for paranoid and nonparanoid patients led to suggestions that paranoid schizophrenia involves overreliance or overactivation of left hemisphere processes, whereas the reverse might be the case for nonparanoid schizophrenia (Gruzelier and Hammond, 1980; Gruzelier, 1981). Gruzulier (1984) subsequently introduced a hemispheric imbalance syndrome model, which hypothesized that schizophrenic patients can be subgrouped according to predominance of active symptoms or withdrawn symptoms. The active syndrome consists of symptoms such as delusions, excitement, cognitive acceleration, and overactivity, and is characterized by left hemisphere activational dominance, whereas the withdrawn syndrome consists of negative symptom features and is characterized by the opposite hemispheric imbalance.

More recent theories have begun to specify anatomic regions that appear to be asymmetric in schizophrenia and may underlie the lateralized cognitive dysfunctions. For instance, Crow (1990) reviewed morphologic evidence of left temporal lobe abnormalities in schizophrenia and hypothesized that schizophrenia involves a disorder of the genetic mechanisms that control the development of cerebral asymmetry. Specifically, Crow suggested that the lateralized abnormality in schizophrenia involves the posterior temporal lobe and includes the planum temporale, a section of the superior temporal gyrus that shows asymmetries in normals adults (Geschwind and Levitsky, 1968; Zatorre et al., 1992). Recent MRI studies have found evidence linking left superior temporal deficits in schizophrenia to positive symptoms of auditory hallucinations (Barta et al., 1990) and thought disorder (Shenton et al., 1992). McCarley and his associates (McCarley et al., 1991; Shenton et al., 1992) have hypothesized that one form of schizophrenia is associated with damage to the posterior superior temporal gyrus and interconnected structures in the limbic system. This is reflected clinically in positive symptoms and physiologically in reduced amplitude of the auditory P3 component. Studies using perceptual asymmetry or ERP asymmetry measures that lend support to this hypothesis of left temporal lobe deficits in schizophrenia are reviewed below.

Dichotic Listening Findings in Schizophrenia

If temporal lobe pathologic changes are a significant feature of schizophrenia, or at least a subtype of schizophrenia, one would expect such changes to affect dichotic listening measures of cerebral dominance. Studies using nonverbal dichotic tests, in which tones or click stimuli are presented to each ear, have agreed in showing a normal right hemisphere (left ear) advantage for schizophrenic patients (Colbourn and Lishman, 1979; Yozawitz et al., 1979; Overby, 1989; Raine et al., 1989). There has been less agreement across studies in findings for verbal tests, which appears to be due to differences in types of dichotic tests and in symptom features of patients in the various studies (see Bruder, 1983, 1988, for reviews).

The earliest studies used dichotic tests in which multiple items are presented simultaneously to the two ears on each trial. For instance, three pairs of digits or words are presented to the two ears and the subject's task is to recall the digits. Five of eight studies using this task found that schizophrenic patients, or a subgroup with paranoid or positive symptoms (hallucinations or delusions), had an abnormally large right ear advantage. This finding has been interpreted as reflecting left hemisphere overactivation in schizophrenia, being more pronounced in paranoid than nonparanoid patients (Nachshon, 1980). A major weakness of the multiple item dichotic test is that it involves a heavy memory load. Since six digits are presented on each trial, three to each ear, the order in which items are encoded and reported is important. If right ear items tend to be reported first, then subjects with a memory deficit are likely to have large right ear advantages. Differences in ear advantages between schizophrenic patients and normals on the multiple item dichotic tests are difficult to interpret because they could be due to language dominance, attentional bias, memory loss, or report order.

These methodologic difficulties can be overcome by using "fused" dichotic syllable or word tests. If subjects perceive and report only one item per trial, the issues of memory load and report order are no longer a problem. With one exception (Raine et al., 1989), studies using fused tests have found reduced or no right ear (left hemisphere) advantage for schizophrenic patients (Colbourn and Lishman, 1979; Kiyota, 1987; Wexler, Giller, and Southwick, 1991). Although schizophrenic patients as a group lacked the normal left hemisphere advantage, the distribution of their perceptual asymmetry scores showed marked individual differences (Colbourn and Lishman, 1979; Wexler et al., 1991). Colbourn and Lishman, for example, reported that about half of their schizophrenic patients displayed evidence of left hemisphere dysfunction. They suggest that individual differences among schizophrenic patients are related to gender, being more abnormal in males, and Wexler et al. (1991) present evidence of an association with the positive vs. negative symptom dimension.

A relationship between reduced left hemisphere dominance for language and positive symptoms would be expected to occur based on recent reports of a correlation between reduced volume of the left superior temporal gyrus and hallucinations (Barta et al., 1990) or thought disorder (Shenton et al., 1992). This region includes the planum temporale, which is thought to be of importance for language dominance (Geschwind and Levitsky, 1968). If the left temporal lobe deficit does influence cognitive *function* mediated by this region, one would predict that reduced right ear advantage for verbal dichotic listening tests would be associated with positive symptoms of schizophrenia. In a preliminary study, we tested 14 psychotic patients from the Schizophrenia Research Unit at New York State Psychiatric Institute on the dichotic fused words test of Wexler et al.(1991). The patients met the following DSM-III-R criteria: 11 schizophrenia, 2 schizoaffective, and 1 schizotype-bipolar disorder (American Psychiatric Association, 1987). Symptom ratings on the Positive and Negative Syndrome Scale (PANSS; Kay, Opler, and Fishbein, 1992) made it possible to correlate the dichotic ear advantages (LQ) of patients (LQ = R − L/R + L × 100) with their scores on positive and negative

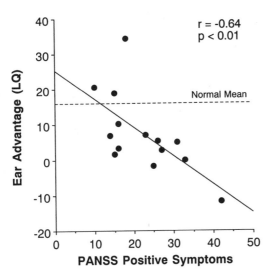

Figure 22.5 Scattergram relating positive symptoms and ear advantages (LQs) for dichotic fused words. PANSS, Positive and Negative Syndrome Scale.

symptoms. As predicted, positive symptom scores were negatively correlated with right ear advantage for dichotic fused words (Pearson $r = -.64$, $P < .01$; Spearman rank order $r = -.61$, $P < .05$). The same correlation held when only the 11 patients having a diagnosis of schizophrenia were included in the analysis ($r = -.73$, $P < .01$). In contrast, there was no significant correlation for negative symptom scores (Pearson $r = .06$, NS). Figure 22.5 plots ear advantages (positive LQ = left hemisphere [right ear] advantage) as a function of scores on the positive symptom scale of the PANSS, and also gives the mean right ear advantage of healthy adults for this test (Wexler et al., 1991). As can be seen, greater positive symptoms were associated with less right ear (left hemisphere) advantage for fused words. The above findings are in accord with the negative correlations between volume of the left superior temporal gyrus and positive symptoms (Barta et al., 1990; Shenton et al., 1992).

Hallucinatory behavior was one of the positive symptoms on the PANSS that was associated with reduced left hemisphere advantage for dichotic fused words. Similarly, Green et al. (in press) reported that hallucinating psychotic patients had no right ear (left hemisphere) advantage for dichotic nonsense syllables, whereas nonhallucinating patients had a normal ear advantage. Also, they found no difference in right ear (left hemisphere) advantage for patients tested in both hallucinating and nonhallucinating states. This is important because it indicates that the left hemisphere abnormality in schizophrenia does not depend on whether or not patients are actively hallucinating during the dichotic tasks, but rather appears to be a state-independent (trait) characteristic. These findings also support the hypothesis that a form of schizophrenia with positive symptoms involves a disturbance of cerebral dominance for language (Crow, 1990).

Bruder: Cerebral Laterality and Psychopathology

Visual Field Asymmetry in Schizophrenia

An important question is whether the reduced left hemisphere advantage in schizophrenia for dichotic words is modality-specific or also occurs for visual half-field tests. The original study by Gur (1978) found results that were in accord with the dichotic listening findings. Schizophrenic patients showed the expected left field (right hemisphere) advantage for a dot localization task, but failed to show a right field (left hemisphere) advantage for a syllable identification task. Schizophrenic patients performed poorer than normal controls for syllables in the right visual field but not the left visual field, which was taken as evidence of left hemisphere dysfunction in schizophrenia. Although two studies did observe a right visual field advantage in schizophrenic patients for word recognition (Colbourn and Lishman, 1979) or letter matching (Eaton, 1979), more recent studies have generally agreed with Gur's finding of no right field advantage in schizophrenic patients (Connolly, Gruzelier, and Manchanda, 1983; Kamali et al., 1991; Min and Oh, 1992). The Kamali et al. study is noteworthy because they recorded both a behavioral laterality measure (reaction time) and ERPs during a verbal half-field task. Normal controls showed the expected right field advantage for reaction time and also had larger amplitudes of late positive ERPs to right than to left field stimuli. In contrast, schizophrenic patients did not show either the behavioral or ERP asymmetry. Schizophrenic patients have consistently been found to show longer reaction times to right than left visual field stimuli, which suggests a slowing of processing stimuli that are initially presented to the left hemisphere (Walker and McGuire, 1982; Min and Oh, 1992).

In summary, the findings for visual half-field tasks provide further evidence of left hemisphere dysfunction in schizophrenia. It is not, however, known whether the abnormal visual field and dichotic listening asymmetries in schizophrenia are related to the same or a different underlying mechanism because studies have not correlated findings for these modalities. Nor do we know if the visual field abnormality in schizophrenia is related to positive or negative symptoms.

ERP Findings in Schizophrenia

Given the involvement of temporal lobe regions in the generation or modulation of auditory ERPs such as N1 and P3 (Näätänen and Picton, 1987; Lovrich, Novick, and Vaughan, 1988; Knight et al., 1989; McCarthy et al., 1989), their measurement may be of particular value in the study of temporal lobe function in schizophrenia. Studies have consistently demonstrated that ERPs to tones, including N1, P2, and P3, are reduced in schizophrenic patients compared to normal controls (for reviews, see Shagass et al., 1977; Pfefferbaum et al., 1989; McCarley et al., 1991). It is, of course, possible that the reduction in amplitude of these components in schizophrenia is not due to temporal lobe deficit, but rather to generalized attentional or cognitive dysfunction or to disruption of other brain regions that modulate these auditory ERPs, e.g., "attention-related" processes in the frontal lobes. There is, however, growing evidence that abnormalities of P3 amplitude and latency in schizophrenia are related to evidence of asymmetric temporal lobe morphology in computed tomography (CT) scans (McCarley et al., 1989) and MRIs (Blackwood et al., 1991; McCarley et al., 1993).

McCarley et al. (1991) reviewed findings from a series of studies, in which auditory ERPs of schizophrenic patients and normal controls were measured in a standard oddball task. P3 amplitude to infrequent target tones was smaller in schizophrenic patients than in normal controls at electrode sites over each hemisphere, but the largest difference in P3 between groups occurred at the left temporal site (T3). They have replicated this finding in three studies (Morstyn et al., 1983; Faux et al., 1988, 1990) and have demonstrated that the P3 asymmetry at temporal lobe sites was present for both medicated and unmedicated schizophrenic patients. P3 over the left temporal region was significantly correlated with positive symptoms of schizophrenia (Shenton et al., 1989) and with widening of the left sylvian fissure in CT scans (McCarley et al., 1989). Most recently, McCarley et al. (1993) measured P3 amplitudes of schizophrenic patients in an auditory oddball task and also measured their gray matter volumes in MRIs of anterior and posterior superior temporal gyrus, hippocampus, amygdala, parahippocampal gyrus, and cingulate gyrus. Volume reduction in the left, but not the right, posterior superior temporal gyrus was significantly correlated with reduced P3 amplitude at left temporal (T3) and central (C3) electrode sites. They also note that their patients were chronic and predominantly positive symptom patients who are likely to show left posterior superior temporal gyrus abnormality (Shenton et al., 1992). These findings support the hypothesis of McCarley et al. (1991) that one form of schizophrenia involves temporal lobe pathologic changes, which are reflected in asymmetric P3 at temporal sites and are related to positive symptom features, including thought disorder, hallucinations, and delusions.

It is, however, important to note that the studies of McCarley and his associates used only male patients. It is not known whether or not these findings generalize to female schizophrenic patients. Also, Pfefferbaum et al. (1989) recorded ERPs of male schizophrenic patients and normal controls in an auditory oddball task and they found an overall reduction of P3 amplitude in schizophrenic patients but no evidence of a hemispheric asymmetry. Although both the Pfefferbaum et al. and McCarley studies used auditory oddball tasks, a comparison of the different characteristics of their tasks suggested the possibility that the McCarley et al. task may have placed greater cognitive demands on the tonal discrimination and memory capacities of patients. There also may have been a difference in the symptom features of the patients in the McCarley et al. and Pfefferbaum et al. studies.

We have begun to measure ERPs of schizophrenic patients during the relatively demanding dichotic Complex Tone Test and our preliminary data do show evidence of an abnormal P3 asymmetry in schizophrenic patients

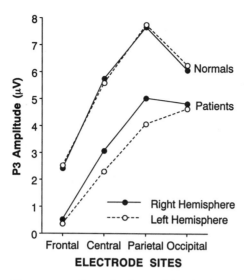

Figure 22.6 P3 amplitude over left and right hemisphere electrode sites.

(Bruder et al., 1992b). ERPs were measured in eight psychotic patients (six males, two females) who met DSM-III-R criteria: five schizophrenia, one schizoaffective, one paranoid delusional, and one schizotype-bipolar disorder (American Psychiatric Association, 1987). Five of the patients were receiving an antipsychotic (haloperidol) and three patients were unmedicated when tested. The comparison group of 20 normal subjects (8 males and 12 females) were from our recent study (Tenke et al., 1993). All but one subject in each group were right-handed, and groups did not differ in age.

Figure 22.6 shows the average P3 amplitude to probe tones recorded at homologous sites over the left and right hemispheres (F3,F4; C3,C4; P3,P4; O1,O2). Patients had overall smaller P3 amplitude than normal controls, which is consistent with prior findings for schizophrenic patients (Shagass et al., 1977; Roth et al., 1986; Pfefferbaum et al., 1989; McCarley et al., 1991). Moreover, the difference in P3 amplitude between patients and normals was greater over the left than over the right hemisphere. As can be seen in figure 22.6, patients had less P3 amplitude over the left than right central and parietal sites, but normals did not. Correlated *t*-tests confirmed that the P3 asymmetry for patients was significant at these sites. It should also be noted that there was no significant difference in overall accuracy or ear advantage between the patient and normal groups. These behavioral data are important because they argue that the abnormal P3 asymmetry in patients was *not* related to their perceptual asymmetry for complex tones.

Because a standard oddball task was not used in this preliminary study, it is not clear if these patients would have shown a similar P3 asymmetry in that paradigm. Nonetheless, our findings are similar to those observed by McCarley et al. (1991) for an auditory oddball task, and support the hypothesis that cognitive demands that challenge tonal discrimination and memory capacities are likely to yield abnormal P3 asymmetries in schizophrenic patients.

CONCLUSIONS AND SUGGESTIONS FOR FURTHER RESEARCH

Although the findings reviewed in this chapter are in general supportive of hypotheses of right hemisphere dysfunction in affective disorders and left hemisphere dysfunction in schizophrenia, not all patients with these disorders show the abnormality. Individual differences in perceptual asymmetry and related hemispheric differences in ERPs are important sources of data for relating abnormalities of cerebral laterality to specific clinical features of affective and schizophrenic disorders. They provide a means of dealing with the heterogeneity of these disorders and could ultimately serve as clinical aids for subtyping of patients into pathologically distinct groups.

Multiple factors appear to be responsible for abnormalities of perceptual and ERP asymmetries in different subtypes of depressive disorder. Asymmetric arousal or attention may result in abnormal asymmetries in bipolar depression, whereas alteration of later cognitive processing appears to be involved in abnormal asymmetries in typical melancholic or simple mood reactive depression. The abnormal asymmetries in these subtypes of depression may stem from the involvement of different subcortical vs. cortical areas in the right temporoparietal region, and the left frontal region may also be involved in some types of depression. It should, however, be stressed that there is as yet little direct morphologic evidence to support the existence of these hypothesized abnormalities of cerebral laterality in depressive disorders.

The perceptual and ERP asymmetry findings in schizophrenia add to the growing evidence of left temporal lobe dysfunction in schizophrenia, which appears to be related to the positive symptoms of thought disorder and hallucinations. The mechanism underlying this abnormality is not, however, well understood. It could involve actual pathologic changes in medial and lateral temporal lobe structures (McCarley et al., 1991) or a lack of development of regions of the superior temporal gyrus that are thought to mediate language dominance (Crow et al., 1989; Crow, 1990).

There are a number of limitations of prior studies in this area that should be addressed in future research. On a behavioral level, there has been a lack of control of attentional asymmetries in dichotic and visual half-field studies in psychiatric patients. The use of directional cues to attend to stimuli on one side or the other could help separate out the contribution of attentional and other cognitive processes to abnormalities of perceptual asymmetry. On an electrophysiologic level, there is a clear need for ERP studies in this area to use larger arrays of recording electrodes. This would provide greater coverage of scalp locations and allow the implementation of advanced techniques for doing topographic mapping of ERPs. The relation of ERP asymmetries to measures of EEG asymmetry (e.g., alpha power) has also not been given sufficient attention.

Most important, further use of imaging techniques (e.g., MRI or PET scans) in conjunction with behavioral or ERP measures should help identify the specific cortical or subcortical regions that may underlie abnormal perceptual or ERP asymmetries in depressive and schizophrenic disorders. The use of perceptual asymmetry tests as "activation tasks" during imaging measurements could be of particular value. Lastly, the relationship of individual differences in laterality among patients to subject variables needs more study. For instance, there is evidence that left temporal lobe deficits in schizophrenia may be particularly likely among males (Bogerts et al., 1990) and yet there has been no systematic study of the effects of gender on laterality in schizophrenia. Similarly, given the hypothesis that schizophrenia involves a left temporal lobe deficit linked to genetic mechanisms for the development of cerebral asymmetry (Crow, 1990), it would seem worthwhile to investigate whether or not laterality abnormalities in schizophrenia are related to familial evidence for the inheritance of the disorder. Investigation of cerebral laterality in family members of patients with schizophrenic or affective disorders is also an area in need of further study.

ACKNOWLEDGMENTS

Preparation of this chapter was supported in part by grant MH-36295 from the National Institute of Mental Health. Findings are reviewed for several studies conducted with the collaboration and help of many people at New York State Psychiatric Institute. My colleagues in the Department of Biopsychology included: James Towey, Craig Tenke, Esther Rabinowicz, Paul Leite, Hulya Erhan, and Martina Voglmaier. My collaborators at the Depression Evaluation Service, including Jonathan Stewart, Frederic Quitkin, Patrick McGrath, Jerry Finkel, Ron Goldman, and Elaine Tricamo, and at the Schizophrenia Research Unit, including Xavier Amador, Allan Brown, Dolores Malaspina, Charles Kaufmann, and Jack Gorman, were responsible for all aspects of the diagnostic evaluation and treatment of patients. I also thank David Friedman for his helpful advice on ERPs and John Sidtis for his help with the complex tone stimuli.

REFERENCES

American Psychiatric Association (1987). *Diagnostic and statistical manual of mental disorders DSM-III-R*, ed 3, revised. Washington, DC: American Psychiatric Association.

Barta, P. E., Pearlson, G. D., Powers, R. E., Richards, S. S., and Tune, L. E. (1990). Auditory hallucinations and smaller superior temporal gyral volume in schizophrenia. *American Journal of Psychiatry, 147,* 1457–1462.

Berlin, C. I., Hughes, L. F., Lowe-Bell, S. S., and Berlin, H. L. (1973). Dichotic right-ear advantage in children 5 to 13. *Cortex 9,* 393–401.

Blackwood, D. H. R., Walley, L. J., Christie, J. E., Blackburn, I. M., St. Clair, D. M., and McInnes, A. (1987). Changes in auditory P3 event-related potential in schizophrenia and depression. *British Journal of Psychiatry, 150,* 154–160.

Blackwood, D. H. R, Young, A. H., McQueen, J. K., Martin, M. J., Roxborough, H. M., Muir, W. J., St. Clair, D. M., and Kean, D. M. (1991). Magnetic resonance imaging in schizophrenia: Altered brain morphology associated with P300 abnormalities and eye tracking dysfunction. *Biological Psychiatry, 30,* 753–769.

Bogerts, B., Ashtari, M., DeGreef, G., Alvir, J. M. J., Bilder, R. M., and Lieberman, J. A. (1990). Reduced temporal limbic structure volumes on magnetic resonance images in first episode schizophrenia. *Psychiatry Research: Neuroimaging, 35,* 1–13.

Bruder, G. E. (1983). Cerebral laterality and psychopathology: A review of dichotic listening studies. *Schizophrenia Bulletin, 9,* 134–151.

Bruder, G. E. (1988). Dichotic listening in psychiatric patients. In K. Hugdahl (Ed.), *Handbook of dichotic listening: Theory, methods and research.* New York, NY: John Wiley & Sons.

Bruder, G. E. (1991). Dichotic listening: New developments and applications in clinical research. *Annals of the New York Academy of Sciences, 620,* 217–232.

Bruder, G. E., Quitkin, F. M., Stewart, J. W., Martin, C., Voglmaier, M. M., and Harrison, W. M. (1989). Cerebral laterality and depression: Differences in perceptual asymmetry among diagnostic subtypes. *Journal of Abnormal Psychology, 98,* 177–186.

Bruder, G. E., Stewart, J. W., Towey, J. P., Friedman, D., Tenke, C. E., Voglmaier, M. M., Leite, P., Cohen, P., and Quitkin, F. M. (1992a). Abnormal cerebral laterality in bipolar depression: Convergence of behavioral and brain event-related potential findings. *Biological Psychiatry, 32,* 33–47.

Bruder, G. E., Stewart, J. W., Voglmaier, M. M., Harrison, W. M., McGrath, P., Tricamo, E., and Quitkin, F. M. (1990). Cerebral laterality and depression: Relations of perceptual asymmetry to outcome of treatment with tricyclic antidepressants. *Neuropsychopharmachology, 3,* 1–10.

Bruder, G. E., Towey, J. P., Malaspina, D., Gorman, J., Tenke, C., and Kaufmann, C. (1992b). Brain potentials to complex tones in schizophrenia. *American Psychiatric Association New Research Abstracts,* NR454.

Bruder, G. E., Towey, J. P., Stewart, J. W., Friedman, D., Tenke, C., and Quitkin, F. M. (1991). Event-related potentials in depression: influence of task, stimulus hemifield and clinical features on P3 latency. *Biological Psychiatry, 28,* 92–98.

Bryden M. D. (1982): Laterality: Functional asymmetry in the intact brain. New York, NY: Academic Press.

Coffey, C. E., Bryden, M. P., Schroering, E. S., Wilson, W. H., and Mathew, R. J. (1989). Regional cerebral blood flow correlates of a dichotic listening task. *Journal of Neuropsychiatry, 1,* 46–52.

Colbourn, C. J., and Lishman, W. A. (1979). Lateralization of function and psychotic illness: A left hemispheric deficit? In J. Gruzelier and P. Flor-Henry (Eds.), *Hemispheric asymmetries of function and psychopathology* (pp 539–559). Amsterdam: Elsevier.

Connolly, J. F., Gruzelier, J. H., and Manchanda, R. (1983). Electrocortical and perceptual asymmetries in schizophrenia. In P. Flor-Henry and J. H. Gruzelier (Eds.), *Laterality and psychopathology* (pp 363–378). Amsterdam: Elsevier.

Crow, T. J. (1990). Temporal lobe asymmetries as the key to the etiology of schizophrenia. *Schizophrenia Bulletin, 16,* 433–443.

Crow, T. J., Ball, J., Bloom, S. R., Brown, R., Bruton, C. J., Colter, N. P., Frith, C. D., Johnstone, E. C., Owens, D. G. C., and Roberts, G. W. (1989). Schizophrenia as an anomaly of the development of cerebral asymmetry. *Archives of General Psychiatry, 46,* 1145–1150.

Davidson, R. J., Chapman, J. P., and Chapman, L. J. (1987). Task-dependent EEG asymmetry discriminates between depressed and non-depressed subjects. *Psychophysiology, 24,* 585.

Davidson, R. J., and Tomarken, A. J. (1989). Laterality and emotion: An electrophysiological approach. In F. Boller and J. Grafman (Eds.), *Handbook of neuropsychology* (pp 419−441). Amsterdam: Elsevier.

Donchin E., and Coles M. G. H. (1988). Is the P300 component a manifestation of context updating? *Behavioral and Brain Science, 11,* 357−374.

Eaton, E. M. (1979). Hemisphere-related visual information processing in acute schizophrenia before and after neuroleptic treatment. In J. H. Gruzelier and P. Flor-Henry (Eds.), *Hemisphere asymmetries of function in psychopathology* (pp 511−526). Amsterdam: Elsevier/North Holland Biomedical Press.

Faux, S. F., Shenton, M. E., McCarley, R. W., Nestor, P. G., Marcy, B., and Ludwig, A. (1990) . Preservation of P300 event-related potential topographic asymmetries in schizophrenia with use of either linked-ear or nose reference sites. *Electreoencephalography and Clinical Neurophysiology, 75,* 378−391.

Faux, S. F., Torello, M., McCarley, R., Shenton, M. E., and Duffy, F. H. (1988). P300 in schizophrenia: Confirmation and statistical validation of temporal region deficit in P300 topography. *Biological Psychiatry, 23,* 776−790.

Flor-Henry, P. (1969). Psychoses and temporal lobe epilepsy: a controlled investigation. *Epilepsia, 10,* 363−395.

Flor-Henry, P. (1976). Lateralized temporal-limbic dysfunction and psychopathology. *Annals of the New York Academy of Sciences, 280,* 777−795.

Geschwind, N., and Galaburda, A. M. (1985). Cerebral lateralization: Biological mechanisms, associations, and pathology: II. A hypothesis and a program for research. *Archives of Neurology, 42,* 521−552.

Geschwind, N., and Levitsky, W. (1968). Left-right asymmetry in temporal speech region. *Science, 161,* 186−187.

Giard, N. H., Perrin, F., Pernier, J., and Bouchet, P. (1990). Brain generators implicated in the processing of auditory stimulus deviance: A topographic event-related potential study. *Psychophysiology, 27,* 627−640.

Green, M. F., Hugdahl, K., Mitchell, S., Gutkind, D., and Christenson, C. (In press). Dichotic listening during auditory hallucinations in schizophrenia. *American Journal of Psychiatry.*

Gruzelier, J. H. (1981). Hemispheric imbalances masquerading as paranoid and nonparanoid syndromes? *Schizophrenia Bulletin, 7,* 662−673.

Gruzelier, J. H. (1984). Hemispheric imbalance in schizophrenia. *International Journal of Psychology, 1,* 227−240.

Gruzelier, J. H., and Hammond, N. V. (1980). Lateralized deficits and drug influences on the dichotic listening of schizophrenic patients. *Biological Psychiatry, 15,* 759−779.

Gruzelier, J. H., and Venables, P. H. (1974). Bimodality and lateral asymmetry of skin conductance orienting activity in schizophrenics: Replication and evidence of lateral asymmetry in patients with depression and disorders of personality. *Biological Psychiatry, 8,* 55−73.

Gur, R. E. (1978). Left hemisphere dysfunction and left hemisphere overactivation in schizophrenia. *Journal of Abnormal Psychology, 87,* 226−238.

Hammond, G. R. (1982). Hemispheric differences in temporal resolution. *Brain and Cognition, 1,* 95−118.

Hellige, J. B., and Wong, T. M. (1983). Hemisphere-specific interference in dichotic listening: Task variables and individual differences. *Journal of Experimental Psychology: General, 112,* 218–239.

Henriques, J. B., and Davidson, R. J. (1990). Regional brain electrical asymmetries discriminate between previously depressed and healthy control subjects. *Journal of Abnormal Psychology, 99,* 22–31.

Henriques, J. B., and Davidson, R. J. (1991). Left frontal hypoactivation in depression. *Journal of Abnormal Psychology, 100,* 535–545.

Heilman, K. M., and Watson, R. T. (1977). Mechanisms underlying the unilateral neglect syndrome. *Advances in Neurology, 18,* 93–106.

Jaeger, J., Borod, J. C., and Peselow, E. (1987). Depressed patients have atypical hemispace biases in the perception of emotional chimeric faces. *Journal of Abnormal Psychology, 96,* 321–324.

Johnson, O., and Crockett, D. (1982). Changes in perceptual asymmetries with clinical improvement of depression and schizophrenia. *Journal of Abnormal Psychology, 91,* 45–54.

Kamali, D., Galderisi, S., Maj, M., Mucci, A., and DiGregorio, M. (1991). Lateralization patterns of event-related potential and performance indices in schizophrenia: Relationship to clinical state and neuroleptic treatment. *International Journal of Psychophysiology, 10,* 225–230.

Kay, S. R., Opler, L. A., and Fishbein, A. (1992). *Positive and negative syndrome scale (PANSS) rating manual.* Toronto, Canada: Multihealth System Inc.

Kim, H., and Levine, S. C. (1992). Variations in characteristic perceptual asymmetry: Modality specific and modality general components. *Brain and Cognition, 19,* 21–47.

Kim, H., Levine, S. C., and Kertesz, S. (1990). Are variations among subjects in lateral asymmetry real individual differences or random error in measurement? Putting variability in its place. *Brain and Cognition, 14,* 220–242.

Kimura, D. (1966). Dual functional asymmetry of the brain in visual perception. *Neuropsychologia, 4,* 275–285.

Kinsbourne, M., and Bemporad, B. (1984). Lateralization of emotion: A model and the evidence. In N. A. Fox and R. J. Davidson, (Eds.), *The psychobiology of affective development.* Hillsdale, NJ: Lawrence Erlbaum Associates.

Kiyota, K. (1987). Dysfunction of intra- and interhemispheric complementarity of recognition in schizophrenics—hierarchy and laterality. In P. Takahashi, P. Flor-Henry, J. Gruzelier, and S. Niwa (Eds.), *Cerebral dynamics, laterality and psychopathology* (pp 333–334). Amsterdam: Elsevier.

Klein, D. F., Gittelman, R., Quitkin, F., and Rifkin, A. L. (1980). *Diagnosis and drug treatment of psychiatric disorders: Adults and children,* ed 2. Baltimore, MD: Williams & Wilkins Co.

Knight, R. T., Hillyard, S. A., Woods, D. L., and Neville, H. J. (1980). The effects of frontal and temporal-parietal lesions on the auditory evoked potentials in man. *Electroencephalography and Clinical Neurophysiology, 50,* 112–124.

Knight, R. T., Scabini, D., Woods, D. L., and Clayworth, C. C. (1989). Contribution of temporal-parietal junction to the human auditory P3. *Brain Research, 502,* 109–116.

Kronfol, Z., Hamsher, K. deS, Digre, K., and Waziri, R. (1978). Depression and hemispheric functions: Changes associated with unilateral ECT. *British Journal of Psychiatry, 132,* 560–567.

Levy, J., Heller, W., Banich, M. T., and Burton, L. A. (1983). Are variations among right-handed individuals in perceptual asymmetries caused by characteristic arousal differences between hemispheres? *Journal of Experimental Psychology: Human Perception and Performance, 9*, 329–359.

Levy, J., and Reid, M. (1976). Variations in writing posture and cerebral organization. *Science, 194*, 337–339.

Liebowitz, M. R., Quitkin, F. M., Stewart, J. W., McGrath, P. J., Harrison, W., Markowitz, J. S., Rabkin, J., Tricamo, E., and Klein, D. F. (1988). Antidepressant specificity in atypical depression. *Archives of General Psychiatry, 45*, 129–137.

Liotti, M., Sava, D., Rizzolatti, G., and Caffarra, P. (1991). Differential hemispheric asymmetries in depression and anxiety: A reaction-time study. *Biological Psychiatry, 29*, 887–899.

Lovrich, D., Novick, B., and Vaughan, H. G., Jr. (1988). Topographic analysis of auditory event-related potentials associated with acoustic and semantic processing. *Electroencephalography and Clinical Neurophysiology, 71*, 40–54.

Luh, K. E., Rueckert, L. M., and Levy, J. (1991). Perceptual asymmetries for free viewing of several types of chimeric stimuli. *Brain and Cognition, 16*, 83–103.

McCarley, R., Faux, S., Shenton, M. E., LeMay, M., Cane, M., Ballinger, R., and Duffy, F. H. (1989). CT abnormalities in schizophrenia: A preliminary study of their correlations with P300/ P200 electrophysiological features and positive/negative symptoms. *Archives of General Psychiatry, 46*, 698–708.

McCarley, R. W., Faux, S. F., Shenton, M. E., Nestor, P. G., and Adams, J. (1991). Event-related potentials in schizophrenia: their biological and clinical correlates and a new model of schizophrenic pathophysiology. *Schizophrenia Research, 4*, 209–231.

McCarley, R. W., Shenton, M. E., O'Donnell, B. F., Faux, S. F., Kikinis, R., Nestor, P. G., and Jolesz, F. A. (1993). Auditory P300 abnormalities and left posterior superior temporal gyrus volume reduction in schizophrenia. *Archives of General Psychiatry, 50*, 190–197.

McCarthy, G., Wood, C. C., Williamson, P. D., and Spencer, D. D. (1989). Task-dependent field potentials in human hippocampal formation. *Journal of Neuroscience, 9*(12), 4253–4268.

McGlone, J., and Davidson, W. (1973). The relation between cerebral speech laterality and spatial ability with special reference to sex and hand preference. *Neuropsychologia, 11*, 105–113.

McGrath, P. J., Stewart, J. W., Harrison, W., Wager, S., and Quitkin, F. M. (1986). Phenelzine treatment of melancholia. *Journal of Clinical Psychiatry, 47*(8), 420–422.

Mesulam, M. M. (1981). A cortical network for directed attention and unilateral neglect. *Annals of Neurology, 10*, 309–325.

Min, S. K., and Oh, B. H. (1992). Hemispheric asymmetry in visual recognition of words and motor response in schizophrenic and depressive patients. *Biological Psychiatry, 31*, 255–262.

Morstyn, R., Duffy, F. H., and McCarley, R. W. (1983). Altered P300 topography in schizoprhenia. *Archives of General Psychiatry, 40*, 729–734.

Moscovitch, M., Strauss, E., and Olds, J. (1981). Handedness and dichotic listening performance in patients with unipolar endogenous depression who received ECT. *American Journal of Psychiatry, 138*, 988–990.

Näätänen, R., and Picton, T. (1987). The N1 wave of the human electric and magnetic response to sound: A review and an analysis of the component structure. *Psychophysiology, 24*(4), 375–425.

Nachshon, I. (1980). Hemispheric dysfunctioning in schizophrenia. *Journal of Nervous and Mental Disease, 168*(4), 241–242.

Otto, M. W., Fava, M., Rosenbaum, J. F., and Murphy, C. F. (1991). Perceptual asymmetry, plasma cortisol, and response to treatment in depressed patients. *Biological Psychiatry, 30,* 703–710.

Overby, L. A., III, Harris, A. E., and Leck, M. R. (1989). Perceptual asymmetry in schizophrenia and affective disorder: Implications from a right hemisphere task. *Neuropsychologia, 27,* 861–870.

Perrin, F., Pernier, J., Bertrand, O., and Echallier, J. F. (1989). Spherical splines for scalp potential and current density mapping. *Electroencephalography and Clinical Neurophysiology, 72,* 184–187.

Pfefferbaum, A., Ford, J. M., White, P. M., and Roth, W. T. (1989). P300 in schizophrenia is affected by stimulus modality, response requirements, medication status, and negative symtoms. *Archives of General Psychiatry, 46,* 1035–1044.

Posner, M. I., Walker, J. A., Friedrich, F. J., and Rafal, R. D. (1984). Effects of parietal injury on covert orienting of attention. *Journal of Neuroscience, 4,* 1863–1874.

Quitkin, F. M., McGrath, P. J., Stewart, J. W., Harrison, W., Wager, S. G., Nunes, E., Rabkin, J. G., Tricamo R. N., Markowitz, P. H., and Klein, D. F. (1989). Phenelzine and imipramine in mood reactive depressives. *Archives of General Psychiatry, 46,* 787–793.

Raine, A., Andrews, H., Sheard, C., Walder, C., and Manders, D. (1989). Interhemispheric transfer in schizophrenics, depressives, and normals with schizoid tendencies. *Journal of Abnormal Psychology, 98,* 35–41.

Robinson, R. G., Kubos, K. L., Starr, L. B., Rao, K., and Price, T. R. (1984). Mood disorders in stroke patients. Importance of location of lesion. *Brain, 107,* 81–93.

Robinson, R. G., and Starkstein, S. E. (1991). Heterogeneity in clinical presentation following stroke neuropathological correlates. *Neuropsychiatry, Neuropsychology, and Behavioral Neurology, 4*(1), 4–11.

Robinson, R. G., and Szetela, B. (1981). Mood change following left hemisphere brain injury. *Annals of Neurology, 9,* 447–453.

Roth, W. T., Duncan, C. C., Pfefferbaum, A., and Timsit-Berthier, M. (1986). Applications of cognitive ERPs in psychiatric patients. In W. C. McCallum, R. Zappoli, and F. Denoth (Eds.), *Cerebral psychophysiology: Studies in event-related potentials,* EEG Suppl 38. Amsterdam: Elsevier.

Ruff, R. M., Hersh, N. A., and Pribram, H. (1981). Auditory-spatial deficits in the personal and interpersonal frames of reference due to cortical lesions. *Neuropsychologia, 19,* 435–443.

Shagass, C., Straumanis, J. J., Roemer, R. A., and Amadeo, M. (1977). Evoked potentials of schizophrenics in several sensory modalities. *Biological Psychiatry, 12,* 221–235.

Shenton, M. E., Faux, S. F., McCarley, R. W., Ballinger, R., Coleman, M., Torello, M., and Duffy, F. M. (1989). Correlations between abnormal auditory P300 topography and positive symptoms in schizophrenia: A preliminary report. *Biological Psychiatry, 25*(6), 710–716.

Shenton, M. E., Kidinis, R., Jolesz, F. A., Pollak, S. D., LeMay, M., Wible, C. G., Hokama, H., Martin, J., Metcalf, D., Coleman, M., and McCarley, R. W. (1992). Abnormalities of the left temporal lobe and thought disorder in schizophrenia. *New England Journal of Medicine, 327,* 604–612.

Sidtis, J. J. (1981). The complex tone test: Implications for the assessment of auditory laterality effects. *Neuropsychologia, 19,* 103–112.

Sidtis, J. J., and Volpe, B. T. (1988). Selective loss of complex-pitch or speech discrimination after unilateral cerebral lesion. *Brain and Language, 34*, 235–245.

Silberman, E. K., Weingartner, H., Stillman, R., Chen, H. J., and Post, R. M. (1983). Altered lateralization of cognitive processes in depressed women. *Amercian Journal of Psychiatry, 140*, 1340–1343.

Speaks, C., Niccum, N., and Carney, E. (1982). Statistical properties of responses to dichotic listening with CV nonsense syllables. *Journal of the Acoustical Society of America, 72*, 1185–1194.

Spitzer, R. L., Endicott, J., and Robins, E. (1978). Research diagnostic criteria. Rationale and reliability. *Archives of General Psychiatry, 35*, 773–782.

Starkstein, S. E., Fedoroff, P., Berthier, M. L., and Robinson, R. G. (1991). Manic-depressive and pure manic states after brain lesions. *Biological Psychiatry, 29*, 149–158.

Stewart, J. W., McGrath, P. J., Quitkin, F. M., Harrison, W., Markowitz, D. P. H., Wager, S., and Leibowitz, M. (1989). Relevance of DMS-III depressive subtype and chronicity of antidepressant efficacy in atypical depression: Differential response to phenelzine, imipramine and placebo. *Archives of General Psychiatry, 46*, 1080–1087.

Stewart, J. W., Quitkin, F., Fyer, A., Rifkin, A., McGrath, P., Leibowitz, M., Rosnick, L., and Klein, D. F. (1980). Efficacy of desipramine in endogenomorphically depressed patients. *Journal of Affective Disorders, 2*, 165–176.

Tenke, C. E., Bruder, G. E., Towey, J., Leite, P., and Sidtis, J. J. (1993). Correspondence between ERP and behavioral asymmetries for complex tones. *Psychophysiology, 30*, 62–70.

Tucker, D. M. (1981). Lateral brain function, emotion, and conceptualization. *Psychological Bulletin, 89*, 19–46.

Tucker, D. M., Stenslie, M. S., Roth, R. S., and Shearer, S. L. (1981). Right frontal lobe activation and right hemisphere performance: Decrement during a depressed mood. *Archives of General Psychiatry, 38*, 169–174.

Walker, E., and McGuire, M. (1982). Intra- and interhemispheric information processing in schizophrenia. *Psychological Bulletin, 92*, 701–725.

Warrington, E. K., and James, M. (1967). Tachistoscopic number estimation in patients with unilateral cerebral lesions. *Journal of Neurology, Neurosurgery and Psychiatry, 30*, 468–474.

Wexler, B. E., Giller, Jr., E. L., and Southwick, S. (1991). Cerebral laterality, symptoms, and diagnosis in psychotic patients. *Biological Psychiatry, 29*, 103–116.

Wexler, B. E., and Halwes, T. (1983). Increasing the power of dichotic methods: The fused rhymed words test. *Neuropsychologia, 21*, 59–66.

Wexler, B. E., and Halwes, T. (1985) . Dichotic listening tests in studying brain-behavior relationships. *Neuropsychologia, 23*, 545–559.

Wexler, B. E., and Heninger, G. R. (1979). Alterations in cerebral laterality during acute psychotic illness. *Archives of General Psychiatry, 6*, 278–288.

Wexler, B. E., and King, G. P. (1990). Within-modal and cross-modal consistency in the direction and magnitude of perceptual asymmetry. *Neuropsychologia, 28*(1), 71–80.

Wexler, B. E., Mason, J. W., and Giller, E. L. (1989). Possible subtypes of affective disorders suggested by differences in cerebral laterality and testosterone: A preliminary report. *Archives of General Psychiatry, 6*, 278–288.

Yozawitz, A., Bruder, G., Sutton, S., Sharpe, L., Gurland, B., Fleiss, J., and Costa, L. (1979). Dichotic perception: Evidence for right hemisphere dysfunction in affective psychosis. *British Journal of Psychiatry, 135,* 224–237.

Zatorre, R. J. (1988). Pitch perception of complex tones and human temporal lobe function. *Journal of the Acoustical Society of America, 84,* 566–572.

Zatorre, R. J. (1989). Perceptual asymmetry on the dichotic fused words test and cerebral speech lateralization determined by the carotid sodium amytal test. *Neuropsychologia, 27,* 1207–1219.

Zatorre, R. J., Evans, A. C., Meyer, E., and Gjedde, A. (1992). Lateralization of phonetic and pitch discrimination in speech processing. *Science, 256,* 846–849.

23 Lateralization of Psychopathology in Response to Focal Brain Injury

Robert G. Robinson and Jack E. Downhill

The role of hemispheric asymmetries in the production of psychopathologic disorders has been a topic of interest to clinicians and researchers for many years. The landmark work of Flor-Henry suggested that the major psychopathologic syndromes of schizophrenia and affective disorders were asymmetrically mediated by the cerebral hemispheres (Flor-Henry, 1976; Flor-Henry and Koles, 1981). According to Flor-Henry's theory, left hemisphere, particularly temporal lobe, processes were prominent in the mediation and pathophysiology of schizophrenia, while affective disorder was produced by mechanisms of the right hemisphere. Since that time, numerous studies have lent support to these hypotheses. Neuropsychological testing has demonstrated greater abnormalities of left hemisphere processing in schizophrenia (Gur, 1978). Electroencephalographic (EEG) studies have demonstrated asymmetries in the electrical activity, particularly of the temporal cortex, of patients with schizophrenia (Morihisa, Duffy, and Wyatt, 1983). Anatomic studies using magnetic resonance imaging (MRI) have also demonstrated abnormalities of the left hemisphere, particularly the temporal lobe, in patients with schizophrenia (Suddath et al., 1989).

Similarly, studies of patients with affective disorder have also demonstrated evidence of asymmetry, although the direction of lateralization has been less clear. Some investigators have reported abnormalities of right hemisphere function including neuropsychological testing and hemispheric processing of emotion (Kronfol et al., 1978), while other investigators have demonstrated left hemisphere abnormalities (d'Elia and Perris, 1973). Metabolic studies of frontal lobe activity have consistently demonstrated a greater degree of hypometabolism in the left compared with the right hemisphere (Baxter et al., 1989; Bench et al., 1992).

These studies, however, have examined patients with no known neuropathologic disorders. They have demonstrated neuropsychological, electrical, or metabolic evidence of asymmetries in brain function which has sometimes been correlated with psychopathologic disorders. For the past 10 years, we have been studying patients with focal neuropathologic injuries in an effort to understand the neural mechanisms of mood disorders and other forms of psychopathologic disorder (Starkstein and Robinson, 1992). These studies have also produced evidence of lateralization of psychopathologic processes in a variety of conditions (Robinson et al., 1984, 1988). This chapter focuses on the research findings of our group as well as other investigators examining patients with focal neuropathologic lesions following cerebral infarction or traumatic head injury. In these studies, the evidence of lateralization is based on differences in psychopathologic manifestation between patients with comparable injury to either the right or left hemisphere. The measurement of psychopathologic changes is verbal report of symptoms elicited through a structured mental status interview. Although some of the lateralized psychopathologic symptoms, each of which occurred following brain injury, are associated with asymmetric changes in brain metabolic activity or receptor binding, the principle measures of lateralization are the patient's report of psychopathologic symptoms. The chapter is organized based on psychopathologic syndromes which show evidence of hemispheric lateralization. The first section focuses on depression for which there is the greatest amount of evidence of lateralized response to hemispheric brain injury.

DEPRESSION

Prevalence

Based on evaluations of 103 consecutive admissions to an acute stroke unit, we found that the frequency of patients who met DSM-III symptom criteria (American Psychiatric Association, 1980) for major depressive disorder was 27% (Robinson et al., 1983). Although this study excluded patients who were not able to respond reliably to a verbal interview because of comprehension deficit or decreased level of consciousness, the finding that approximately 25% of patients with acute stroke have a major depression is consistent with the findings of other investigators (Morris, Robinson, and Raphael, 1990; Sinyor, Jacques, and Kaloupek, 1986). The frequency of minor depression (dysthymic disorder) has been more variable from one study to the next and has been reported to occur in between 10% and 40% of patients with acute stroke (Eastwood et al., 1989; House et al., 1991). Thus, numerous studies have demonstrated that clinically significant depressive disorder following stroke occurs in approximately 30% to 50% of patients. About one half of the patients have major depression and the other half have minor depression.

LATERALIZED RESPONSE TO STROKE

The frequency of major depressive disorder following stroke varies depending upon the hemispheric and intrahemispheric location of the injury. In a study of 45 patients with single stroke lesions restricted to either cortical or subcortical structures of the left or right hemisphere, we found that 7 of 16 of patients (44%) with left cortical lesions had major or minor depression compared with 10% of those of right hemisphere cortical lesions (Starkstein,

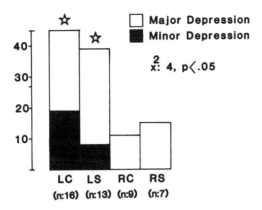

PERCENTAGE OF PATIENTS WITH MAJOR
AND MINOR DEPRESSION

☆

☆ Major Depression
■ Minor Depression

x^2: 4, p<.05

40-
30-
20-
10-

LC   LS   RC   RS
(n:16) (n:13) (n:9) (n:7)

Figure 23.1 The percentage of patients having lesions restricted to either left cortical (LC), right cortical (RC), left subcortical (LS), or right subcortical (RS) brain structures who have either major or minor depression. Patients with lesions restricted to either the left cortical or left subcortical structures had an increased frequency of depression compared to patients with right hemisphere lesions.

Robinson, and Price, 1987b) (figure 23.1). Similarly, in both the previous study (see figure 23.1) and a subsequent study of 25 patients with lesions restricted to subcortical structures (i.e., basal ganglia or thalamus), 7 of 8 patients (88%) with left basal ganglia lesions had major depressive disorder compared with 2 of 7 (14%) with right basal ganglia lesions, 2 of 6 with left thalamic lesions, and none of those with left or right thalamic lesions (Starkstein et al., 1988b) (figure 23.2). Thus, lateralization of depression following stroke was not simply related to hemisphere of injury but was also related to damage of particular structures in the left hemisphere. Left dorsolateral frontal cortical lesions and left basal ganglia lesions produced a significantly higher frequency of major depressive disorder than injury to these structures in the right hemisphere.

Studies that have examined the frequency of depressive disorder in patients with right compared with left hemisphere lesions without examining specific structures of those hemispheres have at times reported a higher frequency with left hemisphere lesions and at other times have not (Robinson and Price, 1982; Folstein, Maiberger, and McHugh, 1977). Thus, it is important to emphasize that not every structure in the left hemisphere is lateralized for depressive disorder. The lateralized response to brain injury is related to specific structures of the left compared to the right hemisphere. Dorsolateral frontal cortex and basal ganglia lesions, particularly of the caudate nucleus, in the left hemisphere appear to be more frequently associated with major depressive disorder than comparable structures of the right hemisphere.

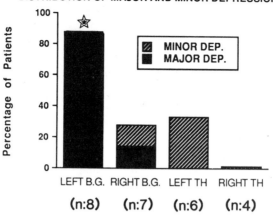

DISTRIBUTION OF MAJOR AND MINOR DEPRESSION

Figure 23.2 The percent of patients with lesions involving the left basal ganglia (left BG), right basal ganglia (right BG), left thalamus (left TH), or right thalamus (right TH) who had major or minor depression. Patients with lesions restricted to the left basal ganglia had a significantly higher frequency of major depression than patients with right basal ganglia lesions or right or left thalamic lesions.

In an effort to identify the clinical factors that are correlated with depression in patients with right hemisphere lesions, we studied 91 patients with single lesions of the right hemisphere (Starkstein et al., 1989b). We found that almost one third of the 17 patients with major depression had a family history of mood disorder. In addition, patients with lesions involving either frontal or parietal cortex were more likely to develop depression than patients with any other lesion location in the right hemisphere (Starkstein et al., 1989b). Other investigators have also reported that both frontal and parietal lesion locations of the right hemisphere are frequently associated with depressive disorder (Sinyor et al., 1986; Finset, 1988).

The logical conclusion to be drawn from these findings is that depressive disorders following brain injury are not a unitary phenomenon. Some depressive disorders appear to be provoked by brain injury in a person with a genetic vulnerability, whereas other depressive disorders may involve psychological response to impairment or lack of social support (Morris et al., 1991). We have hypothesized, however, that there are strategic lesion locations, particularly left dorsolateral frontal cortex and left basal ganglia, which, when injured, are likely to lead to major depressive disorder. When patients with left anterior lesions are compared to patients with similar lesions of the right hemisphere (and no other risk factors for depression), the lateralized nature of major depression is evident.

SPECIFICITY OF DEPRESSIVE SYMPTOMS

Perhaps one of the most fundamental questions about lateralization of psychopathologic symptoms in patients with brain injury is whether the lateralized symptoms could be an indirect consequence of brain injury. For example, patients with acute stroke could have loss of appetite or a sleep disturbance unrelated to depressive disorder but which simply reflects the presence of an acute medical illness. Similarly, patients with syndromes such as neglect or denial might fail to acknowledge or recognize the presence of depressive feelings. These syndromes would lead to an apparent lateralization of depression when, in fact, the findings are simply a consequence of the presence or absence of anosognosia (i.e., an unawareness of a disorder such as depression) in patients with right hemisphere stroke.

We examined this issue in a group of 205 patients with acute stroke who were evaluated in hospital (Fedoroff et al., 1991). Patients were divided into those who acknowledged feelings of depression (n = 85) and those who denied feelings of sadness or depression (n = 120). The frequency of psychological and autonomic symptoms of depression were then examined in the two groups. The psychological symptoms of depression included worrying, brooding, and loss of interest, hopelessness, suicidal plans, social withdrawal, self-depreciation, lack of self-confidence, simple ideas of reference, guilty ideas of reference, pathologic guilt, and irritability. The autonomic symptoms of depression included anxiety, anxious foreboding, morning depression, weight loss, delayed sleep, subjective anergia, early awakening, and loss of libido. Patients who acknowledged depression had a significantly increased frequency of all psychological symptoms and all autonomic symptoms compared to the nondepressed patients with the exception of early-morning awakening. These findings held true even when the depressed and nondepressed groups were controlled for intergroup differences in age, cognitive impairment as measured by Mini-Mental State Exam, and impairment in activities of daily living as measured by the Johns Hopkins Functioning Inventory. Thus, with the exception of early-morning awakening, the frequency of depression-like symptoms in patients who are hospitalized with an acute stroke is significantly less than the frequency of depressive symptoms in patients who acknowledge the existence of depression. This finding also held true even when lesion hemisphere was controlled. We did not find any evidence, for example, that left hemisphere lesions independent of depression produced a higher frequency of vegetative or other symptoms associated with depression.

The mean frequency of autonomic symptoms in the nondepressed group was 0.96 ± 1.12 symptoms compared with a mean frequency of 3.63 ± 1.4 ($P < .001$) in the depressed group (Federoff et al., 1991) (figure 23.3). If the diagnosis of major depression was modified to require the existence of one additional symptom (to account for the nonspecific rate of autonomic symptoms in the nondepressed group), the change in the frequency of major depression was 1.5% (from 24% to 22.5%). Thus, even if it is hypothesized that some patients are overdiagnosed with major depression because of nonspecific symptoms, the frequency of this overdiagnosis appears to be small.

We also examined the issue of whether patients could be denying the existence of depression (Federoff et al., 1991). This is a little more difficult to

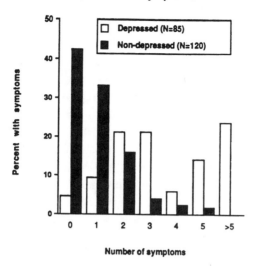

Autonomic Symptoms

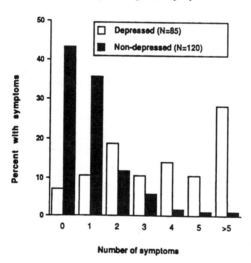

Psychological Symptoms

Figure 23.3 The frequency of autonomic and psychological depressive symptoms among patients with and without depressed mood. Patients without depressed mood had a smooth unimodal distribution while depressed patients had an increased number of psychological and autonomic symptoms which may be bimodal in distribution. Most of the depressed patients with five or more autonomic symptoms had major depression. For both autonomic and psychological symptoms, the mean frequency was more than three times greater in the depressed than the nondepressed groups. (Reprinted with permission from Fedoroff et al., 1991.)

examine because the diagnosis of depression is based on the patient's acknowledgment of specific symptoms, and if patients deny the existence of all symptoms of depression, there is no way to detect the existence of the disorder. We examined the possibility, however, that a patient might acknowledge symptoms of depression but deny feelings of sadness. Of 205 patients included in our study, 10 patients would have fulfilled criteria for major depressive disorder except they denied feelings of depression. All of these patients, however, acknowledged psychological feelings of depression such as hopelessness, self-blame, difficulty with concentration, etc. Thus, we concluded from this study that up to 5% of patients might be underdiagnosed for depression based on their denial of depression even though they acknowledged the presence of other psychological and autonomic symptoms of depression. The only neuropathologic finding associated with denial of depression was the nonexistence of a left hemisphere lesion (i.e., patients who denied depression were significantly less likely to have a left hemisphere lesion than patients who acknowledged depression). Thus, there may be some "masked depressions" following stroke but the number is small (approximately 5%) and the depressions are not completely "masked" since patients acknowledge psychological as well as vegetative symptoms of depression.

Finally, we examined patients specifically for neglect and denial of illness. In a study of 81 patients with acute stroke (a different group than the 205 previously mentioned), we assessed the severity of visual and tactile neglect as well as the existence of anosognosia for either motor symptoms or visual impairment (Starkstein et al., 1992). Although a significant proportion of the patients (22/81, or 27%) were found to have at least a mild degree of anosognosia, the denial of physical symptoms of stroke did not appear to influence the report of psychological symptoms. There were 15 of 54 patients without anosognosia who met criteria for either major or minor depression compared with 8 of 27 with anosognosia who met similar diagnostic criteria. Thus, patients with anosognosia acknowledged feelings of depression just as frequently as patients without anosognosia, suggesting that the denial of physical impairment does not imply that there will be a comparable denial of psychological impairment.

In conclusion, these studies suggest that depressive symptoms are not rampant even in a group of patients with acute medical illness. The number of patients who may be overdiagnosed because of nonspecific symptoms or may be underdiagnosed because of denial of symptoms is relatively small. The use of DSM-III criteria appears to be valid in this brain-injured population. These findings further suggest that the increased frequency of major depressive disorder associated with left dorsolateral frontal cortical or left basal ganglia lesions is not the result of a differential hemispheric effect on symptoms. The finding that patients who fulfilled criteria for major depression but denied feelings of sadness were less likely to have left hemisphere lesions than those who acknowledge depression was present in only a small percentage of mood disorder patients. This is, however, another interesting lateralized phenomenon which is worthy of further investigation.

LATERALIZED BIOCHEMICAL RESPONSE TO BRAIN INJURY AND THE MECHANISM OF POSTSTROKE DEPRESSION

Although the mechanism of lateralized depressive disorders following stroke remains unknown, this lateralized psychopathologic response to focal injury suggests that asymmetries in neurophysiologic or neurochemical processes might be involved in the mechanisms of these disorders. In an effort to investigate some of the neurochemical effects of stroke in living brain, we examined patients with stroke using positron emission tomography (PET) (Mayberg et al., 1988). Seven patients with single lesions of the left hemisphere were compared with eight patients who had single comparable lesions of the right hemisphere. Patient groups were not significantly different in age, sex, previous illnesses, time since stroke, or medications used at the time of the PET study. Patients were studied approximately 1 year following their stroke when both the patients' lesion, as visualized on computed tomography (CT) scan, and their medical status were stable. Patients were given [^{11}C]-N-methylspiperone and quantification of radiotracer uptake was done 1 hour post injection when uptake had reached a steady state. Although spiperone binds to dopamine D2 receptors in the basal ganglia, cortical binding has been demonstrated to be predominantly serotonin S2 receptor binding (Palacios, Niehoff, and Kuhar, 1981). Regions of interest were selected in symmetric areas of frontal temporal and parietal cortex which, based on CT scan visualization of the stroke lesion, were not injured. Spiperone binding was normalized for individual variation in brain uptake by determining the ratio between the number of counts of the radioactive (^{11}C) tracer on the ipsilateral (side of the lesion) compared to the contralateral hemisphere. Patients with right hemisphere lesions were found to have a significantly increased serotonin S2 receptor binding ratio in the right temporal and parietal cortex compared to age-comparable, nonlesion control and left hemisphere lesion patients (figure 23.4). In other words, patients with right hemisphere lesions had a greater amount of spiperone binding (right divided by left hemisphere spiperone counts) in their uninjured temporal and parietal cortex than patients with no lesions or patients with left hemisphere stroke. This suggests that there had been an upregulation of serotonin receptors after right but *not* after left hemisphere stroke.

Although the right hemisphere responded to injury by increasing S2 receptor binding in noninjured areas of the parietal and temporal cortex, severity of depressive symptoms as measured by the Zung depression rating scale was significantly correlated with the amount of S2 receptor binding ratio in the *left* temporal cortex (Palacios et al., 1981) (figure 23.5). The lower the amount of S2 receptor binding in the left compared with the right temporal cortex, the more severe the patient's depressive symptoms.

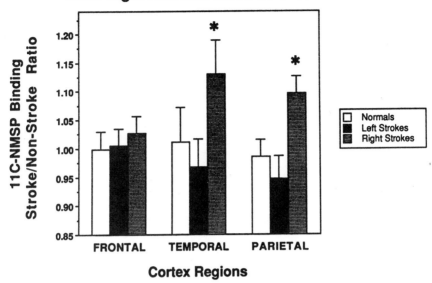

Figure 23.4 *N*-Methylspiperone (IIC-NMSP) binding in the ipsilateral compared with the contralateral hemisphere in noninjured areas of frontal, temporal, and parietal cortex. Based on CT scan, symmetric regions of interest in cortical areas not affected by the stroke were selected. IIC-NMSP binding is primarily serotonin S2 receptor binding in the cortex. Patients with right hemisphere strokes had an increase in S2 receptor binding in the temporal and parietal cortex compared with age-comparable nonlesion controls or patients with left hemisphere stroke. The increase in binding in the right temporal and parietal cortex ratio was due to an increase in binding in these areas rather than a decrease in binding in the left hemisphere. Asterisk, $P < .05$.

Thus, there appeared to be a significant difference in the serotonin receptor response to stroke lesions depending upon which hemisphere was injured. Patients with right hemisphere lesions had an increase in receptor binding in ipsilateral temporal and parietal cortex while patients with left hemisphere lesions showed a significant relationship between the amount of loss of serotonin receptors in the left temporal cortex and the severity of depression.

Studies in rodents have also demonstrated lateralized biochemical responses to brain lesions. Right hemisphere lesions in the rat have been shown to produce a decrease in norepinepherine and dopamine concentrations that does not occur with comparable lesions of the left hemisphere (Robinson, 1979). Either middle cerebral artery ligation or focal suction lesions of the right frontal parietal cortex produced approximately 50% reduction in norepinephrine in the uninjured areas of frontal cortex and locus caeruleus and approximately 40% reduction in dopamine in the substantia nigra. These depletions were evident within 1 to 2 hours after the ischemic lesion and showed a slow recovery over 40 days postoperatively (Robinson, Shoemaker, and Schlump, 1980). Comparable lesions of the right hemisphere produced no measurable changes in norepinephrine or dopamine.

Robinson and Downhill: Lateralization of Psychopathology

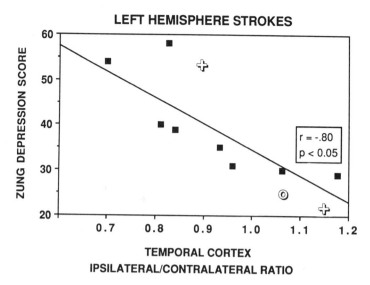

Figure 23.5 *N*-Methylspiperone (NMSP) binding ratio in the left divided by the right temporal cortex was significantly correlated with severity of depressive symptoms. Regions of interest in the temporal cortex which were not affected by the stroke were measured for NMSP binding. NMSP binding is primarily S2 receptor binding in the cortex. There was a significant inverse correlation between Zung depression score and left-to-right-temporal-cortex binding ratio. The lower the S2 receptors in the left temporal cortex, the greater the depression score. Additional patients not included in the original study are indicated by the circle and crosses. The patient indicated by a cross was included in a double-blind treatment study and had a spontaneous remission of depression over a 2-month period. The Zung depression score changed significantly during this time as did the temporal binding ratio. These additional patient data support the original finding of an inverse correlation of depression and S2 receptor binding and demonstrate the changes which can occur in both depression and S2 receptor binding.

In an effort to determine whether the same effect on serotonin receptors as we had previously demonstrated in humans would occur in rats, we examined S2 receptor binding following right vs. left hemisphere lesions (Mayberg, Moran, and Robinson, 1990). We found that right but not left hemisphere lesions produced a bilateral increase in S2 receptor binding in uninjured areas of frontal and parietal cortex which identical left hemisphere lesions did not. This study demonstrated a striking parallel between the biochemical response to unilateral brain injury in humans and rats.

Thus, we have hypothesized that the lateralized psychopathologic response to left hemisphere brain injury in humans may be the result of asymmetries in the biochemical response to brain injury (Mayberg et al., 1991). Right hemisphere lesions produce a decrease in norepinepherine and serotonin, greater in the right hemisphere than the left hemisphere. These depletions of biogenic amines may lead to compensatory upregulation of serotonin receptors in the right temporal and parietal cortex. A left hemisphere lesion causes a relatively smaller depletion of serotonin and norepinephrine which does not trigger upregulation of serotonin receptors. Serotonergic dysfunction, however, results from the left hemisphere lesion and, based on the degree of depletion in the temporal lobe, may ultimately lead to depressive disorder.

MANIA

Mania as defined by DSM-III criteria (American Psychiatric Association, 1980) is a relatively rare consequence of stroke. Although no systematic studies have been done on the prevalence of mania following stroke, we found 3 patients with mania among more than 300 patients examined systematically following stroke. Mania appears to be more common following traumatic brain injury. In a systematic study of 66 patients with traumatic brain injury, 6 patients were found to have mania (Jorge et al., 1993). Because of the relatively low frequency of mania following stroke, most of the patients with poststroke mania included in our studies were identified by admission to a psychiatric hospital and only secondarily found to have a brain lesion (Robinson et al., 1988). Examinations of patients with mania indicate that the symptoms found in patients with brain injury are quite similar to those found in patients without brain injury (Starkstein, Pearlson, and Robinson, 1987a). There were no significant differences in the frequency of any manic symptoms between patients with secondary (post–brain injury) mania and patients with primary (no known neuropathologic lesion) mania (Starkstein et al., 1987a).

Thus, the presentation of mania appears similar whether it is associated with brain injury or not. The cause of secondary mania is unknown, but there are several clinical correlates. Thirteen (39%) of the 33 patients we have studied with secondary mania had a family history of mood or other psychiatric disorder (Robinson et al., 1988). In addition, patients with mania were found to have enlarged ratios of third ventricle and bifrontal ventricle to brain compared with lesion-matched patients without mania (Starkstein et al., 1987a). Thus, many patients that develop secondary mania appear to have some vulnerability, whether it be a genetic loading or a mild degree of subcortical atrophy.

In addition to these clinical correlates of secondary mania, there is a strong lateralized lesion correlate. In a study of 17 patients with secondary mania (Robinson et al., 1988), 12 patients were found to have single lesions involving the right hemisphere. Four had bilateral lesions and only 1 patient had a left hemisphere lesion (figure 23.6). Analysis of CT scans indicated that the lesions associated with secondary mania were limited to several areas of the right hemisphere (Starkstein, Boston, and Robinson, 1988a). These areas included the basotemporal cortex, the orbitofrontal cortex, the basal ganglia, and the thalamus. This association with right hemisphere lesions was confirmed in another series of 8 patients with secondary mania (Starkstein et al., 1990b). Our study of patients with traumatic brain injury and secondary mania indicated that these disorders were also strongly associated with basotemporal lesions (Jorae et al., 1993).

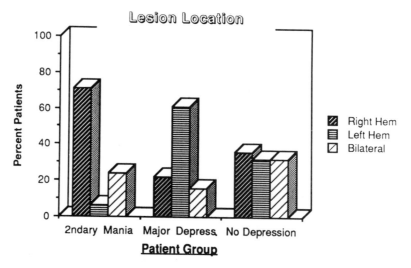

Figure 23.6 The percentage of patients with lesions involving the right hemisphere, left hemisphere, or bilateral brain injury divided by diagnosis. A significantly greater percentage of patients with mania following brain injury had right hemisphere lesions compared with patients with major depression or no mood disturbance ($\chi^2 = 17.5$, $df = 4$, $P < .002$). Likewise, among patients with major depression, there was an increased frequency of left hemisphere lesions compared to patients with mania or no mood disturbance ($\chi^2 = 14.8$, $df = 1$, $P < .001$). Patients with secondary mania had right hemisphere lesions involving the orbitofrontal cortex, basotemporal cortex, thalamus, or basal ganglia. Patients included in the study had the following diagnoses only after stroke (n = 68), trauma (n = 2), or brain tumor (n = 6), mania (n = 17), major depression (n = 31), no mood disturbance (n = 28).

In summary, mania appears to be more common following traumatic than ischemic brain injury. The symptoms of secondary mania are similar to those found in patients with primary mania. There is, however, a strongly lateralized association of lesion location with secondary mania. Lesions of the right hemisphere involving basotemporal cortex, orbitofrontal cortex, basal ganglia, or thalamus have all been associated with secondary mania. This is consistent with our previously reported findings that left hemisphere lesions (frontal and basal ganglia) are associated with major depression. Why right hemisphere lesions lead to mania and left hemisphere lesions lead to depression is an intriguing question which suggests underlying asymmetries of pathophysiologic response to injury.

Mechanisms

Although the mechanism by which lesions of the right hemisphere lead to the development of secondary mania remains unknown, the previously described PET scan studies (Mayberg et al., 1988) suggest the hypothesis that right hemisphere injury leads to an upregulation of S2 serotonin receptors in the parietal and temporal cortex. This increase in serotonergic activity may play a role in the clinical syndrome of mania. In addition to the increased binding of S2 receptors, another PET study examining glucose metabolism ($[^{18}F]$ fluorodeoxygluose) in focal brain regions suggests that lesions may lead to the development of manic symptoms through distant affects on uninjured brain areas (Starkstein et al., 1990b). Three patients who developed mania following focal brain lesions (two stroke and one traumatic injury patients) were examined during the period of their mania. All patients had subcortical lesions involving the basal ganglia or subcortical white matter of the right hemisphere. All three patients were found to have decreased metabolic activity in the right basotemporal cortex compared with age-comparable nonlesion control patients. Since previous studies found that lesions of the right basotemporal cortex may induce mania in some patients (Starkstein et al., 1988a), these findings suggest that subcortical lesions may lead to the development of secondary mania through distant effect of the lesion on right basotemporal cortex. It is unclear whether the previously described change in S2 receptors may be a consequence or a cause of this change in metabolic activity, but this is an issue which deserves further research.

In summary, studies of possible mechanisms of secondary mania have suggested that lateralized biochemical response to right hemisphere brain injury which leads to upregulation of serotonin receptors in uninjured areas of the brain or distant hypometabolic effects in the right basotemporal cortex may play a role in the development of these disorders.

ANXIETY DISORDERS

Anxiety disorders that meet DSM-III criteria for generalized anxiety disorder are common among patients with stroke (Starkstein et al., 1990a). In a study of 309 patients with acute stroke, we found that 27% met criteria for generalized anxiety disorder (GAD) (Castillo et al., 1993). Among these 78 patients with GAD, however, the majority had concomitant depressive disorder and GAD (58/78, or 74%) while a relatively smaller proportion (20/78, 26%) had GAD without depressive disorder. Depressed patients with GAD included both major depression (59%) and minor depression (41%) and 54% had GAD. Although patients with GAD were not significantly different from nonanxious patients in their age, sex, race, socioeconomic status, or any other background or premorbid characteristics, there was a significantly increased frequency of alcohol abuse among the GAD patients without depression (26%) compared with the nonanxious patients (8%) ($P = .037$). In addition, there was also a significant association between anxiety disorder and lesion location. Anxiety plus depression was significantly associated with left cortical lesions while depression without accompanying anxiety disorder was associated with left basal ganglia lesions (Starkstein et al., 1990a) (figure 23.7). Among patients with GAD but without depression, there was a significant association with right hemisphere lesions (Castillo et al., 1993). Analysis of intrahemispheric lesion location indicated that patients with GAD had significantly more posterior lesions of the right hemisphere than patients with

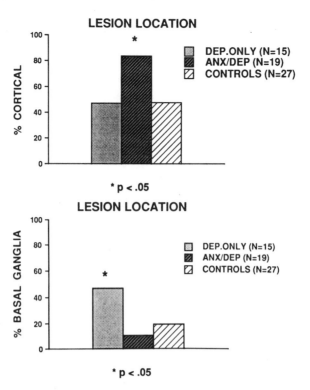

Figure 23.7 The percentage of patients having lesions restricted to the cortex (*top*) divided by diagnostic category. Patients with both major depression and generalized anxiety disorder had a significantly higher frequency of cortical lesions than patients with depression or no mood or anxiety disorder. In contrast, among patients with depression without accompanying anxiety disorder, there was an increased frequency of basal ganglia lesions (*bottom*) compared to anxious and depressed patients or patients with no mood or anxiety disturbance. Patients had the following diagnoses: depression only (n = 24), anxiety and depression (n = 23), no mood or anxiety disorder (n = 45).

right hemisphere lesions but without anxiety disorder (Castillo et al., 1993). Thus, there appears to be a lateralized effect of brain injury on generalized anxiety disorder. Patients with GAD plus depression have left cortical lesions (particularly frontal), while patients with GAD alone have right posterior (particularly parietal) lesions.

In summary, generalized anxiety disorder is common following brain injury. In fact, anxiety disorders may be the second most common emotional disorder (after depression) following stroke. Most anxiety disorders occur in patients with coexisting depression, although a significant number occur without concomitant depressive disorder. Anxiety disorders are associated with both a prior history of alcohol abuse and lesion location. With regard to lesion location, depressive disorder with concomitant anxiety disorder occurs more frequently in patients with left cortical lesions, while anxiety disorder without depression occurs in patients with right hemisphere lesions. Patients with right posterior lesions appear to be particularly vulnerable to developing anxiety disorders. Although human and animal studies have implicated both adrenergic and (γ-aminobutyric acid) GABAergic dysfunction in the mechanism of anxiety disorder (Paul, 1988; Insel et al., 1984), little work has been done to explore the mechanism of these poststroke anxiety disorders. As with depressive disorders, anxiety disorders show a lateralized association with brain lesions, suggesting possible asymmetry of the brain's pathophysiologic response to injury.

PSYCHOTIC DISORDERS

Delusions and hallucinations are a rare consequence of brain injury. Although anecdotal reports have indicated that delusions and hallucinations are associated with a variety of lesion locations (Levine and Finklestein, 1982), there does appear to be some laterality in the association of brain lesions with psychotic disorders (Price and Mesulam, 1985). We examined five patients with delusions or hallucinations following stroke and compared them with five patients matched for size and location of brain lesion but without psychotic disorder (Rabins, Starkstein, and Robinson, 1991). All five patients had lesions of the right hemisphere. Lesions involved cortical areas in four of five patients, and all cortical lesions involved some portion of the temporoparieto-occipital junction. The fifth patient had a basal ganglia lesion. Three of the psychotic patients had a seizure disorder compared with one of the control patients. Seizure disorder is the other clinical variable which has commonly been associated with psychotic symptoms (Levine and Finklestein, 1982). Although there were no significant differences between the psychotic patients and the lesion-control patients in their background characteristics or other clinical variables, the patients with psychotic disorders had significantly larger ventricle-to-brain ratios than the lesion-matched controls (frontal horn ratio $= P < .05$ and third ventricle–brain ratio $= P < .02$) (Rabins et al., 1991). These data suggest that patients who developed poststroke psychotic disorders had significantly more subcortical atrophy than the lesion-matched controls. Because subcortical atrophy was evident in the first CT scans taken after the stroke, it probably preexisted the stroke lesion. Thus, the patients with psychosis may have had a premorbid vulnerability. This slight degree of subcortical atrophy may have made these patients more likely to develop psychotic symptoms following a right parietotemporal brain lesion.

In summary, psychotic disorders are a rare consequence of brain lesions. Although there are insufficient systematic studies to clearly establish whether there is a lateralized response to injury, the anecdotal and few systematic studies of patients with psychotic disorders suggest that they are associated with right hemisphere lesions. Lesions involving the temporoparieto-occipital junction appear to be particularly common sites of injury, although psychotic symptoms can occur following subcortical brain injury. Risk factors for the development of psychotic symptoms appear to be seizure disorder and the existence of subcortical atrophy as indicated by enlarged ventricle-to-brain ratios. There is no work which has suggested possible mechanisms for these disorders. Previous studies describing asymmetric biochemical response to brain injury as well as distant effects of lesions are possible avenues for further investigation of the mechanisms of these disorders.

SUMMARY

Lateralized psychopathologic response to unilateral brain injury occurs with a number of psychiatric disorders and supports early hypotheses proposed by Flor-Henry (1976; Flor-Henry and Koles, 1981). Depressive disorders, manic disorders, generalized anxiety disorder, and psychotic disorders are all more common following injury to one hemisphere than to the other. Left frontal and left basal ganglia lesions lead to an increased frequency of major depression, while right orbitofrontal, basotemporal, basal ganglia, and thalamic lesions are associated with mania. Anxiety disorders without depression and psychotic disorders are also associated with right hemisphere lesions, particularly posterior temporal and parietal lesions. This lateralized effect of brain lesions, however, appears to interact with other factors which can sometimes obscure the lateralized effect or modify its expression. Family history or personal history of depression lead to an increased frequency of depression and may obscure the association of left hemisphere lesions with depression. Enlarged ventricle-to-brain ratio is another factor which seems to play an important role in determining whether patients manifest symptoms of depression, mania, or psychotic disorder. Thus, asymmetry in the brain's response to injury appears to be only one factor in the production of these disorders. Although the lateralized brain response that contributes to the development of these disorders is unknown, there are several studies in both humans and animals which have demonstrated that right and left hemisphere lesions produce different effects on the biogenic amines, particularly serotonin and norepinephrine. These biochemical changes provoked by strategic brain lesions may mediate through asymmetric brain pathways the clinical manifestations of these disorders. Illumination of these brain asymmetries may ultimately lead to targeted and etiologically specific treatments for these disorders.

ACKNOWLEDGMENTS

This work was supported by National Institute of Mental Health Grants Research Scientist Award MH00163 (RGR), MH40355. We acknowledge our collaborators without whom this work would not have been possible: Sergio Starkstein, M.D., Ph.D., J. Paul Fedoroff, M.D., Thomas R. Price, M.D., Helen S. Mayberg, M.D., John R. Lipsey, M.D., Carlos S. Castillo, M.D., and Ricardo E. Jorge, M.D.

REFERENCES

American Psychiatric Association (1980). *Diagnostic and statistical manual of mental disorders DSM-III*, ed 3. Washington, DC: American Psychiatric Association.

Baxter, L. R. Jr., Schwartz, J. M., Phelps, M. E., Mazziotta, J. C., Guze, B. H., Selin, C. E., Gerner, R. H., and Sumida, R. M. (1989). Reduction of prefrontal cortex glucose metabolism common to three types of depression. *Archives of General Psychiatry, 46,* 243–250.

Bench, C. J., Friston, K. J., Brown, R. G., Scott, L. C., Frackowiak, R. S. J., and Dolan, R. J. (1992). The anatomy of melancholia—focal abnormalities of cerebral blood flow in major depression. *Psychological Medicine, 22,* 607–615.

Castillo, C. S., Starkstein, S. E., Fedoroff, J. P., Price, T. R., and Robinson, R. G. (1993). Generalized anxiety disorder following stroke. *Journal of Nervous Mental Disease, 181,* 100–106.

d'Elia, G., and Perris, C. (1973). Cerebral functional dominance and depression. *Acta Psychiatrica Scandinavica, 49,* 191–197.

Eastwood, M. R., Rifat, S. L., Nobbs, H., and Ruderman, J. (1989). Mood disorder following cerebrovascular accident. *British Journal of Psychiatry, 154,* 195–200.

Fedoroff, J. P., Starkstein, S. E., Parikh, R. M., Price, T. R., and Robinson, R. G. (1991). Are depressive symptoms non-specific in patients with acute stroke? *American Journal of Psychiatry, 148,* 1172–1176.

Finset, A. (1988). Depressed mood and reduced emotionality after right hemisphere brain damage. In M. Kinsbourne (Ed.), *Cerebral hemisphere function in depression.* Washington, DC: American Psychiatric Press, Inc.

Flor-Henry P. (1976). Lateralized temporal-limbic dysfunction and psychopathology. *Annals of the New York Academy of Sciences, 280,* 777–797.

Flor-Henry, P., and Koles, Z. J. (1981). Studies in right/left hemisphere energy oscillations in schizophrenia, mania, depression and normals. In C. Perris, D. Kemali, and L. Vacca (Eds.), *Advances in biological psychiatry,* Vol 6. New York, NY: Karger.

Folstein, M. F., Maiberger, R., and McHugh, P. R. (1977). Mood disorder as a specific complication of stroke. *Journal of Neurology, Neurosurgery and Psychiatry, 40,* 1018–1020.

Gur, R. E. (1978). Left hemisphere dysfunction and left hemisphere overactivation in schizophrenia. *Journal of Abnormal Psychology, 87,* 226–238.

House, A., Dennis, M., Mogridge, L., Wanlow, C., Hawton, K., and Jones, L. (1991). Mood disorders in year after stroke. *British Journal of Psychiatry, 158,* 83–92.

Insel, T. R., Ninan, P. T., Aloi, J., Imerson, D. C., Skolnick, P., and Paul, S. M. (1984). A benzodiazepine recetpr—mediated model of anxiety: studies in non-human primates and clinical implications. *Archives of General Psychiatry, 41,* 741–750.

Jorge, R. E., Robinson, R. G., Starkstein, S. E., Arndt, S. V., Forrester, A. W., and Geisler, F. H. (1993). Secondary mania following traumatic brain injury. *American Journal of Psychiatry, 150,* 916–921.

Kronfol, Z., deS Hamsher, K., Digre, K., and Waziri, R. (1978). Depression and hemispheric functions: changes associated with unilateral ECTs. *British Journal of Psychiatry, 132,* 560–567.

Levine, D. N., and Finklestein, S. (1982). Delayed psychosis after right temporoparietal stroke or trauma: relation to epilepsy. *Neurology, 32,* 267–273.

Mayberg, H., Parikh, R., Morris, P., and Robinson, R. (1991). Spontaneous remission of post-stroke depression and temporal changes in cortical S_2-serotonin receptors. *Journal of Neuropsychiatry and Clinical Neurosciences, 3,* 80–83.

Mayberg, H. S., Moran, T. H., and Robinson, R. G. (1990). Remote lateralized changes in cortical ^3H spiperone binding following focal frontal cortex lesions in the rat. *Brain Research, 516,* 127–131.

Mayberg, H. S., Robinson, R. G., Wong, D. F., Parikh, R. M., Bolduc, P., Starkstein, S. E., Price, T. R., Dannals, R. F., Links, J. M., Wilson, A. A., Ravert, H. T., and Wagner, H. N., Jr. (1988). PET imaging of cortical S_2-serotonin receptors after stroke: lateralized changes and relationship to depression. *American Journal of Psychiatry, 145,* 937–943.

Morihisa, J. M., Duffy, F. H., and Wyatt, R. J. (1983). Brain electrical activity mapping (BEAMS) in schizophrenic patients. *Archives of General Psychiatry, 40,* 719–728.

Morris P. L. P., Robinson, R. G., and Raphael, B. (1990). Prevalence and course of depressive disorders in hospitalized stroke patients. *International Journal of Psychiatry in Medicine, 20,* 349–364.

Morris, P. L. P., Robinson, R. G., Ralphael, B., and Bishop, D. (1991). The relationship between the perception of social support and post-stroke depression in hospitalized patients. *Psychiatry: Interpersonal and Biological Processes, 54,* 306–316.

Palacios, J. M., Niehoff, D. L., and Kuhar, M. J. (1981). [^3H] spiperone binding sites in brain: autoradiographic localization of multiple receptors. *Brain, 213,* 277–289.

Paul, S. M. (1988). Anxiety and depression: a common neurobiological substrate? *Journal of Clinical Psychiatry, 49* (Suppl) *10,* 13–16.

Price, B. H., and Mesulam, M. (1985). Psychiatric manifestations of right hemisphere infarctions. *Journal of Nervous and Mental Disease, 173,* 610–614.

Rabins, P. V., Starkstein, S. E., and Robinson, R. G. (1991). Risk factors for deveoping atypical (schizophreniform) psychosis following stroke. *Journal of Neuropsychiatry and Clinical Neuroscience, 3,* 6–9.

Robinson, R. G. (1979). Differential behavior and biochemical effects of right and left hemispheric cerebral infarction in the rat. *Science, 205,* 707–710.

Robinson, R. G., Boston, J. D., Starkstein, S. E., and Price, T. R. (1988). Comparison of mania with depression following brain injury: casual factors. *American Journal of Psychiatry, 145,* 172–178.

Robinson, R. G., Kubos, K. L., Starr, L. B., Rao, K., and Price, T. R. (1984). Mood disorders in stroke patients: importance of location of lesion. *Brain, 107,* 81–93.

Robinson, R. G., and Price, T. R. (1982). Post-stroke depressive disorders: a follow-up study of 103 outpatients. *Stroke, 13,* 635–641.

Robinson, R. G., Shoemaker, W. J., and Schlump, M. (1980). Time course of changes in catecholamines following right hemispheric cerebral infarction in the rat. *Brain Research, 181,* 202–208.

Robinson, R. G., Starr, L. B., Kubos, K. L., and Price, T. R. (1983). A two year longitudinal study of post-stroke mood disorders: findings during the initial evaluaton. *Stroke, 14,* 736–744.

Sinyor, D., Jacques, P., and Kaloupek, D. G. (1986). Post-stroke depression and lesion location: an attempted replication. *Brain, 109,* 537–546.

Starkstein, S. E., Boston, J. D., and Robinson, R. G. (1988a). Mechanisms of mania after brain injury: 12 case reports and review of the literature. *Journal of Nervous and Mental Disease, 176,* 87–100.

Suddath, R. L., Casanova, M. F., Goldberg, T. E., Daniel, D. G., Kelsoe, J. R., and Weinberger, D. R. (1989a). Temporal lobe pathology in schizophrenia: a quantitative magnetic resonance imaging study. *American Journal of Psychiatry, 146*, 464–472.

Starkstein, S. E., Cohen, B. S., Fedoroff, P., Parikh, R. M., Price, T. R., and Robinson, R. G. (1990a). Relationship between anxiety disorders and depressive disorders in patients with cerebrovascular injury. *Archives of General Psychiatry, 47*, 246–251.

Starkstein, S. E., Fedoroff, J. P., Price, T. R., Leiguarda, R., and Robinson, R. G. (1992). Anosognosia in patients with cerebrovascular lesions: a study of causative factors. *Stroke, 23*, 1446–1453.

Starkstein, S. E., Mayberg, H. S., Berthier, M. L., Fedoroff, P., Price, T. R., Dannals, R. F., Wagner, H. N., Leiguarda, R., and Robinson, R. G. (1990b). Mania after brain injury: neuroradiological and metabolic findings. *Annals of Neurology, 27*, 652–659.

Starkstein, S. E., Pearlson, G. D., and Robinson, R. G. (1987a). Mania after brain injury: a controlled study of etiological factors. *Archives of Neurology, 44*, 1069–1073.

Starkstein, S. E., and Robinson, R. G. (1992). Neurospsychiatric aspects of cerebral vascular disorders. In S. G. Yudofsky, and R. E. Hales (Eds.), *Textbook of neuropsychiatry* (pp 449–472). Washington, DC: American Psychiatric Press, Inc.

Starkstein, S. E., Robinson, R. G., Berthier, M. L., Parikh, R. M., and Price, T. R. (1988b). Differential mood changes following basal ganglia versus thalamic lesions. *Archives of Neurology, 45*, 725–730.

Starkstein, S. E., Robinson, R. G., Honig, M. A., Parikh, R. M., Joselyn, R., and Price, T. R. (1989b). Mood changes after right hemisphere lesion. *British Journal of Psychiatry, 155*, 79–85.

Starkstein, S. E., Robinson, R. G., and Price, T. R. (1987b). Comparison of cortical and subcortical lesions in the production of post-stroke mood disorders. *Brain, 110*, 1045–1059.

Contributors

Marie T. Banich
Beckman Institute
University of Illinois
Urbana, Illinois

Brenda E. Berge
Department of Psychology
Brock University
St. Catherines, Ontario, Canada

Carol A. Boliek
Department of Educational
Psychology
University of Arizona
Tucson, Arizona

Halle D. Brown
Department of Psychology
Harvard University
Cambridge, Massachusetts

Gerard E. Bruder
Department of Biopsychology
New York State Psychiatric Institute
New York, New York

Richard J. Davidson
Department of Psychology
University of Wisconsin
Madison, Wisconsin

Marian Cleeves Diamond
Lawrence Hall of Science
University of California
Berkeley, California

Jack E. Downhill
University of Iowa
Department of Psychiatry
Iowa City, Iowa

Jane E. Edmonds
School of Professional Studies
The University of Georgia
Athens, Georgia

Albert M. Galaburda
Department of Behavioral
Neurology
Beth Israel Hospital
Boston, Massachusetts

Josh Hall
School of Professional Studies
The University of Georgia
Athens, Georgia

Anne Harrington
Department of History of Science
Harvard University
Cambridge, Massachusetts

Kenneth Heilman
Department of Neurology
University of Florida College of
Medicine
Gainesville, Florida

Joseph B. Hellige
Department of Psychology
University of Southern California
Los Angeles, California

Merrill Hiscock
Department of Psychology
University of Houston
Houston, Texas

Kenneth Hugdahl
Department of Biological and
Medical Psychology
University of Bergen
Bergen, Norway

George W. Hynd
School of Professional Studies
The University of Georgia
Athens, Georgia

J. Richard Jennings
Western Psychiatric Institute and
Clinic
University of Pittsburgh
Pittsburgh, Pennsylvania

Marcel Kinsbourne
Center for Cognitive Studies
Tufts University
Medford, Massachusetts

Stephen M. Kosslyn
Department of Psychology
Harvard University
Cambridge, Massachusetts

Richard D. Lane
Department of Psychiatry
University of Arizona Health
Sciences Center
Tucson, Arizona

David Warren Lewis
Lawrence Hall of Science
University of California
Berkeley, California

Jacqueline Liederman
Department of Psychology
Boston University
Boston, Massachusetts

Mario Liotti
Research Imaging Center
University of Texas Health Science
Center
San Antonio, Texas

Richard Marshall
Department of Educational
Psychology
University of Texas
Austin, Texas

John E. Obrzut
Department of Educational
Psychology
University of Arizona
Tucson, Arizona

Michael Peters
Department of Psychology
University of Guelph
Guelph, Ontario, Canada

Robert G. Robinson
Department of Psychiatry
University of Iowa
Iowa City, Iowa

Sidney J. Segalowitz
Department of Psychology
Brock University
St. Catherines, Ontario, Canada

Justine Sergent[†]
Cognitive Neuroscience Laboratory
Montreal Neurological Institute
Montreal, Quebec, Canada

[†] Deceased

Don M. Tucker
Department of Psychology
University of Oregon
Eugene, Oregon

Werner Wittling
Department of Biological and
Clinical Psychology
Catholic University Eichstatt
Eichstatt, Germany

Eran Zaidel
Department of Psychology
University of California
Los Angeles, California

Index

Autonomic function
  asymmetries of, 336–337
    sudden cardiac death and, 271–297
  central nervous system regulation of, 278–
    280
  laterality and, 238–239, 341–344
Autonomic nervous system
  asymmetry in heart, 280–281
  in cardiac activity regulation, 323–325
  CNS control of, 292–293
  in conditioning, 244
  in heart, 287
  peripheral, activity level changes in, 222
  psychological stress and, 278
  right hemisphere dominance in, 261
Autonomic-physiologic activity, 305–344
AV conduction time, 324

B cell immunomodulation, 319–320
B cell-specific mitogen, 320
Babbling, 560–561, 563
Balint's syndrome, 410–411, 479
Ball, Benjamin, 17
Barkow, Hans Carl, 9
Basal ganglia
  in affective disorders, 396–397
  dysfunction of, 396
  in depression, 398–399
  injury to, 707, 708
Beck Depression Inventory, 373
Behavior
  asymmetries of
    handedness and, 192–193
    in rodents, 539–540
  callosal anatomy and, 443–444
  complexity of and laterality, 559
  inhibition in infants and children, 378–382
  in language origins, 560–561
  laterality of, 492
    anatomic model of, 492
    in primates, 543–548
Behavioristic tradition, 235–236
Benton, Arthur, 10
Bernard, Claude, 17–18
Bilateral effects, 603–605
Bilateral interhemispheric interaction trials,
  434–435
Biopsychological disease models, 342–344
Birds, asymmetries in, 61, 536–539
Bisexuality theory, 14
Bisymmetry, deviations from, 535–563. See
  also Asymmetry; Lateralization
Bleuler, Eugen, 17

Blood pressure
  hemispheric asymmetry in, 294
  laterality of, 238, 291
  lateralized stimulus effects on, 331–332
Bogen, Joseph, 21
Bon, Gustav le, 13–14
Bonnet, Charles, 4
Bouillaud, Jean-Baptiste, 5
Brain. See also Brain damage; Brain injury;
    specific areas of
  asymmetries of, 8–14
    anatomic, 9–11
    autonomic-physiologic activity, 305–
      344
    in cerebral dominance, 51–69
    frontal, during emotional states, 368–372
    functional, 11–14
    morphologic, 557–558
    ontogeny of, 563
  dopaminergic innervation of, 309–310
  duality of and divided consciousness, 16–
    19
  electrical activity of with emotional states,
    383
  functional units of, 638
  growth of, 557–558
  handedness and structures and functions of,
    193–200
  hemisphere, functional capabilities of, 296
  hemispheric asymmetry of (see Hemispheric
    asymmetry)
  in immunomodulation, 318–322
  intraoperative stimulation of, 286–287
  laterality models of, 19th-century, 3–23
  lateralization of, phylogeny and ontogeny
    of, 535–563
  modular functional organization of, 157–
    158
  morphology of
    future research on, 631–632
    in primates, 543
  "organic" side of, 12
  rodent, 539
  split vs. normal, 527
Brain-behavior relationship studies
  in brain-damaged patients, 159–161
  functional and structural disturbances in,
    165–167
  in normal subjects, 161–163
Brain damage
  cognitive function in, 491–492
  face processing with, 170–171, 176–177
  functional disturbance and, 165–167

Directed attention studies, 644–648

Directionality, 53–55

Disconnection
partial, 494–495
stabilized, 493–494

Disconnection syndromes, 481. *See also* Split-brain syndrome
causes of, 451
symptoms of in callosectomized patient, 468–470

Disinhibition, 397

Dispositional mood, 373–382

Divided visual field studies. *See* Visual half-field studies

Dogs, asymmetries in, 543

Dominance
complementary, 585–586
exclusive, 585, 586
simple, 585, 586
tripartite distinction in, 602–603

Dopamine
in depression, 400–401, 701
imbalance in rodents, 540, 541–542
lateralization of, 309–310, 336
metabolism of, 401
pathways, 400–401

Dot enumeration tests, 670

Double-brain theory, 16, 19

Dreaming, 15

DSM-III criteria
for anxiety disorders, 705
for depression, 699–700

Duchenne smiles, 369–370

Dumontpallier, Amedée, 18–19

Dunn, Th., 10

Dyslexia
atypical cerebral organization in, 641
behavioral symptoms of, 631
brain asymmetry in, 52
brain imaging studies of, 624–625
computed tomographic studies of, 626–627
interhemispheric processing deficit and, 444, 445–446
MRI studies of, 627–630

Dyspraxia, left-sided, 20–21

Ear advantage. *See also* Left ear advantage; Right ear advantage
arousal and, 142–144
change in, 137–141
in depressed patients, 666–668, 674–675
for dichotic fused words in schizophrenia, 679

in dichotic listening, 145–149, 150–151, 663–664
emotionality and, 151
in learning-disabled children, 648
in primates, 547
in rodents, 542
with subarachnoid cysts, 147–149

Ear preference-handedness relation, 193

Eberstaller, O., 10

Electrocardiographic abnormalities, 324–325

Electroconvulsive therapy, 287

Electrodermal activity, 292–294, 335–336

Electrodermal reactivity, 261

Electroencephalographic studies
affective state in infant and, 600
alpha band measurement in, 367
with brain injury, 693
in brain mapping, 288
for central arousal measurement, 222
generator source of, 608
in infants, 555, 600
for learning disability, 641
noninvasiveness of, 366
reliability of, 605–607
resting asymmetry of, 123
signal frequency analysis of, 582
social/attachment challenges and, 601

Electrophysiologic studies
abnormalities of in learning disability, 618
of activation vs. processing, 581–584
advantages of, 580–581
of asymmetries in infancy and childhood, 587–604
cardiac, 289
determining laterality, 584–586
future research questions for, 608–609
generator sources, 608
interpretation of, 607
for learning disability, 641
reliability of, 605–607

Emotion
approach- and withdrawal-related arousal of, 367–372
in asymmetric corticolimbic networks, 389–415
asymmetries in
cerebral, 361–383
frontal, 368–369
hemispheric, 292–295, 297, 336–337
mediation of, 272–273
physiologic, 337
positive and negative regulation of, 390–391

Emotion (cont.)
  biologic substrates of, 361
  brain electrical activity and, 369–372, 383
  cardiovascular effects of, 282–289
  cerebral psychophysiologic asymmetry
    studies of, 365–367
  cortisol in arousal of, 311–315, 317
  facial expression and, 365, 367–369
  laterality of
    in infants and children, 598–602
    in rats, 539
  lateralized stimulus effects on, 328–332
  limbic connections in processing of, 407–
    409
  positive vs. negative, 599–602
  right hemisphere cognition in
    communicating, 391–395
  in right temporal lobe epilepsy, 403
  vulnerability to, 382
Emotional behavior
  disinhibited, 408
  factors affecting, 395–398
Emotional disorders, 11–12
Emotional processing, 362–365, 430–431
Emotional reactivity
  anterior asymmetry differences in, 373–382
  individual differences in, 365
Emotional stress
  cardiovascular effects of, 282–289
  long-term, 274–275
  in sudden cardiac death, 271–278
Emotional surveillance, 404
Emotional vocalizations, 560–561
Emotional words, processing of, 392
Emotionality, 142–143
  ear advantage and, 151
Epidemiologic surveys, for sudden death risk,
  295–296
Epilepsy
  ECGs in seizures of, 292
  emotional changes with, 403
  heart rate changes in, 290–291
  right temporal lobe, 403
  sudden death with, 285–286
Epinephrine release, 276–277
Equipotentiality, 548, 637–638
  argument against, 549–550
  argument for, 551–552
  early asymmetries and, 556
ERPs. See Event-related potentials
Estradiol, 37–38
Estrogen
  in cerebral cortex vs. hypothalamus, 38–39

in cortical growth, 42
  in hypothalamus, 32–33, 38–39
  in male brain, 31
  testosterone conversion to, 36–39
Estrogen receptors
  cortical, 32, 42
  testosterone interactions with, 36–39
Estrone, 37–38
Euphoric mood, 397
Event memory, 460–464
Event-related potentials, 124, 159
  in affective and schizophrenic disorders,
    661, 664–684
  in brain mapping, 288
  with CV syllable stimuli, 583
  in depressed patients, 671–675
  generator source of, 609
  heart rate change and, 332
  in infants, 555, 591
  interpretation of, 607
  for learning disability, 642
  measurement of, 337, 581–582, 664–665
  of nonhuman speech laterality, 595
  PCA-ANOVA analysis of, 583–584
  peak analysis of, 606–607
  in right hemisphere conditioning, 257–260
  in schizophrenia, 680–684
  to speech stimuli, 590–594
  visual
    heart rate and, 332
    for learning disability, 642
  of word processing in infants and children,
    594–598
Explicit transfer. See Information transfer,
  conscious
Extinction
  in facial emotional expression experiments,
    246–247, 251–252
  neuropsychological mechanisms of, 226
  phase of, 237–238
Eye
  movement of in dichotic listening, 144–145
  preference, 193

Face gender categorization, 172–173
Face professional categorization, 172–173
Face recognition, 163–167
  in brain-damaged patients, 170–171
  in different populations, 173–179
  dissociation with facial expression, 392–
    393
  divided-visual-field studies of, 167–170
  of familiar vs. unfamiliar faces, 167–168

DATE DUE

NOV 1 0			